ASPIRIN AND OTHER SALICYLATES

ASPIRIN AND OTHER SALICYLATES

EDITED BY

JOHN R. VANE
Chairman,

and

REGINA M. BOTTING
Information Scientist,

The William Harvey Research Institute
St Bartholomew's Hospital Medical College
London, UK

CHAPMAN & HALL MEDICAL
London · New York · Tokyo · Melbourne · Madras

Published by Chapman & Hall, 2–6 Boundary Row, London SE1 8HN

Chapman & Hall, 2–6 Boundary Row, London SE1 8HN, UK

Blackie Academic & Professional, Wester Cleddens Road,
Bishopbriggs, Glasgow G64 2NZ, UK

Chapman & Hall Inc., 29 West 35th Street, New York, NY10001, USA

Chapman & Hall Japan, Thomson Publishing Japan,
Hirakawacho Nemoto Building, 7F,
1–7–11 Hirakawa–cho, Chiyoda–ku, Tokyo 102, Japan

Chapman & Hall Australia, Thomas Nelson Australia,
102 Dodds Street, South Melbourne, Victoria 3205, Australia

Chapman & Hall India, R. Seshadri,
32 Second Main Road, CIT East, Madras 600 035, India

First edition 1992

© 1992 Chapman & Hall

Typeset in 10 on 12 Palatino by
Falcon Typographic Art Ltd, Fife, Scotland
Printed in Great Britain at the University Press, Cambridge

ISBN 0 412 32370 2

A catalogue record for this book is available from the British Library

Contents

Contents

Contributors

J.R. VANE and R.M. BOTTING
The William Harvey Research Institute, St Bartholomew's Hospital
  Medical College, Charterhouse Square, London EC1M 6BQ, U.K.

K. BRUNE
Department of Pharmacology and Toxicology, University of Erlangen-
  Neurnberg, Universitaetsstrasse 22, Erlangen, Germany.

J.A.CAIRNS
Department of Medicine, McMaster University Medical Centre, Hamilton,
  Ontario, Canada.

W. N. CHARMAN
The School of Pharmaceutics, Victorian College of Pharmacy, Parkville,
  Victoria 3052, Australia.

F. CLIFFORD ROSE
London Neurological Centre, 110 Harley Street, London W1N 1AF,
  U.K.

P.T.G. DAVIES
Department of Neurology, Frenchay Hospital, Bristol, U.K.

M. DE SWIET
Institute of Obstetrics and Gynaecology, Royal Postgraduate Medical
  School, Queen Charlotte's and Chelsea Hospital, Goldhawk Road,
  London W6, U.K.

K. DIETZEL
Byk Gulden Pharmaceuticals, Clinical Research Department, Byk-Gulden-
  Strasse 2, D-7750 Konstanz, Germany.

M.J. DUNN
Division of Nephrology, Department of Medicine, Case Western University and University Hospital, Cleveland, Ohio 44106, U.S.A.

viii

W.S. FIELDS
Cancer Hospital, Box 211, Houston, Texas, 77030 U.S.A.

P. FITSCHA
2nd Department of Internal Medicine, Policlinic, Mariannengasse 10, A-1090 Vienna, Austria.

G.A. FITZGERALD and D.M. KERINS
Centre for Cardiovascular Science, Department of Medicine and Experimental Therapeutics, Mater Misericodiae Hospital, Dublin 7, Ireland.

R.J. FLOWER
St Bartholomew's Hospital Medical College, Charterhouse Square, London EC1M 6BQ, U.K.

R.J. GRYGLEWSKI
Department of Pharmacology, Copernicus Academy of Medicine, Grzegorzecka 16, Cracow, Poland.

G.A. HIGGS
Research Division, Celltech Ltd., 216 Bath Road, Slough, Berkshire, U.K.

E.C. HUSKISSON and J.M.C. AXON
Department of Rheumatology, St Bartholomew's Hospital Medical College,
Charterhouse Square, London EC1M 6BQ, U.K.

M. KUROWSKI
Privat Dozent, Gossler Strasse 6, W–1000 Berlin 41, Germany.

T.W. MEADE
MRC Epidemiology and Medical Care Unit, Wolfson Institute of Preventive Medicine, St Bartholomew's Hospital Medical College, Charterhouse Square, London EC1M 6BQ, U.K.

A.S. MILTON
Department of Pharmacology, University of Aberdeen, Marischal College, Aberdeen, U.K.

A.P. MOWAT
Department of Child Health, King's College Hospital, London, U.K.

J.A. SALMON
Department of Pharmacology, Wellcome Research Labs, Langley Court, Beckenham, Kent, U.K.

Contributors

H. SINZINGER and I. VIRGOLINI
Atherosclerosis Research Group (ASF) Vienna, University of Vienna, Schwarzspanierstrasse 17, Vienna, Austria.

A. SZCZEKLIK
Department of Allergy & Clinical Immunology, Copernicus Academy of Medicine, Skawinska 8, Cracow, Poland.

B.J.R. WHITTLE
Department of Pharmacology, Wellcome Research Labs, Langley Court, Beckenham, Kent, U.K.

D.A. WILLOUGHBY
St Bartholomew's Hospital Medical College, Charterhouse Square, London EC1M 6BQ, U.K.

E.J. ZAMBRASKI
Department of Exercise Science and Sport Studies, Rutgers University, New Brunswick, New Jersey 08903, U.S.A.

Acknowledgements

Grateful thanks are extended to Professor Sergio Ferreira, Professor Gustav Born and Dr Daniela Salvemini for support and helpful discussion and to Josephine and Nina Botting for excellent editing.

Preface

Aspirin is unique as a medicine. Billions of tablets are consumed each year to relieve the common aches and pains suffered by mankind. It has the advantages of being inexpensive to buy and available without the need of a doctor's prescription. It is the most widely used drug in the world thanks partly to its relative lack of toxicity and low addictive liability. Aspirin established the fortunes of Bayer, who originally made it, and is an important product of many other drug companies, who now sell it under other names. Of no less importance than its use as a drug have been the advances aspirin has made possible in the fields of physiology and medicine as a result of the unravelling of its mechanism of action.

Many possible modes of action of aspirin were suggested by various authors, including Harry Collier in the 1960s but the definitive experiments on inhibition of prostaglandin biosynthesis were carried out by John Vane and his group in 1971. This opened the door to further exciting discoveries. Prostacyclin was found in 1976 by Vane and his colleagues working at the Wellcome Laboratories. Inhibition of thromboxane formation in platelets led to an understanding of platelet/blood vessel wall interactions and reinforced the suggested use of aspirin in cardiovascular disease such as myocardial infarction and stroke. Its experimental use to inhibit prostaglandin synthase has made possible the understanding of the metabolism of arachidonic acid in healthy and diseased tissues. As a result, the involvement of prostanoids in allergic and inflammatory diseases such as rheumatoid arthritis and asthma has been clarified.

The elucidation of the mechanism of action of aspirin also allowed the rational development of new therapeutic agents with similar activity to add to the non-steroidal anti-inflammatory drugs already found by empirical means.

This book deals in a comprehensive and definitive way with the pharmacology of aspirin and the scientific discoveries made possible by the use of aspirin and aspirin-like drugs.

JOHN R. VANE and REGINA M. BOTTING

Abbreviations

AA	adjuvant arthritis
ADR	adverse drug reactions
ACTH	adrenocorticotrophic hormone
4Ac	4 acetoamidophenol=acetaminophen=paracetamol
ADP	adenosine diphosphate
ATP	adenosine triphosphate
Ang II	angiotensin II
AMI	acute myocardial infarction
ASA=ASS	aspirin
AUC	area under the curve
AVP	arginine vasopressin
Bk	bradykinin
CNS	central nervous system
CSF	cerebrospinal fluid
cAMP	adenosine 5′-cyclic monophosphate
cGMP	guanosine 5′-cyclic monophosphate
dl	decilitre
DIP	dipyridamole
DAG	diacylglycerol
cDNA	complementary deoxyribonucleic acid
EAE	experimental allergic encephalomyelitis
EP	endogenous pyrogen
EDRF	endothelium-derived relaxing factor
GC/MS	gas chromatography/mass spectrometry
GFR	glomerular filtration rate
GI	gastro-intestinal
g	gram
h	hour
5HT	5-hydroxytryptamine=serotonin
12-HETE	12 hydroxyeicosatetraenoic acid
12-HPETE	12 hydroperoxyeicosatetraenoic acid

HDL	high density lipoprotein
In	indium
INR	international normalized ratio
i.m.	intramuscular
IHD	ischaemic heart disease
IL-1	interleukin-1
i.c.v.	intracerebroventricular
IP	inositol phosphate
i.p.	intraperitoneal
IP_3	inositol 1-4-5 triphosphate
6-keto-$PGF_{1\alpha}$	6-keto-prostaglandin $F_{1\alpha}$=6-oxo-$PGF_{1\alpha}$
LTB_4	leukotriene B_4
LPS	lipopolysaccharide
LDL	low density lipoprotein
min	minute
MI	myocardial infarction
mg	milligram
MDP	muramyl dipeptide
α-MSH	α-melanocyte stimulating hormone
NSAID	non-steroidal anti-inflammatory drug
NAG	N-acetyl-β-glucosaminidase
NK	natural killer
OTC	over-the-counter
OA	osteo-arthritis
OVLT	organum vasculosum laminae terminalis
6-oxo-$PGF_{1\alpha}$	6-oxo-prostaglandin $F_{1\alpha}$=6-keto-$PGF_{1\alpha}$
PG	prostaglandin
PGE_2	prostaglandin E_2
PGG_2	prostaglandin G_2
PGH_2	prostaglandin H_2
PGI_2	prostacyclin
PGE_1	prostaglandin E_1
$PGF_{2\alpha}$	prostaglandin $F_{2\alpha}$
PAI-1	plasminogen activator inhibitor-1
PAH	para-amino hippuric acid
PTFE	teflon
PL	placebo
PTCA	percutaneous coronary angioplasty
PO	preoptic area

Abbreviations

PLA_2	phospholipase A_2
PLC	phospholipase C
PCA	passive cutaneous anaphylaxis
PUFA	polyunsaturated fatty acid
P or p	probability
q.d.s.	four times daily
RA	rheumatoid arthritis
RBF	renal blood flow
mRNA	messenger ribonucleic acid
RTC	randomized controlled trials
RCS	rabbit aorta contracting substance
rh IL-1	recombinant human interleukin-1
sec	second
SA	salicylic acid
SLE	systemic lupus erythematosus
s.c.	subcutaneous
s.e.m.	standard error of mean
TXA_2	thromboxane A_2
tPA	tissue plasminogen activator
t.d.s.=t.i.d.	three times daily
TNF	tissue necrosis factor
vWF	von Willebrand factor

Overview

R.M. BOTTING and J.R. VANE

The story of aspirin has fascinated pharmacologists for almost 100 years. It is probably the most widely used medicinal drug in the world. The British pharmacologist, Harry Collier, encapsulated its history in a fascinating chapter in the book, *Discoveries in Pharmacology* (Collier, 1984). Collier made the important discovery that aspirin antagonized the action of bradykinin in every experimental system he tested. He called aspirin an 'anti-defensive drug'. However, the crucial discovery of the biochemical mechanism of action of aspirin was made by John Vane in 1971. It was against the background of the newly identified prostaglandins (PGs) and the growing understanding that PGs were released by several substances including bradykinin that Vane and his colleagues working at the Royal College of Surgeons in London revealed the true nature by which aspirin produced its diverse effects. These were inextricably linked to the multitudinous effects of the prostaglandins and their synthesis and release by almost all living cells. When Vane proved that aspirin prevented the formation of prostaglandins, he demonstrated the reasons for the anti-inflammatory, analgesic, antipyretic and toxic effects of the most widely used remedy of all time.

This discovery in part coincided with a veritable explosion of aspirin-like drugs, when the pharmaceutical industry took up the development of anti-inflammatory analgesics which were more potent than aspirin and manifested less severe unwanted effects such as stomach bleeding. These drugs, exemplified by phenylbutazone, indomethacin, mefenamic acid, ibuprofen and others were widely used for treating rheumatic conditions. All of them inhibited prostaglandin biosynthesis, but their toxicity remained a problem, probably because it too was caused by the same biochemical intervention. Long acting anti-rheumatics such as benoxaprofen which were slowly degraded by liver enzymes became highly toxic in elderly patients with impaired liver function. The use of these drugs had to be more carefully monitored.

But meanwhile another use for these drugs had also emerged based on their action as analgesics.

Aspirin had been used as a relief for headaches for almost a century, but now its efficacy was acknowledged for other types of pain due to overproduction of PGs in the periphery such as post-operative pain, especially post-operative dental pain, for dysmenorrhoea, for cancer and for other types of clinical pain. The aspirin-like drugs were even more potent in this respect and their use as effective, non-addictive analgesics has accelerated ever since.

More recently, yet another use for aspirin has emerged connected with the discovery of its anti-thrombotic action, which is also based on inhibition of cyclo-oxygenase, the enzyme which produces PGs (and in platelets, thromboxane (TX) A_2). Clinical trials of aspirin for a great variety of thrombotic conditions including secondary prevention of myocardial infarction began in the mid-1970s and are still continuing. The anti-platelet effects of aspirin have been tested in all forms of coronary artery disease, post-operative deep vein thrombosis, graft patency, peripheral artery disease, unstable angina, transient ischaemic attacks and stroke. Because of the infrequency of incidents, individual small scale trials often did not yield conclusive results. However, a meta-analysis of data from all available trials established the usefulness of aspirin as a protection against second heart attacks, transient ischaemic episodes and stroke (Antiplatelet Trialists Collaboration, 1988). Its effectiveness for other thrombotic conditions will be assessed when a second analysis is published in 1992.

The peculiar effectiveness of aspirin in thrombosis is based on its irreversible inhibition of the cyclo-oxygenase enzyme in platelets which makes TXA_2, the potent, pro-aggregatory prostaglandin released from platelets. Of all the aspirin-like drugs, only aspirin permanently inactivates the enzyme (by attaching an acetyl group close to the active site) and thus makes the platelet incapable of synthesizing TXA_2 for the rest of its life (of 8–11 days). The host of other aspirin-like drugs inhibit platelet cyclo-oxygenase weakly and reversibly by occupying the active site and need to be given in much higher doses than the relatively minute amounts (30–50 mg day^{-1}) of aspirin. Regular dosing with low doses of aspirin has a cumulative anti-enzyme effect and inactivates platelet cyclo-oxygenase without affecting the synthesis of prostaglandins in other organs, such as the stomach and blood vessels, which would lead to unwanted side effects. This has partly to do with the pharmacokinetics of aspirin since platelets encounter the highest concentrations of aspirin in the pre-systemic or portal circulation where platelet cyclo-oxygenase is inactivated, before the drug is metabolized by the liver and diluted in the general systemic circulation.

However, acetylation of cyclo-oxygenase does not confer any advantage on aspirin over other aspirin-like drugs as far as its anti-rheumatic and analgesic actions are concerned. In fact, aspirin is actually less potent as an anti-rheumatic and analgesic than other related drugs. The reasons for this are not clear at present. The analgesic and anti-inflammatory effects of aspirin-like drugs are undoubtedly dependent on the inhibition of cyclo-oxygenase. This has been proved in many tests over many years (see Chapters 3, 7 and 8). The actions of sodium salicylate and paracetamol do not sit well in this, but it is possible that sodium salicylate interferes in some other way with PG formation, perhaps by preventing the expression of the mRNA for prostaglandin-synthesizing enzyme.

Taking a forward look at possible new uses for aspirin, some interesting new applications for its therapeutic actions are emerging. One example is the prevention of diabetic and steroid-induced cataracts. Glucose in the plasma of diabetics or steroids administered as drugs react with the special proteins (crystallins) from which the lens is formed, causing them to unfold and aggregate. Thus, the lens becomes opaque and the result is a cataract. Aspirin preferentially acetylates the amino groups of the crystallins and prevents binding of excessive amounts of glucose or of steroid to them *in vitro* (Harding and van Heyningen, 1988; Ajiboye and Harding, 1989). Epidemiological studies have shown that aspirin consumption appears to protect against cataract formation (Harding *et al.*, 1989a,b).

The glycosylation of structural proteins of the aorta and coronary arteries may also lead to the higher incidence of heart disease in diabetic patients and to diabetic retinopathy. In a multicentre, double blind, randomized clinical trial, 1 g daily of aspirin alone or combined with 225 mg of dipyridamole reduced the number of microaneurysms in early diabetic retinopathy (DAMAD Study Group, 1989). It is not certain whether this beneficial effect of aspirin was associated with decreased glycosylation of the basement membrane of retinal blood vessels or with the anti-platelet action of aspirin. Certainly, the platelets of some patients with diabetic retinopathy seem to aggregate more readily than normal platelets.

In addition, a possible anti-cancer action of cyclo-oxygenase inhibitors is under investigation. Activated macrophages release PGE_2, which functions to down-regulate the activity of T-lymphocytes, the major lymphokine-producing cells of the immune system. In cancer, the macrophages produce excessive amounts of PGE_2 which dampens down their own anti-tumour actions together with other forms of anti-tumour activity. Many malignant cells also secrete greater amounts of PGE_2 than their parent tissue. Removal of the inhibitory prostaglandins enhances lymphokine production by T-lymphocytes as well as increasing the activity of other cells of the immune system. Increased release of tumour necrosis factor would enhance the cytotoxic action of macrophages against tumour cells (Wasserman, 1990). Clinical studies carried out with cyclo-oxygenase inhibitors have provided some evidence of anti-tumour effects, but continued studies of these drugs in cancer patients are still needed (Harris and Braun, 1990; Thun *et al.*, 1991).

It is remarkable how the discovery of a mechanism of action not only leads to new, more potent and selective drugs, but also to new uses for the old ones!

REFERENCES

Ajiboye, R. and Harding, J.J. (1989) The non-enzymic glycosylation of bovine lens proteins by glucosamine and its inhibition by aspirin, ibuprofen and glutathione. *Exp. Eye Res.*, **49**, 31–41.

Antiplatelet Trialists Collaboration. (1988) Secondary prevention of vascular disease by prolonged antiplatelet treatment. *Brit. Med. J.*, **296**, 320–31.

Braun, D.P., Bonomi, P.D., Taylor, S. and Harris, J.E. (1987) Modification of the effects of cytotoxic chemotherapy on the immune responses of cancer patients with a nonsteroidal anti-inflammatory drug, piroxicam. *J. Biol. Response Mod.*, **6**, 331–45.

Braun, D.P., Taylor, S.G. and Harris, J.E. (1989) Modulation of immunity in cancer patients by prostaglandin antagonists. *Prog. Clin. Biol. Res.*, **288**, 439–49.

Collier, H.O.J. (1984) The story of aspirin. In *Discoveries in Pharmacology, Vol. 2, Haemodynamics, Hormones and Inflammation*, (eds. M.J. Parnham and J. Bruinvels), Elsevier Science Publishers BV, Amsterdam, pp. 555–93.

Dipyridamole, Aspirin, Microaneurism and Diabetes (DAMAD) Study Group (1989) The effect of aspirin alone and aspirin plus dipyridamole in early diabetic retinopathy. *Diabetes*, **38**, 491–8.

Harding, J.J. and van Heyningen, R. (1988) Drugs, including alcohol, that act as risk factors for cataract, and possible protection against cataract by aspirin-like analgesics and cyclopenthiazide. *Brit. J. Ophthalmol.*, **72**, 809–14.

Harding, J.J., Harding, R.S. and Egerton, M. (1989a) Risk factors for cataract in Oxfordshire: diabetes, peripheral neuropathy, myopia, glaucoma and diarrhoea. *Acta Ophthalmol.*, **67**, 510–17.

Harding, J.J., Egerton, M. and Harding, R.S. (1989b) Protection against cataract by aspirin, paracetamol and ibuprofen. *Acta Ophthalmol.*, **67**, 518–24.

Harris, J. and Braun, D. (1990) The effect of aspirin and other cyclo-oxygenase inhibitors on antitumour immunity. In *Aspirin – towards 2000* (ed. G. Fryers), Royal Society of Medicine Services, London, pp. 45–52.

Thun, M.J., Namboodiri, M.M. and Heath, Jr., C.W. (1991) Aspirin use and reduced risk of colon cancer. *N.Engl. J. Med.*, **325**, 1593–6.

Vane, J.R. (1971) Inhibition of prostaglandin synthesis as a mechanism of action for aspirin-like drugs. *Nature (New Biology)*, **231**, 232–5.

Wasserman, J. (1990) Immunosuppression in irradiated breast cancer patients: *In vitro* effect of cyclo-oxygenase inhibitors. In *Aspirin – towards 2000* (ed. G. Fryers), Royal Society of Medicine Services, London, pp. 39–43.

PART ONE
Introduction

---

1 *The history of aspirin*

J.R. VANE and R.M. BOTTING

The ancestry of aspirin (acetylsalicylic acid) goes back many thousands of years: salicylic acid, or salicylate, from which it is derived is a constituent of several plants long used as medicaments. About 3500 years ago the Ebers papyrus recommended the application of a decoction of the dried leaves of Myrtle to the abdomen and back to expel rheumatic pains from the womb. A thousand years later Hippocrates championed the juices of the Poplar tree for treating eye diseases and those of Willow bark for pain in childbirth and for fever. All contain salicylates.

Celsius (in AD 30) described the four famous signs of inflammation (rubor, calor, dolor and tumor, or redness, heat, pain and swelling) and used extracts of Willow leaves to relieve them. Through the Roman times of Pliny the Elder, Dioscorides and Galen the use of salicylate-containing plants was further developed and Willow bark was recommended for mild to moderate pain. In Asia and China also, salicylate-containing plants were being applied therapeutically. The curative effects of *Salix* and *Spirea* species were even known to primitive races such as the North American Indians and the Hottentots of Southern Africa.

Through the Middle Ages further uses were found, as plasters to treat wounds and various other external and internal applications, including the treatment of painful menstruation and dysentry. However, Willows were needed for basket-making so the women herbalists of those days turned to other related plants. For instance, they grew Meadowsweet (*Spirea ulmaria*) in their herb gardens and made decoctions from the flowers.

The first 'clinical trial' of Willow bark to be published in England was made by a country parson, the Reverend Edward Stone (or Edmund; both names are attributed to him in the text of his original letter to the Royal Society) of Chipping Norton in Oxfordshire (Stone, 1763).

On June 2, 1763, Edward Stone read a report to the Royal Society on the use of Willow bark in fever. He had accidentally tasted it and was surprised by its extraordinary bitterness, which reminded him of the taste of Cinchona bark (containing quinine), then being used to treat malaria. He believed in the 'doctrine of signatures' which dictated that the cures for diseases would be found in the same locations where the malady occurs. Since the 'Willow delights in a moist and wet soil, where agues chiefly abound', he gathered a pound of Willow bark, dried it on a baker's oven for 3 months and pulverized it. His greatest success was with doses of 1 dram, which he reported using in about 50 patients with safety and success.

He concluded his paper by saying, 'I have no other motives for publishing this valuable specific, than that it may have a fair and full trial in all its variety of circumstances and situations, and that the world may reap the benefits occurring from it'.

His wishes have certainly been realized; world production of aspirin has been estimated at many thousands of tons a year, with an average consumption in a developed country of about 100 tablets per person per year. Without the discovery in recent years of a great many replacements for aspirin and its variants, consumption would have surely been very much higher.

However, a further 40 years passed before another group of scientists took up the subject again. It was only during the continental blockade imposed by Napoleon at the beginning of the nineteenth century, when no more quinine could be imported into central Europe, that interest in the properties of the bark of the Willow (*Salix alba vulgaris*) was revived. The first to investigate the components of the bitter-tasting extract of Willow bark was Buchner, Professor of Pharmacy at the University of Munich. In 1828, after extracting the bark with water, precipitating the tannins and other impurities and evaporating the solution, he obtained a yellowish substance that he called 'Salicin', after the Latin name for the Willow. Buchner had no doubts that this substance would prove to be more acceptable than the previous extracts of cortex salicis which contained tannic acid, although he did not manage to produce the bitter ingredient free of all colourants. Only a year later a French pharmacist living in Vitry-le-François, Leroux – inspired by a paper published in 1803 by Wilkinson on 'Cortex salicis latifoliae' – was considering the same problem. By further precipitation he managed to produce salicin in pure crystalline form. In 1830 a study by Academy members Gay-Lussac and Magendie showed that salicin was a non-nitrogenous plant principle, as researchers had suspected. Its glycosidic nature was discovered by Piria, an Italian chemist of a mere 23 years of age. Eight years later Piria continued his work when employed as an assistant at the Sorbonne in Paris. He split salicin into a sugar and an aromatic part and converted the latter by various oxidative processes into an acid consisting of colourless, crystalline needles, 'acide salicylice' or salicylic acid. Shortly after the discovery additional natural sources of salicylic acid were found. As early as 1835, Pagenstecher, a pharmacist from Berne, had extracted a volatile oil from meadow-sweet (*Spirea ulmaria*), from which the German chemist Löwig in Zurich obtained 'Spiersäure' (spiric acid). In fact, as proved by the chemist Dumas in 1839, this acid is identical to salicylic acid. But only when a rich source of salicylic acid was identified in oil of wintergreen extracted from the American plant, *Gaultheria procumbens* in 1843 was it possible to prepare enough of the substance to treat large numbers of patients. The acid rapidly became well known and its use for the relief of pain and to reduce fever spread widely. However, a fresh problem soon arose: how to measure the dosage of a substance accurately when it was not chemically pure. Also, the natural sources of salicylic acid were soon unable to cope with the vast demand for this substance.

It was salicin itself, the glycoside of salicylic acid, which was used in 1876 in an important experiment by T.J. MacLagan, a Dundee physician (MacLagan, 1876). He argued as Stone had done a 100 years before that, since damp climatic conditions give rise to rheumatic fever, the cure for this must come from the Willow which thrives in damp places. He first tried up to 2 g of salicin himself and experiencing no ill effects gave it to his patient. The result of the treatment was a lowering of body temperature and a reduction of the pain and swelling. He thus demonstrated the antipyretic, analgesic and anti-inflammatory effects for which salicylates were used subsequently.

The desire to produce, and thus be able to use, pure salicylic acid provided chemists with the impetus for fresh research. Inspired by the chemical analysis of Carl Gerhardt, who had demonstrated the degradation of salicylic acid on heating into phenol and carbon dioxide, Kolbé, Professor at Marburg University, first managed to identify the structure of salicylic acid as an o-hydroxybenzoic acid. Then in 1859, Kolbé with his colleague Lautemann synthesized it by combining the two decomposition products; passing carbon dioxide through a mixture of melted phenol with sodium. By the time MacLagan's paper was published in the Lancet in 1876, other physicians were using the synthetic compound.

It was another 15 years before von Heyden, a student of Professor Kolbé, made the synthetic process technologically practicable so that the pure active ingredient could be produced industrially, and at one-tenth the cost of the salicylic acid previously obtained from Gaultheria oil. In 1874 he founded the Heyden Chemical Company devoted to the commercial synthesis and distribution of salicylic acid. This led to the liberal use of pure salicylic acid, which reduced fever immediately and relieved pain dramatically, not only rheumatic pain but also neuralgia and headaches. 1876 was also the year when the anti-rheumatic effects of salicylic acid were clinically proven. At Traube's 'Charite' Hospital in Berlin, Dr S. Stricker was the first to introduce salicylic acid as treatment for acute rheumatoid arthritis, almost as a specific agent, and then document its effectiveness (Stricker, 1876).

The sharp, bitter taste of the substance and the side effects of gastric irritation caused by the acid however, made long-term prescribing difficult. A year later Sée tried to replace the acid by a sweet sodium salt. Salts of other metals were also made. Unfortunately, all these manipulations simply improved the taste slightly, but did nothing to alleviate the unpleasant side effects.

On 1st August, 1863 Friedrich Bayer and Johann Weskott had set up a dye production plant in the valley of the River Wupper, close to the centre of a large textile industry. They began with only one worker, the dye smelting initially being done in their own kitchens, but production expanded rapidly and after only 4 years the number of staff had risen to 50. Due to the energy and enterprise of the company's owners, branches opened up in a number of countries in the next 18 years.

The managers of this young limited company were convinced that the company's own research offered the best prospects for profitable expansion. In 1883, several graduate chemists were employed who, to begin with, worked for the company in small science laboratories separate from business concerns or in university departments. One of these chemists was 22 year old Carl Duisberg who was to greatly influence the German chemical industry for the next half century. Soon after his appointment, Duisberg had developed a number of substances that were subsequently patented. In 1884 he invented the dye benzoazurine, an intermediate of which gave rise to the first Bayer pharmaceutical product. Having noted the antipyretic effect of acetanilide described in 1886, Duisberg thought of converting the p-nitrophenol produced in large quantities during dye manufacture into p-acetophenetidine or phenacetin. It was the chemist Oskar Hinsberg who took over this project and had the new substance tested for its fever-reducing properties at Frankfurt University. When phenacetin proved an effective antipyretic and it was decided to manufacture the substance, the company's management found itself entering a totally new area of operations.

In 1888, the then 25 year old company set up a pharmaceutical department, and by 1898 was able to print a 200 page booklet describing its drugs for the Wiesbaden Conference on Internal Medicine. Also by that time, one of the eight chemists working in the company's pharmaceutical laboratory had managed to synthesize a substance that

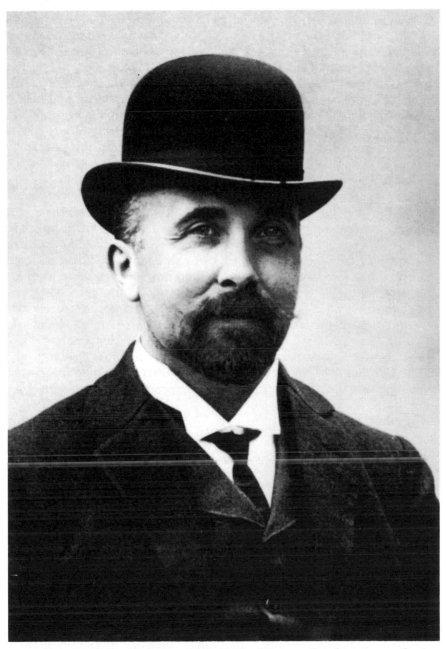

Figure 1.1 Dr Felix Hoffman (1868–1946). He was the first to synthesize acetylsalicylic acid in a pure and stable form.

was to supersede the analgesic salicylic acid and its sodium salt, and ultimately to become the medicine of the century.

The young researcher was Felix Hoffmann (Fig. 1.1). He was born in 1868, the son of a south German factory owner. After a Classical education he at first decided to follow a career in pharmacy. He worked in several pharmacies in Geneva, Hamburg and Neuveville, before studying pharmacy and chemistry at Munich University. In 1881 he passed his state examination in pharmacy with 'magna cum laude', continued his chemistry studies and graduated 2 years later under the tuition of E. Bamberger. He worked for a year in the Munich State Laboratory and then in 1894 joined Friedrich Bayer and Company.

Finding a similar, but better tolerated substitute for salicylic acid, which was associated with some unpleasant side effects, was not part of Bayer's planned research programme. In spite of this, Felix Hoffmann turned his attention to this project. Hoffmann had personal reasons for wanting a more acceptable salicylic acid derivative. His father who had been taking salicylic acid for many years to treat his painful arthritis had recently discovered that he could no longer take the drug without vomiting. Impelled then, by filial affection as well as dedication to his job, Hoffmann searched through the scientific literature. In 1897, he found the answer in the acetylation of salicylic acid. Some 40 years earlier, in 1853, acetylsalicylic acid had been synthesized by the Strasburg chemist, Carl Gerhardt, but in an unstable, impure form and as a result it had received no further attention. In Hoffmann's laboratory records for 10 October 1897, he described the synthesis of acetylsalicylic acid, which he was the first to produce in a chemically pure and stable form (Fig. 1.2).

Together with Bayer's chief pharmacologist, Heinrich Dreser (Fig. 1.3), Hoffman tested the new substance he had made, comparing its therapeutic efficacy and tolerability to products previously used for the treatment of rheumatic pains.

Dreser had studied medicine in Heidelberg and graduated in 1884. Initially, he had worked as an assistant to the physiologist Rudolf Heidenhain in Breslau and later in the Strasbourg Institute of Pharmacology under the direction of Oswald Schmiedeberg. In 1896, he was offered the Chair in Pharmacology at Göttingen University. The same year, however, because of the poor University salary and inadequate equipment, he accepted an offer from the Bayer Company to become Head of its Pharmacology Laboratory and expand it further. It was due to the foresight of Carl Duisberg, then Head of Research, that the Laboratory was fitted with the latest equipment and apparatus, as well as being plentifully supplied with funds. There was hence no problem in starting comprehensive animal studies with the acetylsalicylic acid

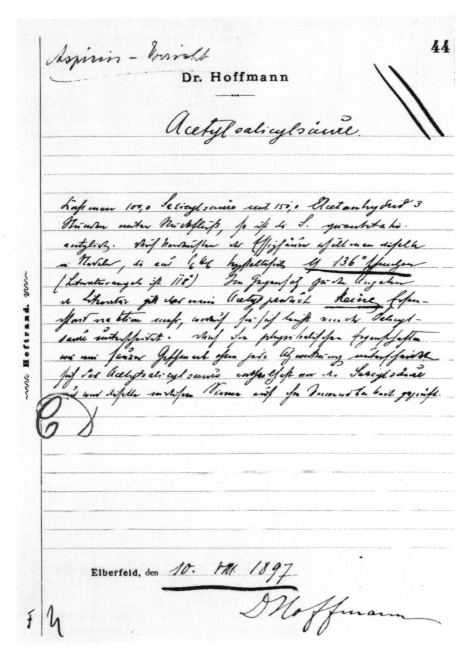

Figure 1.2 Laboratory record of Dr Felix Hoffman for 10 October, 1897.

synthesized by Hoffman – the first ever studies of this kind to be carried out in an industrial laboratory.

Detailed pharmacological and toxicological tests confirmed that the actions of this newly developed drug were very satisfactory. In *Pfluegers Archiv fuer die gesamte Physiologie*, Dreser described the excellent analgesic and antipyretic effects of acetylsalicylic acid at the same time suggesting that aspirin was a convenient way of supplying the body with the active substance, salicylate (Dreser, 1899). Whether aspirin is a pro-drug for salicylate has been debated ever since, but clearly, aspirin has potent actions of its own which are not shared by salicylic acid. Dreser also reported that aspirin had a 'pleasant, acidic taste' and a less damaging effect on the stomach wall than sodium salicylate; a misconception which took many years to refute.

The clinical applications of acetylsalicylic acid were tested in a year-long study by Dr Kurt Wittauer in Halle and the results demonstrated the superior pharmacological properties of the new compound compared to those of salicylic acid. 'The drug has never failed in its effect on pain, inflammation or fever' was the conclusion of Wittauer in his report of the study. He confirmed, 'It has had no adverse effects on heart or stomach even in seriously ill patients.' He also noted how surprisingly good was the appetite of patients when taking acetylsalicylic acid for long periods. It soon became clear that this substance synthesized by Hoffman not only helped rheumatic patients, but also those suffering from headaches, toothache and neuralgic pain.

However, before the company could hand over acetylsalicylic acid to be marketed as an 'over-the-counter' pain killer and anti-rheumatic, a practical, easily pronounceable name had to be found. As recorded in a memorandum of 23 January 1899, the name 'Aspirin' was finally chosen; it contained the root of spiric acid from *Spiraea ulmeria*, chemically identical to salicylic acid, together with 'A' as an abbreviation for 'acetyl'. Interestingly, 'Eûspirin' was suggested in the original documentation as an alternative name (Fig. 1.4). On 1 February of the same year, aspirin was submitted as a trade name to the Patent Office in Berlin and, also in that year, the drug was finally introduced into the German Pharmacopoeia. A circular letter from the company and an advertisement in May notified the medical world of this new analgesic and antipyretic which first came on the market in powder form. A variety of publications appeared in the first decade of its use recommending aspirin not only for rheumatism of the joints and muscles, but for other indications where the pain was mainly caused by inflammation, for instance gout, headaches, neuralgia, dysmenorrhoea and carcinoma. Manufacture of the substance soon swelled to amazing proportions but as a powder, aspirin was poorly soluble in water, so

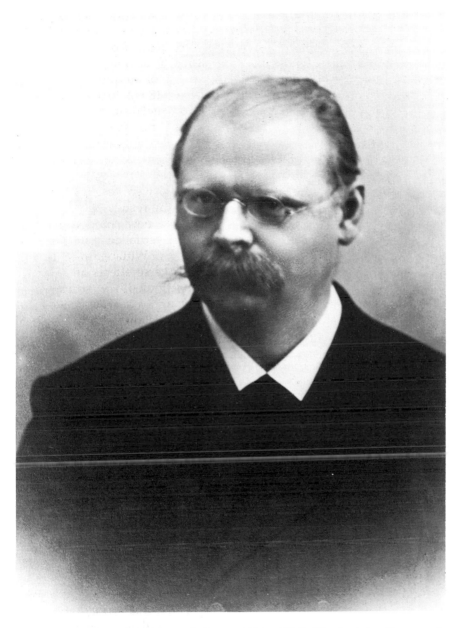

Figure 1.3   Professor Dr Heinrich Dreser (1860–1924). Head of the Pharmacology Laboratory of Farbenfabriken vorm. Friedrich Bayer and Company from 1896 to 1914.

only a year after its launch the company decided to supply the drug in the form of tablets which would immediately disintegrate into powder form in water. So aspirin became the first major medicine to be sold in tablets. Aspirin owed its popularity for the most part to an outstanding ability to relieve even intolerable pain, which was especially valuable in view of the strongly addictive properties of morphine, which was the only alternative treatment available at that time. The US patent for aspirin was granted in February, 1900 and after 1906, it was marketed by the newly founded Bayer Co. Inc. which itself also produced acetylsalicylic acid.

The German Patent Office refused to grant a patent for the acetylation of salicylic acid as they did not consider it a sufficiently novel process. Both Felix Hoffmann and Artur Eichengrün, the head of Bayer's chemical research laboratories, had contracts with Bayer by which they would receive a royalty on any patentable product they invented. Since there was no patent, neither of them received any royalties from the sale of aspirin in Germany. However, Heinrich Dreser had an agreement with Bayer by which he would receive a royalty on any product that he introduced. Thus he received a very substantial royalty for aspirin and was able to retire early as a very rich man.

The Bayer Company enjoyed the profits from aspirin until the outbreak of the First World War. However, in 1918 the US Patent Office cancelled Bayer's patent rights to the name of aspirin because they were considered to be improperly registered. When this decision was challenged by Bayer in the US Supreme Court, the court ruled that Bayer's aspirin had been so widely advertised that it had become a common name (Rainsford, 1984). Bayer's monopoly of aspirin in the USA and Britain was thus effectively broken.

Eleven other companies in the USA started to manufacture aspirin about the turn of the century, but the largest amounts were made by Monsanto Chemical Works which had been founded in 1901 by John Queeny. In 1912, Dr Gaston Dubois of Monsanto visited a chemist in Switzerland and bought from him a very cheap process for the manufacture of aspirin in one operation. By 1917 Monsanto had built a processing plant and were selling large amounts of aspirin. As a result, Bayer accused Monsanto of infringement of tradename rights and the legal battle between the two companies in the US Supreme Court ensued.

Subsequently, Monsanto invested in other manufacturing companies making aspirin, including one in Wales, which was producing aspirin for sale in the UK. Thus, it was able to supply large amounts of aspirin to European countries which did not acknowledge Bayer's patent rights, particularly Great Britain and France. In Australia, when it

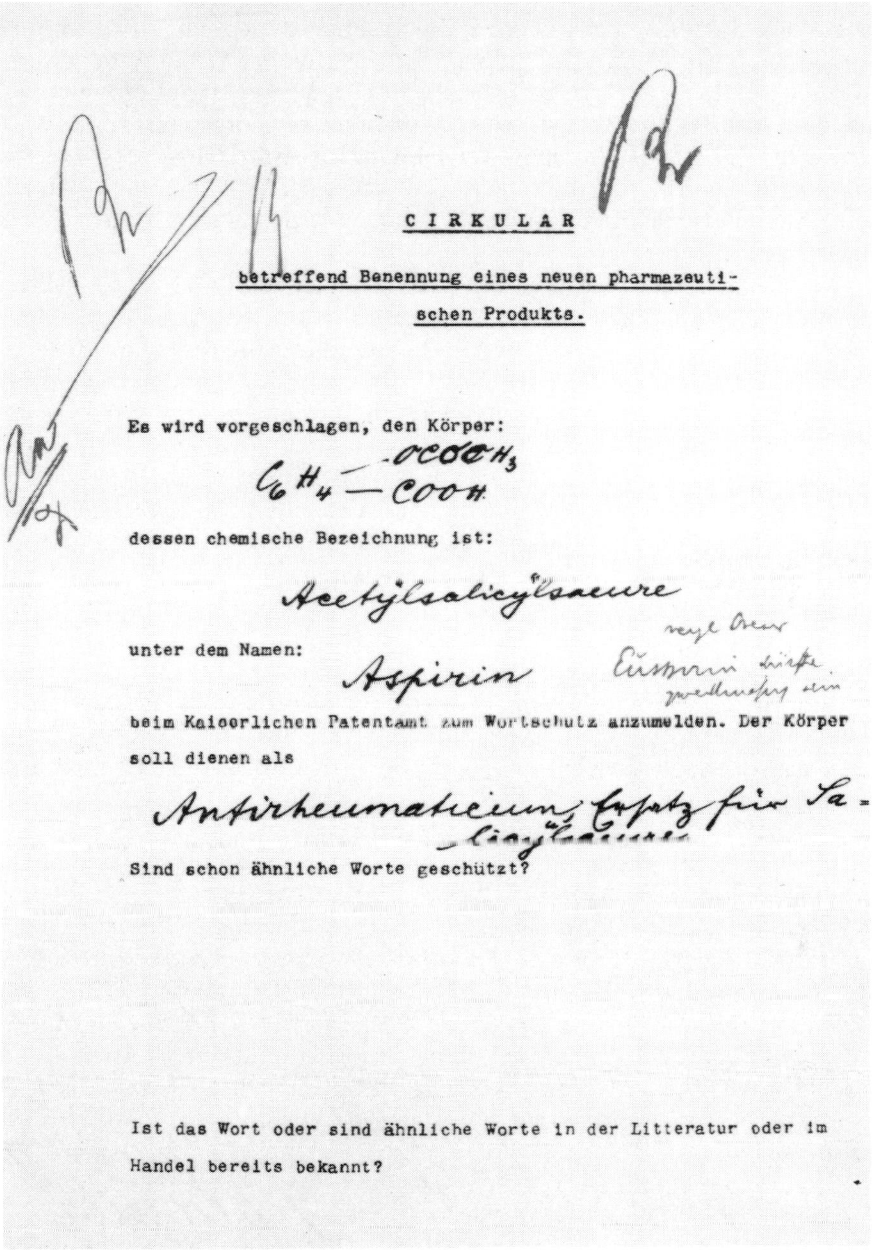

C I R K U L A R

betreffend Benennung eines neuen pharmazeutischen Produkts.

Es wird vorgeschlagen, den Körper:

$C_6H_4 \begin{matrix} -OCOCH_3 \\ -COOH \end{matrix}$

dessen chemische Bezeichnung ist:

Acetylsalicylsaeure

unter dem Namen:

Aspirin

beim Kaiserlichen Patentamt zum Wortschutz anzumelden. Der Körper soll dienen als

Antirheumaticum, Ersatz für Salicylsäure

Sind schon ähnliche Worte geschützt?

Ist das Wort oder sind ähnliche Worte in der Litteratur oder im Handel bereits bekannt?

Figure 1.4 Internal circular of the Bayer Company recording the naming of 'Aspirin'.

Wie ist das Wort entstanden? Ist es ein reiner Phantasiename oder giebt es irgend welchen Anhalt über die Zusammensetzung oder Wirkung des Körpers, für dessen Bezeichnung es bestimmt ist?

[handwritten annotation]

Liegen Bedenken gegen das Wort vor oder haben Sie einen andern Vorschlag zu machen? *[handwritten annotation]*

Cirkuliert bei den Herren:

Direktor Bayer *[signature]*
    "   Dr. Böttinger *[handwritten: Mit Euspirin auch einverstanden]*
    "   König *[signature: König]*
Dr. C. Duisberg *[signature]*
W. Gansser
Karl Hülsenbusch,
Hermann Matthis *[signature: Matthis]*
Prof. Dr. Dreser *[signature: Dreser]*
A. Brestowski *[signature: A. Brestowski]*
Dr. Hoffmann *[signature]*
Fr. Fischer *[signature]*
Dr. Eichengrün *[handwritten annotation]*
Dr. Heymann *[signature: Heymann]*
Dr. Kloeppel *[handwritten: einverst.]*

Zurück an die Juristische Abteilung.

[handwritten: Elberfeld, den 23 Januar 1899]

[signature]

Figure 1.4 cont'd

14

was impossible to obtain supplies of aspirin because of the First World War, the Australian government cancelled Bayer's patent rights. A manufacturing process for producing aspirin was then developed by George Nicholas, a young Australian pharmacist. He later founded the firm of Nicholas Proprietary Ltd and registered their product under the well-known trade name of 'Aspro' (Grenville-Smith and Barrie, 1976). Aspirin manufacturers benefited greatly from the severe influenza epidemics of 1919 and 1920. In Britain the sale of aspirin by the Beecham Pharmaceutical Company supported the famous conductor Sir Thomas Beecham who was part-owner of the firm. He used the profits from aspirin to finance productions by the British Opera Company and to purchase the Covent Garden Opera House in London (Lazell, 1976).

The major producer of aspirin in the USA since the end of the Second World War has been Sterling Drug Inc. During the Asian influenza epidemic at the end of the 1950s, their Trenton works in New Jersey had to operate day and night to satisfy demand for the drug. Such was the popularity of aspirin that the 'mini' pharmacy' on board the space rocket Apollo was supplied with aspirin when it landed on the moon in 1969. Charles Berry, medical director of the American Space Authority at the time attributed the good health of the astronauts to the use of the little white aspirin tablets and forecast that aspirin would 'definitely be used for all eternity'.

By the early years of this century the chief therapeutic actions of aspirin (and sodium salicylate itself) were known as the anti-pyretic, anti-inflammatory and analgesic effects. With the passing of time, several other drugs were discovered which shared some or all of these effects. Amongst these were acetaminophen (paracetamol), phenylbutazone, and more recently the fenamates, indomethacin and naproxen. Because of their similarity of therapeutic action these drugs tended to be regarded as a group and were generally known as the aspirin-like drugs, or because they were clearly distinct from the glucocorticoids (the other major group of agents used in the treatment of inflammation) the non-steroid anti-inflammatory drugs (Flower, 1974). Although this group of drugs is chemically diverse, the fact that most of its members possessed an acidic function suggested yet another name which is still occasionally encountered – the anti-inflammatory acids.

Despite the diversity of their chemical structures, these drugs all share to some extent the same therapeutic properties. In varying doses they alleviate the swelling, redness and pain of inflammation, reduce a general fever and cure a headache. More than that, they also share to a greater or lesser extent a number of similar side effects. Depending on dose, they can cause gastric upset, delay the birth process and in overdose may damage the kidney. A particularly interesting 'side effect', now known as a therapeutic action is the anti-thrombotic effect.

Now, when a chemically diverse group of drugs all share not only the same therapeutic qualities (which in themselves have not much connection with each other) but also the same side effects, it can be fairly certain that the diverse actions of those drugs are based on a single biochemical intervention. For many years pharmacologists and biochemists searched for such a common mode of action without finding a generally acceptable scientific explanation. That is, until 1971, when Vane and his colleagues, working at the Royal College of Surgeons of England discovered that aspirin and similar drugs inhibited the enzyme which generates prostaglandins (Vane, 1971). This mode of action has now been generally accepted.

Nevertheless, despite the satisfaction afforded by such a simple and unifying theory, there are still a few outposts of disaffection, clinging to ambiguous modes of action such as 'stabilization of the cell membrane'. In recent years also, the modulating effects of some prostaglandins on immune mechanisms have led to postulates that the aspirin-like drugs carry with them an inherent pro-inflammatory activity. These points will be discussed later.

REFERENCES

Dreser, H. (1899) Pharmacologisches über Aspirin (Acetylsalicyl-saüre). *Pflüger's Arch. Gesamte Physiol. Menschen Tiere*, **76**, 306–18.

Flower, R.J. (1974) Drugs which inhibit prostaglandin biosynthesis. *Pharmacol. Rev.*, **26**, 33–67.

Grenville-Smith, R. and Barrie, A. (1976) In: *Aspro. How a Family Business Grew Up*. Ebenezer Bayliss, The Trinity Press, Worcester.

Lazell, H.G. (1976) In *From Pills to Penicillin. The Beecham Story*. Heinemann, London.

MacLagan, T.J. (1876) The treatment of acute rheumatism by salicin. *Lancet*, **i**, 342, 383.

Rainsford, K.D. (1984) In *Aspirin and the Salicylates* (ed. K.D. Rainsford). Butterworth & Co Ltd, London, pp 1–12.

Stone, E. (1763) An account of the success of the bark of the willow in the cure of agues. *Phil. Trans. R. Soc. Lond.*, **53**, 195–200.

Stricker, S. (1876) II Aus Traubéschen Klinik. Ueber die Resultate der Behendlung der Polyarthritis rheumatica mit Salicylsaüre. *Berl. Klin. Wochenschr.*, **13**, 1–2, 15–16, 99–103.

Vane, J.R. (1971) Inhibition of prostaglandin synthesis as a mechanism of action for aspirin-like drugs. *Nature (New Biology)*, **231**, 232–5.

2 The prostaglandins

J.R. VANE and R.M. BOTTING

The prostaglandins are among the most prevalent of autacoids and have been detected in almost every tissue and body fluid; their production increases in response to astonishingly diverse stimuli; they produce, in minute amounts, a remarkably broad spectrum of effects that embraces practically every biological function. Inhibition of their biosynthesis by the aspirin-like drugs causes major changes to the pathophysiological functions of the organism.

It all started 60 years ago with an observation made by two American gynaecologists, Kurzrok and Lieb, that strips of human uterus relax or contract when exposed to human semen. A few years later, Goldblatt in England and von Euler in Sweden independently reported smooth muscle-contracting and vasodepressor activity in seminal fluid and accessory reproductive glands, and von Euler identified the active material as a lipid-soluble acid, which he named 'prostaglandin' (von Euler, 1973). More than 20 years were to pass before technical advances allowed the demonstration that 'prostaglandin' was in fact a family of lipid compounds of unique structure. Prostaglandin (PG)E$_1$ and PGF$_{1\alpha}$ were isolated in crystalline form and structures were assigned in 1962 (Bergström and Samuelsson, 1968). Soon, more prostaglandins were characterized and, like the others, proved to be 20-carbon unsaturated carboxylic acids with a cyclopentane ring.

When the general structure of the prostaglandins became apparent, their kinship with essential fatty acids was recognized, and in 1964 Bergström and co-workers and van Dorp and associates independently achieved the biosynthesis of PGE$_2$ from arachidonic acid using enzyme preparations from ram seminal vesicles (Samuelsson, 1972).

Under the influence of Sune Bergström, the Upjohn Company in Kalamazoo, Michigan, USA took a strong interest in prostaglandins, as did the ONO Company in Kyoto, Japan and samples of the precious compounds were distributed widely to biologists around the world. PGE$_1$, PGE$_2$ and PGF$_{2\alpha}$ were found to have a remarkably broad spectrum of activity. For instance, PGE_1 contracted uterine and gastrointestinal smooth muscle, relaxed the airways, caused vasodilatation, inhibited platelet aggregation and caused diarrhoea. The therapeutic potential was clearly there, if only substances could be found which had just one of these actions or even a more selective profile.

Indeed, thousands of analogues of prostaglandins were made in the largely frustrated hope that compounds of therapeutic value with a greater selectivity of action would emerge. However, since 1973, several discoveries have caused a radical shift in emphasis away from the PGEs and PGFs. The first was the isolation and identification of two unstable cyclic endoperoxides, prostaglandin G_2 (PGG$_2$ or 15-OOH PGH$_2$) and prostaglandin H_2 (PGH$_2$; Flower, 1978). Later came the elucidation of the structure of thromboxane A_2 (TXA$_2$) and that of its degradation product, thromboxane B_2 (TXB$_2$; Hamberg et al., 1975), and then the discovery of prostacyclin (PGI$_2$; Moncada et al., 1976). These findings, coupled with the discovery of a different enzymatic pathway (a lipoxygenase), which converts arachidonic acid to compounds such as 12-hydroperoxyeicosatetraenoic acid (12-HPETE) and 12-hydroxyeicosatetraenoic acid (12-HETE), have led to the realization that the 'classical' prostaglandins constitute only a fraction of the physiologically active products of arachidonic acid metabolism.

In 1979, the products of a pathway initiated by the action of a 5-lipoxygenase enzyme were characterized; they were named leukotrienes (LTs) because of their initial discovery in leukocytes and their conjugated triene structure (Samuelsson, 1983). These include a 5,12-dihydroxy compound (LTB$_4$), which has potent chemotactic properties and a 5-hydroxy derivative that is conjugated with glutathione (LTC$_4$). The leukotrienes are believed to have important functions as mediators of inflammation.

Even more recently, several other oxidized products of arachidonic acid have been discovered and named as lipoxins, hepoxilins and trioxilins. Indeed, the latest version of the arachidonic acid cascade contains more than 87 compounds! The rate of discovery has become such that it will take years for the biologist to find out whether some or all of these newly found products of fatty acid peroxidation are of importance to physiology or pathology.

2.1 STRUCTURE AND SYNTHESIS

The families of prostaglandins, leukotrienes, and related compounds are called eicosanoids because they are derived from 20-carbon essential fatty acids. These contain three, four or five double bonds: eicosatrienoic acid (dihomo-γ-linolenic acid), eicosatetraenoic acid (arachidonic acid;

Fig. 2.1) and eicosapentaenoic acid (EPA). In man, arachidonic acid is the most abundant precursor. It is either derived from dietary linoleic acid (octadecadienoic acid) in vegetables or is ingested as a constituent of meat. Arachidonate is then esterified as a component of the phospholipids of cell membranes or is found in ester linkage in other complex lipids.

The enhanced biosynthesis of the eicosanoids that occurs in response to widely divergent physical, chemical or hormonal stimuli involves activation of acyl hydrolases. These release arachidonic acid from cellular stores. The provision of arachidonic acid is the rate limiting step and once released, arachidonic acid and its congeners are rapidly metabolized to oxygenated products by several distinct enzyme systems. Products that contain ring structures (prostaglandins, thromboxanes and prostacyclin) result from the initial action of cyclo-oxygenase, while the hydroxylated derivatives of straight-chain fatty acids (e.g leukotrienes) result from the actions of various lipoxygenases.

2.1.1 Prostaglandins, Thromboxanes and Prostacyclin

The prostaglandins fall into several main classes, designated by letters and distinguished by substitutions on the cyclopentane ring. The main classes are subdivided according to the number of double bonds in the side chains. This is indicated by subscript 1, 2 or 3.

Prostaglandins of the D, E and F_α series are sometimes referred to as the 'primary prostaglandins', even though they are products of the metabolism of prostaglandins of the G and H series. Synthesis of these primary prostaglandins is accomplished in a stepwise manner by a ubiquitous complex of microsomal enzymes, the first of which is 'fatty acid cyclo oxygenase'. The unesterified precursor acids are oxygenated and cyclized to form the cyclic endoperoxide derivatives, prostaglandin G (PGG) and prostaglandin H (PGH). These endoperoxides, which are chemically unstable, are then isomerized enzymatically or non-enzymatically into different products, PGD, PGE or PGF.

The endoperoxide PGH_2 is also metabolized into two unstable and highly biologically active compounds with structures that differ from those of the primary prostaglandins. One of these is thromboxane A_2 (TXA_2), formed by an enzyme, thromboxane synthase, first isolated from platelets (Needleman et al., 1976). TXA_2 has a very short chemical half-life of about 30 s; it breaks down non-enzymatically into the stable and relatively inactive thromboxane B_2 (TXB_2; Fig. 2.1).

The other route of metabolism of PGH_2 is to prostacyclin (PGI_2), yet another unstable compound with a half-life of around 3 min, formed by the enzyme, prostacyclin synthase. PGI_2 has a double-ring

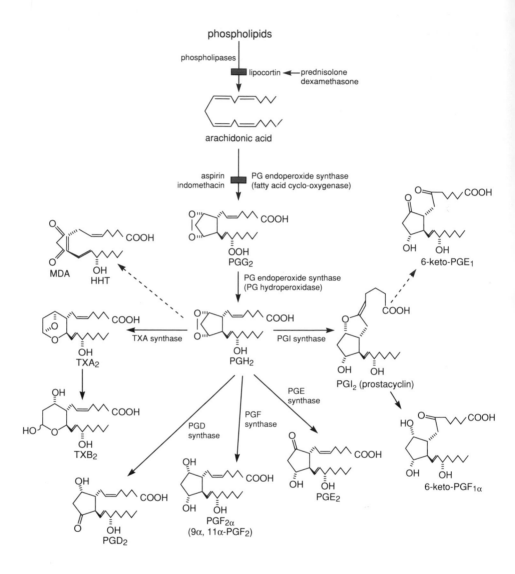

Figure 2.1 Metabolism of arachidonic acid by cyclo-oxygenase. Prostaglandins are formed from arachidonic acid via cyclic endoperoxide intermediates (PGG$_2$ and PGH$_2$). Glucocorticiods (prednisolone and dexamethasone) induce synthesis of the protein lipocortin, which inhibits phospholipase A$_2$ and prevents liberation of arachidonic acid from phospholipids. Aspirin-like drugs inhibit cyclo-oxygenase and prevent prostaglandin generation.

20

structure, closed by an oxygen bridge between carbons 6 and 9. It is hydrolysed non-enzymatically to a much less active, stable compound, 6-keto-$PGF_{1\alpha}$. The presence of the different isomerases varies from tissue to tissue. For example, lung and spleen are able to synthesize the whole range of products, but other tissues cannot; platelets synthesize mainly TXA_2, whereas the blood vessel wall primarily produces PGI_2 (Bunting et al., 1983). PGE_2 is important in the kidney, whereas PGD_2 is made in mast cells (Fig. 2.1).

2.1.2 Products of Lipoxygenases

A number of enzymes have been discovered that peroxidize arachidonic acid in different positions (Nugteren, 1977; Fig. 2.2). The most important of these is a 5-lipoxygenase, which leads to the formation of a complex group of compounds called leukotrienes. Unlike the cyclo-oxygenase, which attacks any available free arachidonic acid, the 5-lipoxygenase needs to be activated, most probably by a rise in intracellular calcium. The first step of the 5-lipoxygenase pathway is the formation of 5-hydroperoxyeicosatetraenoic acid (5-HPETE); this is converted either to the related monohydroxycicosatetraenoic acid (5-HETE) or to the 5,6 epoxide, leukotriene A_4 (LTA$_4$). Leukotriene A_4 may itself be transformed either to 5,12-dihydroxyeicosatetraenoic acid (leukotriene B_4; LTB$_4$), or to leukotriene C_4 (LTC$_4$); the latter is a glutathione derivative, formed by the action of a glutathione-S-transferase. Leukotriene D_4 (LTD$_4$) is made by the removal of glutamic acid from LTC$_4$, and LTE$_4$ results from the subsequent cleavage of glycine (Fig. 2.2). The final step of these transformations produces LTF$_4$ by the reincorporation of γ-glutamic acid into the molecule to form a γ-glutamyl, cysteinyl derivative (Piper, 1983; Samuelsson, 1983). It is now generally accepted that a mixture of LTC$_4$ and LTD$_4$ accounts for the activity originally known as the 'slow-reacting substance of anaphylaxis' (SRS-A).

2.2 METABOLISM OF PROSTAGLANDINS

Efficient mechanisms exist for the catabolism and inactivation of most prostaglandins. For example, about 95% of infused PGE_1, PGE_2 or $PGF_{2\alpha}$ is inactivated during one passage through the pulmonary circulation. Because of the unique position of the lungs between the venous and arterial circulations, the pulmonary vascular bed constitutes an important filter for many substances (including some prostaglandins) that might be released from tissues into the venous circulation. The

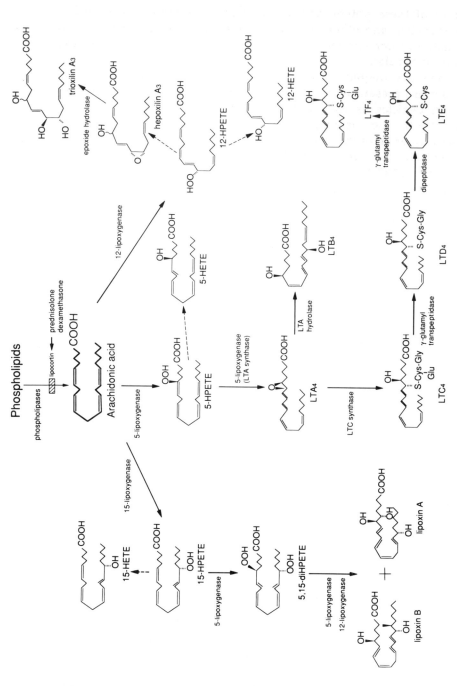

Figure 2.2 Metabolism of arachidonic acid by lipoxygenases. Lipoxygenase enzymes generate hydroperoxyeicosatetraenoic acids (HPETEs) and hydroxyeicosatetraenoic acids (HETEs) from arachidonic acid. 5-hydroperoxyeicosatetraenoic acid (5-HPETE), produced by the action of 5-lipoxygenase, is the precursor of the potent chemotactic and bronchoconstrictor leukotrienes (LTA$_4$, LTB$_4$, LTC$_4$ and LTD$_4$).

clearance of these potent, vasoactive substances protects the cardio-vascular system and other organs from their prolonged effects due to recirculation. Interestingly, prostacyclin survives passage through the pulmonary circulation.

Enzymes that degrade prostaglandins are widely distributed in the body and are present in the spleen, kidney, adipose tissue, intestine, liver and testicles as well as in the lung (Samuelsson *et al.*, 1975; Flower, 1978). The metabolism of TXA_2 in man has been inferred from investigation of the fate of TXB_2. While up to 20 metabolites have been identified in urine, by far the most abundant is 2,3-dinor-TXB_2 (Roberts *et al.*, 1981). The degradation of PGI_2 includes its spontaneous hydrolysis in blood to 6-keto-$PGF_{1\alpha}$ and the main urinary metabolites are 2,3-dinor-6-keto-$PGF_{1\alpha}$ and 6,15-diketo-2,3, dinor-$PGF_{1\alpha}$. The development of sensitive GC/MS methods to measure these metabolites in urine has greatly facilitated our knowledge of the relevance of prostacyclin and TXA_2 in physiology and pathology (Oates *et al.*, 1988a,b).

2.3 PHARMACOLOGICAL ACTIONS

No other autacoids show more numerous and diverse effects than do prostaglandins and other metabolites of arachidonic acid. Not only is the spectrum of actions broad, but also different compounds show different activities, both qualitatively and quantitatively.

2.3.1 Cardiovascular System

In most species and in most vascular beds PGEs and PGAs are potent vasodilators. When injected into the femoral arterial bed in dogs, their potency exceeds that of acetylcholine or histamine, although it is less than that of bradykinin. Responses to $PGF_{2\alpha}$ show species variation, but vasodilatations have been observed following injection into the human brachial artery of $PGF_{2\alpha}$ and PGs A_1, A_2, B_1, E_1, and F_2 (Robinson *el al.*, 1973).

The intravenous administration of PGI_2 causes prominent hypotension in animals, including man. It is about five times more potent than PGE_2 in producing this effect. The compound causes dilatation in various vascular beds, including the coronary, renal, mesenteric and skeletal muscle, and, importantly, the pulmonary circulation. It relaxes essentially all isolated preparations of vascular smooth muscle that have been tested. Its chemical degradation product, 6-keto-$PGF_{1\alpha}$, has less than one thousandth the activity of PGI_2. Because it is not inactivated by the pulmonary circulation, PGI_2 is equipotent as a vasodilator when given either intra-arterially or intravenously (Moncada, 1982; Vane, 1982).

The prostaglandins and related compounds exert powerful actions on platelets. Some of them, like PGE_1 and PGD_2, are inhibitors of the aggregation of human platelets *in vitro* at concentrations around 0.1 μM. PGI_2 is some 30–50 times more potent, inhibiting aggregation at concentrations between 1 and 10 nM. This, together with the observation that PGI_2 is generated by the vascular wall (particularly by the vascular endothelium) has led to the important concept that prostacyclin helps to prevent the aggregation and adhesion of platelets *in vivo*.

The main product of arachidonic acid metabolism in platelets, TXA_2, is a very powerful inducer of platelet aggregation and the platelet release reaction. TXA_2 also potently constricts vascular smooth muscle. The endoperoxides, although active, are much less so than TXA_2. Pathways of platelet aggregation that are dependent on the generation of TXA_2 are sensitive to the inhibitory action of aspirin (Moncada and Vane, 1979) (Chapter 10).

The leukotriene LTB_4 is a potent chemotactic agent for polymorphonuclear leukocytes; other leukotrienes do not share this action (Piper, 1983). Its potency is comparable to that of various chemotactic peptides and platelet-activating factor (PAF). Chemo-attraction of leukocytes appears to be the main effect of LTB_4 in the microvasculature.

2.3.2 Smooth Muscle

Eicosanoids contract or relax many smooth muscles besides those of the vasculature. Again, responses may vary with species, type of prostaglandin, endocrine status of the tissue, and experimental conditions. However, few smooth muscles are uninfluenced, and many display intense and consistent responses.

Prostaglandin endoperoxides and TXA_2 are constrictors of guinea pig tracheal strips *in vitro*. TXA_2 is the more potent and induces bronchoconstriction in guinea pigs when given by aerosol (Hamberg *et al.*, 1976). PGI_2, on the other hand, is without effect or induces slight bronchodilatation; it antagonizes bronchoconstriction produced by other agents in man (Bianco *et al.*, 1978).

The leukotrienes (e.g. LTD_4) contract most smooth muscles. While there is considerable species variation, LTC_4 and LTD_4 are powerful bronchoconstrictors in many species, including man (Piper, 1983). They appear to act directly on smooth muscle, especially that in peripheral airways, and are far more potent than histamine both *in vitro* and *in vivo*.

The intravenous infusion of PGE_2 or $PGF_{2\alpha}$ to pregnant humans produces a dose-dependent increase in the frequency and intensity of uterine contractions. Uterine responsiveness to prostaglandins increases somewhat as pregnancy progresses, but far less than does that to oxytocin.

PGEs, PGAs and PGI_2 inhibit gastric acid secretion stimulated by feeding, histamine or gastrin. Volume of secretion, acidity and content of pepsin are all reduced, probably by an action exerted directly on the secretory cells. In addition, these prostaglandins are vasodilators in the gastric mucosa and PGI_2 is probably involved in the local regulation of blood flow (Whittle, 1987). Mucus secretion in the stomach and small intestine is increased by prostaglandins and there is substantial movement of water and electrolytes into the intestinal lumen. Such effects may underlie the watery diarrhoea noted in animals and man following the oral or parenteral administration of prostaglandins. Inhibition of endogenous prostaglandin production by the aspirin-like drugs may remove their protective effects on the gastric mucosa and lead to damage and ulceration. This is a major disadvantage of the non-steroidal anti-inflammatory agents. The protective action of the prostaglandins is the basis for developing prostaglandin analogues as anti-ulcer drugs.

2.3.3 Afferent Nerves and Pain

In man, PGEs cause pain when injected intradermally and they irritate the mucous membranes of the eyes and respiratory passages. These effects are generally not as immediate or intense as those caused by bradykinin or histamine but they outlast those caused by the other autacoids and are accompanied by tenderness and hyperalgesia. PGEs and PGI_2 sensitize the afferent nerve endings to the effects of chemical or mechanical stimuli; the release of these prostaglandins during the inflammatory process thus serves as an amplification system for the pain mechanism (Moncada et al., 1978; Chapter 8). The actions of the major eicosanoids are summarized in Table 2.1.

2.3.4 Mechanism of Action

In many tissues prostaglandins regulate the synthesis of adenosine 3',5'-monophosphate (cyclic AMP) by activating or inhibiting adenylate cyclase. Moreover, there is a growing body of evidence for the existence of specific membrane-bound receptors for prostaglandins, thromboxanes and leukotrienes in many tissues.

25

Table 2.1 Effects of eicosanoids

PGE_2, PGI_2	$PGF_{2\alpha}$	TXA_2	LTB_4	LTC_4, LTD_4
Vasodilatation	Vasoconstriction or Vasodilatation	Vasoconstriction	Vascular permeability ↑	Bronchoconstriction
Blood pressure ↓	Bronchoconstriction	Blood pressure ↑	Leukocyte chemotaxis ↑	Vascular permeability ↑
Platelet aggregation ↓	Gut smooth muscle contraction	Platelet aggregation ↑	T cell proliferation ↑	Interferon-γ secretion ↑
Gastric secretion ↓	Uterine contraction	Bronchoconstriction	Leukocyte aggregation ↑	
Cytoprotection		Lymphocyte proliferation		
Bronchodilatation				
Hyperalgesia				
T cell proliferation ↓				
Lymphocyte migration ↓				

The mechanism of action of prostaglandins and related substances has been studied intensively in platelets (Mittal and Murad, 1982). The prostaglandin endoperoxides and TXA_2 can cause platelet clumping and facilitate aggregation that has been induced by other agents. These effects are associated with the release of intracellular calcium (Owen and Le Breton, 1981). The increased calcium promotes aggregation and production of additional TXA_2. Platelet aggregation is inhibited by PGI_2 by increasing the concentration of cyclic AMP.

2.3.5 Receptor Antagonists

Several compounds have been designed that selectively antagonize responses to TXA_2 in platelets and smooth muscle from various tissues. The effects of endoperoxides (e.g. PGH_2) are also inhibited, presumably because they interact with the same receptors. The biological and clinical effects of these compounds are currently under investigation, especially with regard to their potential to modify thrombotic phenomena *in vivo* (Humphrey *et al.*, 1990).

Antagonists of the TXA_2 receptor have been found effective in experimental models of myocardial ischaemia, circulatory shock and sudden cardiopulmonary death. These antagonists synergize in their beneficial effects with thromboxane synthetase inhibitors which effectively increase the production of prostacyclin by making platelet endoperoxides available for prostacyclin formation (Lefer and Darius, 1987).

Receptors for LTD_4 have been characterized and a number of selective antagonists to the peptidoleukotrienes are available. They effectively block responses to leukotrienes in models of anaphylaxis but have yet to be proved effective in ameliorating the symptoms of asthma (Musser *et al.*, 1986).

2.4 THE FUNCTIONS OF ENDOGENOUS EICOSANOIDS

Because these substances can be formed by virtually every tissue and cell type, it is not unreasonable to suspect that each pharmacological effect observed may reflect a physiological or pathophysiological function and such suspicions have been nurtured and presented in countless hypotheses bearing on just about every bodily function. Some clarification and simplification have occurred in the last few years, in that it is now generally accepted that PGAs, PGBs and PGCs are not formed endogenously. Furthermore, PGs of the one series, such as PGE_1, are not found in tissues other than semen.

2.4.1 Platelets

Stimulation of platelets to aggregate leads to activation of membrane phospholipases with the consequent release of arachidonic acid and its transformation into prostaglandin endoperoxides and TXA_2. These substances induce platelet aggregation. However, this pathway is not the only one for the induction of platelet aggregation, since, for example, thrombin aggregates platelets without the release of arachidonic acid. The importance of the thromboxane pathway is, however, highlighted by the fact that aspirin inhibits the second phase of platelet aggregation and induces a mild haemostatic defect in humans (Jobim, 1978)(Chapter 10).

Prostacyclin generated in the vessel wall may be the physiological antagonist of this system in platelets. According to this concept, prostacyclin and TXA_2 represent biologically opposite poles of a mechanism for regulating platelet–vessel wall interaction and the formation of haemostatic plugs and intra-arterial thrombi (Moncada and Vane, 1982). Importantly, the formation of prostacyclin is not the only mechanism by which the vascular endothelium defends itself against platelet adhesion and aggregation. Release of endothelium-derived relaxing factor (EDRF) also plays a role, for as well as causing vasodilatation (like prostacyclin) EDRF also inhibits platelet adhesion and aggregation. Indeed, prostacyclin and EDRF (now identified as nitric oxide) act synergistically in this respect (Vane *et al.*, 1990).

2.4.2 Reproduction and Parturition

There has been much interest in the possible involvement of prostaglandins in reproductive physiology. Their very high concentrations in human semen, coupled with the substantial absorption of prostaglandins by the vagina, have encouraged speculation that prostaglandins deposited during coitus may facilitate conception by actions on the cervix, uterine body, fallopian tubes, and transport of semen. While there does seem to be a correlation between lowered concentrations of prostaglandins in semen and some cases of male infertility, the role of the eicosanoids in semen remains obscure.

During pregnancy in the human, the capacity of the foetal membranes to elaborate prostaglandins rises progressively. Concentrations of prostaglandins in blood and amniotic fluid are elevated during labour, but it is not certain whether this is a major determinant of the onset of labour or only serves to sustain uterine contractions that have been initiated by oxytocin. In any event, inhibitors of cyclo-oxygenase such as aspirin can increase the length of gestation, prolong the duration of spontaneous labour, and interrupt premature labour. The last-named effect has prompted clinical investigation of these agents for the prevention of premature delivery. While effective, their potential impact on foetal development (e.g. premature closure of the ductus arteriosus), together with the availability of other tocolytic agents, has limited the use of cyclo-oxygenase inhibitors for this purpose.

$PGF_{2\alpha}$ produced in the uterus is the long-sought luteolytic hormone in some subprimate species. This knowledge has led to the development of prostaglandin analogues for veterinary use in synchronizing oestrus in farm animals such as sheep, cattle, pigs and horses. This method has simplified breeding procedures and is used to provide safe, early abortions before the animals are sent to market. However, a luteolytic prostaglandin analogue for human use has not been developed. The possible roles of prostaglandins in reproductive processes have been reviewed by Karim and Hillier (1979).

2.4.3 Vascular and Pulmonary Smooth Muscle

Local generation of PGE_2 and PGI_2 has been implicated in the maintenance of patency of the ductus arteriosus. This hypothesis has been strengthened by the fact that aspirin-like drugs induce closure of a patent ductus in animals and neonates. Prostaglandins might also play a role in the maintenance of placental blood flow (Rankin, 1978).

A complex mixture of autacoids is released when sensitized lung tissue is challenged by the appropriate antigen. Various prostaglandins and leukotrienes are prominent components of this mixture. While both bronchodilator (PGE_2) and bronchoconstrictor (e.g. $PGF_{2\alpha}$, TXA_2, LTC_4) substances are released, the effects of the peptidoleukotrienes probably dominate during allergic constriction of the airway (Piper, 1983). Evidence to reinforce this conclusion is the ineffectiveness of inhibitors of cyclo-oxygenase and of histamine antagonists in the treatment of human asthma. Moreover, the relatively slow metabolism of the leukotrienes in lung tissue contributes to the long lasting bronchoconstriction that follows challenge with antigen and may be a factor in the high bronchial tone that is observed in asthmatics in periods between acute attacks.

2.4.4 Kidney

Prostaglandins probably modulate renal blood flow and regulate urine formation by both renovascular and tubular effects. Prostacyclin also causes the secretion of renin. The elaboration of PGE_2 and prostacyclin is increased by factors that reduce renal blood flow (e.g. stimulation of sympathetic nerves and angiotensin), and inhibitors of cyclo-oxygenase augment the renal vasoconstriction that is produced by such stimuli (Aiken and Vane, 1973). The effects of antidiuretic hormone on the reabsorption of water may be restrained by the concomitant production and action of PGE_2, and the negative-feedback effects of angiotensin on renin secretion are opposed by the stimulant actions of prostacyclin.

Increased biosynthesis of prostaglandins has been associated with Bartter's syndrome. This is a rare disease characterized by low-to-normal blood pressure, decreased sensitivity to angiotensin, high activity of renin in plasma, hyperaldosteronism, and excessive loss of potassium. There is also an increased granulation of renal medullary interstitial cells and an increased excretion of prostaglandins in the urine. After chronic administration of inhibitors of cyclo-oxygenase, sensitivity to angiotensin, plasma renin values, and the concentration of aldosterone in plasma return to normal. Although plasma potassium rises, it remains low, and urinary potassium wasting persists. Whether an increase in prostaglandin biosynthesis is the cause of Bartter's syndrome or a reflection of a more basic physiological defect is not known (Ferris, 1978).

2.4.5 Inflammation

Prostaglandins and leukotrienes are released by a host of mechanical, thermal, chemical, bacterial and other insults and they contribute importantly to the genesis of the signs and symptoms of inflammation as does another product of phospholipase, 1-alkyl-2-acetyl-sn-glycero-3-phosphocholine or platelet activating factor, now known simply as PAF (Moncada *et al.*, 1978; Larsen and Henson, 1983; Braquet and Rola-Pleszczynski, 1987). The peptidoleukotrienes have powerful effects on vascular permeability, while LTB_4 is a potent chemo-attractant for polymorphonuclear leukocytes and can promote exudation of plasma by mobilizing this source of additional inflammatory mediators. Although prostaglandins do not appear to have direct effects on vascular permeability, both PGE_2 and PGI_2 markedly enhance oedema formation and leukocyte infiltration by promoting blood flow in the inflamed region. Moreover, they potentiate the pain-producing activity of bradykinin and other autacoids.

Since prostaglandins of the E series have potent osteolytic activity, they have been implicated in some types of hypercalcaemia. Other studies have implicated platelet aggregation and the effects of prosta-glandins thereon in the haematogenous metastasis of tumours. While pretreatment of animals with inhibitors of thromboxane synthetase reduces the formation of tumour colonies, the administration of such agents after the injection of tumour cells is without effect. However, the infusion of PGI_2 in rats, either before or after the injection of cells, markedly inhibits the establishment of tumour colonies. These effects have been attributed to inhibition of platelet aggregation, rather than to vasodilatation (Honn et al., 1983) (Chapter 10).

2.4.6 The Immune System

Prostaglandins have also been implicated in the control of the immunological response. PGE_1 has been claimed to influence the functions of B lymphocytes selectively and to act synergistically with procarbazine to depress immune responsiveness. In addition, the humoral antibody response is decreased by PGE_1. Prostaglandins also affect T lymphocytes. The T ('killer') lymphocyte, active in slowing tumour growth and killing malignant cells, is inhibited by PGEs in its ability to reject allogenic thymus cells in vitro.

Some experimental tumours in animals and certain spontaneous human tumours (medullary carcinoma of the thyroid, renal cell adenocarcinoma, carcinoma of the breast) are accompanied by increased concentrations of local or circulating prostaglandins, bone metastasis, and hypercalcaemia. The immunosuppressive activity of certain of these tumours may be related to their ability to produce prostaglandins.

2.5 INHIBITION OF PROSTAGLANDIN BIOSYNTHESIS

Corticosteroids inhibit phospholipase A_2 activity which is necessary for the release of arachidonic acid (Fig. 2.1). Thus, corticosteroids ultimately inhibit the formation of prostaglandins, thromboxane and the leukotrienes, likely explaining their more potent anti-inflammatory properties compared to the non-steroid anti-inflammatory drugs. Anti-inflammatory steroids are thought to inhibit phospholipase A_2 indirectly by inducing the synthesis of an inhibitory protein, termed lipocortin (Flower, 1985, 1988). The lipocortins belong to the same family of cellular proteins as calpactins and a pure, cloned form of lipocortin I with a molecular weight of 37 kDa has become available (Wallner et al., 1986).

A proposed alternative mechanism for the inhibition of prostaglandin formation by steroids is that they prevent synthesis of new cyclo-oxygenase enzyme. Dexamethasone inhibited selectively the enzyme induced with bacterial endotoxin in mouse peritoneal macrophages whereas unstimulated basal cyclo-oxygenase activity was unaffected (Masferrer et al., 1990).

A milestone was passed in prostaglandin research when Vane found

Introduction

in 1971 that aspirin-like drugs inhibit the biosynthesis of prostaglandins. These drugs inhibit the cyclo-oxygenase enzyme which forms the endoperoxides and, as a result, prevent the synthesis of all of the products beyond this step in the metabolic cascade (Flower, 1974). A clear-cut inhibition of prostaglandin synthesis, as measured by a reduction in prostaglandins (or their metabolites) in synovial fluid, urine, or semen, is evident in man treated with conventional doses of these anti-inflammatory agents, and their therapeutic efficacy largely parallels their ability to inhibit fatty acid cyclo-oxygenase. Thus, inhibition of cyclo-oxygenase is the mechanism by which aspirin-like drugs bring about their therapeutic and other effects (see Chapter 3).

Aspirin, in recent extensive clinical trials, had beneficial effects in the prophylaxis of acute myocardial infarction (de Gaetano, 1988) and of a recurrence of infarction. This is attributed to its inhibition of cyclo-oxygenase leading to decreased production of TXA_2. Prostacyclin production is also decreased but the cyclo-oxygenase enzyme in the endothelial cell regenerates so that prostacyclin synthesis is re-established. However, platelets do not form new enzyme and thromboxane synthesis is irreversibly inhibited for their lifetime of 8–10 days in the circulation. In addition, aspirin acetylates cyclo-oxygenase of the platelets in the presystemic circulation before it reaches the general circulation and becomes diluted by peripheral blood. Thus, it should be possible to devise a regimen of aspirin treatment which effectively reduces the aggregability of platelets without greatly affecting the thromboresistance of the vascular endothelial lining. Such a regimen may consist of a slow release tablet of less than 100 mg day^{-1} (Chapters 10 and 12).

REFERENCES

Aiken, J.W. and Vane, J.R. (1973) Intrarenal prostaglandin release attenuates the renal vasoconstrictor activity of angiotensin. *J. Pharmacol. Exp. Ther.*, **184**, 678–87.

Bergström, S. and Samuelsson, B. (1968) The prostaglandins. *Endeavour*, **27**, 109–13.

Bianco, S., Robuschi, M., Ceserani, R. *et al.* (1978) Prevention of a specifically induced bronchoconstriction by prostacyclin (PGI_2) in asthmatic subjects. *Int. Res. Commun. Syst. Med. Sci.*, **6**, 256.

Braquet, P. and Rola-Pleszczynski, M. (1987) Platelet-activating factor and cellular immune responses. *Immunology Today*, **8**, 345–52.

Bunting, S., Moncada, S. and Vane, J.R. (1983) The prostacyclin–thromboxane A_2 balance: pathophysiological and therapeutic implications. *Brit. Med. Bull.*, **39**, 271–6.

De Gaetano, G. (1988) Primary prevention of vascular disease by aspirin. *Lancet*, **i**, 1093–4.

Euler, U.S. von (1973) Some aspects of the actions of prostaglandins. The First Hyemans Memorial Lecture. *Arch. Int. Pharmacodyn. Ther.*, **202** (Suppl.), 295–307.

Ferris, T.F. (1978) Prostaglandins, potassium and Bartter's syndrome. *J. Lab. Clin. Med.*, **92** 663–8.

Flower, R.J. (1974) Drugs which inhibit prostaglandin biosynthesis. *Pharmacol. Rev.*, **26**, 33–67.

Flower, R.J. (1978) Prostaglandins and related compounds. In *Inflammation. Handbook of Experimental Pharmacology, Vol. 50* (eds J.R. Vane and S.H. Ferreira) Springer-Verlag, Berlin, pp. 374–422.

Flower, R.J. (1985) Background and discovery of lipocortins. *Agents Actions*, **17**, 255–62.

Flower, R.J. (1988) Lipocortin and the mechanism of action of the glucocorticoids. *Brit. J. Pharmacol.*, **94**, 987–1015.

Hamberg, M., Svensson, J. and Samuelsson, B. (1975) Thromboxanes: a new group of biologically active compounds derived from prostaglandin endoperoxides. *Proc. Natl Acad. Sci. USA*, **72**, 2994–8.

Hamberg, M., Svensson, J., Hedqvist, P. *et al.* (1976) Involvement of endoperoxides and thromboxanes in anaphylactic reactions. *Adv. Prostaglandin Thromboxane Res.*, **1**, 495–501.

Honn, K.V., Busse, W.D, and Sloane, B.F. (1983) Prostacyclin and thromboxanes: implications for their role in tumor cell metastasis. *Biochem. Pharmacol.*, **32**, 1–11.

Humphrey, P.P.A., Hallet, P., Hornby, E.J. *et al.* (1990) Pathophysiological actions of thromboxane A_2 and their pharmacological antagonism by thromboxane receptor blockade with GR32191. *Circulation*, **81** (Suppl. 1), I-42 – I-52.

Jobim, F. (1978) Acetylsalicylic acid, hemostasis and human thromboembolism. *Semin. Thromb. Hemostas.*, **4**, 199–240.

Karim, S.M.M. and Hillier, K. (1979) Prostaglandins in the control of animal and human reproduction. *Brit. Med. Bull.*, **35**, 173–80.

Larsen, G.L. and Henson, P.M. (1983) Mediators of inflammation. *Ann. Rev. Immunol.*, **1**, 335–59.

Lefer, A.M. and Darius, H. (1987) A pharmacological approach to thromboxane receptor antagonism. *Fed. Proc. Fed. Am. Soc. Exp. Biol.*, **46**, 144–8.

Masferrer, J.L., Zweifel, B.S., Seibert, K. and Needleman, P. (1990) Selective regulation of cellular cyclo-oxygenase by dexamethasone and endotoxin in mice. *J. Clin. Invest.*, **86**, 1375–9.

Mittal, C.K. and Murad, F. (1982) Guanylate cyclase: regulation of cyclic GMP metabolism. In *Cyclic Nucleotides. Handbook of Experimental Pharmacology, Vol. 58* (eds J.A. Nathanson and J.W. Kebabian), Springer-Verlag, Berlin, pp. 225–60

Moncada, S. (1982) Biological importance of prostacyclin. VIII Gaddum Memorial Lecture. *Brit. J. Pharmacol.*, **76**, 3–31.

Moncada, S. and Vane, J.R. (1979) Pharmacology and endogenous roles of prostaglandin endoperoxides, thromboxane A_2 and prostacyclin. *Pharmacol. Rev.*, **30**, 293–331.

Moncada, S. and Vane, J.R. (1982) The role of prostaglandins in platelet-vessel wall interactions. In *Pathobiology of the Endothelial Cell*, (eds H.L. Nossel and H.J. Vogel), Academic Press, New York, pp. 253–85.

Introduction

Moncada, S., Gryglewski, R., Bunting, S. *et al.* (1976) An enzyme isolated from arteries transforms prostaglandin endoperoxides to an unstable substance that inhibits platelet aggregation. *Nature*, **263**, 663–5.

Moncada, S., Ferreira, S.H. and Vane, J.R. (1978) Pain and inflammatory mediators. In *Inflammation. Handbook of Experimental Pharmacology, Vol. 50* (eds J.R. Vane and S.H. Ferreira), Springer-Verlag, Berlin, pp. 588–616.

Musser, J.H., Kreft, A.F. and Lewis, A.J. (1986) New developments concerning leukotriene antagonists: a review. *Agents Actions*, **18**, 332–41.

Needleman, P., Moncada, S., Bunting, S. *et al.* (1976) Identification of an enzyme in platelet microsomes which generates thromboxane A_2 from prostaglandin endoperoxides. *Nature*, **261**, 558–60.

Nugteren, D.H. (1977) Arachidonate lipoxygenase. In *Prostaglandins in Hematology* (eds M. Silver, B.J. Smith and J.J. Kocsis), Spectrum Publications Inc., New York, pp. 11–25.

Oates, J.A., FitzGerald, G.A., Branch, R.A. *et al.* (1988a) Clinical implications of prostaglandin and thromboxane A_2 formation. Part I. *N. Engl. J. Med.*, **319**, 689–96.

Oates, J.A., FitzGerald, G.A., Branch, R.A. *et al.* (1988b) Clinical implications of prostaglandin and thromboxane A_2 formation. Part II. *N. Engl. J. Med.*, **319**, 761–7.

Owen, N.E. and Le Breton, G.C. (1981) Ca^{2+} mobilization in blood platelets as visualized by chlortetracycline fluorescence. *Am. J. Physiol.*, **241**, 613–19.

Piper, P.J. (1983) Pharmacology of leukotrienes. *Brit. Med. Bull.*, **39**, 255–9.

Rankin, J.H.G. (1978) Role of prostaglandins in the maintenance of the placental circulation. *Adv. Prostaglandin Thromboxane Res.*, **4**, 261–9.

Roberts, L.J., Sweetman, B.J. and Oates, J.A. (1981) Metabolism of thromboxane B_2 in man. Identification of twenty urinary metabolites. *J. Biol. Chem.*, **256**, 8384–93.

Robinson, B.F., Collier, J.G., Karim, S.M.M. *et al.* (1973) Effect of prostaglandins A_1, A_2, B_1, E_2 and F_2 on forearm arterial bed and superficial hand veins in man. *Clin. Sci.*, **44**, 367–76.

Samuelsson, B. (1972) Biosynthesis of prostaglandins. *Fed. Proc.*, **31**, 1442–60.

Samuelsson, B. (1983) Leukotrienes: mediators of immediate hypersensitivity reactions and inflammation. *Science*, **220**, 568–75.

Samuelsson, B., Granstrom, E. and Green, K. *et al.* (1975) Prostaglandins. *Ann. Rev. Biochem.*, **44**, 669–94.

Vane, J.R. (1971) Inhibition of prostaglandin synthesis as a mechanism of action for aspirin-like drugs. *Nature (New Biology)*, **231**, 232–5.

Vane, J.R. (1982) Prostacyclin; a hormone with a therapeutic potential. *J. Endocrinol.*, **95**, 3P–43P.

Vane, J.R., Änggård, E.E. and Botting, R.M. (1990) Regulatory functions of the vascular endothelium. *N. Engl. J. Med.*, **323**, 27–36.

Wallner, B.P., Mattaliano, R.J., Hession, C. *et al.* (1986) Cloning and expression of human lipocortin, a phospholipase A_2 inhibitor with potent anti-inflammatory activity. *Nature*, **320**, 77–81.

Whittle, B.J.R. (1987) Protection of the gastric mucosa by prostaglandins and their analogs. *ISI Atlas of Science: Pharmacology*, **1**, 168–72.

3 *The mechanism of action of aspirin*

J.R. VANE, R.J. FLOWER and R.M. BOTTING

3.1 SOME EARLY EXPLANATIONS FOR THE ACTION OF ASPIRIN

Before 1971, little was known about the real mechanism of action of the aspirin-like drugs. They produced an anti-inflammatory effect which was qualitatively and quantitatively different from that of the anti-inflammatory steroids. Their analgesic action too was of a different nature to that produced by the opiates (Chapter 8).

Many biochemical effects of these drugs had been documented, and theories based upon these effects, abandoned. It was observed, for example, that most of the aspirin-like drugs uncoupled oxidative phosphorylation (Whitehouse and Haslam, 1962), that several salicylates inhibited dehydrogenase enzymes especially those dependent upon pyridine nucleotides (Hines and Smith, 1964; Smith *et al.*, 1964). Some amino-transferases (Gould and Smith, 1965a) and decarboxylases (Gould and Smith, 1965b) were also inhibited and so were several key enzymes involved in protein and RNA biosynthesis (Weiss *et al.*, 1962). All these inhibitory actions were at sometime invoked to explain the therapeutic action of aspirin. A problem with most of these ideas was that the concentration of the drugs required for enzyme inhibition was in excess (sometimes greatly in excess) of the concentrations typically found in the plasma after therapy, and there was invariably a lack of correlation between the ability of these drugs to inhibit a particular enzyme, and their activity as anti-inflammatory agents (Whitehouse, 1965). But perhaps the most serious impediment of all to acceptance of any of the above ideas was that their proponents could not provide a convincing reason why inhibition of any of these enzymes should produce the triple anti-inflammatory, analgesic and antipyretic effects of aspirin. Perhaps the most reasonable hypothesis of the time was based upon the observation that the salicylates could inhibit several proteases. Increased extracellular proteolytic activity had been observed in several models of inflammation and was thought to be responsible

35

for the tissue destruction characteristic of such chronic diseases as rheumatoid arthritis (Spector and Willoughby, 1963).

It was, of course, not only biochemists who wondered how these drugs acted; pharmacologists too were intensely interested in their mechanism of action and no one contributed more important observations to this literature in the 1960s than the British pharmacologist Harry Collier. Collier had termed aspirin an 'anti-defensive' drug because of its ability to prevent the physiological defence mechanisms of pain, fever and inflammation from functioning normally (Collier, 1963, 1969). Together with his group he made the important finding that guinea-pigs who had received aspirin were protected from the bronchoconstriction normally elicited in these animals by bradykinin (Collier and Shorley, 1960), ATP (Collier et al., 1966) and SRS-A (slow-reacting substance in anaphylaxis) now identified as a mixture of leukotrienes (Berry and Collier, 1964). Aspirin also prevented the contraction of the guinea-pig isolated tracheobronchial muscle caused by SRS-A and bradykinin (Bhoola et al., 1962) and also the nociceptive response to ATP in mice (Collier et al., 1966).

It was, however, not clear how the bronchoconstrictor response was inhibited by aspirin. Initially, Collier suggested that 'A-receptors' (which could be blocked by aspirin-like drugs) were involved in the spasmogenic response to these agents (Collier and Sweatman, 1968), but later he abandoned this concept and wrote instead that the drugs acted, 'rather by inhibiting some underlying cellular mechanism that takes part to different extents in different responses mediated by different endogenous substances'.

3.2 ASPIRIN AND THE PROSTAGLANDIN SYSTEM

It was then, against this background of knowledge, that the investigation of aspirin's action was taken over by prostaglandin researchers. Priscilla Piper had been working with Harry Collier at the Parke Davis laboratories in Hounslow, Middlesex and came to Vane's laboratory at the Royal College of Surgeons as a graduate student. She had been working on the interactions between bradykinin and aspirin and brought with her an enthusiasm to find out how aspirin worked. Piper and Vane used isolated lungs from sensitized guinea-pigs, perfused with Krebs' solution (Piper and Vane, 1969a). The object was to detect substances released during the anaphylactic reaction, including histamine and SRS-A, both of which had been known for many years as possible mediators of anaphylaxis. They employed the technique of continuous bioassay using the cascade bioassay system (Vane, 1964) developed by Vane in the mid-1960s for use with blood or an artificial salt solution (Fig. 3.1). The method involved perfusing guinea pig isolated lungs with Kreb's solution and using the effluent to superfuse successively strips of gastrointestinal tissues selected for their sensitivity to different substances. Among the tissues used were the rat stomach strip, chick rectum and rat colon, which are specifically contracted by prostaglandins E_2 and $F_{2\alpha}$ (Fig. 3.2).

Piper and Vane found, as expected, the release during anaphylaxis of histamine and SRS-A but they also found some previously unreported substances: prostaglandins (mainly prostaglandin E_2 but with some prostaglandin $F_{2\alpha}$) and another, very ephemeral, substance that, from the assay tissue that picked it up, was called 'rabbit aorta contracting substance' (RCS; the resemblance of these initials to those of the Royal College of Surgeons is not coincidental!). RCS in the lung perfusate had a half-life of about 2 min and even when cooled down to a few degrees above freezing remained stable for no more than 20 min. It was

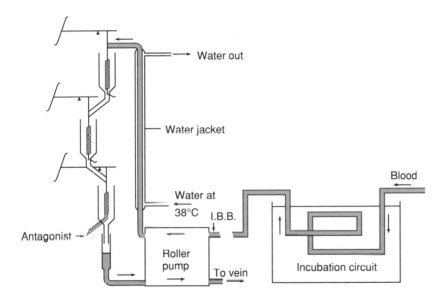

Figure 3.1 Diagram of the blood-bathed organ technique. Blood is continuously withdrawn from a convenient vessel by a roller pump, kept at 37 °C by a water jacket and then allowed to superfuse a series of isolated organs, the longitudinal movements of which are recorded. The blood is then collected in a reservoir and returned to the animal. In some experiments the blood flows through a length of silicone tubing in a water bath (incubating circuit) before superfusing the isolated tissues. Drugs can be applied directly to the isolated tissues by infusions or injections into the bathing blood (IBB) or with a time delay into the incubating circuit (from Vane (1969), Ref. 52, by permission of The Macmillan Press Ltd).

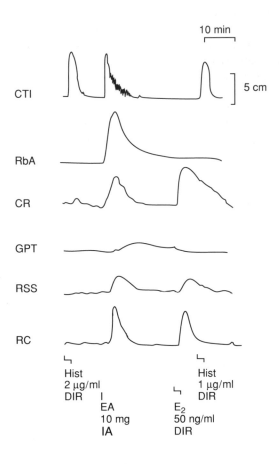

Figure 3.2   Release of mediators from isolated lungs of sensitized guinea pigs. The lungs were perfused through the pulmonary artery with Krebs' solution and the effluent superfused a cat terminal ileum (CTI), rabbit aorta spiral strip (rbA), chick rectum (CR), guinea pig trachea (GPT), rat stomach strip (RSS) and rat colon (RC). All tissues except CTI were blocked with antagonists to 5HT, catecholamines and histamine. Infusions of histamine (2 μg and 1 μg ml^{-1} DIR) and of prostaglandin E$_2$ (E$_2$, 50 ng ml^{-1}DIR) directly to the assay tissues demonstrated the selective sensitivity of the assay system. Anaphylaxis was induced in the lungs by injecting ovalbumen intra-arterially (EA 10 mg IA). Contractions of CTI demonstrated release of histamine, RbA release of RCS, GPT release of SRS–A and CR, RSS and RC release of prostaglandins. Time 10 min; vertical scale 5 cm. (From Vane, 1971a. Reprinted from Ciba Foundation Study No. 38 by permission of The Ciba Foundation.) EA = egg albumin. DIR = directly applied.

identified in 1975 as thromboxane A_2 by Samuelsson's group (Hamberg *et al.*, 1975).

It was RCS that provided the first clue to the relationship between aspirin and the prostaglandins. When Piper was working with Collier, they showed that many effects of bradykinin both *in vitro* and *in vivo* could be reduced by aspirin (Collier *et al.*, 1968a,b). Subsequently, Piper and Vane, in the course of further experiments involving RCS discovered that in some preparations it was released by bradykinin. This raised the possibility that the bradykinin effects previously mentioned were produced not directly by that hormone but via its release of RCS. This, in turn, suggested that aspirin's ability to minimize some effects of bradykinin might be due to its blocking of RCS release. This idea was confirmed when Piper and Vane presented experimental evidence that the release of RCS from guinea-pig isolated lungs during anaphylaxis was blocked by aspirin (Piper and Vane, 1969b).

The next step came from a series of experiments with lung tissue, including whole-body preparations in dogs (Gilmore *et al.*, 1969), guinea-pig isolated lungs (Piper and Vane, 1969b), and chopped lung (Palmer *et al.*, 1970a). Almost any type of stimulus was found to release both RCS and prostaglandins: chemical stimuli such as bradykinin, SRS-A, or arachidonic acid, and mechanical stimuli such as infusing plastic microspheres into the lungs (Palmer *et al.*, 1970b), stroking them, or stirring preparations of chopped lung. In particular, increasing the rate or depth of ventilation of anaesthetized dog lungs released a prostaglandin like substance and RCS activity into the blood which could be detected by the blood-bathed organ technique (Vane, 1969, 1971a). In this *in vivo* situation, aspirin reduced prostaglandin output to a greater degree than it did RCS output.

This contrasted with the *in vitro* experiments on isolated lungs from guinea-pigs where aspirin reduced RCS release much more strikingly (Piper and Vane, 1971). These guinea-pig lung experiments had also indicated that whenever aspirin blocked RCS release there was also a smaller contraction of the tissues which assayed prostaglandins and a reduction in prostaglandin output after aspirin was self-evident.

The natural result of the dog lung experiments was to change the focus of Vane's attention away from RCS and towards prostaglandins. 'While I was writing a review paper over the weekend', he recalled, 'including the results of some of these experiments, a thought occurred to me that perhaps should have been obvious earlier on: in all these experiments (and in those of many other workers), the "release" of prostaglandins must in fact amount to fresh synthesis of prostaglandins. That is, prostaglandin output in these experiments, though very low, was still far higher than the tissues' initial content of the hormones.

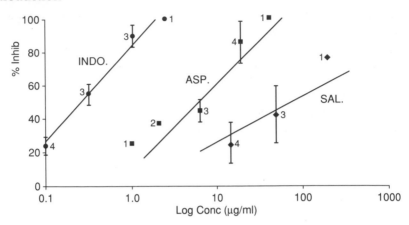

Figure 3.3 Concentration ($\mu g\ ml^{-1}$) of indomethacin (●), aspirin (■) and salicylate (◆) plotted on a log scale against the percentage inhibition of prostaglandin synthesis (assayed as $PGF_{2\alpha}$ on rat colons). The lines are those calculated for best fit. Numbers by the points indicate number of experiments. When three or more estimates were averaged, the standard error of the mean is shown. (From Vane, 1971b, Ref. 6. Reprinted by permission from *Nature*. Copyright © 1971 Macmillan Journals Limited.)

Evidently, then, the various stimuli, mechanical and chemical, which released prostaglandins were in fact "turning on" the synthesis of these compounds. A logical corollary was that aspirin might well be blocking the synthesis of prostaglandins.'

This exciting idea he immediately tested on the Monday morning. In the absence of ram seminal vesicles, from which the synthetase enzyme was normally obtained, he used the supernatant of a broken cell homogenate from guinea-pig lung, the same preparation in which Änggård and Samuelsson in 1965 (Änggård and Samuelsson, 1965) had detected the generation of prostaglandins E_2 and $F_{2\alpha}$. Aliquots of the supernatant were incubated with arachidonic acid and different concentrations of aspirin, indomethacin and sodium salicylate. Prostaglandin $F_{2\alpha}$ generation was estimated by bioassay after 30 min incubation at 37 °C. Figure 3.3 shows the results of Vane's original experiment. There was a dose-dependent inhibition of prostaglandin formation by all three drugs, indomethacin being the most and the sodium salicylate the least, potent. Three other drugs, morphine (an opiate analgesic), hydrocortisone (a steroidal anti-inflammatory) and mepyramine (an anti-histamine) had little or no effect.

Vane published the results of these experiments in *Nature* in 1971 (Vane, 1971b). Two other papers appeared in the same issue which lent support to his finding and also extended it considerably. Both studies originated from the same department and by coincidence one of these stemmed from an entirely independent line of investigation.

Bryan Smith and Jim Willis were investigating the effect of aspirin on platelet behaviour (Smith and Willis, 1971). It had been known for a number of years that aspirin inhibited the aggregation of platelets which occurred in response to certain stimuli such as collagen or ADP, and also prevented the release by aggregating platelets of a smooth muscle contracting substance presumed to be prostaglandin $F_{2\alpha}$. The hypothesis being investigated by these two workers was that the generation of prostaglandins was brought about indirectly by a lysosomal enzyme, phospholipase A_2, released from platelets by aggregation. This enzyme could liberate arachidonic acid from the membrane phospholipids of platelets and thus initiate prostaglandin biosynthesis. Possibly then it was the inhibitory action of aspirin on this phospholipase which was responsible for the effect of this drug.

Once again the experimental protocol was simple: venous blood samples were obtained from three colleagues before and 1 h after taking 600 mg aspirin orally. Platelets were isolated, washed, incubated with the potent aggregating agent thrombin, and the supernatant tested for the presence of released nucleotides, phospholipase and various other enzymes, and of course, prostaglandins. No consistent changes were seen in the release of any of these substances except the prostaglandins, which was substantially inhibited after aspirin. This result was also checked in experiments in which thrombin was added to suspensions of platelets incubated directly with various concentrations of aspirin. Again, there was no clear effect of the aspirin on any parameter other than prostaglandin release. The absence of effect of aspirin on phospholipase release in either experiment suggested that the sole effect of aspirin was on the conversion of arachidonic acid to the prostaglandins.

It was not only aspirin that was active in this respect in the platelet model: indomethacin, but not codeine (another opiate analgesic), also blocked prostaglandin release when taken orally or when added directly to the platelets in vitro.

The importance of this study lay in its demonstration that these drugs were not only active in guinea-pig lungs in vitro but were active in man, in platelets, and following oral administration. In other words the aspirin effect was not restricted to tissue, species or route of administration. All these conclusions derived additional support from the final type of experiment reported in that issue of Nature. John Vane, together with Sergio Ferreira and Salvador Moncada demonstrated that the aspirin-like drugs blocked prostaglandin release from the perfused isolated dog spleen (Ferreira *et al.*, 1971). This organ was known to release large amounts of prostaglandins (mainly E_2 and $F_{2\alpha}$) when subjected to sympathetic nerve stimulation or injections of adrenaline and noradrenaline. In the experiments described by the group, indomethacin and aspirin blocked the release of prostaglandins from the spleen as detected by superfusion bioassay of the effluent. Hydrocortisone was again without effect and so, curiously, was sodium salicylate – much the weakest of the three drugs in all the tests to which it had been subjected.

3.3 CORRELATION OF THE ANTI-ENZYME ACTIVITY OF ASPIRIN WITH ITS THERAPEUTIC ACTIVITY

The major importance of all these findings was, of course, that they provided a simple explanation of the way in which the aspirin-like drugs exerted their therapeutic actions. At the time that the papers were published (1971) there was already some evidence suggesting that prostaglandin E_1 was an extremely potent pyretic agent in several species (Milton and Wendlandt, 1970) and that prostaglandin E_1 or prostaglandin E_2 mimicked the inflammatory response when injected intradermally (Solomon *et al.*, 1968). Prostaglandins had also been detected in inflammatory exudates (Di Rosa *et al.*, 1971) so there were grounds for speculating that prostaglandins might be responsible, at least in part, for the genesis of fever or inflammation and that the aspirin-like drugs might owe their therapeutic activity to their ability to prevent prostaglandin biosynthesis. Certainly, as Vane and his colleagues pointed out, the concentrations of these drugs required to inhibit synthesis were within the plasma levels found during therapy even when protein binding was taken into account (Flower *et al.*, 1972). Of course, only three aspirin-like drugs had been tested so far, but that situation soon changed when the group at the Royal College of Surgeons published data demonstrating that many drugs of the aspirin type blocked prostaglandin generation (Flower, 1974; Table 3.1).

Finally, the discovery that aspirin-like drugs blocked prostaglandin synthesis had another implication. 'These results show' wrote Vane, 'that biologists now have a simple means of preventing prostaglandin synthesis and release and thereby assessing the functions of prostaglandins in individual cells or tissues or in the body as a whole.'

This notion that the aspirin-like drugs could be used as tools was an idea of capital importance. Investigations into the actions of a hormone rested, in 'classical' endocrinology, on deductions based largely upon the deleterious effects observed when the appropriate endocrine organ was removed or ablated. When the hormone in question can be synthesized by virtually every tissue in the body (as is the case with the prostaglandins) then such an experimental design is clearly not possible. By using the aspirin-like drugs however something approaching this type of experiment became possible. This is doubly important because there is still no complete range of antagonists suitable for dissecting out the pharmacological effects of the prostaglandins and achieving the same selectivity of action as has been accomplished so effectively in other branches of pharmacology, for example, with the H_1 and H_2 histamine receptor antagonists, or the α and β adrenoceptor antagonists.

3.4 INHIBITION OF CYCLO-OXYGENASE *IN VITRO*

Inhibition of prostaglandin biosynthesis or release by aspirin or indomethacin was then confirmed in many isolated systems. In acetone-dried powder preparations of sheep vesicular glands (Smith and Lands, 1971), the inhibitory effect of indomethacin was irreversible and was increased by preincubation showing it to be time dependent. Indomethacin was about 2000 times more potent than aspirin as an inhibitor of prostaglandin synthase from bovine seminal vesicles (Tomlinson *et al.*, 1972). In the microsomal fraction of dog spleen (Flower *et al.*,

Table 3.1 Inhibition of prostaglandin formation by anti-inflammatory drugs (assayed on particulate enzyme preparation from dog spleen) (from Flower (1974), with permission)

	Synthetase ID_{50} ($\mu g\ ml^{-1}$)	Rat paw oedema ED_{50} ($mg\ kg^{-1}$)	Peak plasma conc. in man in $\mu g\ ml^{-1}$ (protein binding)
Meclofenamic acid	0.03	15	
Niflumic acid	0.03	47	100 (90%)
Indomethacin	0.06	6	2 (90%)
Mefenamic acid	0.17	68	10 (48%)
Phenylbutazone	2.23	100	150 (98%)
Alclofenac	3.3	approx.100	26 (10%)
Aspirin	6.6	150	55 (80%)
Paracetamol	approx.100.0	inactive	50 (25%)

Conc.=concentrations; approx.=approximately.
Note that the peak plasma concentration of aspirin is expressed as salicylate.

Introduction

1972), aspirin had a similar inhibitory potency as in the guinea-pig lung system, but indomethacin was rather more potent (ID_{50} = 0.06 µg ml^{-1}). Mefenamic acid and phenylbutazone were intermediate in potency between aspirin and indomethacin. Inhibition of prostaglandin formation or release by indomethacin or aspirin also occurred in human semen (Collier and Flower, 1971), dog kidney (Aiken and Vane, 1971, 1973; Herbaczynska-Cedro and Vane, 1972), rabbit kidney (Davis and Horton, 1972), cat spleen (Ferreira and Moncada, 1971), rabbit chopped spleen (Gryglewski and Vane, 1972), rabbit isolated jejunum (Ferreira et al., 1972; Herman et al., 1972), rat uterus (Aiken, 1972; Vane and Williams, 1972), mouse ascites tumour cells (Sykes and Maddox, 1972), and fibrosarcoma cells (Levine, 1972). Several reports also described inhibition of prostaglandin biosynthesis by aspirin or indomethacin in rabbit (Davis, 1972; Tai and Hollander, 1972) and cat kidney (Somova, 1972), cat brain (Milton, 1973), homogenates of human skin (Ziboh, 1973), and guinea-pig uterus (Poyser, 1973).

All non-steroid, anti-inflammatory substances inhibit prostaglandin biosynthesis. Compounds inactive (<10% inhibition at 100 µg ml^{-1}) against prostaglandin synthase include morphine, mepyramine, azathioprine, para- and meta-hydroxybenzoic acid (Flower et al., 1972; Vane, 1971b), phenergan, chloroquine, atropine, methysergide, phenoxybenzamine, propranolol, iproniazid, droperidol, chlorpromazine, and disodium cromoglycate (Flower and Vane, 1972). Inhibition of prostaglandin biosynthesis is, therefore, a unique and general characteristic of aspirin-like drugs. Within 2 years of the discovery that non-steroid anti-inflammatory drugs inhibit prostaglandin synthesis, several classes of inhibitors had been identified (Flower, 1974). One reviewer listed no fewer than 12 major chemical series known directly to affect prostaglandin production and concludes 'It is remarkable that in the short span of time since the first observations with aspirin and indomethacin, such a variety of chemical structures have been identified as inhibitors of prostaglandin synthesis' (Shen, 1979).

This diverse group of chemicals exhibit inhibition of cyclo-oxygenase in a variety of ways which includes both reversible and irreversible mechanisms (Lands, 1981). Examples of reversible competitive inhibitors are fatty acids, closely related to the substrate arachidonic acid, which have a comparable affinity for the enzyme but are not converted to oxygenated products. The anti-inflammatory drug ibuprofen has a binding affinity for cyclo-oxygenase similar to that of the substrate arachidonic acid and this explains why ibuprofen inhibits the enzyme (Rome and Lands, 1975). It is considered that flufenamic acid and sulindac also compete with arachidonic acid for binding to cyclo-oxygenase. This mechanism does not, however, explain the action of other inhibitors.

Indomethacin, meclofenamic acid and flurbiprophen inhibit cyclo-oxygenase activity when 1 molecule of inhibitor binds stereospecifically to 1 molecule of the synthase. The binding is initially rapid and reversible, but the synthase/inhibitor complex then gradually decays to produce a stable form of the cyclo-oxygenase with only 4–10% of the original activity. These inhibitors, therefore, reduce the catalytic capacity of the enzyme probably by producing a selective conformational change in the synthase. It was possible to recover the indomethacin intact after a maximal inhibition of the enzyme had occurred making it unlikely that a covalent interaction had taken place (Kulmacz and Lands, 1985). A more recent theory of indomethacin action is that it produces a conformational change in a protein radical, such as a tyrosyl radical, which is required for the catalytic action of cyclo-oxygenase (Kulmacz *et al.*, 1990).

A model for the active site of cyclo-oxygenase has been proposed, based upon conformational analysis of aryl acidic non-steroid anti-inflammatory drugs (Gund and Shen, 1977). The carboxyl function of these compounds is said to mimic the terminal carboxyl of arachidonic acid and the planar, hydrophobic groups bind to the enzyme to prevent hydrogen abstraction at C13. The presence of an aryl halogen has also been recognized as enhancing this activity (Rome and Lands, 1975). An alternative view is that propionic acids such as naproxen act as structural analogues of the cyclic endoperoxides rather than arachidonic acid itself (Appleton and Brown, 1979). Inhibition by these drugs is stereospecific as a number of α-methyl arylacetic acids with the S(+) configuration are active but their R(−) enantiomers are not (Shen, 1979). This difference also applies to their anti-inflammatory activity *in vivo*. It is generally accepted that the majority of these drugs compete with the substrate for enzyme binding and are competitive irreversible inhibitors.

The induction period required to initiate cyclo-oxygenase activity is reduced by addition of hydroperoxy acids and this has led to the concept that the peroxide tone in inflamed tissues may determine enzyme activity (Lands, 1981). It has been proposed that a continual presence of lipid peroxide induces a free radical chain reaction which sustains cyclo-oxygenase activity. Hydroperoxides, including prosta-glandin G$_2$, generated during the metabolism of arachidonic acid also stimulate cyclo-oxygenase and function as part of a self-amplification mechanism (Marshall *et al.*, 1987). This peroxide tone can be blocked by the addition of radical scavengers or anti-oxidants which act as reversible non-competitive inhibitors. The analgesic drug paracetamol may block prostaglandin synthesis by this mechanism (Lands et al., 1976), although in lower concentrations, it stimulates prostaglandin biosynthesis.

A homogeneous, enzymatically active cyclo-oxygenase or prostaglandin endoperoxide synthase (Hemler et al., 1976) was isolated in 1976. This membrane-bound haemo- and glycoprotein with a molecular weight of around 70 kDa is found in greatest amounts in the endoplasmic reticulum of prostanoid-forming cells (Smith, 1986). It exhibits cyclo-oxygenase activity which both cyclizes arachidonic acid and adds the 15-hydroperoxy group to form prostaglandin G_2. The hydroperoxy group of prostaglandin G_2 is reduced to the hydroxy group of prostaglandin H_2 by a peroxidase that utilizes a wide variety of compounds to provide the requisite pair of electrons. Both cyclo-oxygenase and peroxidase activities are contained in the same dimeric protein molecule (Chapter 2). The amino acid sequence of prostaglandin endoperoxide synthase from sheep vesicular glands was deduced using recombinant DNA methods in 1988 by three laboratories (De Witt and Smith, 1988; Merlie et al., 1988; Yokoyama et al., 1988).

Aspirin selectively acetylates the hydroxyl group of a single serine (Ser530) residue located 70 amino acids away from the C terminus of the enzyme (Roth and Majerus, 1975). Acetylation leads to irreversible cyclo-oxygenase inhibition and thus new enzyme has to be synthesized before more prostanoids are produced. When the purified enzyme is acetylated, only the cyclo-oxygenase but not the hydroperoxidase activity is inhibited. The stoichiometry of this reaction is 1:1, with one acetyl group transferred per enzyme monomer of this dimeric protein. At low concentrations, aspirin acetylates prostaglandin endoperoxide synthase rapidly (within minutes) and selectively. At high concentrations, over longer time periods, aspirin will also acetylate non-specifically a variety of proteins and nucleic acids (Smith, 1989).

By site-directed mutagenesis of the sheep prostaglandin endoperoxide synthase cDNA, De Witt et al. (1990) replaced Ser530 with the amino acid alanine which lacks a hydroxyl group. This mutant enzyme had the same K_m for arachidonate (~8 mM) and the same ID_{50} for the cyclo-oxygenase inhibitor flurbiprophen (~5 mM) but could not be irreversibly inactivated by aspirin. The hydroxyl group of Ser530 is, therefore, not essential for catalysis and substrate binding by prostaglandin endoperoxide synthase. However, substitution of Ser530 with a bulky amino acid such as asparagine removed cyclo-oxygenase but not hydroperoxidase activity, and suggests that acetylation of the enzyme by aspirin places a bulky substituent on the Ser530 oxygen which inhibits binding of arachidonic acid.

Recent evidence indicates that another mechanism by which aspirin inhibits cyclo-oxygenase may be important apart from acetylation. Such a mechanism has been suggested by Wu *et al.* (1991) who demonstrated that in human cultured endothelial cells from the umbilical vein equal concentrations of aspirin or sodium salicylate prevented the expression and *de novo* synthesis of prostaglandin H synthase. Since the concentration of salicylate required to inhibit this synthesis was at least two orders of magnitude lower than that needed to block cyclo-oxygenase activity, this may constitute an important additional mechanism by which the aspirin-like drugs reduce prostaglandin formation *in vivo*. For salicylate, this would also explain why it has little or no effect on platelet aggregation, for platelets do not have the mechanism for expression of cyclo-oxygenase.

The synthesis of prostaglandin endoperoxide synthase can be stimulated by growth factors and tumour promoters and by interleukin-1 (Raz *et al.*, 1988), lipopolysaccharide (Masferrer *et al.*, 1990a) and tumour necrosis factor (Coyne and Morrison, 1990). Interleukin-1 exerts its effect during the transcriptional rather than the translational phase of induced synthesis of prostaglandin synthase (Raz *et al.*, 1989). Induction of prostaglandin endoperoxide synthase gene expression by serum factors occurred after about 2 h in mouse 3T3 cells in which prostaglandins are essential for cell division (De Witt *et al.*, 1990). The inducible synthase is a distinct isoform of cyclo-oxygenase (COX-2) (Sirois and Richards, 1992) encoded by a different gene from the constitutive enzyme (COX-1) (Xie *et al.*, 1991; O'Banion *et al.*, 1991). The amino acid sequence of its cDNA shows only a 60% homology with the sequence of the non-inducible enzyme. Dexamethasone suppresses the induction of cyclo-oxygenase in human monocytes and mouse macrophages but does not affect basal enzyme activity (Fu *et al.*, 1990; Masferrer *et al.*, 1990b).

The termination of the action of cyclo-oxygenase, on the other hand, takes place by a self-catalysed inactivation mechanism rather than when the arachidonic acid substrate becomes exhausted. The substrate appears to act as a 'suicide' substrate to limit the further production of endoperoxides (Marshall *et al.*, 1987). There is controversy about the identity of the intermediates which provide this feedback inhibition to further catalysis. They have variously been identified as oxidizing radicals (Kuehl *et al.*, 1980; Markey *et al.*, 1987) or more recently as protein radicals (Karthein *et al.*, 1988).

The discovery of an inducible form of cyclo-oxygenase changes many aspects of inflammation. For instance, the 'suicide' of cyclo-oxygenase seen *in vitro* (Marshall *et al.*, 1987) becomes less relevant to inflammation for new enzyme will be continuously generated. It also raises the possibility of selective inhibition of the enzyme involved in inflammation (COX-2) as opposed to COX-1.

3.5 INHIBITION OF CYCLO-OXYGENASE *IN VIVO*

In man, aspirin blocks cyclo-oxygenase activity in platelets within an hour of oral administration (Smith and Willis, 1971) and this observation has been confirmed in several species. Because aspirin irreversibly acetylates Ser530 at the active site of the enzyme and platelets are unable to generate new enzyme, inhibition of platelet cyclo-oxygenase lasts for the life-time of the cell. This results in effects on platelet function for several days after a single dose of aspirin (Pedersen and FitzGerald, 1984).

The possibility that aspirin-like drugs influence the release of other substances, such as histamine and bradykinin, was experimentally discounted and further studies were designed to show that the anti-enzyme effect of aspirin-like drugs correlated with their anti-inflammatory effects. Comparing the effects of two optical isomers of naproxen, Tomlinson *et al.* (1972) showed that the one which possesses anti-inflammatory properties (in adjuvant arthritis and carrageenin oedema) was also a potent inhibitor of prostaglandin E_2 synthesis. The other isomer was much less active in all the tests. In a survey of a whole range of non-steroid anti-inflammatory drugs, at therapeutic doses the peak plasma concentrations, even allowing for protein binding, were more than sufficient to inhibit prostaglandin formation in an isolated enzyme preparation (Flower, 1974; Table 3.1).

There is a good correlation between the relative potencies of aspirin-like drugs in reducing prostaglandin concentrations in inflammatory exudates and their inhibition of inflammatory oedema. Using carrageenin to induce inflammation in the rat paw, the release of endogenous prostaglandins was eliminated by aspirin. Then, administration of low doses of exogenous prostaglandin E_2 (1.0 ng) or prostacyclin (10 ng) reversed the effect of aspirin and caused an increase in oedema (Moncada *et al.*, 1973). Furthermore, in groups of patients with arthritis receiving aspirin-like drugs, the mean concentration of a prostaglandin E_2-like substance in synovial fluids was only one tenth of the concentration in fluids from untreated patients (Higgs *et al.*, 1974; Trang *et al.*, 1977) and this was associated with symptomatic relief.

After demonstrating that the anti-inflammatory effects of non-steroid anti-inflammatory drugs are mediated via inhibition of prostaglandin synthesis, it was pertinent to determine whether a similar mechanism underlies the side effect profile of aspirin. This has been addressed with regard to the ulcerogenic potential of aspirin, and it is now known that prostacyclin is an important cytoprotective product of the gastric mucosa (Boughton-Smith and Whittle, 1983). The anti-enzyme activity of several non-steroid anti-inflammatory drugs correlates with their capacity to erode the gastric mucosa (Carson et al., 1987). In the colon, non-steroid anti-inflammatory drugs suppress mucosal prostaglandin formation (Boughton-Smith et al., 1988). However, salicylate decreases prostaglandin concentration in inflammatory exudate without affecting production by the gastric mucosa, and it possesses a very low erosion index (Whittle et al., 1980). It is not known why salicylate differs from other aspirin-like drugs in this manner. Administration of various prostaglandins reverses or prevents experimental gastric ulcers, and some of the recently developed prostaglandin derivatives are now available for clinical use (Roth et al., 1989).

Aspirin-like drugs after long-term administration to rats cause renal papillary necrosis, although they are relatively non-toxic in the healthy human kidney (for review, Patrono and Dunn, 1987). However, in a number of disease states, including congestive heart failure, cirrhosis and renal insufficiency, the local release of a vasodilator prostaglandin helps to maintain renal blood flow. Patients are, therefore, at risk of renal ischaemia when prostaglandin synthesis is diminished by non-steroid anti-inflammatory drugs (Schwartzman et al., 1985).

An anti-proteinuric effect of aspirin-like drugs is easily demonstrable when there is disturbed renal function. In such instances, indomethacin for example, decreases glomerular filtration rate and effective renal plasma flow, possibly via inhibition of prostaglandin synthesis (Arisz et al., 1975; Donker et al., 1975). In experimental models of nephritis, indomethacin affects protein excretion in autologous complex glomerulopathy but not in toxic nephropathy induced by puromycin (Gribnau, 1975). Recent clinical studies found that in patients with mild chronic renal failure, even a brief course of ibuprofen may precipitate acute renal failure (Whelton et al., 1990).

The prolongation and delay in parturition caused by aspirin-like drugs is almost certainly due to inhibition of prostaglandin biosynthesis. Such a conclusion implicates prostaglandin production in the parturition process, and this is most likely through the contractile action of prostaglandins on uterine smooth muscle. A retrospective survey (Lewis and Schulman, 1973) showed that women taking aspirin had an average gestational period a week longer than the control group as well as significantly longer labour, with more blood loss. Prostaglandins may also play a part in the expulsion of uterine contents induced by abortifacients. For instance, Waltman *et al.* (1973) induced abortion by the intra-amniotic instillation of hypertonic saline. The time to abortion for 50 control women was 36.3 ± 2.75 h (mean ± s.e.m.). In women treated with indomethacin this time was prolonged to 68.5 ± 4.8 h. Vane (1971b) suggested that aspirin-like drugs should be tested as a treatment of premature labour. This was done by Wiqvist *et al.* (1976) who concluded that indomethacin is a potent and useful drug in the treatment of premature labour.

The degree to which microsomal prostaglandin synthase preparations from different tissues are inhibited by the aspirin-like drugs varies considerably, and it is possible that the synthase system (or at least one component protein) exists in multiple forms within the organism and that each has its own drug specificity. Results with paracetamol encourage this idea. Paracetamol has analgesic and antipyretic effects but little anti-inflammatory activity. It has only weak activity against most cyclo-oxygenase preparations but is considerably more active in diminishing prostaglandin synthesis within the CNS (Flower and Vane, 1972). However, paracetamol does preferentially reduce synthesis of prostacyclin in healthy volunteers without any obvious effect on thromboxane production (Gréen *et al.*, 1989). Whittle and his colleagues (Whittle *et al.*, 1980) have shown that damage to the gastric mucosa by certain aspirin-like drugs could be correlated with their ability to inhibit mucosal cyclo-oxygenase. In doses which caused reduction of the prostaglandin content of an inflammatory exudate, aspirin and flurbiprofen seemed even more active on the enzyme in rat gastric mucosa. However, sodium salicylate and BW755C did not affect mucosal cyclo-oxygenase activity (Higgs *et al.*, 1979) in doses which reduced prostaglandins in inflammatory exudates. Thus, the well documented variations in gastric side effects of the non-steroidal anti-inflammatory drugs may be based on differential effects on the cyclo-oxygenase enzymes at different sites.

Aspirin is significantly more potent in inhibiting cyclo-oxygenase *in vitro* than salicylate (Vane, 1971b) but the anti-inflammatory potency of the two drugs is similar as is their ability to reduce urinary output of prostaglandin metabolites (Hamberg, 1972). At the high doses of salicylates used to treat rheumatoid arthritis aspirin may be acting as a pro-drug for salicylate. Following large oral doses of aspirin, the drug can be detected in the plasma of peripheral blood and even in the peripheral tissues but aspirin concentrations are rapidly exceeded (50–100 fold) by salicylate concentrations (Higgs *et al.*, 1987). After 1–2 h aspirin is undetectable in the periphery but salicylate persists for more than 6 h. During this time the synthesis of prostaglandins at a peripheral site of inflammation is reduced and this correlates with anti-inflammatory activity. It is likely therefore, that the anti-inflammatory activity of orally dosed aspirin or salicylate is due to the inhibition of prostaglandin production in the inflamed tissues by salicylate (Higgs *et al.*, 1987).

However, this does not explain the difference in potency between aspirin and salicylic acid in inhibiting the cyclo-oxygenase enzyme *in vitro*. The demonstration by Wu *et al.* (1991) that aspirin and salicylate in equal concentrations inhibit the expression of mRNA for prostaglandin endoperoxide synthase, may provide such a unifying solution.

Another hypothesis was put forward by Abramson *et al.* (1983) to explain why similar doses of aspirin and salicylate are used to suppress inflammation *in vivo*, while their *in vitro* potencies are so different. This theory suggests that all non-steroid anti-inflammatory drugs have a common action in inhibiting activation of neutrophils by inflammatory stimuli. High doses of aspirin, sodium salicylate, ibuprofen, piroxicam and indomethacin inhibited aggregation, lyso-somal enzyme release and superoxide generation of neutrophils by preventing movements of calcium and enhancing intracellular levels of adenosine cyclic 3',5'-monophosphate. Whether this suppressant action on neutrophils is relevant to the anti-inflammatory action of non-steroid anti-inflammatory drugs *in vivo* remains to be demonstrated.

Any hypothesis which purports to explain the action of a drug in terms of an anti-enzyme action must satisfy at least two basic criteria. First, the free concentrations achieved in plasma (or at the site of inflammation) during therapy must be sufficient to inhibit the enzyme in question. Second, there must be a reasonable correlation between the level of anti-enzyme activity and the therapeutic potency. Clearly, there is abundant evidence to show that both these criteria are satisfied in the case of aspirin-like drugs and there is also good evidence that therapeutic dosage of these drugs reduces prostaglandin biosynthesis in man (for review, Vane *et al.*, 1982).

3.6 CONCLUSIONS

We have discussed the possible ways in which aspirin-like drugs limit the formation of prostaglandins by interfering with the cyclo-oxygenase activity of prostaglandin endoperoxide synthase.

However, the question remains whether it is beneficial to inhibit prostaglandin production in chronic inflammatory states. Prostaglandin E_2 and prostacyclin have inhibitory effects on immune functions such as secretion from and proliferation of T lymphocytes (Gordon *et al.*, 1979). In a recent experiment where macrophages and lymphocytes were incubated together, indomethacin reduced prostaglandin E_2 production by macrophages and increased release of interleukin-2 which resulted in proliferation of the lymphocytes. Addition of exogenous prostaglandin E_2 reversed this action of indomethacin (Lewis and Barrett, 1986).

Another consequence of removing the suppression of immune processes by prostaglandins may be the enhancement of cartilage breakdown seen with non-steroid anti-inflammatory drugs *in vitro* and *in vivo* (De Brito *et al.*, 1987; Bottomley *et al.*, 1988; Desa *et al.*, 1988; Pettipher *et al.*, 1988). Indomethacin treatment increased lymphocyte infiltration, cartilage degradation and loss of proteoglycan from the knee joints of rabbits with adjuvant-induced arthritis (Pettipher *et al.*, 1988). This may be a result of increased interleukin-1 production by macrophages due to the removal of prostaglandin E_2 which normally inhibits interleukin-1 production (Bahl *et al.*, 1990).

These experiments in rabbits have been confirmed in patients with osteoarthritis of the hip, awaiting arthroplasty. When treated with indomethacin, a potent inhibitor of prostaglandin synthesis, these patients lost joint space more rapidly than when treated with azapropazone, an analgesic with weak cyclo-oxygenase inhibitory activity. The cartilage proteoglycan content remained higher in the azapropazone-treated group and their synovium contained significantly more prostaglandin E_2, thromboxane B_2 and 5-HETE than the indomethacin-treated group (Rashad *et al.*, 1989). Thus, indomethacin appeared to accelerate cartilage breakdown in these patients.

There is, therefore, a great need for drugs which will treat the underlying pathology of chronic inflammatory diseases and not just the superficial symptoms of painful and swollen joints. The aspirin-like drugs will, however, still occupy a unique place as a relatively non-toxic and very effective remedy for headache, fever and acute inflammatory conditions where inhibition of prostaglandin synthesis will relieve the distressing symptoms without necessarily exacerbating an underlying pathological process.

REFERENCES

Abramson, S., Korchak, H., Ludewig, R. *et al.* (1983) Modes of action of aspirin-like drugs. *Proc. Natl Acad. Sci. USA*, **82**, 7227–31.

Aiken, J.W. (1972) Aspirin and indomethacin prolong parturition in rats: Evidence that prostaglandins contribute to expulsion of fetus. *Nature*, **240**, 21–5.

Aiken, J.W. and Vane, J.R. (1971) Blockade of angiotensin-induced prostaglandin release from dog kidney by indomethacin. *The Pharmacologist*, **13**, 564.

Aiken, J.W. and Vane, J.R. (1973) Intra-renal prostaglandin release attenuates the renal vasoconstrictor activity of angiotensin. *J. Pharmac. Exp. Ther.*, **184**, 678–87.

Änggård, E. and Samuelsson, B. (1965) Biosynthesis of prostaglandins from arachidonic acid in guinea-pig lung. *J. Biol. Chem.*, **240**, 3518–21.

Appleton, R.A. and Brown, K. (1979) Conformational requirements at the prostaglandin cyclo-oxygenase receptor site: a template for designing non-steroidal anti-inflammatory drugs. *Prostaglandins*, **18**, 29–34.

Arisz, L., Donker, A.J.M., Brentjens, J.R.H. *et al.* (1975) Het effect van indometacine i op de proteinuri bij het nefrotisch syndroom. *Ned. T. Geneesk.*, **119**, 815.

Bahl, A.K., Foreman, J.C. and Dale, M.M. (1990) The effect of prostaglandin E_2 and non-steroidal anti-inflammatory drugs on cell-associated interleukin-1. *Adv. Prostaglandin Thromboxane Leukotriene Res.*, **21**, 513–15.

Berry, P.A. and Collier, H.O.J. (1964) Bronchoconstrictor action and antagonism of a slow reacting substance from anaphylaxis of guinea-pig isolated lung. *Brit. J. Pharmacol.*, **23**, 201–16.

Bhoola, K.D., Collier. H.O.J., Schachter, M. and Shorley, P.G. (1962) Actions of some peptides in bronchial muscle. *Brit. J. Pharmacol.*, **19**, 190–7.

Bottomley, K.M.K., Griffiths, R.J., Rising, J.J. and Steward, A. (1988) A modified mouse air pouch model for evaluating the effects of compounds on granuloma induced cartilage degradation. *Brit. J. Pharmacol.*, **93**, 627–35.

Boughton-Smith, N.K. and Whittle, B.J.R. (1983) Stimulation and inhibition of prostacyclin formation in the gastric mucosa and ileum *in vitro* by anti-inflammatory agents. *Brit. J. Pharmacol.*, **78**, 173–80.

Boughton-Smith, N.K., Wallace, J.L., Morris, G.P. and Whittle, B.J.R. (1988) The effect of anti-inflammatory drugs on eicosanoid formation in a chronic model of inflammatory bowel disease in the rat. *Brit. J. Pharmacol*, **94**, 65–72.

Carson, J.L., Strom, B.L., Soper, K.A. *et al.* (1987) The association of nonsteroidal antiinflammatory drugs with upper gastrointestinal tract bleeding. *Arch. Intern. Med.*, **147**, 85–8.

Collier, H.O.J. (1963) Aspirin. *Sci. Am.*, **209**, 97–108.

Collier, H.O.J. (1969) A pharmacological analysis of aspirin. *Adv. Pharmacol. Chemother.*, **7**, 333–405.

Collier, H.O.J. and Shorley, P.G. (1960) Analgesic antipyretic drugs as antagonists of bradykinin. *Brit. J. Pharmacol.*, **15**, 601–10.

Collier, H.O.J. and Sweatman, W.J.F. (1968) Antagonism by fenamates of prostaglandin $F_{2\alpha}$ and of slow reacting substance on human bronchial muscle. *Nature*, **219**, 864–5.

Collier, J.C. and Flower, R.J. (1971) Effect of aspirin on human seminal prostaglandins. *Lancet*, **ii**, 852–3.

Collier, H.O.J., James, G.W.L. and Schneider, C. (1966) Antagonism by aspirin and fenamates of bronchoconstriction and nociception induced by adenosine-5'-triphosphate. *Nature*, **212**, 411–12.

Collier, H.O.J., James, G.W.L. and Piper, P.J. (1968a) Antagonism by fenamates and like-acting drugs of bronchoconstriction induced by bradykinin or antigen in the guinea-pig. *Brit. J. Pharmacol.*, **34**, 76–87.

Collier, H.O.J., Dinneen, L.C., Perkins, A.C. and Piper, P.J. (1968b) Curtailment by aspirin and meclofenamate of hypotension induced by bradykinin in the guinea-pig. *NaunynSchmiedebergs Arch. Pharmakol.*, **259**, 159–60.

Coyne, D.W. and Morrison, A.R. (1990) Effects of IL-1 and TNF on PGE_2 production and cyclooxygenase (COX) activity in rat mesangial cells. In *Proceedings 7th International Conference on Prostaglandins and Related Compounds*, Florence, Abstract 116.

Davis, H. and Horton, E.W. (1972) Output of prostaglandins from the rabbit kidney, its increase on renal nerve stimulation and inhibition by indomethacin. *Brit. J. Pharmacol.*, **46**, 658–75.

Davis, H.A. (1972) Output of prostaglandins from the rabbit kidney. In *Advance Abstracts Internationl Conference on Prostaglandins*, Vienna, Abstract 55.

De Brito, F.B., Holmes, M.J.G., Carney, S.L. and Willoughby, D.A. (1987) Drug effects on a novel model of connective tissue breakdown. *Agents Actions*, **21**, 287–90.

Desa, F.M., Chander, C.L., Howat, D.W. *et al.* (1988) Indomethacin and cartilage breakdown. *J. Pharm. Pharmacol.*, **40**, 667.

De Witt, D.L. and Smith, W.L. (1988) Primary structure of prostaglandin G/H synthase from sheep vesicular gland determined from the complementary DNA sequence. *Proc. Natl Acad. Sci. USA*, **85**, 1412–16.

De Witt, D.L., Kraemer, S. A. and Meade, E.A. (1990) Serum induction and superinduction of PGG/H synthase mRNA levels in 3T3 fibroblasts. *Adv. Prostaglandin Thromboxane Leukotriene Res.*, **21**, 65–8.

De Witt, D.L., El-Harith, E.A., Kraemer, S.A. *et al.* (1990) The aspirin and heme-binding sites of ovine and murine prostaglandin endoperoxide synthases. *J. Biol. Chem.*, **265**, 5192–8.

Di Rosa, M., Giroud, J.P. and Willoughby, D.A. (1971) Studies of the mediators of the acute inflammatory response induced in rats in different sites by carrageenin and turpentine. *J. Pathol.*, **104**, 15–29.

Donker, A.J.M., Arisz, L. Brentjens, J.R.H. and Hem, G.K. van der. (1975) Het effect van indometacine i op de glomerulaire filtatie. *Ned. T. Geneesk.*, **119**, 815.

Ferreira, S.H. and Moncada, S. (1971) Inhibition of prostaglandin synthesis augments the effects of sympathetic nerve stimulation on the cat spleen. *Brit. J. Pharmacol.*, **43**, 491P.

Ferreira, S.H., Moncada, S. and Vane, J.R. (1971) Indomethacin and aspirin abolish prostaglandin release from spleen. *Nature*, **231**, 237–9.

Ferreira, S.H., Herman, A. and Vane, J.R. (1972) Prostaglandin generation maintains the smooth muscle tone of the rabbit isolated jejunum. *Brit. J. Pharmacol.*, **44**, 328P.

Flower, R.J. (1974) Drugs which inhibit prostaglandin biosynthesis. *Pharmacol. Rev.*, **26**, 33–67.

Flower, R.J. and Vane, J.R. (1972) Inhibition of prostaglandin synthetase in brain explains the antipyretic activity of paracetamol (4-acetamidophenol). *Nature*, **240**, 410–11.

Flower, R., Gryglewski, R., Herbaczynska-Cedro, K. and Vane, J.R. (1972) The effects of anti-inflammatory drugs on a cell-free prostaglandin synthetase system from dog spleen. *Nature*, **238**, 104–6.

Fu, J.-Y., Masferrer, J.L., Seibert, K. *et al.* (1990) The induction and suppression of prostaglandin H_2 synthase (cyclooxygenase) in human monocytes. *J. Biol. Chem.*, **265.**, 16737–40.

Gilmore, N., Vane, J.R. and Wyllie, J.H. (1969). Prostaglandin release by the spleen in response to infusion of particles. In *Prostaglandins, Peptides and Amines*, (eds P. Mantegazza and E.W. Horton) Academic Press, London, New York, pp. 21–9.

Gordon, D., Henderson, D.C. and Westwick, J. (1979) Effects prostaglandins E_2 and I_2 on human lymphocyte transformation in the absence and presence of inhibitors of prostaglandin biosynthesis. *Brit. J. Pharmacol.*, **67**, 17–22.

Gould, B.J. and Smith, M.J.H. (1965a) Salicylate and aminotransferases. *J. Pharm. Pharmacol.*, **17**, 83–8.

Gould, B.J. and Smith, M.J.H. (1965b) Inhibition of rat brain glutamate decarboxylase activity by salicylate *in vitro*. *J. Pharm. Pharmacol.*, **17**, 15–18.

Gréen, K., Drvota, V. and Vesterqvist, O. (1989) Pronounced reduction of *in vivo* prostacyclin synthesis in humans by acetaminophen (paracetamol). *Prostaglandins*, **37**, 311–15.

Gribnau, F.W.J. (1975) Studies in Heymann-type nephritis and in puromycin aminonucleoside nephropathy. In *Indomethacin in Experimental Nephritis* (ed. F.W.J. Gribnau), Drukkerij Brakkenstein, Netherlands.

Gryglewski, R. and Vane, J.R. (1972) The release of prostaglandins and rabbit aorta contracting substance (RCS) from rabbit spleen and its antagonism by anti-inflammatory drugs. *Brit. J. Pharmacol.*, **45**, 37–47.

Gund, P. and Shen, T.Y. (1977) A model for the prostaglandin synthetase cyclo-oxygenation site and its inhibition by anti-inflammatory arylacetic acids. *J. Med.*, **20**, 1146–52.

Hamberg, M. (1972) Inhibition of prostaglandin synthesis in man. *Biochem. Biophys. Res. Commun.*, **49**, 720–6.

Hamberg, M., Svensson, J. and Samuelsson, B. (1975) Thromboxanes: a new group of biologically active compounds derived from prostaglandin endoperoxides. *Proc. Natl Acad. Sci. USA*, **72**, 2994–8.

Hemler, M., Lands, W.E.M. and Smith, W.L. (1976) Purification of the cyclooxygenase that forms prostaglandins. Demonstration of two forms of iron in the holoenzyme. *J. Biol. Chem.*, **251**, 5575–9.

Herbaczynska-Cedro, K. and Vane, J.R. (1972) An intra-renal role for prostaglandin production. In *Proceedings V International Congress on Pharmacology*, San Francisco, Abstract 596.

Herman, A.G., Eckenfels, A., Ferreira, S.H. and Vane, J.R. (1972) Relationship between tone of isolated smooth muscle preparations and production of prostaglandins, In *Proceedings V International Congress on Pharmacology*, San Francisco, Abstract 597.

Higgs, G.A., Vane, J.R., Hart, F.D. and Wojtulewski, J.A. (1974) Effects of anti-inflammatory drugs on prostaglandins in rheumatoid arthritis. In *Prostaglandin Synthetase Inhibitors* (eds H.J. Robinson and J.R. Vane), Raven Press, New York, pp. 165–73.

Higgs, G.A., Flower, R.J. and Vane, J.R. (1979) A new approach to antiinflammatory drugs. *Biochem. Pharmacol.*, **28**, 1959–61.

Higgs, G.A., Salmon, J.A., Henderson, B. and Vane, J.R. (1987) Pharmacokinetics of aspirin and salicylate in relation to inhibition of arachidonate cyclo-oxygenase and anti-inflammatory activity. *Proc. Natl Acad. Sci. USA*, **84**, 1417–20.

Hines, W.J.W. and Smith, M.J.H. (1964) Inhibition of dehydrogenases by salicylate. *Nature*, **201**, 192.

Karthein, R., Dietz, R., Nastainczyk, W. and Ruf, H.H. (1988) Higher oxidation states of prostaglandin H synthase. EPR study of a transient tyrosyl radical in the enzyme during the peroxidase reaction. *Eur. J. Biochem.*, **171**, 313–20.

Kuehl, F.A., Humes, J.L., Hamm, E.A. *et al.* (1980) Inflammation: the role of peroxidase-derived products. *Adv. Prostaglandin Thromboxane Res.*, **6**, 77–86.

Kulmacz, R.J. and Lands, W.E.M. (1985) Stoichiometry and kinetics of the interaction of prostaglandin H synthase with anti-inflammatory agents. *J. Biol. Chem.*, **23**, 12572–8.

Kulmacz, R.J., Ren, Y., Tsai, A-L. and Palmer, G. (1990) PGH synthase: interaction with hydroperoxides and indomethacin. *Adv. Prostaglandin Thromboxane Leukotriene Res.*, **21**, 137–40.

Lands, W.E.M. (1981) Actions of anti-inflammatory drugs. *Trends Pharmacol. Sci.*, **2**, 78–80.

Lands, W.E.M., Cook, H.W. and Rome, L.H. (1976) Prostaglandin biosynthesis: Consequences of oxygenase mechanism upon *in vitro* assays of drug effectiveness. *Adv. Prostaglandin Thromboxane Res.*, **1**, 7–17.

Levine, L. (1972) Prostaglandin production by mouse fibrosarcoma cells in culture: inhibition by indomethacin and aspirin. *Biochem. Biophys. Res. Commun.*, **47**, 888–96.

Lewis, L.B. and Schulman, J.D. (1973) Influence of acetylsalicylic acid, an inhibitor of prostaglandin synthesis, on the duration of human gestation and labour. *Lancet*, **ii**, 1159–61.

Lewis, G.P. and Barrett, M.L. (1986) Immunosuppressive actions of prostaglandins and the possible increase in chronic inflammation after cyclooxygenase inhibitors. *Agents Actions*, **19**, 59–65.

Markey, C.M., Alward, A., Weller, P.E. and Marnett, L.J. (1987) Quantitative studies of hydroperoxide reduction by prostaglandin H synthase. Reducing substrate specificity and the relationship of peroxidase to cyclooxygenase activities. *J. Biol. Chem.*, **262**, 6266–79.

Marshall, P.J., Kulmacz, R.J. and Lands, W.E.M. (1987) Constraints on prostaglandin biosynthesis in tissues. *J. Biol. Chem.*, **262**, 3510–17.

Masferrer, J.L., Zweifel, B.S. and Needleman, P. (1990a) The biochemical and pharmacological manipulation of cellular cyclooxygenase (COX) activity. *Adv. Prostaglandin Thromboxane Leukotriene Res.*, **21**, 45–51.

Masferrer, J.L., Zweifel, B.S., Seibert, K. and Needleman, P. (1990b) Selective regulation of cellular cyclooxygenase by dexamethasone and endotoxin in mice. *J. Clin. Invest.*, **86**, 1375–9.

Merlie, J.P., Fagan, D., Mudd, J. and Needleman, P. (1988) Isolation and characterization of the complementary DNA for sheep seminal vesicle prostaglandin endoperoxide synthase (cyclooxygenase). *J. Biol. Chem.*, **263**, 3500–53.

Milton, A.S. (1973) Prostaglandin E_1 and endotoxin fever, and the effects of aspirin, indomethacin, and 4-acetamidophenol. *Adv. Biosci.*, **9**, 495–500.

Milton, A.S. and Wendlandt, S. (1970) A possible role for prostaglandin E_1 as a modulator of temperature regulation in the central nervous system of the cat. *J. Physiol.*, **207**, 76–7.

Moncada, S., Ferreira, S.H. and Vane, J.R. (1973) Prostaglandins, aspirin-like drugs and oedema of inflammation. *Nature*, **246**, 217–19.

O'Banion, M.K., Sadowski, H.B., Winn, V. and Young, D.A. (1991) A serum- and glucocorticoid-regulated 4-kilobase mRNA encodes a cyclooxygenase-related protein. *J. Biol. Chem.* **266**, 23261–7.

Palmer, M.A., Piper, P.J. and Vane, J.R. (1970a) The release of RCS from chopped lung and its antagonism by anti-inflammatory drugs. *Brit. J. Pharmacol.*, **40**, 581P.

Palmer, M.A., Piper, P.J. and Vane, J.R. (1970b) Release of vaso-active substances from lungs by injection of particles. *Brit. J. Pharmacol.*, **40**, 547P.

Patrono, C. and Dunn, M.J. (1987) The clinical significance of inhibition of renal prostaglandin synthesis. *Kidney Int.*, **32**, 1–12.

Pedersen, A.K. and FitzGerald, G.A. (1984) Dose-related kinetics of aspirin. Presystemic acetylation of platelet cyclo-oxygenase. *N. Engl. J. Med.*, **311**, 1206–11.

Pettipher, E.R., Henderson, B., Edwards, J.C.W. and Higgs, G.A. (1988) Indomethacin enhances proteoglycan loss from articular cartilage in antigen-induced arthritis. *Brit. J. Pharmacol.*, **94**, 341P.

Piper, P.J. and Vane, J.R. (1969a) Release of additional factors in anaphylaxis and its antagonism by anti-inflammatory drugs. *Nature*, **223**, 29–35.

Piper, P.J. and Vane, J.R. (1969b) The release of prostaglandins during anaphylaxis in guinea-pig isolated lungs. In *Prostaglandins, Peptides and Amines* (eds P. Mantegazza and E.W. Horton) Academic Press, London, New York, pp. 15–19.

Piper, P.J. and Vane, J.R. (1971) The release of prostaglandins from lung and other tissues. *Ann. NY Acad. Sci. USA*, **180**, 353–85.

Poyser, N.L. (1973) The formation of prostaglandins by the guinea-pig uterus and the effect of indomethacin. *Adv. Biosci.*, **9**, 631–4.

Rashad, S., Hemingway, A., Rainsford, K. *et al.* (1989) Effect of non-steroidal anti-inflammatory drugs on the course of osteoarthritis. *Lancet*, **ii**, 519–22.

Raz, A., Wyche, A., Siegel, N. and Needleman, P. (1988) Regulation of fibroblast cyclooxygenase synthesis by interleukin-1. *J. Biol. Chem.*, **263**, 3022–8.

Raz, A., Wyche, A. and Needleman, P. (1989) Temporal and pharmacological division of fibroblast cyclooxygenase expression into transcriptional and translational phases. *Proc. Natl Acad. Sci. USA*, **86**, 1657–61.

Rome, L.H. and Lands, W.E.M. (1975) Structural requirements for time dependent inhibition of prostaglandin biosynthesis by anti-inflammatory drugs. *Proc. Natl Acad. Sci. USA*, **72**, 4863–5.

Roth, G.J. and Majerus, P.W. (1975) The mechanism of the effect of aspirin on human platelets. 1. Acetylation of a particulate fraction protein. *J. Clin. Invest.*, **56**, 624–32.

Roth, S., Agrawal, N., Mahowald, M. *et al.* (1989) Misoprostol heals gastroduodenal injury in patients with rheumatoid arthritis receiving aspirin. *Arch. Intern. Med.*, **149**, 775–9.

Schwartzman, M., Carroll, M.A., Ibraham, N.G. *et al.* (1985) Renal arachidonic acid metabolism. The third pathway. *Hypertension*, **7**, 136–44.

Shen, T.Y. (1979) Prostaglandin synthetase inhibitors. In *Anti-Inflammatory*

Drugs (eds J.R. Vane and S.H. Ferreira), Springer Verlag, Berlin, pp. 305–47.

Sirois, J. and Richards, J.S. (1992) Purification and characterisation of a novel, distinct isoform of prostaglandin endoperoxide synthase induced by human chorionic gonadotropin in granulosa cells of rat preovulatory follicles. *J. Biol. Chem.*, **267**, 6382–8.

Smith, J.B. and Willis, A.L. (1971) Aspirin selectively inhibits prostaglandin production in human platelets. *Nature*, **231**, 235–7.

Smith, M.J.H., Bryant, C. and Hines, W.J.W. (1964) Reversal by nicotinamide adenine dinucleotide of the inhibitory action of salicylate on mitochondrial malate dehydrogenase. *Nature*, **202**, 96–7.

Smith, W.L. (1986) Prostaglandin biosynthesis and its compartmentation in vascular smooth muscle and endothelial cells. *Ann. Rev. Physiol.*, **48**, 251–62.

Smith, W.L. (1989) The eicosanoids and their biochemical mechanisms of action. *Biochem. J.*, **259**, 315–24.

Smith, W.L. and Lands, W.E.M. (1971) Stimulation and blockade of prostaglandin biosynthesis. *J. Biol. Chem.*, **246**, 6700–3.

Solomon, L.M., Juhlin, L. and Kirschbaum, M.B. (1968) Prostaglandins in cutaneous vasculature. *J. Invest. Derm.*, **51**, 280–2.

Somova, L. (1972) Inhibition of prostaglandin synthesis in the kidneys by aspirin like drugs. *Adv. Biosci.*, **9**, 335–9.

Spector, W.G. and Willoughby, D.A. (1963) Anti-inflammatory effects of salicylate in the rat. In *Salicylates. An International Symposium* (eds A. St J. Dixon, B.K. Martin, M.J.H. Smith, and P.H.N. Wood), Little Brown, Boston, MA, pp. 141–7.

Sykes, J.A.C. and Maddox, I.S. (1972) Prostaglandin production by experimental tumours and effects of anti-inflammatory compounds. *Nature*, **237**, 59–61.

Tai, H.H. and Hollander, C.S. (1972) Regulation of prostaglandin synthetase activity in rabbit kidney medulla: a possible mechanism of hormonal and drug action. In *Advance Abstracts International Conference on Prostaglandins*, Vienna, Abstract 5.

Tomlinson, R.V., Ringold, H.J., Qureshi, M.C. and Forchielli, E. (1972) Relationship between inhibition of prostaglandin synthesis and drug efficacy: support for the current theory on mode of action of aspirin-like drugs. *Biochem. Biophys. Res. Commun.*, **46**, 552–9.

Trang, L.E., Granstrom, E. and Lovgren, O. (1977) Levels of prostaglandin $F_{2\alpha}$ and E_2 and thromboxane B_2 in joint fluid in rheumatoid arthritis. *Scand. J. Rheumatol.*, **6**, 151–4.

Vane, J.R. (1964) The use of isolated organs for detecting active substances in the circulating blood. *Brit. J. Pharmacol. Chemother.*, **23**, 360–73.

Vane, J.R. (1969) The release and fate of vaso-active hormones in the circulation. *Brit. J. Pharmacol.*, **35**, 209–42.

Vane, J.R. (1971a) Mediators of the anaphylactic reaction. In *Identification of Asthma. Ciba Foundation Study No. 38*, Churchill Livingstone, Edinburgh, London, pp. 121–31.

Vane, J.R. (1971b) Inhibition of prostaglandin synthesis as a mechanism of action for aspirin-like drugs. *Nature (New Biology)*, **231**, 232–5.

Vane, J.R. and Williams, K.I. (1972) Prostaglandin production contributes to the contractions of the rat isolated uterus. *Br. J. Pharmacol.*, **45**, 146P.

Vane, J.R., Flower, R.J. and Salmon, J.A. (1982) Inhibitors of arachidonic acid metabolism, with especial reference to the aspirin-like drugs. In *Prostaglandins and Related Lipids, Vol. 2, Prostaglandins and Cancer* (eds T.J. Powels, R.S. Bockman, K.V. Honn, and P. Ramwell), Alan R. Liss, Inc., New York, pp. 21–45.

Waltman, R., Tricomi, V. and Palav, A.B. (1973) Aspirin and indomethacin: effect on instillation abortion time of mid-trimester hypertonic saline-induced abortion. *Prostaglandins*, **3**, 47–58.

Weiss, W.P., Campbell, P.L., Diebler, G.E. and Sokoloff, L. (1962) Effects of salicylate on amino acid incorporation into protein. *J. Pharmacol. Exp. Ther.*, **136**, 366–71.

Whelton, A., Stout, R.L., Spilman, P.S. and Klassen, D.K. (1990) Renal effects of ibuprofen, piroxicam, and sulindac in patients with asymptomatic renal failure. A prospective, randomized, crossover comparison. *Ann. Intern. Med.*, **112**, 568–76.

Whitehouse, M.W. (1965) Some biochemical and pharmacological properties of anti-inflammatory drugs. *Prog. Drug Res.*, **8**, 321–429.

Whitehouse, M.W. and Haslam, J.M. (1962) Ability of some antirheumatic drugs to uncouple oxidative phosphorylation. *Nature*, **196**, 1323–4.

Whittle, B.J.R., Higgs, G.A., Eakins, K.E. *et al.* (1980) Selective inhibition of prostaglandin production in inflammatory exudates and gastric mucosa. *Nature*, **284**, 271–3.

Wiqvist, N., Lundström, V. and Gréen, K. (1976) Indomethacin and premature labour. *Adv. Prostaglandin Thromboxane Res.*, **2**, 998.

Wu, K.K., Sanduja, R., Tsai, A.-L. *et al.* (1991) Aspirin inhibits interleukin-1-induced prostaglandin H synthase expression in cultured endothelial cells. *Proc. Natl Acad. Sci. USA*, **88**, 2384–7.

Xie, W. Chipman, J.G. Robertson, D.L. *et al.* (1991) Expression of a mitogen-responsive gene encoding prostaglandin synthase is regulated by mRNA splicing. *Proc. Natl. Acad. Sci. USA* **88**, 2692–6.

Yokoyama, C., Takai, T. and Tanabe, T. (1988) Primary structure of sheep prostaglandin endoperoxide synthase deduced from cDNA sequence. *FEBS Lett.*, **231**, 347–51.

Ziboh, V.A. (1973) Biosynthesis of prostaglandin E_2 in human skin: subcellular localization and inhibition by unsaturated fatty acids and antiinflammatory agents. *J. Lipid. Res.*, **11**, 377–84.

PART TWO
Pharmacokinetics of aspirin and salicylates

4 Is aspirin a pro-drug for salicylate?

G.A. HIGGS and J.A. SALMON

4.1 INTRODUCTION

Aspirin is the drug which launched the Pharmaceutical Industry as we know it today and it remains the most widely used drug of all time. By the end of the nineteenth century salts of salicylic acid were being used to remedy the aches and pains associated with rheumatic fever. At this time the science of pharmacy was slowly emerging from the traditional empiricism of the herbalist and the search was on for a synthetic substitute for the analgesic properties of quinine.

Salicylic acid itself was precluded from use because of its gastric toxicity and the large doses of sodium salicylate required for efficacy led to problems with salt loading. The successful chemical synthesis of acetylsalicylic acid from salicylic acid in 1899, led Dreser to propose that this compound, known as aspirin, would act as a pro-drug for salicylic acid. In fact, aspirin lived up to its expectations as an analgesic and was soon widely used. The analgesic, antipyretic and anti-inflammatory actions of aspirin were recognized and it soon became regarded as a panacea. The administration of aspirin in a variety of diseases became established with clear indications of therapeutic benefit and relatively few adverse effects. All of this happened with very little knowledge of what exactly aspirin was doing or whether it really could be explained as a pro-drug for salicylate.

It took almost a century of medical experience with aspirin before its mechanism of action began to be unravelled. We now know considerably more about aspirin and as a result there is a rational basis for the use of aspirin in different pathologies. This understanding has also revealed new indications for aspirin which would otherwise not have been obvious. In the light of our understanding of the molecular mechanism of action of aspirin, we shall review in this chapter Dreser's original proposal that aspirin is a pro-drug for salicylate.

4.2 THE FATE OF ASPIRIN IN THE BODY

Although it was assumed that aspirin would be rapidly hydrolysed to salicylate in the gut, it was soon reported that the pharmacology of aspirin is sufficiently different from salicylate to indicate that the differences in action are due in part to undecomposed acetylsalicylic acid. The improved analgesia seen with aspirin is one of the most marked clinical differences from salicylate and it was suggested that this property is attributable to a direct effect of aspirin. Experiments *in vitro* showed that salicylic acid is liberated from aspirin in conditions of acidity and alkalinity which mimic the gastric and intestinal juices (Hanzlik and Presko, 1923). It was found, however, that considerable amounts of aspirin remained unchanged in buffers close to neutral pH. Hanzlik and Presko predicted that significant absorption of unchanged aspirin would occur and in a small clinical study they found that 8.8–36.6% of the aspirin administered appeared in the urine.

With advances in the field of pharmacokinetics and drug metabolism the techniques for measuring drugs and metabolites in biological fluids became more sophisticated and the question of absorption of unchanged aspirin was re-addressed. Hanzlik and Presko (1923) had used a colorimetric method to distinguish between the salicyl and acetylsalicyl groups which depended upon ferric alum as the indicator. It is now evident from the work of Kapp and Coburn (1942) that what they were actually determining was the glycuronide fractions. Using colorimetric methods to determine free salicylate, Smith, (1946) found that after oral administration of aspirin to patients, the only detectable form of salicylate in the plasma was free salicylate. They reported similar findings after intravenous administration of aspirin to dogs.

Further investigations confirmed that acetylsalicylic acid is rapidly hydrolysed after absorption but, up to a period of 1–2 h after oral administration, as much as a quarter of the salicylate in the plasma may be in the acetylated form (Lester, 1946). Refinement of the assays for aspirin and salicylate to enable measurements following low-dose administration also indicated that up to 30% of salicylates in the plasma are present as unchanged aspirin up to 1 h after oral dosing (Smith, 1951). Furthermore, evidence was reported that plasma proteins assert a stronger binding action on salicylate than aspirin. This work revitalized the view that the analgesic action of aspirin is due to the unhydrolysed acetylated fraction in the plasma.

In 1972, Rowland and his colleagues conducted a comprehensive study of the absorption kinetics of aspirin in man following oral administration of an aqueous solution. Plasma samples were assayed for aspirin using gas–liquid chromatography and salicylic acid was determined fluorimetrically. The drug was given in solution to avoid the effects of varying dissolution rates from tablets.

Concentrations of aspirin rise rapidly in the plasma to a peak of approximately 25 μg ml^{-1} 20 min after oral administration of 650 mg aspirin in solution. These levels decline to less than 5 μg ml^{-1} after 2 h. Plasma salicylate concentrations rise equally rapidly reaching a peak of approximately 45 μg ml^{-1} 1 h after administration. Salicylate levels declined far more slowly than aspirin levels and after 2 h the plasma salicylate concentration was still above 40 μg ml^{-1}.

Although the decline of aspirin in the plasma was rapid, it was always longer after oral than after intravenous administration, presumably due to continued absorption from the gut following the oral route. The peak of salicylate concentrations up to 1 h after the aspirin peak is consistent with aspirin being the precursor of salicylate. Rowland and his colleagues concluded that the absorption of aspirin in man follows first order kinetics with a half-life in the region of 10 min. They showed that less than 70% of the administered aspirin reached the peripheral circulation intact by oral or intravenous routes. They also proposed that a two-compartment model for both aspirin and salicylate, in which there is a constant hydrolysis of aspirin to salicylate, explains the resultant plasma levels of aspirin and salicylate.

These finding have been confirmed in a number of other studies in man and animals (Pedersen and Fitzgerald, 1984; Cerletti et al., 1985; Higgs et al., 1987). In rats, aspirin appears briefly in the peripheral circulation following an oral dose of 200 mg kg^{-1} but is undetectable after 1 h (Fig. 4.1). Peak plasma salicylate concentrations are ten times higher than peak plasma aspirin concentrations and only decline by half after 6 h (Fig. 4.1). The clearance of salicylate from the plasma after aspirin administration follows a similar time course to that seen after administration of salicylate (Fig. 4.1).

4.3 MECHANISM OF ACTION OF ASPIRIN

Until the 1970s, the pharmacokinetics of aspirin could only be related to therapeutic and toxic effects. It was known that aspirin is a more potent analgesic agent than salicylate but that their anti-inflammatory effects are similar. Relatively large doses of aspirin or salicylate are required for anti-inflammatory effects in arthritic diseases whereas aspirin is an effective analgesic at low doses. Similarly, Hanzlik and Presko (1923) noted that asprin caused toxic signs such as oedema of the lower eyelids, and other anaphylactoid effects at lower doses than salicylate. There was no explanation, however, of the specific mechanism of action of aspirin or salicylate which could be used as an index of drug activity.

65

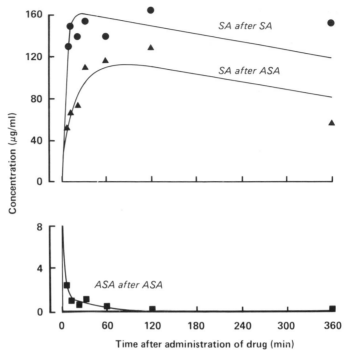

Figure 4.1 Concentration of salicylate and aspirin in plasma after oral doses of salicylate or aspirin at 200 mg kg^{-1} to rats. The upper panel shows concentration of salicylate after salicylate (●) and after aspirin (▲). The lower panel shows concentrations of aspirin after aspirin (■). Each point represents the mean of values from five animals. The curves were fitted by least squares to a pharmacokinetic model similar to that reported by Rowland (1972) but with zero-order salicylate elimination. The data are from Higgs *et al.* (1987).

In 1971, Vane and his colleagues (Ferreira *et al.*, 1971; Smith and Willis, 1971; Vane, 1971) showed that aspirin and a number of other related non-steroid anti-inflammatory and analgesic drugs are specific inhibitors of prostaglandin synthesis. They proposed that this activity explains the therapeutic and toxic side effects of aspirin.

4.4 BIOSYNTHESIS OF PROSTAGLANDINS

Prostaglandins were initially thought to come from the prostate (von Euler, 1937) but are now known to be produced by most mammalian tissues when appropriately stimulated. Prostaglandins are cyclic fatty acids derived from the 20 carbon polyunsaturated fatty acid,

66

arachidonic acid, which is widely distributed in cell membranes as an esterified component of phospholipids. When tissues are stimulated by a wide variety of stimuli including mechanical, chemical or immunological challenge, arachidonic acid is released from phospholipids by the action of phospholipase A_2 and may then be oxygenated by the microsomal enzyme cyclo-oxygenase. Cyclo-oxygenase is present in all cell types with the possible exception of erythrocytes. Cyclo-oxygenase incorporates molecular oxygen into arachidonic acid through the formation of unstable cyclic endoperoxides which are intermediates in the formation of a number of products, including prostaglandins (PGs). The biochemical mechanisms involved in these pathways have been extensively reviewed by Samuelsson (1978) and his colleagues.

4.5 INFLAMMATORY PROPERTIES OF CYCLO-OXYGENASE PRODUCTS

Inflammation is the response of living tissue to injury. Prostaglandin synthesis always accompanies inflammation because phospholipase A_2 is activated when tissues are damaged or stimulated. Prostaglandin E_2 is the predominant product of arachidonic acid metabolism detected in inflammatory conditions ranging from experimental acute oedema and sunburn through to chronic arthritis in humans (Higgs et al., 1990). Because inflammation is one of the few conditions in which PGE_2 is a major product of cyclo-oxygenase, it is possible that the process of inflammation directs the enzymatic pathway towards this product.

Prostaglandin E_2 is a potent dilator of vascular smooth muscle, accounting for the characteristic vasodilation and erythema (redness) seen in acute inflammation. The effect of vasodilatation is to increase the flow of blood through inflamed tissues and this augments the extravasation of fluid (oedema) caused by agents which increase vascular permeability such as bradykinin and histamine (Williams and Peck, 1977). Prostaglandin E_2 also acts synergistically with other mediators to produce inflammatory pain. Without having any direct pain-producing activity, PGE_2 sensitizes receptors on afferent nerve endings to the actions of bradykinin and histamine (Ferreira, 1972). Thirdly, PGE_2 is a potent pyretic agent and its production in bacterial and viral infection contributes to the fever associated with these diseases (Saxena et al., 1979). The pyrexia induced by endogenous pyrogen, now known to be interleukin-1, is reduced by cyclo-oxygenase inhibitors and is principally mediated by PGE_2 (Bernheim et al., 1980).

Many other cyclo-oxygenase products have been detected in inflammatory lesions. These include $PGF_{2\alpha}$, PGD_2, prostacyclin and TXB_2, but

67

usually they are present at less than a quarter the concentrations of PGE_2. Of these products, prostacyclin is probably the most important in terms of inflammatory signs. Prostacyclin has a similar vasodilator potency to PGE_2 and is a more potent hyperalgesic agent than PGE_2 (Higgs et al., 1978). It is likely, therefore, that both PGE_2 and prostacyclin contribute to the development of inflammatory erythema, oedema and pain. Inhibition of the formation of these products of cyclo-oxygenase by aspirin and salicylate accounts for their anti-inflammatory, analgesic and anti-pyretic actions (Vane, 1971).

4.6 THE ROLE OF CYCLO-OXYGENASE PRODUCTS IN CARDIO-THROMBOTIC DISEASES

In the absence of inflammation, the cyclic endoperoxide products of cyclo-oxygenase activity are converted to thromboxane A_2 (TXA_2) or prostacyclin. The isolation and identification of endoperoxides and thromboxanes arose from the study of arachidonic acid metabolism in platelets (Samuelsson, 1978). The unstable TXA_2 was found to be a potent aggregator of platelets and it was proposed, therefore, that it was a key factor in the development of thrombosis. The discovery of TXA_2 led to a search for thromboxane-producing cells in blood vessel walls in the expectation that in disease, arteries may actually contribute to thrombosis formation.

The search revealed, however, that vascular endothelial cells produce predominantly prostacyclin, which is a potent inhibitor of platelet aggregation and acts as a protective mechanism to prevent platelet and leukocyte adherence to blood vessel walls. Thromboxane A_2 and prostacyclin also have opposing effects on vascular smooth muscle; TXA_2 is a potent vasoconstrictor and prostacyclin is a potent vasodilator. It has been proposed that the balance between prostacyclin and TXA_2 production is an important factor in the maintenance of homeostasis (Moncada and Vane, 1978).

The involvement of cyclo-oxygenase products in cardiovascular physiology and pathology provides a rational basis for the clinical investigation of aspirin in cardio-thrombotic diseases. In situations in which platelet activation or vasospasm may contribute to the pathology, the inhibition of TXA_2 production should be beneficial. In well controlled clinical trials, aspirin prevents transient ischaemic attacks and stroke, death and non-fatal myocardial infarction in unstable angina and coronary graft occlusion. The analysis of combined data from these trials indicated a 21% reduction in reinfarction rate and a 16% reduction in cardiovascular mortality rate in patients treated with aspirin (Mustard et al., 1983).

4.7 INHIBITION OF CYCLO-OXYGENASE

The inhibition of prostaglandin synthesis by aspirin has been demonstrated in a wide variety of cell types and tissues ranging from whole animals and humans to microsomal enzyme preparations. Cyclo-oxygenase is inhibited by preventing the abstraction of hydrogen from C13 in arachidonic acid and, therefore, blocking peroxidation at C11 and C15. This action is highly specific, since similar abstraction and peroxidation reactions at other points in the fatty acid are not inhibited (Higgs and Vane, 1989). Furthermore, aspirin does not prevent the generation of prostaglandins from cyclic endoperoxides.

There is a diverse group of chemicals which inhibit cyclo-oxygenase and they are generally known as the non-steroid anti-inflammatory drugs (NSAIDs) or aspirin-like drugs. These drugs have been broadly classified to exhibit three types of inhibition; reversible competitive, irreversible and reversible non-competitive (Lands, 1981). Aspirin itself is an irreversible inhibitor, which covalently acetylates a serine residue in the active site of the enzyme (Roth and Majerus, 1975).

4.8 INHBITION OF CYCLO-OXYGENASE *IN VIVO*

In humans, aspirin blocks cyclo-oxygenase activity in platelets within 1 h of oral administration (Smith and Willis, 1971) and this observation has been confirmed in several species. Because aspirin irreversibly acetylates the enzyme and platelets are unable to generate new enzyme, inhibition of platelet cyclo-oxygenase lasts for the lifetime of the cell. This results in effects on platelet function for several days after a single dose of aspirin.

The anti-thrombotic effect of aspirin is due to its inhibition of platelet thromboxane production but as aspirin prevents the generation of cyclic endoperoxides from arachidonic acid, the production of prostacyclin in other tissues will also be blocked. Certain factors, however, indicate that aspirin may inhibit TXA_2 production at doses that do not impair prostacyclin production by the vascular endothelium. First, the vascular endothelium, unlike the platelets, is able to synthesize new enzyme and so inhibition can be overcome more rapidly. Second, the platelet cyclo-oxygenase appears to be more sensitive to aspirin than the endothelial cyclo-oxygenase (Burch *et al.*, 1978). Third, studies using a deuterated aspirin analogue have shown that platelets passing through the gut capillaries while an oral dose of aspirin is undergoing presystemic hydrolysis can be exposed to higher concentrations of aspirin than platelets present in the peripheral circulation (Pedersen and Fitzgerald, 1984). Thus, serum thromboxane concentrations can be significantly reduced by oral doses of aspirin prior to the drug's appearance in the systemic circulation. Attempts have been made to titrate the dose of aspirin down to one which will achieve inhibition of TXA_2 formation in man without affecting prostacyclin production. The chances of achieving this differential effect on platelet and endothelial cyclo-oxygenase will depend on the demonstration of a lack of effect on prostacyclin production of the relatively high concentrations of salicylate which are known to exist in the systemic circulation following aspirin administration. It can be said, however, that in the cardio-thrombotic diseases aspirin is being used as a drug in its own right and not as a pro-drug for salicylate. This is further supported by

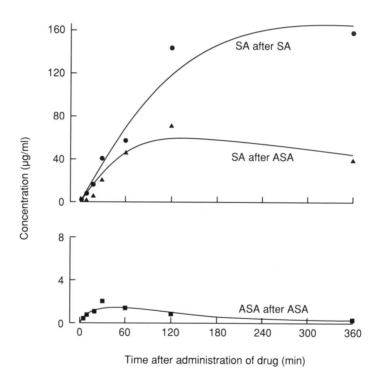

Figure 4.2 Concentrations of salicylate and aspirin in inflammatory exudates after oral doses of salicylate or aspirin at 200 mg kg^{-1}. The upper panel shows concentrations of salicylate after salicylate (●) and after aspirin (▲) and the lower panel shows concentrations of aspirin after aspirin (■). All the exudates were collected 6 h after the subcutaneous implantation of sponges in rats. Each point is the mean of values from five animals. The curves were fitted by least squares to a pharmacokinetic model similar to that reported by Rowland (1972); the exudate was considered to be another compartment linked to the central plasma compartment. The data are from Higgs *et al.* (1987).

the apparent lack of effect of salicylate on TXA_2 production by platelets (Vargaftig, 1977).

Aspirin is significantly more potent in inhibiting cyclo-oxygenase *in vitro* than salicylate (Vane, 1971), but the anti-inflammatory potency of the two drugs is similar, as is their ability to reduce urinary output of prostaglandin metabolites (Hamberg, 1972). Both drugs cause a dose-dependent reduction in the concentration of PGE_2 in inflammatory exudates in experimental inflammation and their ED_{50} values are not significantly different (Higgs and Vane, 1989).

Following the oral administration of aspirin, only very low concentrations of aspirin itself are detected in inflammatory exudates induced by subcutaneous irritants in rats (Higgs *et al.*, 1987). Salicylate concentrations are up to fifty times higher and are detectable for several hours (Fig. 4.2). Furthermore, the synthesis of PGE_2 by explants in inflamed tissues was almost completely inhibited by concentrations of salicylate which could be found in exudates after oral dosing (Fig. 4.3). These experiments indicate that the anti-inflammatory activity of aspirin is through the inhibition of prostaglandin synthesis by salicylate and that aspirin is a pro-drug for salicylate in inflammatory diseases. Interestingly, Salmon *et al.*, (1983), reported that aspirin was approximately five times more potent in reducing thromboxane concentrations in

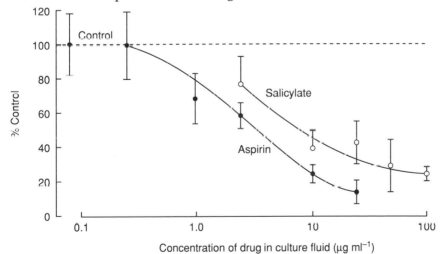

Figure 4.3 The effect of aspirin (●) or salicylate (○) on PGE_2 synthesis by explants of acutely inflamed tissue from rats. Explants (30–60 mg) were incubated in non-proliferative culture for 24 h and then the PGE_2 content of the medium was assayed by specific radioimmunnoassay. Each point is the mean of 4–12 values and the bars represent ± 1 SEM. The data are from Higgs *et al.* (1987).

inflammatory exudates than PGE_2 concentrations. This would appear to be a direct effect of aspirin on leukocyte cyclo-oxygenase in the pre-systemic circulation since the thromboxane found in inflammatory exudates is all produced by leukocytes infiltrating the inflamed tissues from the blood stream (Higgs et al., 1983).

SUMMARY

Aspirin is a widely used drug which is rapidly hydrolysed to salicylate after administration to man or animals. The therapeutic effects of aspirin itself are probably confined to a direct and irreversible inhibition of cyclo-oxygenase in blood cells such as platelets and leukocytes which are exposed to aspirin in the pre-systemic portal circulation. The effects of aspirin on peripheral tissues in inflammatory diseases are due to conversion to salicylate which also inhibits cyclo-oxygenase but is less potent.

REFERENCES

Bernheim, H.A., Gilbert, T.M. and Stitt, J.T. (1980) Prostaglandin E levels in third ventricular cerebrospinal fluid of rabbits during fever and changes in body temperature. *J. Physiol.*, **301**, 69–78.

Burch, J.W., Baenziger, N.L., Stanford, N. and Majerus, P.W. (1978) Sensitivity of fatty acid cyclo-oxygenase from human aorta to acetylation by aspirin. *Proc. Natl. Acad. Sci. USA*, **75**, 5181–4.

Cerletti, C., Latini, R., Dejana, E. *et al.* (1985) Inhibition of human platelet thromboxane generation by aspirin in the absence of measurable drug levels in peripheral blood. *Biochem. Pharmacol.*, **34**, 1839–41.

Dreser, H. (1899) Pharmakologisches über Aspirin (Acetylsalicyl-saüre). *Pfluegers Arch. gesamte Physiol. Menchen Tiere.*, **76**, 306–18.

Ferreira, S.H. (1972) Prostaglandins, aspirin-like drugs and analgesia. *Nature*, **240**, 200–3.

Ferreira, S.H., Moncada, S. and Vane, J.R. (1971) Indomethacin and aspirin abolish prostaglandin release from the spleen. *Nature*, **231**, 237–9.

Hamberg, M. (1972) Inhibition of prostaglandin synthesis in man. *Biochem. Biophys. Res. Commun.*, **49**, 720–6.

Hanzlik, P.J. and Presko, E. (1923) The salicylates. XIV. Liberation of salicyl from and excretion of acetylsalicylic acid. *J. Pharmacol.*, **21**, 247–61.

Higgs, G.A. and Vane, J.R. (1989) Inhibitors of enzymes of the arachidonic acid metabolic pathways. In *Design of Enzyme Inhibitors as Drugs* (eds M. Sandler and H.J. Smith), Oxford University Press, Oxford, pp. 314–42.

Higgs, E.A., Moncada, S. and Vane, J.R. (1978) Inflammatory effects of prostacyclin (PGI_2) and 6-oxo-$PGF_{1\alpha}$ in the rat paw. *Prostaglandins*, **16**, 153–62.

Higgs, G.A., Moncada, S. Salmon, J.A. and Seager, K. (1983) The source of prostaglandins and thromboxanes in experimental inflammation. *Brit. J. Pharmacol.*, **79**, 863–8.

Higgs, G.A., Salmon, J.A., Henderson, B. and Vane, J.R. (1987) Pharmaco-kinetics of aspirin and salicylate in relation to inhibition of arachidonate cyclo-oxygenase and anti-inflammatory activity. *Proc. Natl Acad. Sci., USA*, **84**, 1417–20.

Higgs, G.A., Higgs, E.A. and Moncada, S. (1990) The arachidonic acid cascade. In *Comprehensive Medicinal Chemistry, Vol. 2* (ed. P.G. Sammes), Pergamon Press, Oxford, pp. 147–73.

Kapp, E.M. and Coburn, A.F (1942) Urinary metabolites of sodium salicylate. *J. Biol. Chem.*, **145**, 549–65.

Lands, W.E.M. (1981) Actions of anti-inflammatory drugs. *Trends Pharmacol. Sci.*, **2**, 78–80.

Lester, D. (1946) The fate of acetylsalicylic acid. *J. Pharmacol.*, **87**, 329–42.

Moncada, S. and Vane, J.R. (1978) Pharmacology and endogenous roles of prostaglandin endoperoxides, thromboxane A_2 and prostacyclin. *Pharmacol. Rev.*, **30**, 293–331.

Mustard, J.F., Kinlough-Rathbone, R.L. and Packham, M.A. (1983) Aspirin in the treatment of cardiovascular disease: a review. *Am. J. Med.*, **74**, 43–9.

Pedersen, A.K. and Fitzgerald, G.A. (1984) Dose-related kinetics of aspirin. *N. Eng. J. Med.*, **311**, 1206–11.

Roth, G.J. and Majerus, P.W. (1975) The mechanism of the effect of aspirin on human platelets. 1. Acetylation of a particulate fraction protein. *J. Clin. Invest.*, **56**, 624–32.

Rowland, M. (1972) Absorption kinetics of aspirin in man following oral administration of an aqueous solution. *J. Pharm. Sci.*, **61**, 379–85.

Salmon, J.A., Simmons, P.M. and Moncada, S. (1983) The effects of BW755C and other anti-inflammatory drugs on eicosanoid concentrations and leukocyte accumulation in experimentally-induced acute inflammation. *J. Pharm. Pharmacol.*, **35**, 808–13.

Samuelsson, B. (1978) Prostaglandins and thromboxanes. *Ann. Rev. Biochem.*, **47**, 997–1029.

Saxena, P.N., Beg, M.M.A., Singhal, K.C. and Ahmad, M. (1979) Prostaglandin-like activity in the cerebrospinal fluid of febrile patients. *Indian J. Med. Res.*, **79**, 495–8.

Smith, J.B. and Willis, A.L. (1971) Aspirin selectively inhibits prostaglandin production in human platelets. *Nature*, **231**, 235–7.

Smith, M.J.H. (1951) Plasma-salicylate concentration after small doses of acetysalicylic acid. *J. Pharm. Pharmacol.*, **3**, 409–14.

Smith, P.K. (1946) Studies on the pharmacology of salicylates. *J. Pharmacol.*, **87**, 237–55.

Vane, J.R. (1971) Inhibition of prostaglandin synthesis as a mechanism of action for aspirin-like drugs. *Nature*, **231**, 232–5.

Vargaftig, B.B. (1977) Salicylic acid fails to inhibit generation of thromboxane A_2 activity in platelets after *in vivo* administration to the rat. *J. Pharm. Pharmacol.*, **30**, 101–4.

Von Euler, U.S. (1937) On the specific vaso-dilating and plain muscle stimu-lating substance from accessory genital glands in man and certain animals (prostaglandin and vesiglandin). *J. Physiol.*, **88**, 213–17.

Williams, T.J. and Peck, M.J. (1977) Role of prostaglandin-mediated vasodilation in inflammation. *Nature*, **270**, 530–2.

5 Aspirin: pharmacokinetics and pharmacodynamic effects on platelets and vascular function

W.N. CHARMAN, D.M. KERINS and G.A. FITZGERALD

5.1 INTRODUCTION

The impact of aspirin on cardiovascular therapeutics has been both substantial and recent. In an impressive monograph of some 300 pages entitled *Aspirin and the Salicylates* which was published in 1984 (Rainsford, 1984), the use of this drug in thrombo-embolic disease merited three pages. Some 6 years later, the use of aspirin in the prevention of stroke, myocardial infarction and vascular death is well established and accepted by medical practitioners. The purpose of this chapter is to review the progress – in pharmacology, biochemistry, molecular biology and epidemiology – which has encouraged this evolution in the use of aspirin and the consequent reduction in cardiovascular morbidity and mortality.

5.2 PHARMACOKINETIC ASPECTS

5.2.1 Absorption

Aspirin and salicylate are rapidly and extensively absorbed by a first order process following oral administration of solution formulations to man (Rowland *et al.*, 1972; Miaskiewicz *et al.*, 1982). The absorption half-life of aspirin is less than that of salicylate, however, values for both compounds can be quite variable (Rowland *et al.*, 1972; Miaskiewicz *et al.*, 1982). Differences in the rate and extent of absorption are a function of inter-related and dependent factors which include pH, pre-absorptive hydrolysis and first-pass effects.

Aspirin and salicylate are both weak acids with pK_a values of 3.6 and 3.0, respectively. As would be expected, both exhibit a pH dependency of absorption, being slowest from an alkaline medium (Dotevall and Ekenved, 1976). Notwithstanding this feature, both aspirin and salicylate are more rapidly absorbed from the duodenum than from the stomach due to its relatively greater surface area (Rowland et al., 1972). However, the intestinal absorption of both compounds is still dependent upon the rate at which the stomach empties. It has been reported that large doses of salicylate can decrease gastric emptying and thereby lead to a decreased rate of drug absorption (Matthew et al., 1966).

Although aspirin is extensively absorbed following oral administration, the fraction of the administered dose reaching the systemic circulation ranges from 50 to 75% (Rowland et al., 1972; Pedersen and FitzGerald, 1984). The presystemic loss of a drug can be a function of luminal degradation, gut wall metabolism and hepatic extraction. However, the relative contribution of these different mechanisms to the first-pass effect of aspirin in man has not been quantitatively analysed.

The pre-absorptive hydrolysis of aspirin, which includes both chemical and enzymatic components, is difficult to estimate. The chemical hydrolysis of aspirin at 37 °C is unlikely to account for significant loss due to the relatively slow reaction rate and short residence time of aspirin solutions in the GI tract. Enzymatic hydrolysis of aspirin could occur either in the lumen or be associated with brush-border esterase activity. Such esterase activity has been demonstrated in rat, rabbit, dog and human GI tracts (Levy et al., 1967; Levy and Angelino, 1968) so it would appear reasonable that some enzymatic hydrolysis of aspirin would occur. Although studies have suggested negligible luminal hydrolysis of aspirin in man (Rowland et al., 1972), such conclusions must be tempered by the problems associated with aspiration of representative samples of luminal and brush-border fluid. In the same study, everted rabbit gut demonstrated substantial esterase activity hydrolysing up to 30% of an aspirin dose in 1 h. Although difficult to quantitate, pre-absorptive hydrolysis of aspirin is most likely the result of enzymatically mediated hydrolysis.

Gut wall metabolism plays a role in aspirin hydrolysis (Spenney, 1978), although it is not readily differentiated from possible brush-border effects. In the dog, Harris and Riegelman (1969) estimated that approximately 20% of doses ranging between 250 and 500 mg aspirin were metabolized by the gut wall. This calculation was based upon the relative areas under the plasma aspirin concentration–time profiles (AUC) following administration by the oral route relative to infusion of aspirin into the hepatic portal vein. In this same study, aspirin AUC values following administration into the hepatic portal vein and vena cava, respectively, indicated the percentage metabolism of aspirin occurring on first-pass through the liver to be in the range of 22–46%. Although the contribution of luminal, gut wall or liver metabolism of aspirin is difficult to quantitate, it does account for up to 25–50% of the administered dose. These estimates compare quite well with the systemic availability of aspirin in man (section 5.3.1). In man, the variability in the first-pass effect of aspirin between subjects is high, although the magnitude of the effect is generally constant within the same subjects (Levy, 1980).

5.2.2 Disposition

Aspirin and salicylate are rapidly and extensively distributed throughout body fluids following oral administration. The plasma concentration-time profiles for both compounds can be described with bi-exponential equations fitted to a two-compartment open model system. Table 5.1 describes selected estimates of the volume of distribution and the terminal elimination half-lives for aspirin and salicylate taken from the limited intravenous data available in the literature. The steady state volumes of distribution, derived from statistical moment calculations for aspirin and salicylate appear to be independent of sex (Aarons et al., 1989). The volume of distribution for aspirin, from an administered dose of 650 mg, was marginally greater than the salicylate value. This is thought to result from the higher binding of salicylate to albumin (Davidson and Smith, 1961; Rowland and Riegelman, 1968). Physicochemical properties and lipophilicity are also likely to play a role in the slightly different volumes of distribution (Rowland and Riegelman, 1968). The volume of distribution for salicylate has been shown to increase with increasing doses of aspirin which has been attributed to dose-related alterations in plasma protein binding (Dromgoole and Furst, 1986).

The initial distribution phase for both aspirin and salicylate following intravenous administration is rapid with half-life values in the range of 2–5 min (Rowland and Riegelman, 1968; Aarons et al., 1989). In contrast, the elimination half-life for aspirin ranges from 14 to 19 min while that of salicylate is considerably longer being in the range of 230–300 min. The elimination half-life of aspirin is essentially dose independent, while the elimination of salicylate is non-linear and dose dependent (see section 5.2.3).

The binding of aspirin and salicylate to serum proteins plays a role in their distribution throughout the body. The binding of salicylate to albumin is reversible, and occurs through two primary high affinity binding sites and a number of secondary sites (Davidson and Smith, 1961; Borga et al., 1976). In the normal therapeutic concentration

Table 5.1 Selected pharmacokinetic parameters following intravenous administration of aspirin or salicylate

Subjects		Vol. of distribution (l/kg)		Half-Life (min)[a]		Reference
		ASA	SA	ASA	SA	
Male	(*n*=9)	0.221[b]		16.3		Aarons
Female	(*n*=9)	0.218[b]		14.5		*et al.* (1989)
Male	(*n*=6)		0.18[c]		300	Miaskiewicz
Female	(*n*=6)		0.18[c]		276	*et al.* (1982)
Male	(*n*=4)	0.16[d]	0.13[d]	14.9	238	Rowland
						et al. (1972)

[a] Terminal elimination half-life.
[b] Calculated as V_{dss} from statistical moment analysis.
[c] Calculated as V_d = dose/b.AUC, where b = the slope of the terminal elimination phase.
[d] Calculated as $V_d = V_c ((k_{12} + k_{21})/k_{21})$, where V_c = volume of the central compartment, and k_{12} and k_{21} are first order rate constants. A body weight of 70 kg was assumed.

range, the protein binding of salicylate is approximately 80–90% (Wanwimolruk *et al.*, 1982). However, the free fraction of salicylate is concentration dependent, subject to wide inter-subject variability and affected by disease (Ekstrand *et al.*, 1979; Levy *et al.*, 1980; Dromgoole and Furst, 1986). The interaction of aspirin with plasma proteins is more complex than that observed with salicylate. This is due partly to the inherent propensity of aspirin to acetylate proteins, which is also considered a major determinant of both its mechanism of action and toxicity. The acetylation of various proteins, glycoproteins and lipids in the stomach, kidney, liver and bone marrow by aspirin has been demonstrated (Rainsford *et al.*, 1983).

Aspirin and salicylate readily distribute into synovial fluid. The maximal concentration of salicylate in synovial fluid is less than that observed in plasma and is consistent with the decreased albumin concentration in synovial fluid relative to plasma (Needs and Brooks, 1985). Not surprisingly, aspirin concentrations in synovial fluid peak later and are significantly less than maximum concentrations in plasma. However, the clearance of aspirin from synovial fluid proceeds less rapidly than from plasma (Soren, 1979). Results of a similar nature were reported by Higgs *et al.* (1987) who studied the pharmacokinetics of aspirin and salicylate in inflammatory exudate fluid in rats. They found the salicylate concentrations to be much greater and more sustained than the corresponding aspirin levels.

Pharmacokinetics of aspirin and salicylates

Salicylate distributes into breast milk, although the amount transferred into the milk after a single oral dose of aspirin is small (Findlay *et al.*, 1981). Placental transfer is quantitatively more important as neonatal plasma concentrations of salicylate at birth are higher than concurrent maternal plasma concentrations. The extent of salicylate binding and the relative neonatal/maternal albumin concentrations contribute to these plasma concentration differences (Garretson *et al.*, 1975; Levy *et al.*, 1975).

Salicylate is also distributed into saliva and the resulting concentrations have been found to be proportional to plasma concentrations (Graham and Rowland, 1972; Roberts *et al.*, 1978). However, the effect of saliva pH on the observed salicylate concentration, and the inherent inter- and intra-subject variability preclude the clinical application of this technique for routine estimation of plasma salicylate concentrations (Levy, 1980).

5.2.3 Metabolism and Excretion

Following oral administration, aspirin is rapidly absorbed and is subject to first-pass clearance to form salicylate as described in section 5.2.1. The elimination half-life of aspirin from the plasma is in the range of 15–20 min (Table 5.1). The hydrolytic conversion of aspirin to salicylic acid is quantitative and independent of dose and is due to a variety of esterases found in various body tissues (Ali and Kaur, 1983). Red blood cell aspirin esterase appears to be responsible to a significant extent for aspirin hydrolysis in the systemic circulation (Costello and Green, 1983). Furthermore, studies in sheep suggest that extrahepatic metabolism of aspirin can occur in the hind legs and other vascular beds (Cossum *et al.*, 1986). Intact aspirin is the major form of drug in plasma for the first 20–30 min following oral administration and is readily detectable before salicylate levels can be measured. As the clearance of aspirin is rapid and the first-pass effect is substantial, the resultant plasma concentrations of aspirin are highly dependent upon the rate of absorption. Dose form effects for the control/manipulation of aspirin plasma levels are discussed in section 5.3.2.

The metabolism and excretion of salicylic acid is complex, dose dependent and, therefore, non-linear. There are five parallel pathways (three first order and two non-linear pathways) which quantitatively account for the metabolism and excretion of salicylic acid (and aspirin) from the body (Levy *et al.*, 1972). All metabolites are excreted via the kidney, only a small fraction of salicylic acid being excreted unchanged in the urine. The metabolic products of salicylate biotransformation are salicyluric acid (SU, a glycine conjugate), salicyl phenolic glucuronide

78

and salicyl acyl glucuronide (SPG and SAG, respectively, glucuronic acid conjugates), and gentisic acid (GA, an oxidation product) (Levy and Tsuchiya, 1972). Gentisuric acid (GU) may be formed from GA via glycine conjugation or from SU via microsomal oxidation (Wilson et al., 1978). There can be considerable inter-subject variability in the relative contribution of the five parallel metabolic pathways to the biotransformation of salicylic acid (Levy, 1979; Caldwell et al., 1980; Dromgoole and Furst, 1986).

Figure 5.1 describes the metabolic transformation of aspirin and salicylate. The formation of SU and SPG from salicylic acid is saturable and can be described by Michaelis–Menten kinetics, whereas both the formation of SU and GA and the renal elimination of free salicylic acid are linear first order processes (Levy, 1979). The V_{max} and K_m values (Michaelis–Menten parameters) describing the salicylate to SU transformation are 60.3 mg h^{-1} and 338 mg, respectively, and are 32.3 mg h^{-1} and 629 mg, respectively, for SPG formation from salicylate (Levy et al., 1972). From consideration of the capacity limited nature of the biotransformation of salicylate to SU and SPG, it is apparent that the proportional renal excretion of the five metabolic products will be dose dependent. For example, doses of aspirin less than 300 mg result in approximately 90% being excreted as SU or SPG with the kinetics of elimination being reasonably linear (Tsuchiya and Levy, 1972a). However, for comparison, a 3.0 g aspirin dose (above the respective K_m values for SU and SPG) results in a marked change in the metabolite excretion profile: SU accounts for 50% of the dose, SPG for 20%, 10% as SAG, 14% as salicylic acid, and 3.1% as GU (Levy et al., 1972; Tsuchiya and Levy, 1972b).

A further complication with chronic salicylate therapy is that it appears to have the potential to induce its own metabolism by increasing the production of SU (Furst et al., 1977; Rumble et al., 1980) which leads to a decrease in the steady state plasma levels of salicylate. Day et al. (1983) found that the production of SU increased approximately 73% and occurred within 2 weeks of chronic aspirin therapy in patients with rheumatoid arthritis. A similar increase was observed in the V_{max} value for SU formation.

The renal excretion of salicylate, a first order process, involves glomerular filtration, active tubular secretion and partial passive tubular back-diffusion (Levy, 1979). Only the non-ionic form of salicylate undergoes tubular re-absorption and therefore, the renal clearance of salicylic acid (pK$_a$ 3.0) is sensitive to urine pH. A change in urine pH from 5 to 8 results in a twenty-fold increase in the renal clearance of free salicylate (Smith et al., 1946). For doses of salicylate greater than the K_m for SU and SAG formation, changes in urine pH have a profound

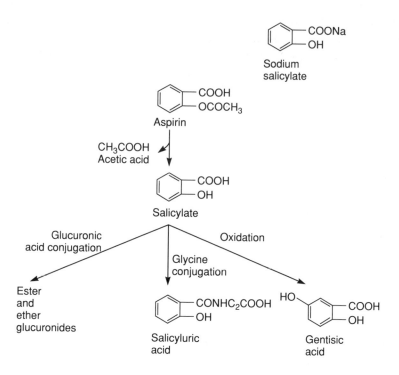

Figure 5.1 Metabolic pathways of aspirin and salicylate biotransformation. (Reproduced from FitzGerald, G.A. and Sherry, S. (1982).)

effect as free salicylate excretion accounts for a greater proportion of the dose than observed with lower doses. Although these changes in free salicylate excretion are most marked at high plasma levels of salicylate, they are still observed after administration of low doses of aspirin (Levy and Leonards, 1971).

The pharmacokinetic manifestation of the saturable metabolism and clearance of salicylate is that the observed plasma levels of salicylate are not proportional to the administered dose of aspirin. This non-linearity between dose and plasma levels has implications with regard to drug accumulation in the body, the choice of dosing intervals and the time taken to reach steady state plasma levels of salicylate.

The primary factor controlling the potential for non-linearity in salicylate excretion is the choice of administered dose of aspirin. For example, in contemporary anti-thrombotic therapy where the administered daily dose of aspirin is generally less than 350 mg, the elimination of salicylate is not dose dependent and drug and/or metabolite accumulation is unlikely to occur. However, dose dependent metabolism of salicylate will occur with high dose chronic aspirin therapy as often prescribed for arthritic and associated conditions. The potential for dose dependent salicylate excretion must be evaluated when considering chronic therapy with aspirin at doses in excess of 500 mg day^{-1}.

5.3 BIOPHARMACEUTICAL PROFILE

5.3.1 Bioavailability of Orally Administered Aspirin

Historically, plasma salicylate concentration–time profiles have been utilized as a bioavailability index of aspirin formulations. This practice has been suitable for evaluating the bioavailability (of salicylate) from high dose aspirin formulations as the plasma concentrations of salicylate were readily quantified and salicylate was generally considered the active form of the drug for arthritic conditions. These assessment procedures are, however, inappropriate for assessing the bioavailability of aspirin from lower dose formulations (e.g. less than 300 mg). Recent improvements in analytical methodology have enabled routine assessment of aspirin plasma concentrations and thereby evaluation of aspirin bioavailability from lower dose formulations (Pedersen and FitzGerald, 1984, 1985; Brandon et al., 1985; Siebert and Bochner, 1987).

Pedersen and FitzGerald (1984) evaluated the oral bioavailability of aspirin in the dose range of 20–1300 mg administered as standard gelatin capsules. Deuterium labelled aspirin was administered intravenously to healthy male subjects who simultaneously ingested unlabelled aspirin orally. The absolute oral bioavailability of aspirin was calculated from the ratio of the plasma aspirin concentration–time profiles for the labelled and unlabelled drug. The systemic bioavailability of aspirin ranged from 46 to 51% after single oral doses of either 20, 40, 325 or 1300 mg aspirin. Furthermore, the bioavailability of 325 mg aspirin was similar after a single dose or following repeated long term administration. In accord with these results, Bochner et al. (1988) estimated the oral bioavailability of an oral solution of aspirin (50 mg) to be approximately 50% and Aarons et al. (1989) found the oral bioavailability of 1000 mg aspirin administered as a solution to be 54%.

These data indicate the oral bioavailability of aspirin to be dose independent and approximately 50% of the administered dose. However, this statement requires clarification – the formulation or dose form in which aspirin is orally administered can be a crucial determinate

81

of the drug's oral bioavailability and should always be specified and adequately described.

5.3.2 Dose Form Effects on Bioavailability

The dose form in which aspirin is orally administered can have a significant effect upon the aspirin plasma concentration–time profiles. Although many different formulations of aspirin and salicylate have been developed for different routes of administration (e.g. rectal, intramuscular, oral), only the oral route will be considered in the context of this chapter. As discussed in section 5.2.1, aspirin is rapidly absorbed, is subject to extensive first-pass metabolism and is rapidly cleared from the plasma. Due to these factors, the systemic plasma levels of aspirin and resulting bioavailability of different aspirin dose forms are a function of the absorption rate of aspirin from the GI tract.

Historically, the development and evaluation of the majority of enteric coated aspirin preparations has been predicated upon the evaluation of salicylate plasma concentration–time profiles. Consequently, limited data are available in the literature concerning the aspirin plasma concentration–time profiles of enteric coated formulations, relative to appropriate intravenous standards, as these data have been dependent upon the availability of suitable assay methodology.

Table 5.2 lists examples of aspirin bioavailability data for solution, compressed tablet and enteric coated aspirin formulations in the dose range 20–1300 mg. Enteric coated formulations, which can be either monolithic or multi-particulate in nature, delay the release of drug until the formulation empties from the stomach into the small intestine. In the newer enteric coated systems, the pH change encountered by the dose form upon gastric emptying initiates dissolution of a pH sensitive polymer system (which is coated on the formulation) which leads to drug release. Enteric coated formulations are generally not considered to be a controlled release dose form.

The pharmaceutical characteristics of either the solution or the enteric coated dose form have a pronounced effect upon the pharmacokinetic characteristics of orally administered aspirin and are reflected in the plasma concentration–time profiles. The maximum plasma aspirin concentration is dramatically reduced by administering the enteric coated formulations relative to either a solution or a compressed tablet. For example, in the work of Bochner *et al.* (1988) the maximum plasma aspirin concentration after administration of the enteric coated formulation was 16%, relative to an oral solution, and reflected the slower release of aspirin from the enteric coated formulation. More significantly, in terms of the pharmacodynamics of aspirin (section 5.4), the absolute bioavailability of the 50 mg aspirin dose was reduced from 42% to 24% by administering the enteric coated formulation rather than the solution.

There are a number of explanations for the decreased bioavailability of aspirin after administration of the enteric coated formulation. However, the study of Bochner *et al.* (1988) was sufficiently well designed to rule out the possibility of incomplete drug absorption. Assessment of the urinary recovery of salicylate and the area under the plasma salicylate–time profile (relative to an intravenous aspirin standard) revealed complete drug release and absorption from both the solution and enteric coated formulations.

These data are consistent with the hypothesis that the enteric coated aspirin formulation, which decreased the absorption rate of aspirin from the GI tract and led to a lower absolute bioavailability of aspirin, did so by increasing the pre-systemic clearance of the drug. Such increased pre-systemic clearance is unlikely to be a function of increased luminal hydrolysis and must therefore represent an increased extraction occurring between, and including, the gut wall and the liver.

Table 5.2 Selected maximum plasma aspirin concentrations (C_{max}, ng ml^{-1}) and bioavailability data from different formulations and doses of orally administered aspirin

Dose (mg)	Formulation	C_{max} (ng ml^{-1})	% Bioavail. (relative to i.v. standard)	Reference
50	Solution	1323	42	Bochner
50	Enteric coated	221	24	et al. (1988)
20	Capsule	n.a.[a]	49	Pedersen and
40	Capsule	n.a.	48	FitzGerald
325	Capsule	n.a.	51	(1984)
300	Solution	7650	no i.v admin.	Roberts
300	Enteric coated	610	28[b]	et al. (1984)
1000	Solution	20255	54	Aarons et al. (1989)

[a] Data not available.
[b] Value based upon comparison of salicylate AUC values following oral administration of solution and enteric coated formulation. The low value reflects problems due to limited assay sensitivity, but nevertheless indicates reduced bioavailability.

Pharmacokinetics of aspirin and salicylates

Recent studies in our laboratory (FitzGerald *et al.*, 1991) where a solution of aspirin was administered at different rates via a nasogastric tube into the duodenum of healthy subjects, confirm and extend the data of Bochner *et al.* (1988). In our studies, the bioavailability of aspirin was reduced, relative to an oral solution, when the infusion rate of aspirin into the duodenum was decreased. However, the increase in pre-systemic clearance of aspirin which was achieved by decreasing the intra-duodenal infusion rate appeared to plateau at slower infusion rates.

The significance of the pre-systemic clearance of aspirin following administration of oral aspirin for anti-thrombotic therapy is discussed in section 5.5.

5.3.3 Effects of Food

The mechanism(s) by which food can affect the bioavailability of drugs are generally inadequately characterized as the endpoints of such studies are often the plasma levels of the administered drug. In the case of aspirin, most food effect studies have utilized salicylate plasma levels as the pharmacokinetic endpoint which makes it difficult to extrapolate the data to the likely effect of food upon the plasma levels of aspirin. Of the limited studies in which aspirin levels have been studied, ingestion of food generally decreased the maximum aspirin plasma concentrations by approximately 50% and delayed the overall appearance of aspirin in the plasma. Koch *et al.* (1978) reported no statistically significant difference in plasma aspirin AUC values after administration of 650 mg aspirin in either the fed or fasted state. In terms of lower aspirin doses, there have been no reported data to assess the effect of food on aspirin plasma profiles.

The co-administration of food has been demonstrated to increase the oral availability of drugs undergoing extensive first-pass metabolism, such as propranolol and labetalol (Melander *et al.*, 1977; Melander and McLean, 1983). These effects are presumed to be a function of a decreased pre-systemic clearance of these drugs after co-administration of food (Welling, 1984). Although the metabolic profiles of these beta blockers are different from aspirin, the potential effect of food on the bioavailability of low dose aspirin assumes significance when considering the pharmacodynamic hypothesis for increasing the pre-systemic clearance of aspirin following oral administration.

Food effects on the pharmacokinetic profile of high dose enteric coated aspirin preparations have been extensively studied using salicylate plasma levels as an index of bioavailability. Enteric coated aspirin products have been associated with variable onset of action and erratic drug absorption (Leonards and Levy, 1965; Paull et al., 1976). Bogentoft et al. (1978) found that food intake decreased the plasma salicylate levels from enteric coated aspirin products and that drug absorption was variable. In some patients, plasma salicylate levels were not observed until 4 h after dosing.

Recent studies of enteric coated aspirin preparations in dogs (Lui et al. 1986) and man (Mojaverian et al., 1987) have indicated that the observed inter-subject variability in plasma levels is often a function of the gastric emptying profile of the formulation. The study of Lui et al. (1986) also identified the time for the dissolution of the enteric coating in the intestine to be a contributory factor in the delayed plasma levels of drug.

5.3.4 Age and Sex Differences

There are numerous reports concerning the effect of gender on the disposition and pharmacokinetics of aspirin and salicylate (Miaskiewicz et al., 1982; Trnavska and Trnavsky, 1983; Ho et al., 1985; Montgomery et al., 1986). Miaskiewicz et al. (1982) administered sodium salicylate (9 mg kg^{-1}) to male and female subjects and found that the maximum plasma concentration of salicylate was similar between males and females, although the time taken to reach maximum concentrations was longer in females. Furthermore, there were no observed gender-dependent differences in the volume of distribution or clearance of salicylate. In contrast, in a study where male and female subjects ingested a compressed aspirin tablet, Trnavska and Trnavsky (1983) found that the maximum plasma salicylate levels were lower in males and the time taken to reach the maximum plasma concentrations was longer in males than females. Ho et al. (1985) administered 600 mg of aspirin as a solution to males and females and found, in accordance with the results of Trnavska and Trnavsky (1983), that the maximum plasma levels of both aspirin and salicylate were lower in males than females. However, there were no gender dependent differences in either the time taken to reach peak concentrations or the respective volumes of distribution for aspirin and salicylate.

Montgomery et al. (1986), in a comprehensive study involving 44 subjects, found negligible gender-dependent differences in the kinetics of salicylate after single dose administration of 900 mg aspirin. The values for the maximum plasma concentrations of salicylate, time to reach maximum plasma concentrations, clearance of salicylate and the volume of distribution were not statistically different between males and females. In addition, the urinary recovery of selected salicylic acid metabolites was similar between males and females in terms of rate of excretion and extent of recovery.

Aarons *et al.* (1989) evaluated the disposition of 1000 mg of aspirin (administered as the lysinate salt) in males and females after intravenous and oral administration. Their data indicated that the disposition of aspirin, assessed by measurement of plasma aspirin and salicylate concentrations, was independent of gender as there were no statistically significant differences in the elimination kinetics, clearance or volume of distribution of aspirin. After oral administration of 1000 mg of aspirin to males and females, the systemic bioavailability of aspirin was similar between sexes (54%), although the absorption of aspirin was most rapid in females.

Although the effect of gender on the pharmacokinetics of orally administered aspirin is controversial, it appears that the major difference (if it does exist) is a more rapid absorption of aspirin in females (Aarons *et al.*, 1989). The pharmacokinetic manifestations of the more rapid absorption of aspirin in females are that plasma aspirin concentrations may be higher and peak earlier.

The effect of age on the pharmacokinetics of aspirin and salicylate is also a contentious issue. It is difficult to evaluate clearly the effect of age on the pharmacokinetics of aspirin due to the problems in differentiating between age and disease state-induced changes in metabolic function. Cuny *et al.* (1979), Ho *et al.* (1985) and Netter *et al.* (1985) have all reported decreased plasma clearance of aspirin in elderly bedridden patients. Montgomery and Sitar (1981) reported increased levels of the salicylate metabolites, SU and GA, in patients greater than 60 years of age.

These observed age-dependent changes in the kinetics of aspirin are possibly a function of the patient's clinical history rather than a reflection of the ageing process. Montgomery *et al.* (1986) conducted a study of the kinetics and metabolism of salicylate in healthy men and women across a broad age range and found no major difference in salicylate disposition as a function of age between 20 and 78 years old.

It appears that advanced age has no major intrinsic effect upon the pharmacokinetics of aspirin and salicylate, and that any alteration in the kinetics of aspirin in the aged is likely to be a function of an underlying pathophysiological condition (Netter *et al.*, 1986).

5.4 MECHANISM OF ACTION

The development of the platelet aggregometer (Born, 1962) permitted the detection of the antiplatelet actions of aspirin, first *in vitro*, then *ex vivo* (Weiss and Aledort, 1967; O'Brien, 1968). Subsequent

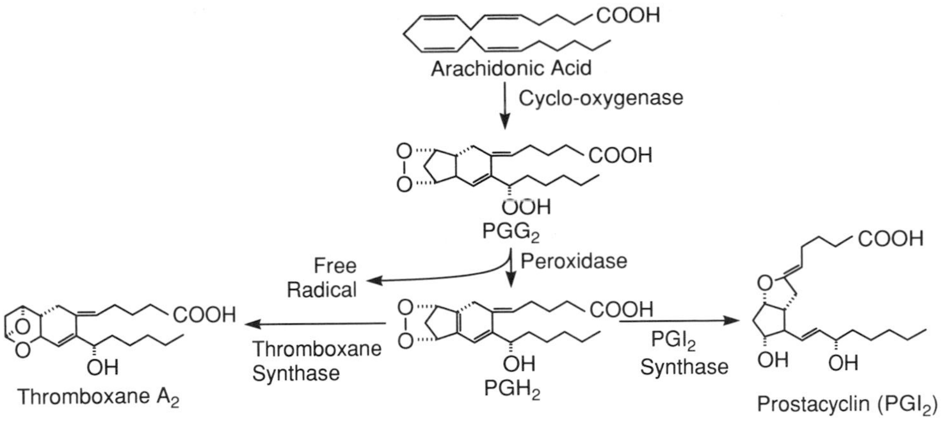

Figure 5.2 Metabolism of arachidonic acid: the site of action of aspirin.

to these observations, the elegant studies of Vane (1971) and Smith and Willis (1971), employing bioassay techniques, demonstrated that aspirin might influence a wide variety of biological processes, including platelet function, by inhibiting the metabolism of arachidonic acid by the cyclo-oxygenase component of the enzyme, prostaglandin (PG) G/H synthase (Fig. 5.2).

The mechanism of aspirin's interaction with the cyclo-oxygenase was first characterized at the biochemical level by van der Ouderaa *et al.* (1980) who demonstrated that aspirin acetylated the enzyme, leaving the hydroperoxidase component of the prostaglandin G/H synthase activity intact. Roth and Majerus and their colleagues (Roth and Majerus, 1975; Roth and Siok, 1978; Roth *et al.*, 1978) extended these observations, providing biochemical evidence that aspirin irreversibly acetylates Ser530 in platelet cyclo-oxygenase. It appears that a haeme-induced conformational change, correlated with the protection of the Arg253–Gly254 peptide bond from tryptic cleavage, facilitates the acetylation of the serine residue by aspirin (Chen and Marnett, 1989). Furthermore, as the platelet is anucleate and incapable of *de novo* protein synthesis, repeated exposure of platelets *in vitro* to submaximally effective concentrations of aspirin leads to cumulative inhibition of the enzyme (Fig. 5.3).

Classical non-steroidal anti-inflammatory drugs, such as indomethacin and ibuprofen (Ferreira and Vane, 1979) were shown to inhibit cyclo-oxygenase reversibly. Interestingly, the deacetylation product of aspirin, salicylate, was shown to compete with aspirin for the active site of cyclo-oxygenase *in vitro*; prior exposure to salicylate protected platelets from aspirin action *in vitro*. Although infusion experiments demonstrated that a similar effect was demonstrable *in vivo* in rats (Dejana *et al.*, 1981), it is thought unlikely that such an effect is relevant to the relative plasma concentrations of aspirin and salicylate attained after even chronic administration of high doses of aspirin in man.

Information on the site of action of aspirin in platelets has recently been extended to the molecular level. De Witt and Smith (1988) have cloned the ram seminal vesicle cyclo-oxygenase and expressed the enzyme in NIH 3T3 cells (DeWitt *et al.*, 1989). Interestingly, deletion of the target for aspirin action, Ser530, and its replacement with an Ala residue had no detectable effect on cyclo-oxygenase activity. Whereas the mutant was still inhibited by flurbiprofen, aspirin was inactive. It was concluded from these observations that the Ser residue was adjacent to, rather than within, the active site and that the action of aspirin derived from steric hindrance of substrate access to the active site by the bulky aspirin moiety (DeWitt *et al.*, 1990). Genomic cloning revealed only a single copy of the cyclo-oxygenase gene in the sheep, but biochemical studies by Raz *et al.* (1989) and molecular studies by Bailey and Verma (1990) in human lung suggest the possibility of isozymes. The pharmacological studies in support of this hypothesis have been

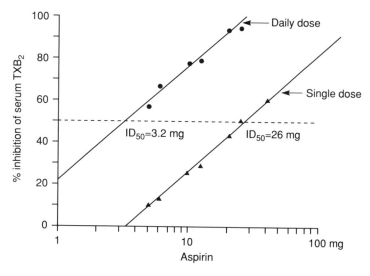

Figure 5.3 Dose dependence of the inhibition of platelet TXB_2 production by aspirin. Serum TXB_2 was measured before and after single (▲) or daily (●) dosing with aspirin in four healthy subjects. Individual data are expressed as percentage inhibition, with each subject serving as his or her own control. Daily dosing values represent measurements obtained at steady-state inhibition ID_{50} = 50% inhibitory dose. (Reproduced with permission from Patrono *et al.* (1985))

similarly conflicting. Thus, differences in the sensitivity of platelet and coronary vessel microsomal cyclo-oxygenase to aspirin have been reported (Burch et al., 1978) whereas others (Jaffe and Weksler, 1979) have failed to confirm these observations. We have recently employed the polymerase chain reaction to clone the cyclo-oxygenase from human platelets (Funk et al., 1991). This approach has been employed successfully to amplify the vestigial amounts of mRNA that remain in platelets (Newman et al., 1988). The platelet enzyme is the same gene product as that cloned from ram seminal vesicles (COX-1). A second gene (COX-2) has recently been cloned from chick fibroblasts. The message has been detected in a variety of tissues and initial studies with the expressed recombinant enzymes suggest that they may differ in their sensitivity to inhibition by aspirin and other NSAIDs (Xie et al., 1991). The other arachidonic acid metabolizing enzyme in platelets, the 12-lipoxygenase, also appears to differ from that in other human tissues. Thus, the human platelet enzyme is only 70% homologous with that in porcine leucocytes (Funk et al., 1990; Yoshimoto et al., 1990). Although human leucocytes do not possess 12-lipoxygenase activity, the porcine leucocyte enzyme is immunologically identical to that in human tracheal cells and brain and distinct from that in platelets.

5.5 ASPIRIN AND THROMBOXANE A_2

The biochemical product of the cyclo-oxygenation of arachidonic acid was characterized by Hamberg and Samuelsson (Hamberg and Samuelsson, 1974; Hamberg et al., 1974, 1975). PGH_2 aggregates platelets and constricts smooth muscle. It is further metabolized by thromboxane synthase to form thromboxane $(TX)A_2$ which has similar biological properties. The conventional interpretation of existing data has been that both PGH_2 and TXA_2 act at a shared receptor on platelets although there is some disagreement as to whether they have a similar affinity for this binding site or that TXA_2 is the more potent (Bhagwat et al., 1985; Mayeux et al., 1988). Recently, we have discriminated two functionally distinct binding sites for PG endoperoxide analogues on human platelets (Takahara et al., 1990) with the antagonist ligand GR 32191 (Lumley et al., 1989). It is unclear whether these sites represent two distinct receptor sites or varied degrees of post-translational modification of a single site. It is possible that they differ in their respective affinities for PG endoperoxides and TXA_2, a proposition which was originally formulated on the basis of pharmacological experiments (Carmo et al., 1985). Pharmacological and biochemical characterization of receptors in vascular smooth muscle suggest that they are likely to represent subtypes distinct from those observed in platelets (Mais *et al.*, 1985; Hanasaki *et al.*, 1988).

Platelet aggregation by endoperoxide analogues, such as U46619 (Wilson and Jones, 1985), results from activation of a phospholipase C linked to the receptor site irreversibly bound by GR32191 (Takahara *et al.*, 1990) via an uncharacterized, pertussis toxin insensitive, G protein (Brass *et al.*, 1987). Liberation of diacylglycerol is accompanied by activation of protein kinase C and influx of calcium from extracellular stores. Although the bulk of the analogue-evoked rise in calcium is derived from intracellular stores, liberation of calcium in this way is via activation of the site bound reversibly by GR 32191 and results in platelet shape change (Takahara *et al.*, 1990). Recently Dorn (1989) has reached similar conclusions, discriminating receptor-induced shape change from aggregation with the agonist ligand I-BOP.

The metabolism of TXA_2 is well understood. Following its rapid hydrolysis to the biologically inactive TXB_2 at physiological pH, TXA_2 is metabolized by two major pathways involving beta oxidation and dehydrogenation at the hemiacetal at C-11 (Roberts *et al.*, 1981). The predominant urinary metabolites of these pathways, 2,3-dinor-TXB_2 and 11-dehydro-TXB_2 are used as non-invasive indices of TX biosynthesis (Catella and FitzGerald, 1987). Despite concerns that the metabolism of TXA_2 might differ from that of TXB_2 (Granström *et al.*, 1982), recent experiments in non-human primates indicate that the major urinary products formed from both eicosanoids are identical (Patrignani *et al.*, 1989).

The concentration of TXB_2 in serum has been utilized as a convenient marker of the capacity of platelets to form TXA_2. Patrignani *et al.* (1982) demonstrated that repeated administration of submaximally effective doses of aspirin caused cumulative inhibition of serum TXB_2 formation *ex vivo*. A second feature of the irreversible inhibition of the platelet enzyme by aspirin is that, once inhibited, recovery occurs as a function of platelet turnover time. Thus, following complete inhibition of both serum TXB_2 (Patrignani *et al.*, 1982) and excretion of TX metabolites (Catella and FitzGerald, 1987) by aspirin, recovery of these indices takes 10–14 days. The effects of aspirin on TX synthesis appear similar irrespective of sex (Patrignani *et al.*, 1982; FitzGerald *et al.*, 1983), age (Reilly and FitzGerald, 1986) or the presence of atherosclerotic disease (Knapp *et al.*, 1988).

The relationship between inhibition of the capacity of platelets to form TXA_2 and TXA_2-dependent platelet function is non-linear. Thus, it appears that capacity must be inhibited by 95% or more before function is markedly inhibited (Reilly and FitzGerald, 1987; Lands *et al.*, 1985). It also appears that the rate of aspirin administration, as well

90

as dose, may influence the efficiency of inhibition of cyclo-oxygenase. Thus, using submaximally effective doses of aspirin, the degree of inhibition was greater if the same dose was infused over time rather than administered as a bolus (Pedersen *et al.*, 1985). This property may provide an advantage when selecting the lowest dose sufficient to inhibit the platelet enzyme acutely, a theoretically desirable objective in a patient presenting with an acute ischaemic syndrome.

5.6 EFFECTS OF ASPIRIN ON OTHER PROSTAGLANDINS

A second situation where rate as well as dose of aspirin administration has pharmacodynamic relevance is in its 'biochemical selectivity'; that is, the design of a form of aspirin which blocks the biosynthesis of TXA_2, but not other prostaglandins. Specifically, concern has related to prostacyclin (PGI_2), the predominant product of the cyclo-oxygenase reaction in macrovascular endothelial cells. PGI_2 inhibits platelet function and relaxes vascular smooth muscle (Moncada and Vane, 1978). Originally, it was believed that PGI_2 circulated in sufficient quantities to function as a vasodilator, platelet inhibitory hormone. It is now recognized that this is not so; the quantities of this eicosanoid which circulate fall considerably below the threshold for demonstrable effects on either blood pressure or platelet function (FitzGerald *et al.*, 1979, 1981). However, the arguments for the biological importance of PGI_2 extend beyond the teleological. PGI_2 is formed in biologically active concentrations at the site of vascular injury in man (Nowak and FitzGerald, 1989). Many of the stimuli to PGI_2 production by endothelial cells *in vitro* are platelet products or are themselves procoagulant. Consistent with this eicosanoid serving a local homeostatic role *in vivo*, PGI_2 biosynthesis is increased in syndromes of platelet activation in man (FitzGerald *et al.*, 1984, 1986; Reilly *et al.*, 1986). Finally, there is evidence from animal models that pharmacological augmentation of PGI_2 formation may serve an antithrombotic role *in vivo*. Thus, thromboxane synthase inhibitors, which increase PGI_2 formation at the site of vascular injury in man (Nowak and FitzGerald, 1989) are only modestly effective in preventing circumflex coronary artery thrombosis induced by vascular injury in the dog, as, indeed, are thromboxane receptor antagonists. However, the effects of these compounds are synergistic when combined together. Thus, the antagonists block the effects of the endoperoxides which accumulate during thromboxane synthase inhibition, permitting expression of the efficacy of the latter drugs. That this is dependent on prostaglandins, such as PGI_2, is indicated by the abolition of this synergism by preadministration of aspirin (Fitzgerald *et al.*, 1988a). Similar results were obtained by measuring the bleeding time in humans following acute administration of thromboxane synthase inhibitors and receptor antagonists alone and in combination with each other (Gresele *et al.*, 1987).

Given these observations, it seemed intuitively desirable to minimize the inhibition of PGI_2 which would occur coincident with that of TXA_2 by varying the dose and/or rate of administration of aspirin. Experiments *in vitro* suggested that this might be a simple matter. Recovery of thrombin-stimulated PGI_2 formation by bovine endothelial cells occurred within hours of exposure to aspirin in concentrations sufficient to inhibit completely endothelial cyclo-oxygenase (Jaffe and Weksler, 1979). However, subsequent experiments *in vitro* suggested that there might be components of the recovery with a slower turnover time (Pash and Bailey, 1988) and excretion of the major prostacyclin metabolite was depressed over 3 days after an 8 week course of ascending doses of aspirin by volunteers (FitzGerald *et al.*, 1983). As referred to above, some pharmacological studies had suggested that the endothelial enzyme might be less susceptible than that in the platelet to inhibition by aspirin, thus it was hypothesized that lower doses of aspirin might spare PGI_2 formation. However, measurements of urinary metabolite excretion in volunteers given ascending doses of aspirin suggested that any such dose-related selectivity was relative, not absolute (FitzGerald *et al.*, 1983) and even doses of aspirin less than 100 mg administered acutely prior to coronary artery bypass grafting were shown to reduce significantly the capacity of human coronary vessels to form PGI_2 (Weksler *et al.*, 1985). Finally, chronic administration of aspirin 20 mg twice per day (Ciabattoni *et al.*, 1987) and of aspirin 325 mg on alternate days (Clarke *et al.*, 1991) led to a progressive reduction in PGI_2 metabolite excretion. Although bradykinin-evoked PGI_2 formation *in vivo* recovers rapidly after a single high (650 mg) dose of aspirin (Heavey *et al.*, 1985; Barrow *et al.*, 1986), the possibility of cumulative inhibition of this index of stimulated production has not been addressed.

An alternative approach to sparing PGI_2 formation is to take advantage of the kinetics of aspirin, as described above. Conventionally formulated low doses of aspirin exhibit distinct components of action on platelets in the presystemic and systemic circulations (Pedersen and FitzGerald, 1984). Formulation of aspirin in a controlled release tablet formulation which releases it at a rate which facilitates hepatic extraction, markedly reduces the systemic bioavailability of the drug (FitzGerald *et al.*, 1991). Despite this, inhibition of platelet TXA_2 production is maximal, as is achieved with higher doses formulated conventionally. A modest depression of basal PGI_2 formation is observed on chronic administration of this preparation (Clarke *et al.*, 1991), probably accounted for by the effects of aspirin on the presystemic vasculature (Cerletti *et al.*, 1986). However, the increase in PGI_2 formation evoked in volunteers by systemic infusion of bradykinin is not suppressed by the controlled release preparation, in contrast to the same dose of aspirin, conventionally formulated (Clarke *et al.*, 1991). This preparation of aspirin is likely to provide a useful tool with which to explore the functional significance of sparing the capacity to synthesize prostaglandins by the systemic vasculature.

5.7 CLINICAL EFFECTS OF ASPIRIN IN CARDIOVASCULAR DISEASE

The observation that aspirin inhibited platelet function prompted retrospective reviews of the incidence of thrombotic events in patients who had been taking aspirin for other reasons, mostly for the treatment of arthritic disease. The most celebrated of these case control analyses was performed by the Boston Collaborative Drug Surveillance Group (1974) and suggested that the prevalence of non-fatal myocardial infarction was lower in those patients taking aspirin. This prompted the initiation of multiple prospective studies designed to explore the efficacy of aspirin in the secondary prevention of myocardial infarction. The results were disappointing. Although several of the studies suggested a trend in favour of aspirin, this did not attain statistical significance. Enthusiasm for research into the cardiovascular therapeutics of aspirin waned. This perception was changed by a landmark study by Lewis *et al.* (1983) performed in patients with unstable angina. Angiographic (DeWood *et al.*, 1980), angioscopic (Sherman *et al.*, 1986) and biochemical (Fitzgerald *et al.*, 1986) studies indicate that the ischaemic events in patients with this syndrome are directly precipitated by platelet-dependent vascular occlusion. This perception has been confirmed by the performance of elegant post-mortem studies of individuals who had suffered this prodrome to sudden death (Falk, 1985; Davies and Thomas, 1984). Besides focussing their interest on a population much more likely to be susceptible to intervention with aspirin than survivors of a myocardial infarction, Lewis *et al.* accomplished initiation of therapy (aspirin/placebo) within 51 h of presentation in hospital. The previous studies had been initiated in some patients years after their index infarct (Reilly and FitzGerald, 1988). In this study, aspirin reduced the incidence of both myocardial infarction and death by about 50%. Similar effects were subsequently obtained in three other controlled trials of aspirin in unstable angina in doses ranging from 75 to 1300 mg day^{-1} (Cairns *et al.*, 1985; Theroux *et al.*, 1988; Wallentin, 1990). Thus, in accordance with the biochemical pharmacology of aspirin, the benefit remained evident as the dose was reduced.

Pharmacokinetics of aspirin and salicylates

In the light of these observations, it seemed possible that the populations studied post myocardial infarction might have been dilute with respect to a potential benefit from aspirin. If this were true, then the sample sizes would have been inadequate to detect an effect of a magnitude that one might reasonably expect. Consistent with this hypothesis, an overview of six such trials suggested that, while failing to demonstrate the benefit of the data when taken individually, the grouped data provided sufficient information to detect an average reduction in the incidence of a second myocardial infarction or death by about 20% (Antiplatelet Trialists Collaboration, 1988).

The appreciation of the importance of sample size in the design of clinical trials in cardiovascular disease owes much to Peto and Collins who continue to coordinate the data deriving from ongoing trials of aspirin. This point was amplified by the rapid performance of the ISIS-2 study which demonstrated that the effect of aspirin was additive to and of similar magnitude to that of streptokinase in reducing cardiac mortality in patients presenting acutely with myocardial infarction (ISIS-2 Collaborative Group, 1988). Biochemical studies had demonstrated that coronary thrombolysis with streptokinase is accompanied by a marked increase in thromboxane biosynthesis (Fitzgerald et al., 1988b), a phenomenon which is also observed in patients treated with tissue plasminogen activator (rt-PA; Kerins et al., 1989). Experiments with rt-PA in a canine model of occlusion–reperfusion have demonstrated the functional importance of thromboxane synthesis, platelet activation and thrombin formation in the re-occlusion which complicates this process (Gold et al., 1986; Golino et al., 1988; Fitzgerald et al., 1989; Fitzgerald and FitzGerald, 1989).

The impact of aspirin is best summarized by the overview of the Antiplatelet Trialists' Collaboration of 1990 (to be published) of the 189 controlled secondary prevention studies of antiplatelet drugs in cardiovascular disease. These studies involved almost 10 000 events in more than 90 000 individuals. Compared with placebo, the incidence of the combined endpoint of myocardial infarction, stroke and vascular death was reduced by 25% on average in the actively treated group, a highly significant ($2p<0.000\,01$) effect. Although some other drugs were included in this analysis, the overwhelming bulk of the data were obtained on aspirin.

In addition to patients who have suffered a myocardial infarction or an episode of unstable angina, a transient ischaemic attack or stroke, this approach (Antiplatelet Trialists Collaboration, 1990) has established the efficacy of the drug in the prevention of deep venous thrombosis and pulmonary embolism in patients who have undergone surgery. Aspirin also prevents occlusion of coronary bypass grafts (Cheseboro et al., 1984; Goldman et al., 1988), periprocedural myocardial infarctions in patients undergoing angioplasty (but not late reocclusion; Schwartz et al., 1988) and stroke in patients with non-valvular atrial fibrillation (Stroke Prevention in Atrial Fibrillation Study Group Investigators, 1990). Small studies have demonstrated its ability to prevent haemodialysis shunt occlusion. The most recent overview (Antiplatelet Trialists Collaboration, 1990) has clarified two controversial issues which have pertained to the use of aspirin in the secondary prevention of cardiovascular disease. First, in patients with transient ischaemic attacks, the small increase in absolute risk of haemorrhagic stroke in patients treated with aspirin is overwhelmed by the larger reduction in the risk of thrombotic stroke. Second, in accordance with biochemical and pharmacological studies of aspirin action, sufficient information has been accumulated to permit confirmation of the efficacy of aspirin in certain subgroups. Its effectiveness in reducing the incidence of myocardial infarction, stroke and vascular death does not appear to vary as a function of age, sex or the presence or absence of diabetes or hypertension.

The utility of aspirin in the primary prevention of cardiovascular disease remains unproven (Kerins and FitzGerald, 1992). Although there was a significant reduction in the incidence of myocardial infarction in a large controlled study of US male physicians, the relationship between benefit and risk is unclear (Steering Committee of the Physicians Health Study Research Group, 1989). There was a non-significant tendency towards an increase in stroke in the aspirin-treated group and total mortality did not differ between the groups. Furthermore, the magnitude of the beneficial impact on myocardial infarction may have been exaggerated by the premature cessation of the trial. A further concern has been the degree to which the cardiovascular study population was representative of the population at large. The death rate in the control group was only 15% of that expected in a general population of males in that age group. This has been attributed to an unusual degree of cardiovascular risk modification; smoking was roughly a third of that expected, regular aerobic exercise more common. Finally, the participants were screened for the development of aspirin-related side effects prior to entry into the study (Patrono and FitzGerald, 1989). An unblinded, smaller study of British physicians failed to detect a beneficial effect of aspirin on the incidence of myocardial infarction (Peto et al., 1988). While the case for aspirin in this setting remains unproven, the results of the US Physicians' study certainly provide the basis for pursuing the potential for this type of intervention in the primary prevention of cardiovascular disease in controlled trials in more representative populations.

95

Another potential indication for the use of aspirin is in the prevention or amelioration of pregnancy-induced hypertension. Thromboxane biosynthesis is increased in normal pregnancy and the increment mainly derives from platelets (Fitzgerald *et al.*, 1987). In patients with moderately severe pregnancy induced hypertension, there is a further increase in thromboxane formation which correlates with independent indices of the severity of the condition (Fitzgerald *et al.*, 1990). This may contribute to the reduction in placental blood flow which is the hallmark of the disease. Thromboxane A_2 reduces placental blood flow in a receptor-dependent manner in the human placental cotyledon, where it is a more potent and efficacious vasoconstrictor than angiotensin II (Fitzgerald and FitzGerald, 1990). Platelet activation may occur in the placental bed secondary to vascular damage, perhaps of immunological origin. In any event, there have been a series of small studies which suggest the potential benefit – both foetal and maternal – of administering aspirin to women at demographic risk of developing the disease (Beaufils *et al.*, 1985; Wallenburg *et al.*, 1986; Benigni *et al.*, 1989; Schiff *et al.*, 1989). These have prompted the initiation of three large scale multicentre trials to address this issue. Although the existing studies are much too small to assess the risk to the foetus, there has been one disturbing observation. In a study where the women were given aspirin 60 mg day^{-1}, TXA_2 formation by foetal platelets was inhibited by roughly 60% (Benigni *et al.*, 1989). In this regard, a preparation of aspirin such as that described above, in which maternal platelets were inhibited but systemic bioavailability was minimized might have particular utility.

The development of biochemical indices of thromboxane biosynthesis has facilitated the identification of novel potential clinical indications for aspirin, amongst them the vasospasm which complicates subarachnoid haemorrhage, progressive renal disease and drug induced nephrotoxicity. Given this progress, it is perhaps worth remembering that aspirin inhibits just one pathway of platelet activation and that one in a less than theoretically optimal manner. Perhaps its effect is sufficient to be detected by so crude an instrument as a clinical trial because of the role TXA_2 plays as an amplifying signal for other platelet agonists (Murray and FitzGerald, 1989). The success of aspirin in clinical trials which confirmed the promise defined by basic studies of its pharmacology should encourage, rather than deter, comparative evaluation of the safety and efficacy of theoretically more effective interventions. There is no reason to expect that a reduction in cardiovascular events by a fifth to a quarter cannot be improved upon. In an era when the rapid performance of clinical trials of requisite size has become demonstrably feasible at reasonable cost, it would be unfortunate if pharmaceutical companies did not rise to the 'aspirin challenge'.

5.8 CONCLUSION

It is almost 100 years since the therapeutic possibilities of aspirin were first appreciated. Its effects on platelets were first described 30 years ago. Since that time, our understanding of its mechanism of action has been extended to the molecular level and its utility in the treatment of cardiovascular disease clearly established. As epidemiological studies continue to confirm the experimental concepts of aspirin action, this inexpensive drug is likely to be used ever more widely, at doses which are more readily tolerated and perhaps, more effective, in the coming decade than in the last one.

REFERENCES

Aarons, L., Hopkins, K., Rowland, M. *et al.* (1989) Route of administration and sex differences in the pharmacokineticss of aspirin, administered as its lysinate salt. *Pharm. Res.*, **6**, 660–6.

Ali, B. and Kaur, S. (1983) Mammalian tissue acetylsalicylic acid esterase(s): Identification, distribution and discrimination from other esterases. *J. Pharmacol. Exp. Ther.*, **226**, 589–94.

Antiplatelet Trialists Collaboration (1988) Secondary prevention of vascular disease by prolonged antiplatelet treatment. *Br. Med. J.*, **296**, 320–31.

Bailey, J.M. and Verma M. (1990) Identification of a highly conserved 3'UTR in the translational regulated mRNA for prostaglandin synthase. *Prostaglandins*, **40**, 585–90.

Barrow, S.E., Dollery, C.T., Heavey, D.J. *et al.* (1986) Effect of vasoactive peptides on prostacyclin synthesis in man. *Brit. J. Pharmacol.*, **87**, 243–7.

Beaufils, M., Uzan, S., Donsimoni, R. and Colau, J.C. (1985) Prevention of pre-eclampsia by early antiplatelet therapy. *Lancet*, **i**, 840–2.

Benigni, A., Gregorini, G., Frusca, T. *et al.* (1989) Effect of low-dose aspirin on fetal and maternal generation of thromboxane by platelets in women at risk of pregnancy induced hypertension. *N. Engl. J. Med.* **321**, 357–62.

Bhagwat, S.S., Hamann, P.R., Still, W.E. *et al.* (1985) Synthesis and structure of the platelet aggregation factor thromboxane A_2. *Nature*, **315**, 511–13.

Bochner, F., Williams, D,B., Morris, P.M.A. *et al.* (1988) Pharmacokinetics of low dose oral modified release, soluble and intravenous aspirin in man, and effects on platelet function. *Eur. J. Clin. Pharmacol.*, **35**, 287–94.

Bogentoft, C., Carlsson, I., Ekenved, G. and Magnusson, A. (1978) Influence of food on the absorption of acetylsalicylic acid from enteric coated dosage forms. *Eur. J. Clin. Pharmacol.*, **14**, 351–5.

Borga, O., Odar-Lederlof, I., Ringberger, V-A. and Norlin, A. (1976) Protein binding of salicylate in uraemic and normal plasma. *Clin. Pharmacol. Ther.*, **20**, 464–75.

Pharmacokinetics of aspirin and salicylates

Born, G.V.R. (1962) Aggregation of blood platelets by adenosine diphosphate and its reversal. *Nature*, **194**, 927.

Boston Collaborative Drug Surveillance Group (1974) Regular aspirin intake and myocardial infarction. *Brit. Med. J.*, **1**, 440–3.

Brandon, R.A., Eadie, M.J. and Smith, M.T. (1985) A sensitive liquid chromatographic assay for plasma aspirin and salicylate concentrations after low doses of aspirin. *Ther. Drug Monit.*, **7**, 216–21.

Brass, L.F., Shaller, C.C. and Belmonte, E.J. (1987) Inositol 1, 4–5-triphosphate induced granule secretion in platelets. Evidence that the activation of phospholipase C mediated by platelet thromboxane receptors involves a guanine nucleotide binding protein–dependent mechanism distinct from that of thrombin. *J. Clin. Invest.*, **791**, 1269–75.

Burch, J.W., Stanford, N. and Majerus, P.W. (1978) Inhibition of platelet prostaglandin synthase by oral aspirin. *J. Clin. Invest.*, **61**, 314–19.

Cairns, J.A., Gent., M., Singer, J. *et al.* (1985) Aspirin, sulfinpyrazone, or both in unstable angina: results of a Canadian multicenter trial. *N. Engl. J. Med.*, **313**, 1369–75.

Caldwell, J., O'Gorman, J, and Smith, R.L. (1980) Inter-individual differences in the glycine conjugation of salicylic acid. *Brit. J. Clin. Pharmac.*, **9**, 114.

Carmo, L.G., Hatmi, M., Rotilio, D. and Vargaftig, B.B. (1985) Platelet desensitization induced by arachidonic acid is not due to cyclo-oxygenase inactivation and involves the endoperoxide receptor. *Brit. J. Pharmac.*, **85**, 849–59.

Catella, F. and FitzGerald, G.A. (1987) Paired analysis of urinary thromboxane B_2 metabolites in humans. *Throm. Res.*, **47**, 647–56.

Cerletti, C., Gambino, M.C., Garattini, S. and de Gaetano, G. (1986) Biochemical selectivity of oral versus intravenous aspirin in rats. Inhibition by oral aspirin of cyclooxygenase activity in platelets and presystemic but not systemic vessels. *J. Clin. Invest.*, **78**, 323–6.

Chen, Y-N. P. and Marnett, L.J. (1989) Heme prosthetic group required for acetylation of prostaglandin H synthase by aspirin. *FASEB J.*, **3**, 2294–7.

Chesebro, H.J., Fuster, V., Elveback, L.R. *et al.* (1984) Effect of dipyridamole and aspirin on late vein-graft patency after coronary bypass operations. *N. Engl. J. Med.*, **310**, 209–14.

Ciabattoni, G., Boss, A.H., Daffonchio, L. *et al.* (1987) Radioimmunoassay measurement of 2, 3-dinor metabolites of prostacyclin and thromboxane in human urine. *Adv. Prostaglandins Thromboxane Leukotrienes Res.*, **17**, 598–602.

Clarke, R.J., Mayo, G., Price, P. and FitzGerald, G.A. (1991) Suppression of thromboxane A_2 but not of systemic prostacyclin by controlled release aspirin. *N. Engl. J. Med.*, **325**, 1137–41.

Cossum, P.A., Roberts, M.S., Kilpatrick, D. and Yong, A.C. (1986) Extrahepatic metabolism and distribution of aspirin in vascular beds of sheep. *J. Pharm. Sci.*, **75**, 731–7.

Costello, P.B. and Green, F.A. (1983) Identification and partial purification of the major aspirin hydrolysing enzyme in human blood. *Arthrit. Rheumatol.*, **26**, 541–7.

Cuny, G., Royer, R.J. and Mur, J.M. (1979) Pharmacokinetics of salicylates in elderly. *Gerontol*, **25**, 49–55.

Davidson, C. and Smith, P.K. (1961) The binding of salicylic acid and related substances to purified proteins. *J. Pharmacol. Exp. Ther.*, **133**, 161–70.

Davies, M.J. and Thomas, A. (1984) Thrombosis and acute coronary artery lesions in sudden cardiac ischemic death. *N. Engl. J. Med.* **310**, 1137–40.

Day, R.O., Shen, D.D. and Azarnoff, D.L. (1983) Induction of salicyluric acid formation in rheumatoid arthritis patients treated with salicylates. *Clin. Pharmacokin.*, **8**, 263–71.

Dejana, E., Cerletti, C., De Castellarnau, C. *et al.* (1981) Salicylate–aspirin interaction in the rat. Evidence that salicylate accumulating during aspirin administration may protect vascular prostacyclin from aspirin–induced inhibition. *J. Clin. Invest.*, **68**, 1108–12.

DeWitt, D.L. and Smith, W.L. (1988) Primary structure of prostaglandin G/H synthase from sheep vesicular gland determined from the complementary DNA sequence. *Proc. Natl Acad. Sci. USA.*, **85**, 1412–16.

DeWitt, D.L., El-Harith, E.A. and Smith, W.L. (1989) Prostaglandin endoperoxide G/H synthase as a regulatory enzyme in prostaglandin biosynthesis. In *Platelets and Vascular Occlusion* (eds. C. Patrono and G.A. FitzGerald), Raven Press, New York, pp. 109–18.

DeWitt, D.L., El-Harith, E.A., Kraemer, S.A., *et al.* (1990) The aspirin and heme binding sites of *ovine* and *murine* prostaglandin endoperoxide synthases. *J. Biol. Chem.*, **265**, 5192–8.

DeWood, M.A., Spres, J. and Notske, R. (1980) Prevalence of total coronary occlusion during the early hours of transmural myocardial infarction. *N. Engl. J. Med.*, **303**, 897–902.

Dorn, G.W., II (1989) Distinct platelet thromboxane A_2/prostaglandin H_2 receptor subtypes. A radioligand binding study of human platelets. *J. Clin. Invest.*, **84**, 1883–91.

Dotevall, G. and Ekenved, G. (1976) The absorption of aspirin from the stomach in relation to intragastric pH. *Scand. J. Gastroent.*, **11**, 801–5.

Dromgoole, S.H. and Furst, D.E. (1986) Salicylates. In *Applied Pharmacokinetics*, 2nd edn, (eds. W.E. Evans, J.J. Schentag and W.E. Jusko), Applied Therapeutics, Inc, Vancouver, pp. 944–77.

Ekstrand, R., Alvan, G. and Borga, O. (1979) Concentration dependent plasma protein binding of salicylate in arthritis patients. *Clin. Pharmacokin.*, **4**, 137–43.

Falk, E. (1985) Unstable angina with fatal outcome: dynamic coronary thrombosis leading to infarction and/or sudden death. *Circulation*, **71**, 699–708.

Ferreira, S.H. and Vane, J.R. (1979) Mode of action of anti-inflammatory agents which are prostaglandin synthetase inhibitors. In *Antiinflammatory Drugs* (eds J.R. Vane and S.H. Ferreira) Springer-Verlag, Berlin, pp. 348–98.

Findlay, J.W., DeAngelis, R.W., Kearney, M.F. *et al.* (1981) Analgesic drugs in breast milk and plasma. *Clin. Pharmacol. Ther.*, **29**, 625–33.

Fitzgerald, D.J. and FitzGerald, G.A. (1989) The role of thrombin and thromboxane A_2 in vascular reocclusion following coronary thrombolysis with tissue type plasminogen activator. *Proc. Natl Acad. Sci. USA*, **86**, 7585–9.

Fitzgerald, D.J. and FitzGerald, G.A. (1990) Eicosanoids in pregnancy-induced hypertension. In *Hypertension: Pathophysiology, Diagnosis and Management* (eds J. Laragh and B.M. Brenner), Raven Press, New York, pp. 1789–808.

Fitzgerald, D.J., Catella, F. and FitzGerald, G.A. (1986). Platelet activation in unstable coronary disease. *N. Engl. J. Med.*, **315**, 983–9.

Fitzgerald, D.J., Mayo, G., Catella, F. *et al.* (1987) Increased thromboxane biosynthesis in pregnancy derives largely from platelets. *Am. J. Obstet. Gynecol.*, **157**, 325–30.

Fitzgerald, D.J., Fragetta, J. and FitzGerald, G.A. (1988a) Prostaglandin endoperoxides modulate the response to thromboxane synthase inhibition during coronary thrombosis. *J. Clin. Invest.*, **82**, 1708–13.

Fitzgerald, D.J., Catella, F., Roy, L. and FitzGerald, G.A. (1988b) Marked platelet activation *in vivo* after intravenous streptokinase in patients with acute myocardial infarction. *Circulation*, **77**, 142–50.

Fitzgerald, D.J., Wright, F. and FitzGerald, G.A. (1989) Increased thromboxane biosynthesis during coronary thrombolysis: Evidence that platelet activation and thromboxane A_2 modulate the response to tissue-type plasminogen activator *in vivo*. *Circ. Res.*, **65**, 83–94.

Fitzgerald, D.J., Rocki, W., Murray, R. *et al.* (1990) Thromboxane A_2 synthesis in pregnancy induced hypertension. *Lancet*, **335**, 751–4.

FitzGerald, G.A. and Sherry, S. (1982) The pharmacology and pharmacokinetics of platelet-active drugs under clinical investigation. *Adv. Prostag. Thrombox. Leuk. Res.*, **10**, 107–72.

FitzGerald, G.A., Friedman, L.A., Miyamori, I. *et al.* (1979) A double blind placebo controlled evaluation of prostacyclin in man. *Life Sci.*, **25**, 665–72.

FitzGerald, G.A., Brash, A.R., Falardeau, P. and Oates, J.A. (1981) Estimated rate of prostacyclin secretion into the circulation of normal man. *J. Clin. Invest.*, **68**, 1272–5.

FitzGerald, G.A., Oates, J.A., Hawiger, J. *et al.* (1983) Endogenous synthesis of prostacyclin and thromboxane and platelet function during chronic aspirin administration in man. *J. Clin. Invest.*, **71**, 676–88.

FitzGerald, G.A., Smith, B., Pedersen, A.K. and Brash, A.R. (1984) Increased prostacyclin biosynthesis in patients with severe atherosclerosis and platelet activation. *N. Engl. J. Med.*, **310**, 1065–8.

FitzGerald, G.A., Lupinetti, M., Charman, S.A. and Charman, W.N. (1991). Presystemic acetylation of platelets by aspirin: Reduction in the rate of drug delivery to improve biochemical selectivity for thromboxane A_2. *J. Pharmacol. Exp. Ther.*, **259**, 1043–9.

Funk, C.D., Furci, L. and FitzGerald, G.A. (1991) Polymerase chain reaction cloning and expression of eicosanoid metabolizing enzymes from blood cells. In, *Adv. Prostaglandin, Thromboxane Leukotriene Res.*, **21A**, 33–6.

Funk, C., Furci, L. and FitzGerald, G.A. (1990b), Molecular cloning, primary structure and expression of the human platelet/erythroleukemia cell 12-lipoxygenase. *Proc. Natl Acad. Sci. USA*, **87**, 5638–42.

Furst, D.E., Gupta, N. and Paulus, H.E. (1977) Salicylate metabolism in twins; Evidence suggesting a genetic influence and induction of salicylurate formation. *J. Clin. Invest.*, **60**, 32–42.

Garrettson, L.K., Procknal. J.A. and Levy, G. (1975) Fetal acquisition and neonatal elimination of a large amount of salicylate. *Clin. Pharmacol. Ther.*, **17**, 98–103.

Gold, H.K., Leinbach, R.C., Garabedian, H.D. *et al.* (1986). Acute coronary reocclusion after thrombolysis with recombinant human tissue-type plasminogen activator: prevention by a maintenance infusion. *Circulation*, **73**, 347–52.

Goldman, S., Copeland, J., Moritz, T. *et al.* (1988) Improvement in early saphenous vein graft patency after coronary artery bypass surgery with antiplatelet therapy: results of a Veterans Administration Cooperative study. *Circulation*, **77**, 1324–32.

Golino, P., Ashton, J.H., Glas-Greenwalt, P. *et al.* (1988) Mediation of reocclusion by thromboxane A_2 and scrotonin after thrombolysis with tissue-type plasminogen activator in a canine preparation of coronary thrombosis. *Circulation*, **77**, 678–84.

Graham, G.G. and Rowland, M. (1972) Application of salivary salicylate data to biopharmaceutical studies of salicylates. *J. Pharm. Sci.*, **61**, 1219–22.

Granström, E., Diczfalusy, U., Hamberg, M. *et al.* (1982) Thromboxane A_2: Biosynthesis and effects on platelets. In *Prostaglandins and the Cardiovascular System, Vol. 10* (ed. J.A. Oates), Raven Press, New York, pp. 15–58.

Gresele, P., Arnout, J., Deckmyn, H. *et al.*. (1987) Role of proaggregatory and antiaggregatory prostaglandins in hemostasis. Studies with combined thromboxane synthase inhibition and thromboxane receptor antagonism. *J. Clin. Invest.*, **80**, 1435–45.

Hamberg, M. and Samuelsson, B. (1974) Prostaglandin endoperoxides – novel transformations of arachidonic acid in human platelets. *Proc. Natl Acad. Sci. USA*, **71**, 3400–4.

Hamberg, M., Svensson, J., Wakabayski, T. and Samuelsson, B. (1974) Isolation and structure of two prostaglandin endoperoxides that cause platelet aggregation. *Proc. Natl, Acad. Sci. USA*, **71**, 345–9.

Hamberg, M., Svensson, J. and Samuelsson, B. (1975); Thromboxanes: a new group of biologically active compounds derived from prostaglandin endoperoxides. *Proc. Natl Acad. Sci. USA*, **72**, 2994–8.

Hanasaki, K., Nakano, K., Kasai, H. *et al.* (1988) Identification of thromboxane A_2 receptors in cultured vascular endothelial cells of rat aorta. *Biochem. Biophys. Res. Comm.*, **151**, 1352–7.

Harris, P.A. and Riegelman, S. (1969) Influence of the route of administration on the area under the plasma concentration–time curve. *J. Pharm. Sci.*, **58**, 71–5.

Heavey, D.J., Barrow, S.E., Hickling, N.E. and Ritter, J.M. (1985) Aspirin causes short-lived inhibition of bradykinin-stimulated prostacyclin production in man. *Nature*, **318**, 186–8.

Higgs, G.A., Salmon, J.A., Henderson, B. and Vane, J.R. (1987) Pharmacokinetics of aspirin and salicylate in relation to inhibition of arachidonate cyclooxygenase and antiinflammatory activity. *Proc. Natl Acad. Sci. USA*, **84**, 1417 20.

Ho, P.C., Triggs, E.J., Bourne, D.W.A. and Heazlewood, N.J. (1985) The effect of age and sex on the disposition of acetylsalicylic acid and its metabolites. *Brit. J. Clin. Pharmac.*, **19**, 675–84.

ISIS-2 (Second International Study Group of Infarct Survival) Collaborative Group. (1988) Randomised trial of intravenous streptokinase, oral aspirin, both, or neither, among 17,187 cases of suspected acute myocardial infarction: ISIS-2. *Lancet*, **ii**, 349–60.

Jaffee, E.A. and Weksler, B.B. (1979) Recovery of endothelial cell prostacyclin production after inhibition by low doses of aspirin. *J. Clin. Invest.* **63**, 532–5.

Kerins, D.M. and FitzGerald, G.A. (1992) Arachidonic acid metabolism, platelets and thromboembolic disease. In *Handbook of Experimental Pharmacology, Vol. 101, Biochemical Pharmacology of Blood and Blood-Forming Organs* (ed. J.W. Fisher), Springer-Verlag, New York (in press).

Kerins, D.M., Roy, L., FitzGerald, G.A. and Fitzgerald, D.J. (1989) Platelet activation and thromboxane formation during coronary thrombolysis with tissue-type plasminogen activator. *Circulation*, **80**, 1718–25.

Knapp, H.R., Healy, C., Lawson, J. and FitzGerald, G.A. (1988) Effects of low-dose aspirin on endogenous eicosanoid formation in normal and atherosclerotic men. *Throm. Res.*, **50**, 377–86.

Koch, P.A., Schuitz, C.A., Wills, R.J. *et al.* (1978) Influence of food and fluid ingestion on aspirin bioavailability. *J. Pharm. Sci.*, **67**, 1533–5.

Lands, W.E.M., Culp, B.R., Hirai, A. and Gorman, R. (1985). Relationship of thromboxane generation to the aggregation of platelets from humans: effects of eicosapentaenoic acid. *Prostaglandins*, **30**, 819–25.

Leonards, J.R. and Levy, G. (1965) Absorption and metabolism of aspirin administered in enteric coated tablets. *J. Am. Med. Assoc.*, **193**, 93–8.

Levy, G. (1979) Pharmacokinetics of salicylate in man. *Drug Met. Rev.*, **9**, 3–19.

Levy, G. (1980) Clinical pharmacokinetics of salicylates: A re-assessment. *Brit. J. Clin. Pharmac.*, **10**, 2855–905.

Levy, G. and Angelino, N.J. (1968) Hydrolysis of aspirin by rat small intestine. *J. Pharm. Sci.*, **57**, 1449–50.

Levy, G. and Leonards, J.R. (1971) Urine pH and salicylate therapy. *J. Am. Med. Assoc.*, **217**, 81.

Levy, G. and Tsuchiya, T. (1972) Salicylate accumulation kinetics in man. *N. Engl. J. Med.*, **287**, 430–2.

Levy, G., Angelino, N.J. and Matsuzawa, T. (1967) Effect of certain nonsteroidal antirheumatic drugs on active amino acid transport across the small intestine. *J. Pharm. Sci.*, **56**, 681–3.

Levy, G., Tsuchiya, T. and Amsel, L.P. (1972) Limited capacity for salicyl phenolic glucuronide formation and its effects on the kinetics of salicylate in man. *Clin. Pharmacol. Ther.*, **13**, 258–68.

Levy, G., Procknal, J.A. and Garrettson, L.K. (1975) Distribution of salicylate between neonatal and maternal serum at diffusion equilibrium. *Clin. Pharmacol. Ther.*, **18**, 210–14.

Levy, G., Procknal, J.A., Olufs, J.A. and Pachman, L.M. (1980) Relationship between saliva salicylate concentration and free or total salicylate concentration in serum of children with juvenile rheumatoid arthritis. *Clin. Pharmacol. Ther.*, **27**, 619–27.

Lewis, H.D., Davis, J.W., Archibald, D.G. *et al.* (1983) Protective effects of aspirin against acute myocardial infarction and death in men with unstable angina, *N. Engl J. Med.*, **309**, 396–403.

Lui, C.Y., Oberle, A., Fleisher, D. and Amidon, G.L. (1986) Application of a radiotelemetric system to evaluate the performance of enteric coated and plain aspirin tablets. *J. Pharm. Sci.*, **75**, 469–74.

Lumley, P., White, B.P. and Humphrey, P.P.A. (1989) GR32191, a highly potent and specific thromboxane A_2 receptor blocking drug on platelets and vascular and airways smooth muscle *in vitro*. *Brit. J. Pharmacol.*, **97**, 783–94.

Mais, D.E., Saussy, D.L., Jr, Chaikhouni, A. *et al.* (1985) Pharmacologic characterization of human and canine thromboxane A₂/prostaglandin H₂ receptors in platelets and blood vessels: Evidence for different receptors. *J. Pharm. Exp. Ther.*, **233**, 418–24.

Matthew, H., Mackintosh, T.F., Tompsett, S.L. and Cameron, J.C. (1966). Gastric aspiration and lavage in acute poisoning. *Brit. Med. J.*, **1**, 1333–7.

Mayeux, P.R., Morton, H.E., Gillard, J. *et al.* (1988) The affinities of prosta-glandin H₂ and thromboxane A₂ for their receptor are similar in washed human platelets. *Biochem. Biophys. Res. Comm.*, **157**, 733–9.

Melander, A., Danielson, K., Scherstein, B. and Wahlin, E. (1977) Enhance-ment of the bioavailability of propranolol and metoprolol by food. *Clin. Pharmacol. Ther.*, **22**, 108–12.

Melander, A. and McLean, A. (1983) Influence of food intake on presystemic clearance of drugs. *Clin. Pharmacokin.*, **8**, 286–96.

Miaskiewicz, S.L., Shively, C.A. and Vesell, E.S. (1982) Sex differences in absorption kinetics of sodium salicylate. *Clin. Pharmacol. Ther.*, **31**, 30–7.

Mojaverian, P., Rocci, M.L., Conner, D.P. *et al.* (1987). Effect of food on the absorption of enteric-coated aspirin; Correlation with gastric residence time. *Clin. Pharmacol. Ther.*, **41**, 11–17.

Moncada, S. and Vane, J.R. (1978) Unstable metabolites of arachidonic acid and their role in haemostasis and thrombosis. *Br. Med. Bull.*, **34**, 129–35.

Montgomery, P.R. and Sitar, D.S. (1981) Increased serum salicylate metabolites with age in patients receiving chronic aspirin therapy. *Gerontol.*, **27**, 329–33.

Montgomery, P.R., Berger, L.G., Mitenko, P.A. and Sitar, D.S. (1986) Salicylate metabolism: Effects of age and sex in adults. *Clin. Pharmacol. Ther.*, **39**, 571–6.

Murray, R. and FitzGerald, G.A. (1989) Regulation of thromboxane receptor activation in human platelets. *Proc. Natl Acad. Sci. USA*, **86**, 124–8.

Needs, C.J. and Brooks, P.M. (1985) Clinical pharmacokinetics of the salicylates. *Clin. Pharmacokin.*, **10**, 164–77.

Netter, P., Faure, G., Regent, M.C. *et al.* (1985) Salicylate kinetics in old age. *Clin. Pharmacol. Ther.*, **38**, 6–11.

Newman, P.J., Gorski, J., White, G.C. *et al.* (1988) Enzymatic amplification of platelet-specific messenger RNA using the polymerase chain reaction. *J. Clin. Invest.*, **82**, 739–43.

Nowak, J. and FitzGerald, G.A. (1989) Redirection of prostaglandin endo-peroxide metabolism at the platelet–vascular interface in man. *J. Clin. Invest.*, **83**, 380–5.

O'Brien, J.R. (1968) Effects of salicylates on human platelets. *Lancet*, **i**, 779.

Ouderra van der, F.J., van der Buytenhek, M., Nugteren, D.H. and Van Dorp, D.A. (1980) Acetylation of prostaglandin endoperoxide synthetase with acetylsalicylic acid. *Eur. J. Biochem.*, **109**, 1–8.

Pash, J.M. and Bailey, J.M. (1988). Inhibition by corticosteroids of epidermal growth factor-induced recovery of cyclooxygenase after aspirin inactiva-tion. *FASEB J.* **2**, 2613–18.

Patrignani, P., Filabozzi, C. and Patrono, C. (1982) Selective cumulative inhibition of platelet thromboxane production by low-dose aspirin in healthy subjects. *J. Clin. Invest.*, **69**, 1366–72.

Patrignani, P., Morton, H., Cirino, M. *et al.* (1989). Fractional conversion of thromboxane A_2 and B_2 to urinary 2,3–dinor-thromboxane B_2 and 11–dehydrothromboxane B_2 in the cynomolgus monkey. *Biochim. Biophys. Acta*, **992**, 71–7.

Patrono, C. and FitzGerald, G.A. (1989) Physicians' health study: Aspirin and primary prevention of coronary heart disease (ll). *N. Engl. J. Med.*, **321**, 1826.

Patrono, C. Ciabattoni, G. Patrignani, P. *et al.* (1985) Clinical pharmacology of platetet cyclo oxygenase inhibition. *Circulation*, **72**, 1177–84.

Paull, P., Day, K., Graham, G. and Champion, D. (1976). Single dose evaluation of a new enteric coated aspirin preparation. *Med. J. Aust.*, **1**, 617–19.

Pedersen, A.K. and FitzGerald, G.A. (1984) Dose related pharmacokinetics of aspirin: Presystemic acetylation of platelet cyclooxygenase in man. *N. Engl. J. Med.*, **311**, 1206–11.

Pedersen, A.K. and FitzGerald, G.A. (1985) Preparation and analysis of deuterium labelled aspirin: Application to pharmacokinetic studies. *J. Pharm. Sci.*, **74**, 188–92.

Pedersen, A.K., Nowak, J. and FitzGerald, G.A. (1985) Slow administration of low dose aspirin: Enhanced inhibition of platelet cyclooxygenase. *Circulation*, Part II, III-193 (abstract).

Peto, R., Gray, R., Collins, R. *et al.* (1988) Randomised trial of prophylactic daily aspirin in British male doctors. *Brit. Med. J.*, **296**, 13–16.

Rainsford, K.D. (1984) *Aspirin and the Salicylates*, Butterworths, London.

Rainsford, K.D., Schweitzer, A. and Brune, K. (1983) Distribution of the acetyl compared with the salicyl moiety of acetylsalicylic acid. *Biochem. Pharmacol.*, **32**, 1301–8.

Raz, A., Wyche, A. and Needleman, P. (1989) Temporal and pharmacological division of fibroblast cyclooxygenase expression into transcriptional and translational phases. *Proc. Natl Acad. Sci. USA*, **86**, 1657–61.

Reilly, I.A.G. and FitzGerald, G.A. (1986). Eicosanoid biosynthesis and platelet function with advancing age. *Thromb. Res.*, **41**, 545–54.

Reilly, I.A.G. and FitzGerald, G.A. (1987) Inhibition of thromboxane formation *in vivo* and *ex vivo*: Implications for therapy with platelet inhibitory drugs. *Blood*, **69**, 180–6.

Reilly, I.A.G. and FitzGerald, G.A. (1988) Aspirin in cardiovascular disease. *Drugs*, **35** 154–76.

Reilly, I.A.G., Roy, L. and FitzGerald, G.A. (1986) Thromboxane biosynthesis is increased in systemic sclerosis with Raynaud's phenomenon. *Brit. Med. J.* **292**, 1087–9.

Roberts, M.S., Rumble, R.H. and Brooks, P.M. (1978) Salivary salicylate secretion and flow rate. *Brit. J. Clin. Pharmac.*, **6**, 429.

Roberts, L.J., ll, Sweetman, B.J. and Oates, J.A. (1981) Metabolism of thromboxane B_2 in man: Identification of twenty urinary metabolites. *J. Biol. Chem.*, **256**, 8384–93.

Roberts, M.S., McLeod, L.J., Cossum, P.A. and Vial, J.H. (1984) Inhibition of platelet function by a controlled release acetylsalicylic acid formulation – single and chronic dosing studies. *Eur. J. Clin. Pharmacol.*, **27**, 67–74.

Roth, G.J. and Majerus, P.W. (1975) The mechanism of the effect of aspirin on human platelets. I. Acetylation of a particulate fraction protein. *J. Clin. Invest.*, **56**, 624–32.

Roth, G.J. and Siok, C.J. (1978) Acetylation of the NH_2-terminal serine of prostaglandin synthase by aspirin. *J. Biol. Chem.*, **253**, 3782–4.

Roth, G.J., Stanford, N. and Majerus, P.W. (1978) Acetylation of prostaglandin synthetase by aspirin. *Proc. Natl Acad. Sci. USA*, **72**, 3073–6.

Rowland, M. and Riegelman, S. (1968) Pharmacokinetics of aspirin and salicylic acid after intravenous administration in man. *J. Pharm. Sci.*, **57**, 1313–19.

Rowland, M., Riegelman, S., Harris, P.A. and Sholkoff, S.D. (1972) Absorption kinetics of aspirin in man following oral administration of an aqueous solution. *J. Pharm. Sci.*, **61**, 379–85.

Rumble, R.H., Brooks, P.M. and Roberts, M.S. (1980) Metabolism of salicylate during chronic aspirin therapy. *Brit. J. Clin. Pharmac.*, **9**, 41–5.

Schiff, E., Peleg, E., Goldenberg, M. *et al.* (1989). The use of aspirin to prevent pregnancy-induced hypertension and lower the ratio of thromboxane A_2 to prostacyclin in relatively high risk pregnancies. *N. Engl. J. Med.*, **321**, 351–6.

Schwartz, L., Bourassa, M.G., Lesperance, J. *et al.* (1988) Aspirin and dipyridamole in the prevention of restenosis after percutaneous transluminal coronary angioplasty. *N. Engl. J. Med.*, **318**, 1714–19.

Sherman, C.T., Litvack, F. and Grundfest, W. (1986) Coronary angioscopy in patients with unstable angina pectoris. *N. Engl. J. Med.*, **315**, 913–19.

Siebert, D.J. and Bochner, F. (1987) Determination of plasma aspirin and salicylate concentrations after low aspirin doses by HPLC with post column hydrolysis and fluorescence. *J. Chromatogr.*, **20**, 425–31.

Smith, J.H. and Willis, A.L. (1971) Aspirin selectively inhibits prostaglandin production in human platelets. *Nature (New Biology)*, **231** 235–7.

Smith, P.K., Gleason, H.L., Stoll, C.G. and Ogorzalek, S. (1946) Studies on the pharmacology of salicylates. *J. Pharmacol. Exp. Ther.*, **87**, 237–55.

Soren, A. (1979) Kinetics of aspirin in blood and joint fluid. *J. Clin. Pharmacol.*, **16**, 279–85.

Spenncy, J.G. (1978) Acetylsalicylic acid hydrolase of gastric mucosa. *Am. J. Physiol.*, **234**, E606–10.

Steering Committee of the Physicians' Health Study Research Group (1989) Final report on the aspirin component of the ongoing physicians' health study. *N. Engl. J. Med.*, **321**, 129–35.

Stroke Prevention in Atrial Fibrillation Study Group Investigators (1990) Preliminary report of the stroke prevention in atrial fibrillation study. *N. Engl. J. Med.*, **322**, 863–8.

Takahara, K., Murray, R., FitzGerald, G.A. and Fitzgerald, D.J. (1990) The response to thromboxane A_2 in human platelets: discrimination of two binding sites linked to distinct effector systems. *J. Biol. Chem.*, **265**, 6836–44.

Theroux, P., Quimet, H., McCans, J. *et al.* (1988) Aspirin, heparin, or both to treat acute unstable angina. *N. Engl. J. Med*; **319**, 1105–11.

Trnavska, Z. and Trnavsky, K. (1983) Sex differences in the pharmacokinetics of the salicylates. *Eur. J. Clin. Pharmacol.*, **25**, 679–82.

Pharmacokinetics of aspirin and salicylates

Tsuchiya, T. and Levy, G. (1972a) Biotransformation of salicylic acid to its acyl and phenolic glucuronides in man. *J. Pharm. Sci.*, **61**, 800–1.

Tsuchiya, T. and Levy, G. (1972b) Relationship between dose and plateau levels of drugs eliminated by parallel first-order and capacity-limited kinetics. *J. Pharm. Sci.*, **61**, 541–4.

Vane, J.R. (1971) Inhibition of prostaglandin synthesis as a mechanism of action for aspirin-like drugs. *Nature (New Biol.)*, **231**, 232–5.

Wallenburg, H.C., Dekker, G.A., Makovitz, J.W. and Rotmans, P. (1986), Low-dose aspirin prevents pregnancy-induced hypertension and pre-eclampsia in angiotensin-sensitive primigravidae. *Lancet* **i**, 1–3.

Wallentin, L. for the RISC Study Group (1990) Risk of myocardial infarction and death during treatment with low dose aspirin and intravenous heparin in men with unstable coronary disease. *Lancet*, **336**, 827–30.

Wanwimolruk, S., Birkett, D.A. and Brooks, P.M. (1982) Protein binding of some non-steroidal anti-inflammatory drugs in rheumatoid arthritis. *Clin. Pharmacokin.*, **7**, 85–92.

Weiss, H.J. and Aledort, L.M. (1967) Impaired platelet connective tissue reaction in man after aspirin ingestion. *Lancet*, **ii**, 495.

Weksler, B.B., Tack-Goldman, K., Subramanian, V.A. and Gray, W.A., Jr (1985) Cumulative inhibitory effect of low-dose aspirin on vascular prostacyclin and platelet thromboxane production in patients with atherosclerosis. *Circulation*, **71**, 332–40.

Welling, P.G. (1984) Interactions affecting drug absorption. *Clin. Pharmacokin.*, **9**, 404–34.

Wilson, N.H. and Jones, R.L. (1985) Prostaglandin endoperoxide and thromboxane A_2 analogs. *Adv. Prostaglandin Thromboxane Leukotriene Res.*, **14**, 393–426

Wilson, J.T., Howell, R.L., Holladay, M.W. *et al.* (1978) Gentisuric acid: Metabolic formation in animals and identification as a metabolite of aspirin in man. *Clin. Pharmacol. Ther.*, **23**, 635–43.

Xie, W.L., Chipman, J.G., Robertson, D.L. *et al.* (1991) Expression of a mitogen-responsive gene encoding prostaglandin synthase is regulated by mRNA splicing. *Proc. Natl Acad. Sci. USA*, **88**, 2692–6.

Yoshimoto, T., Suzuki, H., Yamamoto, S. *et al.* (1990) Cloning and sequence analysis of the cDNA for arachidonate 12-lipoxygenase of porcine leukocytes. *Proc. Natl Acad. Sci. USA*, **87**, 2142–6.

106

6 Differential pharmacokinetics of different salicylates

K. DIETZEL and K. BRUNE

6.1 INTRODUCTION

Salicylates are very important drugs for the treatment of fever, pain and various types of arthritis. More than 150 years ago salicylic acid was first isolated from the bark of the willow in the form of the glycoside called salicin which is converted to salicylic acid *in vivo*. At the end of the last century, acetylsalicylic acid was introduced. Salicin may be considered as the natural, and aspirin as the first, synthetic pro-drug of salicylic acid.

Problems associated with the use of aspirin and salicylic acid, like the poor water solubility and the side effects in the gastro-intestinal tract, have been the reason for the synthesis of different derivatives with apparently improved properties in these respects. To increase the solubility, salts of both salicylic acid and aspirin, e.g. sodium, potassium, magnesium and choline salts, were synthesized. To improve the gastric tolerability, different esters were prepared such as the methyl, ethyl or phenolic esters. Substitution in the 3- and 5-positions of the salicylate molecule yields derivatives (e.g. 5-chlorosalicylic acid, 3-methylsalicylic acid) with modified physicochemical properties. Triglycerides of aspirin with 1,3-didecanoylglycerol and 1,3-dipalmitoylglycerol have been synthesized, the idea being that aspirin would be released by lipases following absorption of the compounds. Other developments include the condensation of two molecules of salicylic acid to form salicylsalicylic acid and the condensation of one molecule of aspirin and one molecule of paracetamol to form benorylate and eterylate. Prodrugs of 5-chlorosalicylic acid are meseclazone and seclazone. These compounds break down prior to or after absorption. Salicylic acid amide (salicylamide) was the parent compound for the synthesis of several derivatives such as 2-carbamoylphenoxy acetic acid, salacetamide, ethoxybenzamide, aspirin phenylalanine amide or aspirin phenylalanine ethyl ester.

The modern salicylic acid derivative diflunisal must be considered separately because it is not metabolized to salicylic acid and, hence, it is not a prodrug.

The objective of this contribution is to review the pharmacokinetics of different salicylic acid derivatives mainly in terms of absorption, metabolism and availability of salicylate or salicylamide which are considered as active compounds in most cases. Table 6.1 summarizes the availability of the active compounds after oral administration of the prodrugs to humans. Only salicylic acid derivatives with antipyretic and analgesic properties have been included. This chapter deals with the pharmacokinetics of aspirin and salicylic acid only very briefly, because this subject is addressed in detail in another chapter of this book.

6.2 SALICYLIC ACID AND ITS PRO-DRUGS

6.2.1 Salicylic Acid

The chemical structures of salicylic acid and some of its pro-drugs are summarized in Fig. 6.1.

Salicylic acid has been quoted in all textbooks on pharmacology and pharmacokinetics due to its unusual pharmacokinetic behaviour. As Levy (1965) pointed out, 'the pharmacokinetics of salicylate elimination were found to be unusual both qualitatively and quantitatively'. The pharmacokinetics of salicylic acid depend largely on the administered dose. With increasing dose the apparent half-life of the drug becomes longer due to saturable metabolic processes. The kinetics can no longer be described by first order processes.

Due to its physicochemical properties, absorption of salicylic acid already begins in the stomach by passive diffusion. Although there are optimum pH conditions in the stomach (assuming pH 2.5–4) absorption occurs mainly in the intestine due to the much greater surface area (Rowland *et al.*, 1972). Taken as tablets or capsules the drug can only be absorbed after disintegration of the solid form and dissolution. The absorption is even more delayed if an enteric coated tablet is administered. Very fast absorption can be achieved by the use of liquid dosage forms which contain salts of salicylic acid. Taking these aspects into account, the rate of absorption which finds its expression in the time necessary to reach maximum plasma concentrations depends largely on the stomach emptying time and the nature of the administered dosage form. The bioavailability, however, which is usually described by the area under the plasma concentration–time curve is mainly independent of these parameters. It is usually

Table 6.1 Salicylic acid derivatives and important pharmacokinetic parameters of the active compounds after oral administration to humans if not otherwise noted (see text for references). ASA, aspirin; SA, salicylic acid; PAR, paracetamol; SAM, salicylamide; ?, either no data available or data insufficient

Compound	Active compound	Bioavailability of active compound		t_{max} (h) of active compound
Salicylic acid (SA)	SA	100%		1–2
I. Salts of salicylic acid (SA)				
Sodium	SA	100%	(solution)	0.5–1.0
Choline	SA	100%	(solution)	0.3–0.5
Magnesium	SA	100%		?
Choline magnesium trisalicylate	SA	100%		?
II. Prodrugs of salicylic acid				
Aspirin	SA	100%		0.3–2.0
Lysine acetyl salicylate	SA	100%	(parenteral)	1.0–1.2?
Methyl SA	SA	12–20%	(cutan)	?
Salsalate	SA	65–85%		2 7
Benorylate	SA	85–95%		2–3
	PAR	75–90%		4–5
Eterylate	SA	90%?		3–4
	PAR	90%?		?
Fosfosal	SA	100%	(rat, dog)	?
III. Other salicylates				
3-methyl-SA	3 methyl-SA	?		?
3-methyl-ASA	3-methyl-SA	?		?
	3-methyl-ASA	?		?
5-chloro-SA	5 chloro-SA	?		?
Seclazone	5-chloro-SA	55–80%		16
Meseclazone	5-chloro-SA	60–90% ?		12–13?
Diflunisal	diflunisal	100%		1–4
IV. Salicylamide and derivatives				
Salicylamide-	SAM	Strongly dose-		0.3–1.0
sodium salt	SAM	dependent		0.1–0.5
Salacetamide	SAM	?		?
Ethoxybenzamide	SAM	50% ?		0.5–1 ?

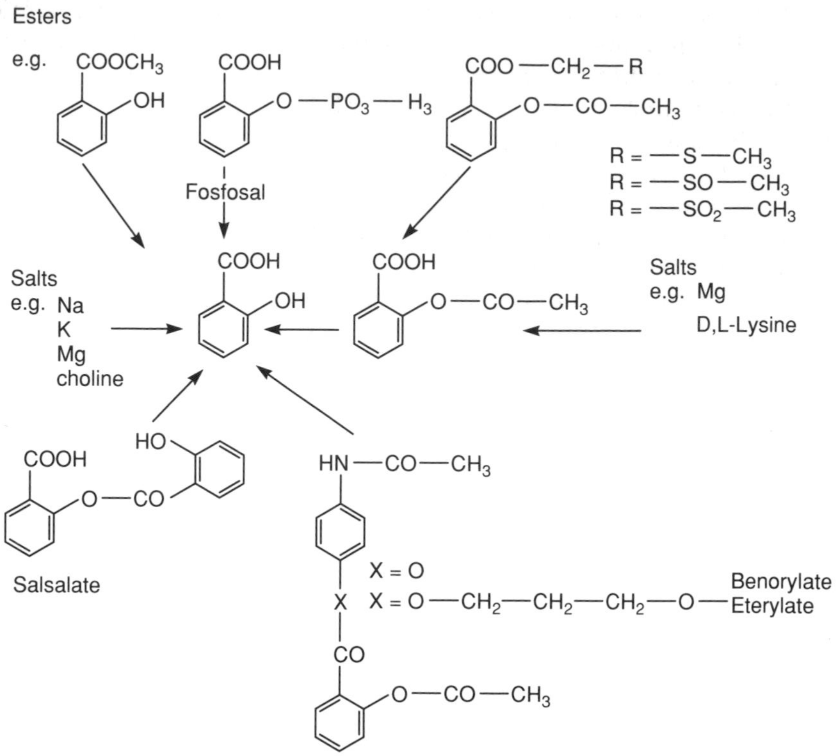

Figure 6.1 Salicylic acid pro-drugs.

determined in comparison to an intravenously administered dose or an orally administered solution. After oral administration the absorption is considered to be complete. After rectal administration, however, the bioavailabilty was found to be only 59% of that achieved from oral ingestion of aspirin (Superstine *et al.*, 1978).

Salicylic acid and other acidic anti-inflammatory drugs are not distributed equally throughout the body. It could be shown using rat whole body autoradiography that high concentrations in the inflamed tissue, blood, bone marrow, liver, kidney and the stomach wall were present (Brune, 1974; Brune *et al.*, 1976). The two different parts of the rat stomach, i.e. the glandular and the non-glandular tissues, showed a strikingly different pattern of drug concentrations after oral administration. In the non-glandular part, there was a slow increase in concentration reaching a maximum after about 45 min. In the glandular part, the mucosa of which is comparable to that found in humans, highest concentrations were found only 1 min after administration and declined rapidly thereafter (Brune *et al.*, 1977).

Salicylic acid shows a concentration-dependent plasma protein binding. At low (therapeutic) concentrations (< 100 μg ml^{-1}) about 90% is bound. In higher (toxic) concentrations (400 μg ml^{-1}) only 76% is bound (Dromgoole et al., 1981). Since only unbound drug is available for distribution, metabolism and elimination, this increase in free drug concentration leads to an increase in the volume of distribution. The extent of protein binding can be influenced by changes in the pH or by changes in the plasma protein concentration. It could be shown that the decrease of albumin concentration from 5 to 2 g per 100 ml leads to an increase in free salicylate from 10% to 50% (Woislait, 1976; Ekstrand et al., 1979). This binding characteristic to plasma proteins is supposed to be the reason for interactions with other highly protein bound drugs. It has been observed that phenytoin is displaced from albumin binding sites, increasing free phenytoin concentrations and enhancing phenytoin clearance. This phenomenon is accompanied by a depletion of serum folate, which is essential for the metabolism of phenytoin. Consequently, phenytoin clearance decreases and intoxication occurs (Furst, 1988). On concomitant administration of salicylate and other NSAIDs (diflunisal, flurbiprofen, ibuprofen, isoxicam, ketoprofen, naproxen, tolmetin), these drugs are displaced by salicylate leading to an increase in the incidence of side effects (Brune and Lanz, 1985; Furst, 1988). Concentrations of both fenoprofen and indomethacin were reduced significantly when administered with salicylate (Rubin et al., 1973).

Salicylic acid is metabolized by linear and saturable processes (Fig. 6.2). On the one hand it is conjugated with glucuronic acid to form phenolic (SPG) or acyl glucuronides (SAG) and with glycine to salicyluric acid (SU). On the other hand oxidation yields gentisic acid (GA) which, in turn, is eliminated either free or conjugated with glycine (gentisuric acid, GSA). Although the formation of salicyluric acid is the preferred metabolic pathway, the capacity for the formation of SPG and SU is limited leading to an increasing elimination of the other metabolites if the amount of salicylate in the body exceeds 600 mg. The effect of the salicylate dose on the metabolic pattern is presented in Fig. 6.3. The overall elimination of salicylate proceeds by first order kinetics at low doses, and by parallel zero and first order processes at higher doses. Consequently, the elimination plasma half-life increases with dose and the plasma levels increase disproportionately. This disproportionality is more pronounced with respect to unbound plasma salicylate, due to the decreased plasma protein binding with increasing concentrations (Levy, 1980). Levy and Leonards (1966) and Paulus et al. (1971) have shown that such capacity-limited metabolism can increase salicylic acid 'half-life' from about 3.5 h to 30 h or more.

Pharmacokinetics of aspirin and salicylates

This non-linearity in salicylate metabolism is of special importance in the case of long-term high dose therapy with aspirin or other salicylates. However, it has been observed that salicylic acid is likely to induce its own metabolism associated with a decrease in salicylate plasma levels and an increase in urinary elimination of salicyluric acid by approximately 50% after 3 days of therapy (Dromgoole *et al.*, 1981).

Salicylate and metabolites are mainly eliminated into the urine by filtration and tubular secretion. The renal elimination is strongly pH dependent (MacPherson *et al.*, 1955; Levy and Leonards, 1971). Raising the pH (e.g. with bicarbonate) leads to an increase in salicylate elimination because only the unionized molecules can be reabsorbed. When sodium hydroxide is added to an aspirin regimen leading to an increase in urinary pH by 1 pH unit, steady state salicylate concentrations are decreased by about 40% (Levy, 1978; Furst, 1988). This alkalizing effect on the urine can also be achieved by the use of magnesium/aluminium hydroxide combination antacids (Furst, 1988) or even by alkali salts of salicylate itself.

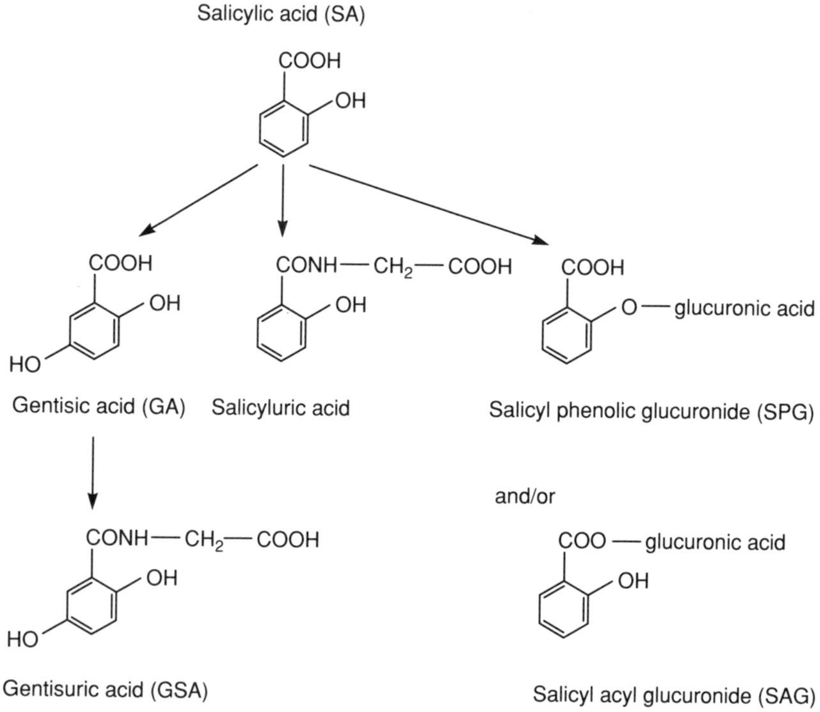

Figure 6.2   Pathways of salicylic acid metabolism.

112

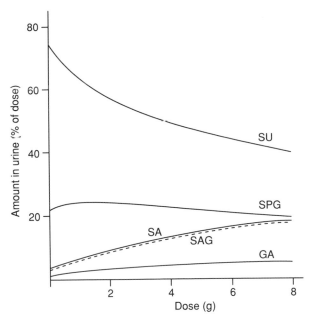

Figure 6.3 Urinary elimination pattern of salicylic acid and metabolites after different doses in man (from Gibaldi and Perrier, 1982). Abbreviations in text.

6.2.2 Salts of Salicylic Acid

The absolute bioavailabilty of sodium salicylate was found to be 100% after oral administration of a solution in a dose of 9 mg kg^{-1} bodyweight (Miaskiewicz *et al.*, 1982). Maximum salicylate plasma concentrations were reached after 32 and 54 min in male and female subjects, respectively. The choline salt of salicylic acid is absorbed completely after oral administration. Maximum plasma levels of salicylate are reached after 20–30 min, i.e. faster than after aspirin (Broh-Kahn, 1960; Davis *et al.*, 1960; Leary, 1960; Wolf and Aboody, 1960). In these studies, however, choline salicylate was administered as a solution whereas aspirin was used as a solid. The availability of salicylic acid is comparable to that of an equimolar dose of aspirin (Wilson *et al.*, 1982).

In another study plasma salicylate and urine salicylurate levels were compared following solid dosage forms of aspirin, magnesium salicylate and choline magnesium trisalicylate (Mason, 1980). There were no significant differences in the rate and extent of absorption of salicylate following the three dosage forms tested, and the elimination kinetics of salicylic acid were not altered by these dosage forms.

6.2.3 Acetylsalicylic Acid

The synthesis of the acetic acid ester of salicylic acid, i.e. aspirin, was the first attempt to create a safer salicylate with a more amenable taste (Dreser, 1907). Aspirin is absorbed from the stomach at about one-half to one-third of the rate of salicylic acid (Rainsford, 1984). This difference was attributed to the higher lipophilicity of salicylic acid compared with aspirin. Aspirin is still absorbed rapidly (absorption half-life: 5–16 min) and completely after oral administration (Rowland et al., 1972). It could be shown in rats that intestinal aspirin absorption increased as the concentration of hydrogen ions, bile salts and ascorbic acid in the perfusate increased. Aspirin was not absorbed by the stomach at pH 6.5 (Hollander et al., 1981). Peak plasma levels of aspirin and salicylate are reached after 10–40 min and 20–120 min, respectively, depending on the dose and pharmaceutical preparation (Soren, 1977; Mason and Winer, 1981; Proost et al., 1983; Roberts et al., 1983; Rainsford, 1984; Spahn et al., 1985). Maximum levels in joint fluid of aspirin but mainly of salicylic acid occurred after 50–110 min and 120–145 min, respectively (Soren, 1977). The average peak levels of aspirin and salicylic acid in joint fluid were about 75% and 60% of the maximum respective drug level in blood. Systemic bioavailability of aspirin in man was found to be 50–70% after single oral doses ranging from 20 to 1300 mg (Rowland et al., 1972; Pedersen and Fitzgerald, 1984). The absorption half-life from suppositories was found to be much longer (about 3 h) than the oral absorption half-life (Dromgoole et al., 1981). Therefore the bioavailability after rectal administration depends largely on the retention time of the suppository. A retention time of 4–5 h results in about 60% of the dose being absorbed (Nowak et al., 1974).

The non-enzymatic hydrolysis of aspirin varies largely with pH, having a minimum at a pH of 2. Raising the pH to values above 8 causes a considerable increase in hydrolysis rate (Martin, 1971). The mean half-lives of aspirin at 37 °C in gastric and duodenal juices were found to be 16 and 17 h, respectively (Rowland et al., 1972). Approximately 28–35% of an oral dose of aspirin 650 mg is hydrolysed during absorption in man (Rowland et al., 1972). The major portion of salicylate is generated from aspirin by the action of esterases in the gastrointestinal tract, blood, liver, kidney and other organs. The binding of aspirin (about 85%) to plasma proteins is less compared to salicylic acid. The half-life in plasma is approximately 15–20 min (Rowland and Riegelman, 1968; Rowland et al., 1972; Levy and Giacomini, 1978).

The lysine salt of aspirin is much more water soluble than aspirin and is used primarily for parenteral administration (von Voss et al., 1978).

6.2.4 Methylsalicylate

Methylsalicylate (Fig. 6.1) is mainly used externally in a number of liniments and ointments for the relief of minor muscular aches and pains. Skin permeability and systemic availability of different preparations were evaluated by applying 0.65–2.5 g methlysalicylate to the forearm (area 50 cm^2) of healthy subjects (Roberts *et al.*, 1982) for 10 h and measuring the urinary elimination of salicylate for 48 h. The application site was covered with a sheet of aluminium foil and greaseproof paper. On average, 12–20% of the dose was absorbed. However, the individual variability was fairly great. Calculated steady-state plasma levels of salicylate were highest after the 2.5 g dose (7.6 μg ml^{-1}) but certainly not sufficient to produce a systemic effect. A probable interaction between topically administered methylsalicylate and warfarin has been reported (Chow *et al.*, 1989). The percutaneous absorption could be enhanced by exercise and heat exposure due to an increased skin temperature, hydration and blood flow (Danon *et al.*, 1986).

6.2.5 Fosfosal

Fosfosal, 2-phosphonoxy-benzoic acid (Fig. 6.1), is the phosphate ester of salicylic acid. It is highly soluble in water. In solution, however, fosfosal is hydrolysed into salicylic acid. The pharmacokinetic properties of the compound in rats and dogs are reported by Ramis *et al.* (1989). After intravenous administration, fosfosal plasma levels decreased rapidly with a half-life of 2.7 min in rats and 6.7 min in dogs. In rat plasma, fosfosal is rapidly hydrolysed producing maximum levels of salicylate 15 and 60 min after intravenous and oral administration, respectively. In the dog, absorption and/or hydrolysis seems to be much slower, because maximum salicylate plasma concentrations were not reached until 2–3.5 h after administration. After oral administration, only salicylic acid was found in the plasma, indicating that hydrolysis occurs already during absorption. However, since the AUC of salicylate was equal after intravenous and oral administration, absorption seems to be complete in both species.

6.2.6 Salsalate (Salicylsalicylic Acid)

Salsalate consists of two molecules salicylic acid linked by an ester bond (Fig. 6.1). Like salicylic acid, salsalate is soluble in the acidic stomach milieu only very poorly (Singleton, 1980). Therefore, the major site of absorption is the small intestine (Singleton, 1980). After oral administration, the absorption seems to be essentially complete. The major portion of the dose is already hydrolysed into two molecules of salicylic acid prior to or during absorption. The drug that reaches the circulation unchanged is cleaved very rapidly. Salsalate peak concentrations in plasma are reached after approximately 1–5 h. Maximum levels of salicylate are measured 2–7 h after oral administration (Harrison *et al.*, 1981; Dromgoole *et al.*, 1984). Between 65% and 85% of the area under the total radioactivity curve in plasma was due to salicylic acid. In comparison to an equivalent dose of aspirin the AUC of salicylate was approximately 15% lower after salsalate, probably due to incomplete hydrolysis (Dromgoole *et al.*, 1983). The volume of distribution was reported to be $0.31 \, l \, kg^{-1}$ (Nordquist, 1976), and the half-life as 1.0–1.5 h (Harrison *et al.*, 1981; Williams *et al.*, 1986). Salsalate is mainly hydrolysed into salicylic acid (Fig. 6.1) and, consequently, eliminated as salicylate and its metabolites. Approximately 7–13% of the dose is excreted renally as unchanged salsalate or glucuronide (Dromgoole *et al.*, 1983, 1984). The fraction found in the stools was less than 1% (Dromgoole *et al.*, 1984). The phenomenon that salicylate concentrations in plasma after administration of salsalate are essentially lower than after equivalent doses of aspirin is caused by incomplete hydrolysis of salsalate which, in turn, is eliminated very rapidly in the urine. Depending on the dose this reduced availability of salicylate may lead to a more than proportional decrease in salicylate plasma levels (Dromgoole *et al.*, 1984).

6.2.7 Benorylate

Benorylate (4-acetamidophenyl-2-acetoxybenzoate) is the acetaminophen ester of aspirin (Fig. 6.1). Four grams of benorylate is equivalent to 2.4 g of aspirin (Dromgoole *et al.*, 1981).

In the rat, benorylate absorption was found to be relatively slow. High concentrations of unchanged benorylate were found in the lower section of the small intestine 4 h after oral administration (Liss and Robertson, 1975). *In-vitro* incubation of benorylate with gastric and intestinal fluids at 37 °C caused only negligible degradation (2% h^{-1}). Upon incubation in fresh human plasma at 37 °C, benorylate was hydrolysed enzymically with a half-life of 2–10 min (Robertson *et al.*, 1972), indicating a complete availability of salicylic acid and paracetamol after absorption. It could be shown in *ex-vivo* experiments that during passage through the rat small intestine wall benorylate is completely hydrolysed (Humphreys and Smy, 1975). It was concluded from urinary recovery data that at least 90% of an oral dose is absorbed in man (Robertson *et al.*, 1972). The rate of absorption, however, is slower but of longer duration than either aspirin or paracetamol. Hämäläinen *et al.* (1973)

have shown the presence of benorylate *per se* in synovial membrane and synovial fluid in patients undergoing synovectomy indicating that the benorylate molecule is absorbed intact. These results were confirmed by Manz and Glynn (1975) in six patients with rheumatoid arthritis after treatment with 8 g day^{-1} benorylate for 9–14 days. Benorylate was found in the synovial tissue in concentrations ranging from 2–5 μg ml^{-1} and was not detectable in blood. The salicylate concentrations in synovial tissue, however, were between 10 and 60 μg ml^{-1}, the acetaminophen levels were 1–5 μg ml^{-1}. Aylward *et al.* (1976) reported that synovial fluid levels of benorylate and salicylic acid persisted above 0.5 μg ml^{-1} and 50 μg ml^{-1}, respectively, for at least 7 h after a single oral 4 g dose of benorylate. After i.v. administration of ^{14}C-benorylate (labelled on the acid chloride carbonyl atom) the radioactivity was eliminated from plasma with a half-life of approximately 1.9 h.

Total salicylic acid metabolites recovered in the urine accounted for 85–95% of the administered aspirin dose and 75–90% was recovered as total paracetamol metabolites. About 14% of the administered dose was found in the faeces (Robertson *et al.*, 1972).

6.2.8 Eterylate

Eterylate, 2-(4'-acetamidophenyloxy)-ethyl-2-acetoxy-benzoate (Fig. 6.1), differs from benorylate only by an additional ethyloxy group introduced to link the parent molecules, aspirin and acetaminophen (Sunkel *et al.*, 1978). The metabolism of eterylate in rat, dog and man was summarized by Wood *et al.* (1983) (Fig. 6.4). Oral doses of ^{14}C-eterylate (10 mg kg^{-1}) were well absorbed by rat and man. Peak plasma concentrations of ^{14}C were generally reached after 1–3 h. *In-vitro* stability studies demonstrated that eterylate is rapidly deacetylated in plasma followed by further hydrolysis into salicylic acid and 2-(4'-acetylaminophenoxy)-ethanol with a half-life of about 4 h. In humans, only two metabolites, salicylic acid and 4-acetamido-phenoxyacetic acid were detected in plasma. Maximum salicylate concentrations of 10–20 μg ml^{-1} were reached after 3–4 h and declined with an initial half-life of 2–3 h.

Plasma 4-acetamido-phenoxyacetic acid concentrations reached a peak (4–10 μg ml^{-1}) after 2–3 h and declined with a half-life of about 1 h. Highest radioactivity levels in dogs and rats were found in the liver and kidneys after 3 and 1 h, respectively. Very high ^{14}C concentrations were found in dog bile (50–100 times higher than in plasma). The major metabolites in human urine were salicyluric acid and 4-acetamidophenoxyacetic acid. Minor metabolites were salicylic acid, gentisic acid and acetaminophen. Dog urine also contained an essential portion of relatively non-polar, unspecified components. Over

117

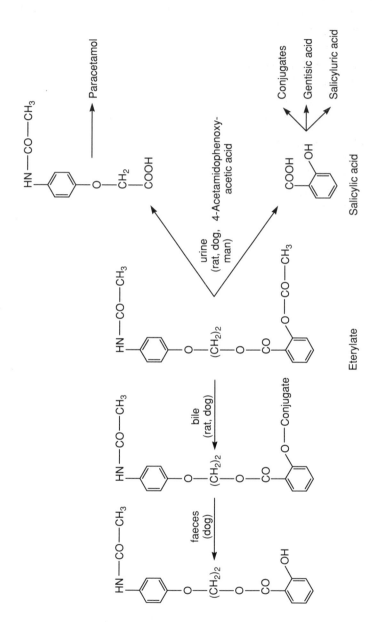

Figure 6.4 Metabolic fate of eterylate in rat, dog and man (modified after Wood *et al.*, 1983).

a period of 3 days, rats excreted a mean of 93.7% of the dose via the urine. Bile duct-cannulated rats eliminated about 22% of an oral dose into the bile within 48 h. In dogs, biliary elimination seems to be even higher. Humans eliminated about 91% of the dose via urine and 4% via faeces within 5 days.

6.3 RING SUBSTITUTED SALICYLIC ACID DERIVATIVES AND THEIR PRO-DRUGS

6.3.1 3-Methylsalicylic Acid and its Acetyl Derivative

3-Methylsalicylic acid and 3-methylacetylsalicylic acid are the respective ring substituted homologues of salicylic acid and acetylsalicylic acid. In rats, the absorption of 3-methylsalicylic acid is slower after oral administration compared to salicylic acid (Rainsford *et al.*, 1980). The blood salicylate levels are approximately one-third of those reached after salicylic acid administration. In therapeutically active concentrations, 80–85% of 3-methylsalicylic acid is bound to whole bovine plasma proteins (Stafford, 1962). The pharmacokinetics of these derivatives in man were investigated by Cummings and Martin (1965). Based on plasma and urinary excretion data, the half-life of 3-methylsalicylic acid was calculated to be about 18 h. No increase in half-life with increasing dose has been observed up to 1 g twice daily for 3 days. However, it is likely that after higher doses metabolic processes become saturated and non-linear pharmacokinetics become evident. The metabolic scheme is identical to that of salicylic acid, major metabolites being 3-methylsalicyluric acid and 3-methylsalicylic acid glucuronides.

Within 7 h after administration of 3-methylacetylsalicylic acid, 6–17% of the dose is excreted unchanged in the urine with a maximum about 2 h after dosage, indicating its superior hydrolytic stability to aspirin.

6.3.2 5-Chlorosalicylic Acid and its Pro-drugs

The plasma protein binding of 5-chlorosalicylic acid (Fig. 6.5) in humans, monkeys and dogs was found to be between 97 and 99.4% (Edelson *et al.*, 1975). Pharmacokinetic data are not available.

Data are available on the pharmacokinetics of seclazone, 7-chloro-3,3a-dihydro-2H, 9H-isoxazolo (3,2-b) (1,3) benzoxazin-9-one (Fig. 6.5), in rats, dogs, monkeys and man (Edelson *et al.*, 1973, 1974). After oral administration of ^{14}C labelled seclazone, maximum levels of radioactivity in plasma are reached after 4–5 h in animals and after 16 h in man. Plasma radioactivity declined with a half-life of approximately 6 (rhesus monkey), 8.5 (beagle dog), 10 (rat), and 14 h (man). Seclazone

Pharmacokinetics of aspirin and salicylates

is broken down in the animal body almost completely, since only negligible amounts of unchanged drug are eliminated via the urine. It has been shown in rats that hydrolysis occurs primarily on passage through the intestinal wall during absorption. After the ingestion of 1 g of seclazone no unchanged drug could be detected at any time. In man, 55–77% and 0.2–7.2% of dose were found in urine and in the faeces, respectively, within 48 h after drug intake. Essentially all of the urinary radioactivity (90–95%) was accounted for as 5-chlorosalicylic acid either free or in the form of its conjugates with glycine and glucuronic acid (Fig. 6.5). A portion less than 1% was excreted as unchanged seclazone. The three carbons of the isoxazolo moiety are metabolized mainly to malonic acid and carbon dioxide.

Meseclazone, 7-chloro-3,3a-dihydro-2-methyl-2H, 9H-isoxazolo (3,2-b) (1,3) benzoxazin-9-one (Fig. 6.5), differs from seclazone only by an additional methyl group at C-2. The pharmacokinetics in animals and man have been described by Edelson et al. (1975) and Dromgoole et al. (1978).

Ex-vivo studies using rat intestine showed that the dissolved drug is absorbed rapidly by first order processes with a half-life of about

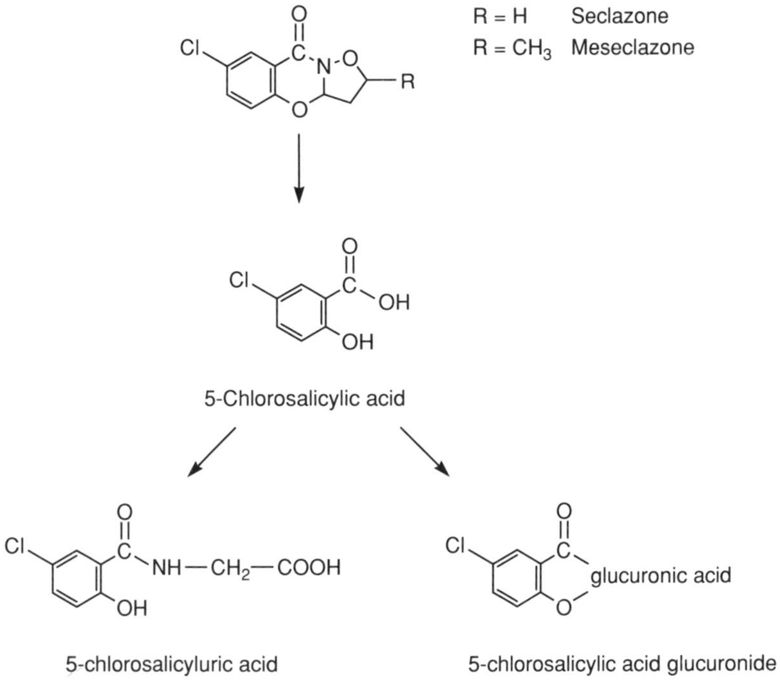

Figure 6.5 Bioactivation and metabolism of seclazone and meseclazone (after Edelson et al., 1973, 1975).

120

6 min. Since substantial amounts of 5-chlorosalicylic acid were found in the hepatic portal vein, the hydrolysis is already likely to take place during the passage through the intestinal wall. Since meseclazone was not degraded by incubation with whole rat blood for 4 h, the unaltered drug that is absorbed is probably degraded by liver enzymes.

In contrast to these *ex-vivo* results, peak radioactivity levels in plasma were not reached before 2.5, 5 and 13 h in rat, dog and man, respectively, after oral administration of ^{14}C-labelled meseclazone. The absorption half-life in man was calculated as 6.3 h (Dromgoole *et al.*, 1978). This apparent slow absorption is probably due to the dissolution step of meseclazone, since it is only poorly soluble in water (Dromgoole *et al.*, 1978). The half-life of blood radioactivity was about 12 and 18 h in the beagle dog and the rat, respectively. In human subjects, no intact drug was detected in the plasma. The active metabolite, 5-chlorosalicylic acid, was cleared from the plasma with a half-life of about 33 h. As in the case after administration of seclazone, the major excretion products were 5-chlorosalicylic acid (9% of total urinary elimination products) and its conjugates with glycine (5%) and glucuronic acid (82%) (Fig. 6.5). The elimination in urine and stools accounted for 91% of the dose. The isoxazole moiety was converted into β-hydroxybutyric acid and its metabolites carbon dioxide and fumaric, citric, α-ketoglutaric, succinic and malonic acids. It is interesting to note that meseclazone is primarily eliminated by conjugation of 5-chlorosalicylic acid with glucuronic acid, whereas salicylic acid elimination procceds via a capacity-limited conjugation with glycine (Dromgoole *et al.*, 1978). The binding of meseclazone to plasma proteins was about 80% in humans, monkeys and dogs in a concentration of 80 μg ml^{-1} and was, thus, substantially lower than the protein binding of 5-chlorosalicylic acid.

6.4 SALICYLAMIDE AND ITS DERIVATIVES

The chemical structures of salicylamide and its prodrugs are presented in Fig. 6.6.

6.4.1 Salicylamide

Salicylamide possesses only weak analgesic and antipyretic rather than anti-inflammatory properties (Rainsford, 1984). According to Podder *et al.* (1988) 65–75% of an oral dose is absorbed by dogs. The pharmacokinetics of salicylamide elimination in man has been described by Levy and Matsuzawa (1967). Biotransformation products in man are the ether glucuronide and the ester sulphate of salicylamide and gentisamide and its glucuronide (Fig. 6.7). The fraction of the dose

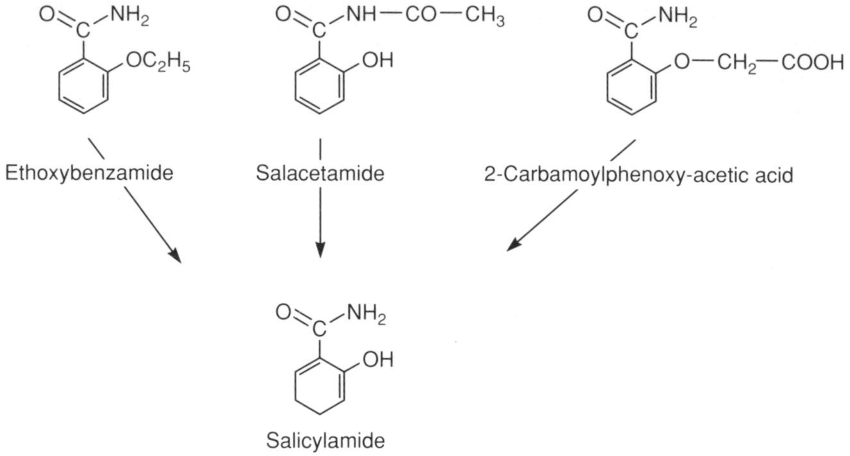

Figure 6.6 Prodrugs of salicylamide.

which is excreted as salicylamide sulphate decreases with increasing dose (Fig. 6.8). The elimination rate of salicylamide sulphate approaches a limiting value when 0.6–1.0 g of salicylamide is administered orally in solution, i.e. in a rapidly absorbable form. If salicylamide is administered in a slowly absorbed form, larger amounts of the sulphate are eliminated. The limiting factor seems to be the availability of sulphate, since concomitant administration of sulphate or sulphate precursors (L-cysteine) increases the maximum excretion rate and the total amount excreted as salicylamide sulphate. Gentisamide glucuronide is a minor biotransformation product which is produced only in significant quantities when the salicylamide sulphate formation is saturated, i.e. after relatively high and rapidly absorbed doses. Other sources of non-linear salicylamide metabolism appear to be saturable oxidation reactions, depletion of cosubstrates, extensive extraction in the intestinal wall and the liver and, possibly, end-product inhibition (Waschek *et al.*, 1984; Tozer *et al.*, 1989). Only a very small portion of the dose was excreted unchanged in urine (<1%).

The plasma concentration profiles of salicylamide and conjugates have been reported by Fleckenstein *et al.* (1976). Little free salicylamide was found in plasma after a 650 mg oral dose. The major fraction was present in the form of conjugates. It has been described that conjugation with glucuronic acid and sulphuric acid occurs already in the intestine (Podder *et al.*, 1988) and that the first-pass metabolism after small oral doses (<1 mg kg^{-1}) is almost exclusively intestinal (Waschek, 1986). Maximum plasma levels were reached after 20–60 min. After administration of a sodium salt solution, significantly higher plasma concentrations of free salicylamide were obtained much earlier (10–30 min). Increasing the dose of sodium salicylamide to 1.3, 1.95 and 2.6 g caused a more than proportional increase in the AUC of free, not conjugated, salicylamide probably due to saturable conjugation processes. The AUC of total salicylamide (free + conjugates) increased in a linear fashion with dose.

In dogs, dose-dependent first pass metabolism caused an increase in bioavailabilty from 0.24 ± 0.14 to 0.76 ± 0.20 after 5 and 40 mg kg^{-1}, respectively. Clearance decreased from 3.4 ± 1.0 to 0.60 ± 0.11 l min^{-1} and half-life increased from 5.0 ± 1.2 to 23.5 ± 6.1 min (Waschek *et al.*, 1984).

Concurrent administration of salicylamide and ascorbic acid increases salicylamide half-life and the AUC and decreases its clearance due to competition for available sulphate and consequent inhibition of sulphate conjugate formation. There was no influence of ascorbic acid on the total amount of drug and metabolites eliminated via the urine. However, the fraction of the dose eliminated as sulphate decreased significantly. This interaction is most pronounced when both drugs are administered orally, possibly due to their high concentrations in the intestinal wall and liver during the first-pass (Houston and Levy, 1975, 1976).

6.4.2 Salacetamide

Salacetamide, N-acetylsalicylamide, is transformed *in vivo* into salicylamide (Fig. 6.6). The pharmacokinetic data are not available.

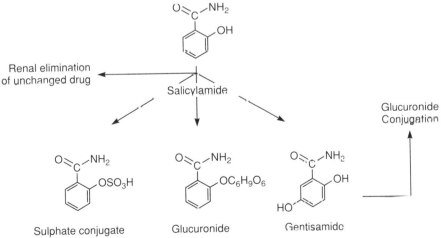

Figure 6.7 Metabolism of salicylamide.

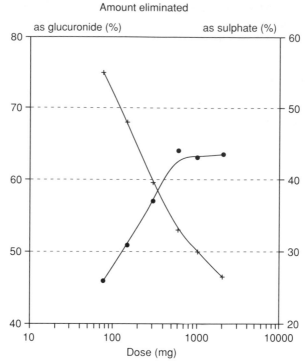

Figure 6.8 Effect of salicylamide dose (75–2000 mg orally) on the formation of salicylamide conjugates (+ = sulphate, ● = glucuronide) in humans (after Levy and Matsuzawa, 1967).

6.4.3 Ethoxybenzamide

After oral administration, ethoxybenzamide (2-ethylsalicylamide) (Fig. 6.6) is absorbed rapidly, leading to maximum plasma concentrations 30–60 min after administration (Davison *et al.*, 1962). The half-life is approximately 1 h. The major fraction seems to be converted to salicylamide. In rats, 82% of the dose was present as salicylamide in the systemic circulation (Shibasaki *et al.*, 1984). In dogs, the first-pass metabolism of ethoxybenzamide was found to be higher than that of salicylamide (Podder *et al.*, 1988). The absorption seems to be complete, since equal amounts were found in the urine (70–80% of dose) after intravenous as well as after oral administration. In contrast to salicylamide, ethoxybenzamide is absorbed unchanged. No conjugation has been observed in the intestine. In humans, no unchanged ethoxybenzamide could be detected in the urine. Only one-half of the dose could be recovered as either the ethereal sulphate

(34%) or the glucuronide (15%) of salicylamide (Davison *et al.*, 1962) indicating a low bioavailability of ethoxybenzamide or the formation of metabolites which could not be detected by the methods used.

6.4.4 2-Carbamoylphenoxyacetic Acid

No data are available on the pharmacokinetics of 2-carbamoylphenoxyacetic acid (Fig. 6.6).

6.5 DIFLUNISAL

Diflunisal, 5-(2,4-difluorophenyl)salicylic acid (Fig. 6.9), differs from the compounds described above in that it is not metabolized to salicylic acid. The difluorophenyl group at C5 is preferably rotated approximately 50° from the plane of the salicylic acid moiety. This reduces the conjugation of the two phenyl rings and preserves the electronic characteristics of the salicylic acid portion (Shen, 1983). This substitution causes a stereochemical configuration and the lipophilicity generally preferred by non-steroidal anti-inflammatory drugs. In healthy volunteers, diflunisal is absorbed slowly, but probably almost completely after oral administration (Davies, 1983; Nuernberg and Brune, 1989). Maximum plasma levels after a single dose of 500 mg are reached after 1–4 h. After intravenous administration of 500 mg, the terminal elimination half-life was found to be 12.8 h. Steady-state plasma levels are reached dose-dependently after 3–4 days (125 mg p.o. twice daily) or after 7–9 days (500 mg twice daily) (Brogden *et al.*, 1980). Diflunisal is eliminated from plasma after a dose of 500 mg with a half-life of 7–16 h (Brogden *et al.*, 1980; Davies, 1983; Nuernberg, 1986; Nuernberg and Brune, 1989). In plasma, 98–99% of diflunisal is bound to proteins (Brogden *et al.*, 1980). It could be shown that the binding to rat plasma proteins is concentration-dependent. At a diflunisal concentration of 5 μg ml^{-1} only 0.22% were unbound, whereas at 100 μg ml^{-1} 0.50% of the total concentration was free (Lin *et al.*, 1985). After oral administration of 500 mg to young, healthy volunteers, maximum plasma concentrations were between 60 and 100 μg ml^{-1} (Brogden *et al.*, 1980; Davies, 1983; Nuernberg and Brune, 1989; Verbeeck *et al.*, 1979a). The bioavailability of diflunisal in fasted subjects is significantly decreased (20–50%) by the concomitant ingestion of aluminium containing antacids (Verbeeck *et al.*, 1979b), while magnesium hydroxide antacids increase total diflunisal absorption by about 10% (Furst, 1988). In fed subjects these antacids caused a reduction of peak plasma levels by approximately 20% but no influence on the AUC was evident (Verbeeck *et al.*, 1979b).

125

Pharmacokinetics of aspirin and salicylates

It could be shown in rats that diflunisal is not distributed equally in the body. High concentrations have been found in the kidneys, the lungs, the stomach and in the inflamed tissue (Brune and Schneider, 1982). The apparent volume of distribution is 7.3 ± 0.41 in subjects with normal renal function. It is significantly increased to 16.2 ± 2.21 in patients with renal impairment (Verbeeck et al., 1979a). In lactating women, the concentration of diflunisal in milk is 2–7% of that in their plasma (Brogden et al., 1980).

The difluorophenyl substituent in diflunisal is metabolically very stable. It cannot be converted into salicylic acid, and there is no evidence of fluoride release in vivo (Shen, 1983). The principal metabolite is the phenolic glucuronide of diflunisal (Fig. 6.9) which accounts for about 64% of the radioactivity found in urine after a single 50 or 500 mg dose. The sulphate conjugate accounts for up to 44% and the ester glucuronide for up to 20% of the urinary radioactivity (Tocco et al., 1975; Loewen et al., 1986). The elimination of free diflunisal is less than 5% (Davies, 1983; Nuernberg, 1986; Nuernberg and Brune, 1989). There are hints that some saturable metabolism is involved in diflunisal biotransformation as well. Tocco et al. (1975) reported that the AUC after a 500 mg dose was approximately 18 times higher compared to the AUC after a 50 mg dose. Moreover, the half-life after administration of 50 mg in this study was found to be only 5.6 h compared to 7–16 h after 500 mg. After doses ranging from 125 to 500 mg, a non-linear increase of C_{max} and AUC_{0-60h} was observed (Davies, 1983). Up to 10% of the administered diflunisal is found in the bile of patients (Nuernberg, 1986). Since the elimination via

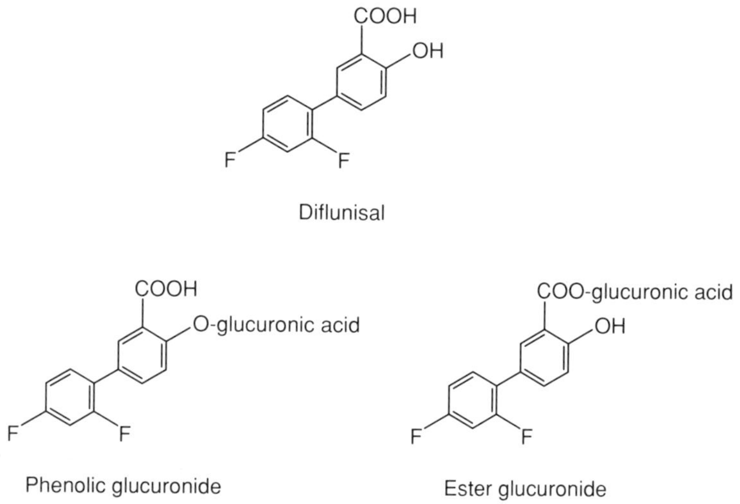

Diflunisal

Phenolic glucuronide

Ester glucuronide

Figure 6.9 Metabolism of diflunisal.

the faeces is less than 5%, enterohepatic circulation of diflunisal is likely to occur in man (Davies, 1983; Brogden et al., 1980). In rats, within 26 h after an intravenous 10 mg dose, approximately 42% of the dose was eliminated via the bile. On average, approximately 65% of the amount of drug and its glucuronides excreted in bile was reabsorbed (Lin et al., 1985).

In terminal renal impairment (creatine clearance < 2 ml min⁻¹) the terminal elimination half-life increases to 115–189 h (Brogden et al., 1980). In these patients only 2.7 ± 0.9% of a dose could be recovered in the 72 h urine sample as parent drug and glucuronides (Verbeeck et al., 1979a). It has been speculated, that in severe renal impairment, the biliary elimination of diflunisal and conjugates might be enhanced accompanied by reabsorption after hydrolysis in the intestine because of the molecular size of the diflunisal glucuronides. This hypothesis is supported by the existence of this pathway in animals, and the small amount eliminated in the faeces of volunteers (Levy, 1979). Diuresis and alkalization of the urine by antacids increased the renal clearance rate of free drug (Davies, 1983). Pharmacokinetic interactions between concomitantly administered drugs and diflunisal summarized by Davies (1983) and Tempero et al. (1979) include oral anticoagulants (increase in free warfarin plasma levels), aspirin (decrease in diflunisal levels), naproxen (urinary excretion of naproxen and its glucuronide metabolite decreased), indomethacin (indomethacin plasma levels increased), sulindac (plasma levels of the active sulindac sulphide metabolite decreased), hydrochlorothiazide (hydrochlorothiazide plasma levels increased) and acetaminophen (acetaminophen plasma levels increased).

6.6 OTHER SALICYLATE DERIVATIVES

6.6.1 Triglycerides of Aspirin

The idea behind the development of aspirin triglycerides is that the triglycerides would pass through the stomach unchanged and that aspirin would be released by lipases prior to or following absorption of the drug (Rainsford, 1984).

In rats, 1,3-dipalmitoyl-2(2'-acetoxy-carboxylbenzoyl) glycerol (Fig. 6.10a) is absorbed through the intestine mainly as 2-aspirin monoglyceride, some 20% of which is transported through the thoracic duct chyle and about 30% through the portal system (Kumar and Billimoria, 1978). Compared to an equimolar dose of aspirin the availabilty of salicylate is approximately 50% (calculated from the plasma salicylate concentrations). In the stomach, almost no breakdown of the

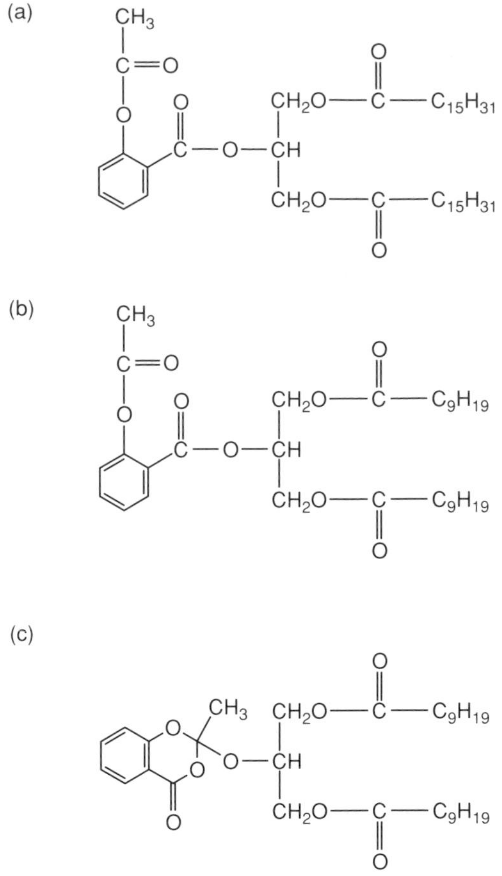

Figure 6.10 Aspirin triglycerides.

triglyceride occurs. In the intestine, the compound is cleaved mainly to the aspirin monoglyceride which is absorbed as such and is cleaved in the mucosa and the blood to free salicylate, which accounts for 90–95% of blood radioactivity. Since obviously very little absorption takes place in the stomach, and due to the digestion process necessary to release salicylate, peak plasma concentrations are not reached before 6–8 h.

In (2-(1,3-didecanoyl-oxy)-propyl) 2-acetyloxybenzoate (Fig. 6.10b), aspirin is incorporated in the 2-position of a triglyceride containing decanoic acid at the 1- and 3-positions. After oral administration to rats, the compound releases salicylate leading to maximum salicylate levels after 3–6 h. By comparison of the plasma salicylate AUCs (0–24 h), the availability of salicylate was found to be approximately 75% that of aspirin (Carter *et al.*, 1980). Obviously, marked species differences

128

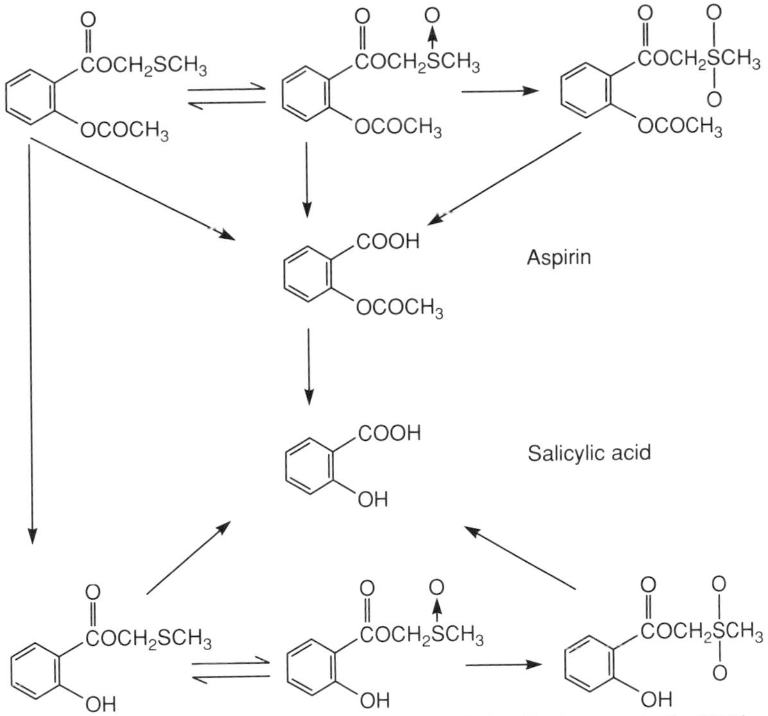

Figure 6.11 Bioactivation of aspirin thioesters (after Loftsson *et al.*, 1981).

exist in the ability to liberate the aspirin moiety, e.g. the availability of salicylate was only 6% that of aspirin in the monkey. In man, mean peak plasma levels were found to be approximately 80% those of aspirin. Since availability of salicylate after intravenous administration was much lower compared to oral administration, the cleavage of the glyceride occurs probably in the gastrointestinal tract before and/or during absorption.

Paris *et al.* (1979) reported about cyclic aspirin triglycerides, such as 1,3-didecanoyl-2-2(2-methyl-4-oxo-1,3-benzodioxan-2-yl)glyceride (Fig. 6.10c). Preliminary results suggest that the plasma salicylate level, obtained 5 h after administration, was approximately 70% of that after an equimolar dose of aspirin.

6.6.2 Methylthiomethyl Ester of Aspirin

The methylthiomethyl, methylsulphinylmethyl and methyl-sulphonyl-methyl esters of aspirin were cleaved *in vitro* in plasma to form aspirin rather than the corresponding salicylates (Fig. 6.11). In the beagle dog,

Pharmacokinetics of aspirin and salicylates

the methylsulphinylmethyl derivative was found to be a true aspirin prodrug, since aspirin was detected in the blood after prodrug administration. Following intravenous administration of the compounds, peak salicylic acid concentrations in plasma occurred after 10–30 min. After oral administration, absorption and/or hydrolysis was delayed resulting in maximum salicylate levels after 5–6 h (Loftsson *et al.*, 1981).

6.6.3 Phenylalanine Derivatives of Aspirin

The phenylalanine ethyl ester and its amide, and the phenylacetate ester of aspirin (Fig. 6.12) have been designed as substrates of digestive enzymes to release aspirin *in vivo* (Banerjee and Amidon, 1981). These prodrugs were tested *in vitro* with regard to substrate activity for the enzymes carboxypeptidase A and chymotrypsin. It could be shown that aspirin phenylalanine ethyl ester was the best substrate for chymotrypsin, while aspirin phenylacetic acid was the best substrate for the carboxypeptidase.

6.7 CONCLUSION

More than 100 years of the use of salicylic acid and more than 90 years of clinical application of aspirin have not exhausted the therapeutic potential of these relatively simple chemical molecules. Following

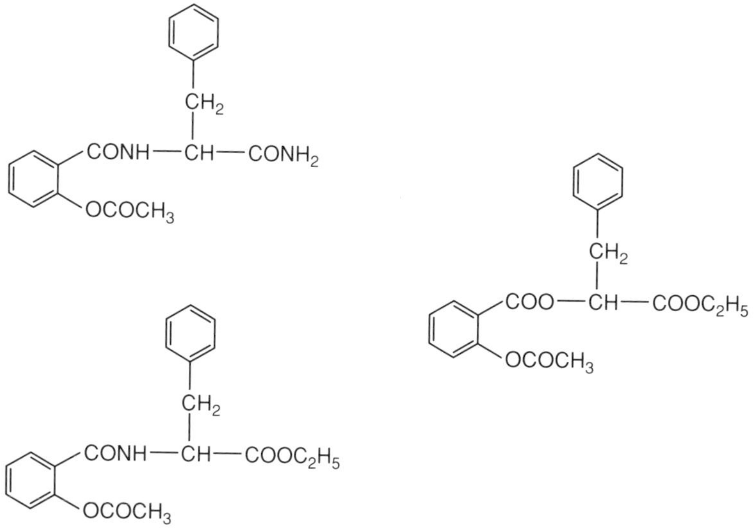

Figure 6.12 Phenylalanine derivatives of aspirin.

130

the administration of salicylic acid and its salts as anti-rheumatic anti-inflammatory compounds, aspirin was recently introduced as an analgesic and anti-thrombotic agent. Most of the latest discoveries and apparent improvements on the basic molecule may be related to pharmacokinetic differences. Dreser, the first pharmacologist who investigated aspirin, came to the conclusion that aspirin is a prodrug of salicylic acid which should be better tolerated. His insight was based on rather imaginative experiments employing the fins of goldfish (Dreser, 1907). Hoffmann's synthesis of acetylsalicylic acid was not aimed at improving the gastric toxicity of salicylic acid or its salts, but rather because Hoffmann's father, who suffered from chronic rheumatic diseases, could no longer stand the aversive taste of large quantities of salicylic acid or its salts. At that time galenic 'tricks' were not on hand, so that the patient had to swallow several grams of bad-tasting powder every day. Under these circumstances, acetylsalicylic acid, owing to its much better taste, was a major improvement. Regrettably, later text books misquoted Hoffmann's observations and claimed aspirin to be a substance much more amenable to the stomach, despite the fact that this theory is not backed by experimental data. We conclude that even the lower toxicity of aspirin as compared to salicylic acid towards goldfish fins was related to the lower acidity of aspirin in comparison to salicylic acid and not to the sustained release of salicylic acid from aspirin.

Later improvements were aimed to either enhance absorption in order to achieve faster pain relief or retard absorption in order to reduce gastric and duodenal toxicity, and enhance lipophilicity in order to reduce the overall gastrointestinal toxicity. All these attempts led to only limited success. Retarded absorption by either the formulation of non-acidic prodrugs or lipophilic substitution of the original molecule may lead to somewhat less gastrointestinal toxicity, but this is achieved at the expense of a delayed onset of action, one of the major merits of aspirin and salicylic acid as compared to more modern NSAIDs. The success of attempts to load the human body with chemical combinations (esters) of either two molecules of salicylates (salsalate) or paracetamol plus aspirin (benorylate) was also rather limited. Either the addition of paracetamol did not improve upon the analgesic effect of aspirin (Lee et al., 1976) or the resulting overall effectiveness and toxicity were comparable. Finally, aspirin salts produced to either improve the absorption or the solubility of aspirin for parenteral administration, were hampered by their limited stability.

In conclusion, it may be stated that one may assume a good galenic preparation of salicylic acid or a suitable salicylic acid salt should still be a good analgesic/anti-phlogistic drug. Aspirin may now have found its final indication, i.e. prevention of unwanted blood-clotting. All other

131

Pharmacokinetics of aspirin and salicylates

derivatives of salicylic acid or other salicylates appear not to have major advantages qualifying them for specific indications at least on the basis of our present knowledge.

REFERENCES

Aylward, M., Maddock, J., Rees, P. et al. (1976) Simultaneous pharmacokinetics of benorylate in plasma and synovial fluid of patients with rheumatoid arthritis. Scan. J. Rheumatol., Suppl. 13, 9–12.

Banerjee, P.K. and Amidon, G.L. (1981) Physicochemical property modification strategies based on enzyme substrate specificities I: Rationale, synthesis, and pharmaceutical properties of aspirin derivatives. J. Pharm. Sci., 70, 1299–303.

Brogden, R.N., Heel R.C., Pakes, G.E. et al. (1980) Diflunisal: A review of its pharmacological properties and therapeutic use in pain and musculoskeletal strains and sprains and pain in osteoarthritis. Drugs, 19, 84–106.

Broh-Kahn, R.H. (1960) Choline salicylate: A new, effective, and well-tolerated analgesic, anti-inflammatory, and anti-pyretic agent. Intern. Rec. Med., 173, 217–33.

Brune, K. (1974) How aspirin might work: A pharmacokinetic approach. Agents Actions, 4, 230–2.

Brune K. and Schneider, E. (1982) Entzündungsreaktionen und ihre Beeinflussung durch antiphlogistisch-analgetische Pharmaka. In Diflunisal, Profil einer neuen Substanz (ed. G. Nuki), Zucherschwerdt Verlag, München, pp. 31–50.

Brune, K. and Lanz, R. (1985) Pharmacokinetics of non-steroidal anti-inflammatory drugs. In Handbook of Inflammation, Vol. 5, The pharmacology of inflammation, (eds I.L. Bonta, M.A. Bray and M.J. Parnham), Elsevier Science Publishers B.V., Amsterdam, pp. 413–49.

Brune, K., Glatt, M. and Graf, P. (1976) Mechanism of action of antiinflammatory drugs. Gen. Pharmacol., 7, 27–33.

Brune, K., Schweitzer, A. and Eckert, H. (1977) Parietal cells of the stomach trap salicylates during absorption. Biochem. Pharmacol., 26, 1735–40.

Carter, G.W., Young, P.R., Sweet, L.R., and Paris, G.Y. (1980) Pharmacological studies in the rat with (2-(1,3-didecanoyl-oxy)-propyl)2-acetyloxy-benzoate (A-45474): An aspirin prodrug with negligible gastric irritation. Agents Actions, 10, 240–5.

Chow, W.H., Cheung, K.L., Ling, H.M. and See, T. (1989) Potentiation of warfarin anticoagulation by topical methylsalicylate ointment. J.R.Soc. Med., 82, 501–2.

Cummings, A.J. and Martin, B.K. (1965) A kinetic study on the elimination of 3-methylsalicylic acid and its acetyl derivative in man. Brit. J. Pharmacol., 25, 470–80.

Danon, A., Ben-Shimon, S. and Ben-Zevi, Z. (1986) Effect of exercise and heat exposure on percutaneous absorption of methyl salicylate. Eur. J. Clin. Pharmacol., 31, 49–52.

Davies, R.O. (1983) Review of the animal and clinical pharmacology of diflunisal. Pharmacotherapy, 3, 9S–22S.

Davis, G.M., Moore, P.T., Siemsen, J.K. *et al.* (1960) A preliminary study on the clinical use of choline salicylate. *Am. J. Med. Sci.*, **239**, 273–7.

Davison, C., Wangler, J. and Smith, P.K. (1962). On the metabolism of o-ethoxybenzamide. *J. Pharmacol. Exp. Ther.*, **136**, 226–31.

Dreser, H. (1907) Ueber modifizierte Salicylsäuren. *Med. Klin.*, **14**, 390–3.

Dromgoole, S.H., Nyman, K.E., Furst, D.E. *et al.* (1978) Metabolism of meseclazone in man. *Drug Metab. Dispos.*, **6**, 102–4.

Dromgoole, S.H., Furst, D.F. and Paulus, H.E. (1981) Rational approaches to the use of salicylates in the treatment of rheumatoid arthritis. *Sem. Arthrit. Rheumat.*, **11**, 257–83.

Dromgoole, S.H., Cassell, S., Furst, D.E. and Paulus, H.E. (1983) Availability of salicylate from salsalate and aspirin. *Clin. Pharmac. Ther.*, **34**, 539–45.

Dromgoole, S.H., Furst, D.E. and Paulus, H.E. (1984) Metabolism of salsalate in normal subjects. *J. Pharm. Sci.*, **73**, 57–9.

Edelson, J., Douglas, J.F. and Ludwig, B.J. (1973) Absorption, distribution and metabolic fate of seclazone (7-chloro-3,3a-dihydro-2H,9H-isoxazolo(3,2-b) (1,3)-benzoxazine-9-one). *J. Pharm. Sci.*, **62**, 229–32.

Edelson, J., Schuster, E., Shahinian, S. and Dougles, J.F. (1974) The Metabolic fate of seclazone in man. *Arch. Int. Pharmacodyn.*, **209**, 66–74.

Edelson, J., Douglas, J.F., Ludwig, B.J. *et al.* (1975) Absorption, distribution and metabolic fate of seclazone (7-chloro-3,3a-dihydro-2-methyl-2H,9H-isoxazolo(3,2-b) (1,3)-benzoxazine-9-one) in rats, dogs, and humans. *J. Pharm. Sci.*, **64**, 1316–21.

Ekstrand, R., Alvyn, G. and Borga, O. (1979) Concentration dependent plasma protein binding of salicylate in rheumatoid patients. *Clin. Pharmacokin.*, **4**, 137–43.

Fleckenstein, L., Mundy, G.R., Horovitz, R.A. and Mazzullo, J.M. (1976) Sodium salicylamide: Relative bioavailability and subjective effects. *Clin. Pharmacol. Ther.*, **19**, 451–8.

Furst, D.E. (1988) Clinically important interactions of nonsteroidal anti-inflammatory drugs with other medications. *J. Rheumatol.*, **15** (Suppl. 17), 58–62.

Gibaldi, M. and Perrier, D. (1982) *Pharmacokinetics*, 2nd ed, Marcel Dekker, Inc., New York, Basel.

Hämäläinen, M., Laine, V.A., Penn, R.G. and Vainio, K. (1973) The passage of benorylate into the synovial fluid and tissue of rheumatoid patients. *Rheumatol. Rehabil.*, Suppl., 85–91.

Harrison, L.I., Funk, M.L., Re, O.N. and Ober, R.E. (1981) Absorption, biotransformation and pharmacokinetics of salicylsalicylic acid in humans. *J. Clin. Pharmacol.* **21**, 401–4.

Hollander, D., Dadufalza, V.D. and Fairchild, P.A. (1981). Intestinal absorption of aspirin: Influence of pH, taurocholate, ascorbate, and ethanol. *J. Lab. Clin. Med.*, **98**, 591–8.

Houston, J.B. and Levy, G. (1975). Modification of drug transformation by vitamin C in man. *Nature*, **225**, 78–9.

Houston, J.B. and Levy, G. (1976). Effect of route of administration on competitive drug biotransformation interaction: Salicylamide–ascorbic acid interaction in rats. *J. Pharmacol. Exp. Ther.*, **198**, 284–94.

Pharmacokinetics of aspirin and salicylates

Humphreys, K.J. and Smy, J.R. (1975). The absorption of benorylate from everted sacs of rat intestine. *J. Pharm. Pharmacol.*, **27**, 962–4.

Kumar, R. and Billimoria, J.D. (1978). Gastric ulceration and the concentration of salicylate in plasma in rats after administration of ^{14}C-labelled aspirin and its synthetic triglyceride, 1,3,-dipalmitoyl-2(2-acetoxy-(^{14}C)carboxylbenzoyl)glycerol. *J. Pharm. Pharmacol.*, **30**, 754–8.

Leary, J.F. (1960) Preliminary pharmacological comparison of choline salicylate with acetylsalicylic acid. *Internat. Rec. Med.*, **173**, 259–61.

Lee, P., Anderson, J.A., Miller, J., Webb, J. and Buchanan, W.W. (1976) Evaluation of analgesic action and efficacy of antirheumatic drugs. *J. Rheumatol.*, **3**, 283–93.

Levy, G. (1965) Pharmacokinetics of salicylate elimination in man. *J. Pharm. Sci.* **54**, 959–67.

Levy, G. (1978) Clinical pharmacokinetics of aspirin. *Pediatrics*, **62** (Suppl.), 867–72.

Levy, G. (1979) Decreased body clearance of diflunisal in renal insufficiency – an alternative explanation. *Brit. J. Clin. Pharmacol.*, **8**, 601.

Levy, G. (1980) Clinical pharmacokinetics of salicylates: a re-assessment. *Brit. J. Clin. Pharmac.*, **10**, 285S–90S.

Levy, G. and Leonards, J.R. (1966). Absorption, metabolism and excretion of salicylates. In *The Salicylates*, (eds M.J.H. Smith and P.K.Smith), John Wiley, New York, pp. 5–48.

Levy, G. and Matsuzawa, T. (1967). Pharmacokinetics of salicylamide elimination in man. *J. Pharmacol. Exp. Ther.*, **156**, 285–93.

Levy, G. and Leonards, J.R. (1971). Urine pH and salicylate therapy. *J. Am. Med. Assoc.*, **217**, 81.

Levy, G. and Giacomini, K.M. (1978). Rational aspirin dosage regimens. *Clin. Pharmacol. Ther.*, **23**, 247–52.

Lin, J.H., Yeh, K.C. and Duggan, D.E (1985). Effect of enterohepatic circulation on the pharmacokinetics of diflunisal in rats. *Drug Metab. Dispos.*, **13**, 321–6.

Liss, E. and Robertson, A. (1975). The distribution and elimination of radioactivity in the rat after administration of ^{14}C-4-acetamidophenyl-2-acetoxy-benzoate (benorylate). *Arzneim.-Forsch. (Drug Res.)*, **25**, 1792–3.

Loewen, G.R., McKay, G. and Verbeeck, R.K. (1986). Isolation and identification of a new major metabolite of diflunisal in man. The sulfate conjugate. *Drug Metab. Dispos.*, **14**, 127–31.

Loftsson, T., Kaminski, J.J. and Bodor, N. (1981). Improved delivery through biological membranes VIII: Design, synthesis, and *in vivo* testing of true prodrugs of aspirin. *J. Pharm. Sci.*, **70**, 743–9.

MacPherson, C.R., Milne M.D. and Evans, B.M. (1955). The excretion of salicylate. *Brit.J.Pharmacol.*, **20**, 484–9.

Manz, G. and Glynn, J.P. (1975). Die Verteilung von Benorilat in Plasma, Synovialflüssigkeit und Synovialgewebe bei rheumatoider Arthritis. *Z. Rheumatol.*, **34**, 400–7 (in German).

Martin, B.K. (1971) The formulation of aspirin. *Adv. Pharmaceut. Sci.*, **3**, 107–71.

Mason, W.D. (1980). Comparative plasma salicylate and urine salicylurate levels following administration of aspirin, magnesium salicylate, and choline magnesium trisalicylate, *J. Pharm. Sci.*, **69**, 1355–6.

Mason, W.D. and Winer, N. (1981). Kinetics of aspirin, salicylic acid, and salicyluric acid following oral administration of aspirin as a tablet and two buffered solutions. *J. Pharm. Sci.* **70**, 262–5.

Miaskiewicz, S.L., Shively, C.A. and Vesell, E.S. (1982). Sex differences in absorption kinetics of sodium salicylate, *Clin. Pharmacol. Ther.*, **31**, 30–7.

Nordquist, P. (1976). Disalicylsäure. *Akt. Goront.*, **6**, 31–6.

Nowak, M.M., Grundhofer, B. and Gibaldi, M. (1974). Rectal absorption from aspirin suppositories in children and adults. *Pediatrics*, **54**, 23–6.

Nuernberg, B. (1986), PhD. thesis, University Erlangen-Nuernberg, FRG.

Nuernberg, B. and Brune, K. (1989). Buffering the stomach contents enhances the absorption of diflunisal in man. *Biopharm. Drug Dispos.*, **10**, 377–87.

Paris, G.Y., Garmaise, D.L. and Cimon, D.G. (1979). Glycerides as prodrugs. 2. 1,3-Dialkanoyl-2-2(2-methyl-4-oxo-1,3-benzodioxan-2-yl)glycerides (cyclic aspirin triglycerides) as antiinflammatory agents. *J. Med. Chem.*, **23**, 79–82.

Paulus, H.E., Siegel, M. and Morgan, E. (1971). Variation of serum concentrations and half-life of salicylate in patients with rheumatoid arthritis. *Arthritis. Rheum.*, **14**, 527–32.

Pedersen, A.K. and Fitzgerald, G.A. (1984). Dose-related kinetics of aspirin. *N. Engl. J. Med.*, **311**, 1206–11.

Podder, S.K., Nakamura, T., Nakashima, M. *et al.* (1988). Comparison of salicylamide and acetaminophen and their prodrug disposition in dogs. *J. Pharmacobio-Dyn.*, **11**, 324–9.

Proost, J.H., Van Imhoff, G.W. and Wesseling, H. (1983). Plasma levels of acetylsalicylic acid and salicylic acid after oral ingestion of plain and buffered acetylsalicylic acid in relation to bleeding time and thrombocyte function. *Pharm. Weekbl. (Sci.)*, **5**, 22–7.

Rainsford, K.D. (1984) *Aspirin and the Salicylates*, Butterworths, London.

Rainsford, K.D., Schwcitzer, A., Green, P. *et al.* (1980). Bio-distribution in rats of some salicylates with low gastric ulcerogenicity. *Agents Actions*, **10**, 457–64.

Ramis, J., Mis, R. and Forn, J. (1989). Pharmacokinetics of fosfosal in rats and dogs. *Arzneim.-Forsch./Drug Res.*, **39**, 74–7.

Roberts, M.S., Favretto, W.A., Meyer, A. *et al.* (1982). Topical bioavailability of methyl salicylate. *Aust. N.Z. J. Med.*, **12**, 303–5.

Roberts, M.S., Rumble, R.H., Wanwimolruk, S., *et al.*, (1983). Pharmacokinetics of aspirin and salicylate in elderly subjects and in patients with alcoholic liver disease. *Eur. J. Clin. Pharmacol.*, **25**, 253–61.

Robertson, A., Glynn, J.P. and Watson, A.K. (1972). The absorption and metabolism in man of 4-acetamidophenyl-2-acetoxybenzoate (benorylate). *Xenobiotica*, **2**, 339–47.

Rowland, M. and Riegelman, S. (1968). Pharmacokinetics of acetylsalicylic acid and salicylic acid after intravenous administration in man. *J. Pharm. Sci.*, **57**, 1313–19.

Rowland, M., Riegelman, S., Harris, P.A. and Sholkoff, S.D. (1972). Absorption kinetics of aspirin in man following oral administration of an aqueous solution. *J. Pharm. Sci.*, **61**, 379–86.

Rubin, A., Rodda, B.E., Warrick, P., Gruber, C.M. Jr. and Ridolfo, A.S. (1973). Interactions of aspirin with nonsteroidal antiinflammatory drugs in man. *Arthritis Rheum.*, **16**, 635–45.

Pharmacokinetics of aspirin and salicylates

Shen, T.Y. (1983). Chemical and pharmacological properties of diflunisal. *Pharmacotherapy*, **3** (Suppl.1), 3S-8S.

Shibasaki, J., Konishi, R., Takemura, M. *et al.* (1984). Comparison of the first-pass metabolism of ethenzamide and salicylamide in rats. *J. Pharmacobio-dyn.*, **7**, 804.

Singleton, P.T. (1980). Salsalate: Its role in the management of rheumatic disease. *Clin. Ther.*, **3**, 80–102.

Soren, A. (1977). Dissociation of acetylsalicylic acid in blood and joint fluid. *Scand. J. Rheumatol.*, **6**, 17–22.

Spahn, H., Altmayer, P., Cattarius-Korb, S. *et al.*, (1985). Untersuchungen zur Bioverfügbarkeit eines Kombinationspräparates von Acetylsalicylsäure und Codeinphosphat. *Arzneim.-Forsch./Drug Res.*, **35**(1), 973–6.

Stafford, W.L. (1962). The binding by bovine plasma and plasma fractions of salicylic acid and some of its 3-alkyl analogues. *Biochem. Pharmacol.*, **11**, 685–92.

Sunkel, C., Cillero, F., Armijo, M., *et al.* (1978). Synthesis and pharmacological properties of eterylate, a new derivative of acetylsalicylic acid. *Arzneim.-Forsch./Drug Res.*, **28**, 1692–4.

Superstine, S.Y., Superstine, E. and Penchas, S. (1978). Comparison of the bioavailiability of aspirin tablets and suppositories. *Isr. J. Med. Sci.*, **14**, 292–4.

Tempero, K.F., Cirillo, V.J. and Steelman, S.L. (1979). Diflunisal: chemistry, toxicology, experimental and human pharmacology. In *Diflunisal: New perspectives in Analgesia* (eds E.C. Huskisson and A.D.S. Caldwell), Royal Society of Medicine, Academic Press, London, pp. 1–20.

Tocco, D.J., Breault, G.O., Zacchei, A.G., Steelman, S.L. and Perrier, C.V. (1975) Physiological disposition and metabolism of 5-(2,4-difluorophenyl)salicylic acid, a new salicylate. *Drug Metab. Dispos.*, **3**, 453–66.

Tozer, T.N., Callaway, J., Hellgeth, M. *et al.* (1989) Concurrent determination of hepatic bioavailabilty of salicylamide by three techniques in the dog. *J. Pharm. Sci.*, **78**, 462–4.

Verbeek, R., Tjandramaga, T.B., Mullie, A. *et al.* (1979a) Biotransformation of diflunisal and renal excretion of its glucuronides in renal insufficiency. *Brit. J. Clin. Pharmac.*, **7**, 273–82.

Verbeek, R., Tjandramaga, T.B., Mullie, A. *et al.* (1979b) Effect of aluminium hydroxide on diflunisal absorption. *Brit. J. Clin. Pharmacol.*, **7**, 519–22.

von Voss, H., Gobel. U., Petrich, C. and Putter, J. (1978) Pharmacokinetic investigations in adult humans after parenteral administration of the lysine salt of acetyl-salicylic acid. *Klin. Wschr.* **56**, 1119–23.

Waschek, J.A., Rubin, G.M., Tozer, T.N. *et al.* (1984) Dose-dependent bioavailability and metabolism of salicylamide in dogs. *J. Pharmacol. Exp. Ther.*, **230**, 89–93.

Waschek, J.A., Fielding, R.M., Tozer, T.N. *et al.* (1986) Availability of plasma sulfate for conjugation of salicylamide in dogs. *Biochem. Pharmacol.*, **35**, 544–6.

Williams, M.E., Weinblatt, M., Rosa, R.M. *et al.* (1986) Salsalate kinetics in patients with chronic renal failure undergoing hemodialysis. *Clin. Pharmacol. Ther.*, **39**, 420–4.

Wilson, J.T., Brown, D.B., Bochini, J.A. and Kearns, G.L. (1982) Efficacy, disposition and pharmacodynamics of aspirin, acetaminophen and choline salicylate in young febrile children. *Therapeut. Drug Monit.* **4**, 147–80.

Woislait, W.D. (1976). Theoretical analysis of the binding of salicylate by human serum albumin: The relationship between free and bound drug and therapeutic levels. *Eur. J. Clin. Pharmacol.*, **5**, 285–90.

Wolf, J. and Aboody, R. (1960). Choline salicylate: A new and more rapidly absorbed drug for salicylate therapy. *Int. Rec. Med.*, **173**, 234–41.

Wood, S.G., John, B.A., Chasseaud, L.F. *et al.* (1983) The metabolism of the anti-inflammatory drug eterylate in rat, dog and man. *Xenobiotica*, **13**, 731–42.

PART THREE
Pharmacology of aspirin and salicylates

7 The anti-inflammatory action of the salicylates

D. A. WILLOUGHBY and R. J. FLOWER

7.1 INTRODUCTION

When considering the anti-inflammatory effects of compounds such as aspirin and the salicylates it is important to define what type of inflammation is targeted. In the case of acute non-immune inflammation this is associated with a predominantly vascular response brought about by the sequential release of pharmacologically active mediators (Di Rosa et al., 1971). The initial mediators are the amines, histamine and 5-hydroxytryptamine followed by the vasoactive polypeptide bradykinin, the process of oedema formation being maintained by release of the prostanoids. This process of increased vascular permeability is associated with the adhesion of leucocytes to the endothelial cells and the migration firstly of the polymorphonuclear leucocytes and ultimately the mononuclear phagocytes which transform into macrophages. This process is brought about by the expression of adhesion molecules on the appropriate cell type followed by the generation and release of chemotactic factors.

In this simple type of inflammation an agent will be considered anti-inflammatory if it exerts an effect on the leakage of the plasma protein from the microcirculation or by stopping the locomotion of the leucocytes.

In long lasting or chronic inflammation, the dominant feature is usually the accumulation of mononuclear phagocytes at a site of injury or irritation. In this type of inflammation the leakage of plasma protein is not so prominent. Unlike acute inflammation this process does not readily resolve. For the inflammation to persist, cells must remain at the site of injury and there are various mechanisms which may contribute to this. In the first instance there is the question of the persistence of the irritant and also there is the possibility of tissue injury subsequent to the initial insult. This may result in the development of modified tissue proteins, in other words an endogenous antigen. Such an antigen could

141

then act as a stimulus for an ongoing autoimmune type of inflammation (Willoughby and Ryan, 1970).

At least three mechanisms have been identified which contribute to the persistence of macrophages at the inflamed site. An experimental granuloma may be variously maintained by: (1) constant migration of mononuclear cells from the circulation; (2) proliferation of cells at the inflamed site (high turnover) with little or no long-term contribution from the cells of the circulation; (3) the formation of a population of long lived cells, which do not depend on more migration or on proliferation; (4) a mixture of all three processes (Spector and Willoughby, 1968). It follows that if a drug prevents one of these activities, say proliferation, and is tested against a low turnover granuloma which is maintained by on-going migration it would be deemed to have no anti-inflammatory activity. Testing this same substance against a high turnover granuloma, it would be classified as an anti-inflammatory.

Further aspects involved in chronic inflammation would include control of the growth of new blood vessels. This is particularly important in the control of large granulomatous masses such as the pannus in rheumatoid arthritis.

It is self-evident that if blood vessel growth or angiogenesis can be controlled then growth developing tissue will be arrested. It is suggested that at least one disease-modifying anti-rheumatic drug, gold, may act in this way. Certainly it has been shown to inhibit endothelial cell proliferation (Matsubara and Ziff, 1987). Such an effect is anti-inflammatory yet not all would consider angiostatic drugs anti-inflammatory *per se*.

Immunological inflammation presents a complex picture and it follows that suppression of the immune response, be it at the level of antigen uptake, lymphocyte proliferation, production of antibody or sensitized cells, or ultimately exposure to antigen, can result in a reduction of the inflammatory response. The reduction of cytokine output will similarly attenuate the response (Desa *et al.*, 1989).

The antigen/antibody mediated type of inflammation resembles acute non-immune inflammation although there are some differences. The sequential release of mediators is essentially the same, however there is a much larger early release of histamine (Willoughby, 1975). There is often an involvement of the complement system and the suppression or depletion of this system will lead to a dramatic reduction in both oedema and accumulation of leucocytes. Curiously a wide variety of non-immune inflammatory stimuli will activate the complement system by way of the alternative pathway. Classical examples are carrageenin and thermal injury (Willoughby *et al.*, 1968).

Cell-mediated immune inflammation is characterized by a slower reaction and in contrast to antigen/antibody reactions which involve large numbers of polymorphonuclear leucocytes (PMNs), it is characterized by an accumulation of mononuclear phagocytes. Once again the cytokines play an important role in the establishment of the inflammatory response, apart from bringing it to fruition, the secretion of lymphokines, such as 'macrophage inhibition factor' ensure that cells move to the inflamed site when they are required. Other lymphokines will contribute towards a proliferation of the macrophages at the site. However, looking at oedema formation it can be shown that this is mediated by the same sequential release of pharmacologically active substances as with the other types of inflammation (Willoughby and Di Rosa, 1972; Doherty, 1989). Hence inhibition of the oedema associated with this type of inflammation could theoretically be induced by the same drugs as those which suppress non-immune inflammation.

In more recent work there is now a concerted effort towards the discovery of 'chondroprotective drugs', that is drugs which afford protection against destruction of cartilage, a prominent feature of the arthropathies (Di Rosa et al., 1972; Doherty, 1989). There appears to be a certain amount of confusion as to whether such agents already exist. Certain cytokines have been proposed as potential destructive agents of cartilage as they 'instruct' chondrocytes to break down cartilage (Dingle et al., 1987).

Cartilage is essentially in a kinetic state with a balance being maintained between synthesis and breakdown of proteoglycan. It has recently been suggested that certain non-steroidal anti-inflammatory drugs (NSAIDs) exert an action on either the catabolic or anabolic process (Lewis, 1978). Additionally, certain NSAIDs have been shown to promote the loss of proteoglycan from cartilage (Desa et al., 1988).

There are a number of models in which to test these different types of activity; in this chapter we will look at the effects of aspirin/salicylates on a variety of such models. It is urged that a suppressive effect or lack of effect in particular needs to be interpreted with great caution.

7.2 ASPIRIN/SALICYLATE IN DIFFERENT MODELS

Non-steroidal anti-inflammatory drugs have been examined for their effect on a wide variety of models often with little idea as to what significance or relevance these may have to human disease. In this brief introduction to the more commonly used models of inflammation we will attempt to outline the underlying mechanisms of the models.

Carrageenin paw oedema was widely used following its introduction in 1962 by Winter et al., and indeed its use contributed to the discovery of indomethacin. In this model carrageenin is injected into the hind paw of rats, and the resultant swelling is measured usually with the aid of a plethysmograph. This model was used for a number of years with little understanding of the release of mediators or pattern of cell migration that followed the injection of the irritant. Finally the mechanism was unravelled and shown to be as described in the general introduction with a sequential release of mediators starting with histamine followed by 5HT during the first 90 mins. These amines were then followed by a short release of bradykinin and the increased leakage of plasma protein was ultimately maintained by the prostaglandins. It was also found that depletion of circulating complement would cause a suppression of foot swelling. This finding was due to serendipity in that attempts were made to study the role of polymorphonuclear leucocytes (PMNs) in bringing about leakage of plasma protein. In the experiments PMNs were depleted using an antibody which resulted in suppression of paw oedema.

Depletion of PMNs using chemical methods failed to affect the oedema. Subsequently complement titres were measured and it was found that the original experiment using an antibody led to a striking depletion of complement. This drop in complement could be reproduced using a variety of methods all of which reduced paw oedema.

It is important to have an appreciation of the mechanisms underlying a particular model of inflammation to avoid misleading results, e.g. if a potential anti-inflammatory agent suppressed this model at 1 h post injection of irritant it is likely to be an antihistamine, whereas if it suppressed at 4–6 h it is more likely to be an inhibitor of the arachidonic acid pathway.

Table 7.1 shows the effect of aspirin and salicylate on models of carrageenin paw oedema. In these models aspirin was more effective during the later phase of the inflammation. This is consistent with the effect being on the prostaglandin-mediated phase of the oedema. Much of this work was actively being pursued prior to the classical demonstration by Vane and his colleagues (1971) that aspirin inhibited the prostaglandin-forming cyclo-oxygenase enzyme. It is interesting that attention was given to the inhibition of migration of mononuclear cells into the inflamed site. Needless to say migration of the mononuclear cells which followed the locomotion of the PMNs was coincident with the release of prostaglandins. Indeed this migration of mononuclear cells could have contributed to the release of prostaglandins. This effect of salicylates on mononuclear cell migration could also be demonstrated *in vitro* (Table 7.1).

One of the early researchers into the effects of salicylates on hind paw oedema was Keleman (1957a,b) who used 5HT or testicular extract as the inflammatory stimulus and observed suppression by salicylates.

Table 7.1 Summary of some of the models in which salicylates have been tested

Model	Result	Ref.
Osteoarthritis in rabbit	Increased $^{35}SO_4$ in cartilage but didn't affect fixed charge density	Marcelon *et al.*, 1975
Cotton pellet granuloma		Domenjoz, 1971
Ocular response to bad endotoxin	Asprin prevents permeability change	Howes and MacKay, 1976
Cartilage destruction in septic arthritis in rabbit	Salicylate failed to protect against cartilage breakdown	Boyer *et al.*, 1977
Endotoxic shock in primates	Unlikely that patients with established shock would benefit from aspirin	Rao *et al.*, 1981
Cerebral vasospasm in dogs	Some benefit in reducing signs	White and Robertson, 1983
Endotoxin shock in rats	Aspirin reduced mortality	Schaper *et al.*, 1988
Ag-induced synovitis in rabbits (Arthus)	Aspirin suppressed exudate and infiltrate	Goldlust *et al.*, 1977
E. coli-induced inflammation in rabbit skin	Aspirin reduced hyperaemia, vascular permeability and leucocyte infiltration	Issekutz and Bhimji, 1982a
Immune complex (RPA) and chemotactic factor inflammation ZAP, $C5_a$ des Arg.	Reduced blood flow infiltration and permeability	Issekutz and Bhimji, 1982b
Arthus reaction in rabbits	Local injection of aspirin reduced blood flow, infiltration and haemorrhage	Crawford, 1988
EAE and adjuvant arthritis	Aspirin and phenylbutazone only effective in adjuvant not in EAE whereas cortisone and 6 MP inhibited both	Rosenthale and Nagra, 1967
Response of AA spleen cells to CON A	Neither aspirin nor indomethacin had an effect	Binderup *et al.*, 1982

Table 7.1 cont.

Model	Result	Ref.
Thermal injury		
Thermal injury in rats	Salicylate suppressed later phase and venular carbon leakage	Spector *et al.*, 1965
Thermal injury in rabbits	Suppressed oedema, improved renal function	Ono *et al.*, 1989
Thermal injury microvasculature; review	Discussion of mediators and mechanisms	Shea *et al.*, 1973
Thermal injury in rats	Salicylate suppressed	Spector and Willoughby, 1959b
Pleural inflammation		
Turpentine pleurisy	Salicylate suppressed later stages of pleurisy	Spector and Willoughby, 1959a
Turpentine pleurisy	Salicylate suppressed pleurisy but only leakage from venules not capillaries	Hurley and Spector, 1965
Dextran pleurisy	Inhibition by aspirin of mononuclear cell migration	Di Rosa *et al.*, 1972
Calcium pyrophosphate inflammation	Acetylsalicylic acid reduced inflammation with no effect on IL1 levels	Paegelow and Werner, 1989
Carrageenin pleurisy	Aspirin suppressed exudate and PGE_2 levels using GC/MS	Harada *et al.*, 1982
Evans blue/ carrageenin pleurisy	Aspirin suppressed increased permeability	Sancilio, 1968
Paw oedema		
Traumatic paw oedema	Sodium salicylate effective	Riesterer and Jacques, 1970
Kaolin paw oedema Cu aspirinate vs aspirin	Little difference	Lewis, 1978
PAF induced paw oedema	Aspirin and salicylate both inhibit	Cordeiro *et al.*, 1986
Carrageenin paw oedema	Showed variability in plasma concentration of aspirin and anti-inflammatory effect also variation due to ambient temperature	Green *et al.*, 1971

Model	Result	Ref.
Carrageenin paw oedema and gastric ulceration in rat	No absolute correlation but also reach the variability of response	Walz et al., 1970
5HT paw oedema	Suppressed by salicylates	Keleman, 1957b
Testicular extract paw oedema	Suppressed by salicylates	Keleman, 1957a
Carrageenin paw oedema	Sequential release of mediators, PG phase susceptible to cyclo-oxygenase inhibitors	Di Rosa et al., 1971
Carrageenin paw oedema	Inhibition of oedema by aspirin and other NSAIDs correlates with inhibition of monocyte migration	Di Rosa and Willoughby, 1971
Carrageenin paw oedema	Showed anti-inflammatory effect on bone marrow precursor cells	Di Rosa et al., 1971
Carrageenin paw oedema	Suppressed with topical Cu salicylate and Cu salicylate mixture	Walker et al., 1980 Korolkiewicz et al., 1989
Carrageenin paw oedema	Salicylate and aspirin equally effective in suppressing oedema and cells	Smith et al., 1975
Carrageenin paw oedema	Suppressed by aspirin and glutamine but increased together	Jain et al., 1988
Cell Migration Dextran pleurisy	Stronger effect on migration of mononuclear cells rather than PMNs	Di Rosa et al., 1972
Carrageenin paw oedema	Migration of mononuclear cells suppressed	Di Rosa and Willoughby, 1971
Carrageenin paw oedema	Migration of mononuclear cells and cytotoxic effect of other NSAIDS	Di Rosa et al., 1971
Leucocyte migration *in vitro*	NSAIDs inhibited leucocyte migration	Meacock and Kitchen, 1975
Leucocyte migration	NSAIDs inhibit	Willoughby and Di Rosa, 1972

Table 7.1 cont.

Model	Result	Ref.
Adjuvant arthritis		
Adjuvant arthritis (rats)	Acetylsalicylic acid reduced paw volumes both injected and non-injected	Walz *et al.*, 1971 Sofia *et al.*, 1973
	Reduced paw oedema and body weight. No effect on articular damage	Martel *et al.*, 1984
	Ethanolic Cu salicylate preparations applied topically suppressed established polyarthritis	Walker *et al.*, 1980
Adjuvant	Topical application of aspirin (6%) reduced oedema and weight loss	Walz *et al.*, 1971
Adjuvant	Compared potency of various drugs: aspirin had lowest activity	Winter and Nuss, 1966
Adjuvant/EAE	Aspirin effective in AA but not EAE	Rosenthale and Nagra, 1967
Adjuvant	Aspirin and other NSAIDs effective on this model	Van Arman *et al.*, 1973
Modified adjuvant		
(1) Adjuvant plus carrageenin at 6 days	Aspirin effective against foot swelling	Mizushima *et al.*, 1972
(2) Early phase adjuvant 4 days	Aspirin slowed development of disease	Wax *et al.*, 1975
Sponge model		
Sponge implant	Aspirin suppresses inflammation but does not increase effect of other NSAIDs	Garrett *et al.*, 1983
Sponge implant	Aspirin suppresses inflammation but is not enhanced by other NSAIDs	Jain *et al.*, 1988

For abbreviations see text.

Injection of carrageenin into the pleural cavity appeared to afford a model which was susceptible to finer analysis of the underlying mechanisms. Although the response is very acute, inflammation in a closed body cavity enables analysis of the whole inflammatory exudate for mediators, protein content, total and differential cell counts. In fact the pleural model confirmed the results of the paw oedema studies with the same sequential release of mediators as described above although much of the analysis of mediators was originally performed using a different irritant, turpentine, injected into the pleural cavity. This irritant unfortunately was cytotoxic so their cell counts were difficult if not nearly impossible to evaluate.

Majno and Palade (1961) and Majno et al. (1961) injected colloidal carbon intravenously to elucidate which vessels were contributing to increased vascular permeability, i.e. venules or capillaries. Their studies showed that all mediators of vascular permeability studied by them affected venules and not capillaries. Using this method Hurley and Spector (1965) found that after intrapleural turpentine only venules leaked carbon initially but that capillary leakage could be observed later (2 h) when venular leakage had ceased. At 5 h venular leakage became intense, with capillary leakage persisting. From 16 to 48 h leakage from venules persisted whereas capillary permeability had returned to normal.

Systemic salicylate which inhibited the major part of exudate formation suppressed the second sustained wave of carbon leakage from the venules but failed to affect the capillary leakage. The early phase of venular leakage could only be suppressed by systemic antihistamines. This supported the view that exudate formation was a consequence of mediators acting sequentially on the venules.

Subsequently other workers showed that treatment with aspirin led to a reduction of prostaglandins in the exudate. Once again it was noted that aspirin would suppress the migration of mononuclear cells into the pleural cavity following either carrageenin or dextran injection (Table 7.1). It is worth remarking that dextran pleurisy has a different pattern of mediators to those hitherto described and is predominantly brought about by histamine and 5HT and it is therefore of interest that mononuclear cells are inhibited by aspirin in this model.

A further model which was also used in the search for non-steroidal anti-inflammatory drugs was thermal injury. This has been well reviewed by Shea et al. (1973). Once again the model of acute inflammation has been shown to be brought about by the same sequential release of mediators described above for carrageenin paw

oedema or carrageenin pleurisy and although the mediators participate in the same sequence their release is faster; thus histamine
and 5HT are released in the first few minutes rather than the
first hour and so on. In striking contrast it has been remarked
that following irradiation injury the release of mediators becomes
even more protracted, with histamine appearing during the first
24 h, then 5HT and ultimately the prostaglandin phase on about
day 3. Once again systemic treatment with salicylate suppresses
the venular leakage of colloidal carbon after thermal injury, with no
effect on the capillaries. This effect of salicylate becomes enhanced
by concomitant treatment with antihistamines. A more recent study
on thermal injury has been performed by Ono and his colleagues
(1989) who not only measured the inhibitory effect of aspirin on
oedema but also noted an improved renal function after treatment
with the drugs.

A model which would seem to have more relevance in the search for
potential anti-rheumatic therapy is adjuvant arthritis. This model was
introduced by Pearson and Wood (1959) who found that following the
subcutaneous injection of complete Freund's adjuvant into the hind
paws of rats, the animals would subsequently develop a generalized
disease with swelling of joints. The inflammation is essentially fairly
acute in the injected paw but with secondaries appearing in the
contralateral paw at about 12 days. This disease would persist for
about 3 weeks. The reaction is a cell-mediated immune reaction and
maybe passively transferred by T-lymphocytes. It is not identical to
human arthritis; the histology differs in the joints and the disease will
finally regress completely. Nevertheless it is a model of more chronic
inflammation driven by T-lymphocytes.

It is of interest that whereas aspirin reduces swelling in both the
injected paw and in the secondary lesions it is without effect on articular
damage. Interestingly, aspirin will protect against the characteristic
weight loss that occurs during the development of the disease. It has
been reported that topical aspirin will reduce the paw swelling although
in some of the experiments the vehicle was ethanol which is itself an
anti-inflammatory agent. Evidence has been produced to suggest that
aspirin is not acting as an immunosuppressant in this model, but is
acting on the released mediators. Indeed, in a comparison between
adjuvant arthritis (AA) and experimental allergic encephalomyelitis,
(EAE) Rosenthale and Nagra (1967) found aspirin only to be effective
against adjuvant arthritis, yet both their models are examples of
cell mediated immunity and both may be passively transferred by
sensitized T cells. In contrast, cortisone and 6-mercaptopurine (6MP)
inhibited inflammation in both models.

Aspirin has been shown to be effective in a variety of Arthus-type reactions which are mediated by released prostaglandins; a classical model is the antigen-induced synovitis in rabbits. Similarly the Arthus reaction in the skin of rabbits showed a reduction in blood flow, permeability, infiltration of cells and haemorrhage after local injection of aspirin. In these models it is apparent that authors invariably report an effect of aspirin or salicylates on cell migration; Issekutz and Bhimji (1982a,b) showed a reduction of cell infiltration following the reverse passive arthus (RPA) reaction and injection of chemotactic factors. Caution must be applied when looking at the effect of the aspirin-like drugs on chemotaxis *in vitro*; many of these drugs are acidic and subsequently cytotoxic for cells (see below) and what is often taken as a dose-response effect on chemotaxis is in effect a dose-response effect on viability of cells.

A model which was widely used to examine the effects of potential NSAIDs was the cotton pellet granuloma model. In this model cotton pellets are implanted subcutaneously and then removed at various times up to 10 days, and the 'wet' and 'dry' weights are measured as an indication of granulation tissue. It is not generally recognized that this model is once again dependent upon T-cells and can be shown to be essentially a cell-mediated immune type reaction. Thus normal thymectomy will suppress the response to cotton pellets in adult rats. Extracts of granulation tissue mixed with adjuvant will lead to a marked increase in the formation of granulation tissue. Conversely, extracts of the granulation tissue injected into neonates will lead to a failure in adult rats to develop granulation tissue around the implanted pellet (Willoughby and Ryan, 1970). This curious reaction appears to be dependent upon the formation of an endogenous antigen. Domenjoz (1971) found a suppression of this reaction in rats following treatment with salicylates (Table 7.1).

In conclusion aspirin/salicylate appear to exert an anti-inflammatory effect in most models of acute and even chronic inflammation. In most of these model systems there is clear evidence for a role for the prostanoids which is often associated with the migration of mononuclear cells. This phenomenon warrants further investigation in view of the more recent identification of adhesion molecules. Aspirin may possibly have a subtle effect on the expression of these molecules in addition to inhibition of the formation of prostanoids. It would also be of interest to look at the effect of aspirin on some of the more chronic models of exudate and cell migration, e.g. carrageenin air pouch model where the exudate persists not merely for 12–24 h but for 4 6 weeks, with a similar migration of cells.

7.3 MECHANISTIC ASPECTS

Throughout their venerable history many theories and hypotheses have been advanced to explain the mechanism of anti-inflammatory, antipyretic and analgesic activity of the aspirin-like drugs. A detailed examination of all of these early ideas is beyond the scope of this chapter but some deserve mention, for whilst they proved unsatisfactory as explanations of the therapeutic activity of these drugs they often proved of value in understanding the side effects or the toxicity. The subject has been extensively reviewed by several authors, Gryglewski (1979) and Smith and Dawkins (1971) have provided particulary useful surveys of this area.

7.3.1 Some Theories from the 'Pre-prostaglandin' Era

Aspirin itself, the salicylates in general and indeed the vast majority of all NSAIDS are acidic in nature and as such can bind to many enzymatic as well as non-catalytic proteins. This phenomenon has been observed by many groups (for example Whitehouse et al. (1971)) and was at one time considered important for their therapeutic effects.

The binding of aspirin and aspirin-like drugs in general to proteins was found to produce many effects; for example these drugs could compete with other low molecular weight substances at their binding sites on proteins thus increasing the free plasma concentration of other substances such as warfarin (Solomon and Schrogie, 1967), barbiturates (Chaplin et al., 1973), urate (Whitehouse et al., 1971) and tryptophan (MacArthur and Dawkins, 1969) to name but a few. Indeed at one time an entire theory concerning the mechanism of action of these drugs was built around their ability to liberate tryptophan from plasma albumin: it was suggested that a peptide inhibitor of inflammation, normally bound to plasma proteins at the tryptophan binding site, was released in the presence of the aspirin-like drugs thus explaining their anti-inflammatory effect (MacArthur et al., 1971). A similar type of mechanism, the displacement of corticosteroids from their binding sites in plasma apparently does not occur (Stenlake et al., 1971).

The ability of aspirin and the other non-steroidal anti-inflammatory agents to bind to proteins has other effects as well. It is said that these agents can unmask 'cryptic' sulphydryl groups within proteins and it has been hypothesized that some of these exposed sulphydryl groups could be important in regulating inflammation (Famaey and Whitehouse, 1975).

Most aspirin-like drugs also protect proteins (e.g. albumin) against chemical or physical denaturation and at one time this test was used as a way of predicting the anti-inflammatory potencies of these drugs (Wagner-Jauregg et al., 1969) although the correlations obtained ultimately proved disappointing.

It has been known for a long while that the aspirin-like drugs have fibrinolytic properties (Gryglewski, 1966) presumably a further consequence of binding to sensitive sites on proteins. Unfortunately many agents which possess fibrinolytic properties are devoid of anti-inflammatory action (Desnoyers et al., 1972) and conversely there are examples of potent acidic aspirin-like drugs which do not possess fibrinolytic activity (Hansch and von Kaulla, 1970; De Clerk et al., 1975). These findings unfortunately mean that this theory has little validity.

In addition to their ability to interact with proteins themselves, many workers have demonstrated that aspirin, salicylates and other related drugs can interact with biological membranes although whether this is a true interaction with the lipid bilayer or with proteins embedded in the bilayer is not clear. Also unclear is the result of such an interaction: some authors maintain that these drugs can stabilize membranes (Miller and Smith, 1966) whilst others report a labilization (Brown and Schwartz, 1969).

Many workers seem to have looked at the effect of these drugs on erythrocyte membranes. Red blood cells from dogs, rats and humans have been reported to be protected against the injurious action of several stimuli by aspirin-like drugs at concentrations in the 'high therapeutic range' (Brown et al., 1967; Inglot and Wolna, 1968; Glenn and Bowman, 1969). This protective effect appears to be dependent upon various other factors such as the pH and the temperature of the assay and indeed a labilizing action may be seen if the temperature is altered.

Disappointingly, there is no strict correlation between the anti-inflammatory and membrane stabilizing properties of the most common aspirin-like drugs, indeed aspirin itself is amongst the weakest of the protecting agents in this group (Tanaka et al., 1973). In addition a great many other drugs display similar types of erythrocyte-stabilizing effects (for example Mikikits et al., 1970).

A major theory to explain the activity of aspirin-like drugs, and indeed other anti-inflammatory drugs was centred about their ability to stabilize the membranes of lysosomes. By preventing the release of hydrolytic and other tissue-degrading enzymes these drugs were supposedly able to reduce chronic inflammation and minimize tissue destruction.

Many groups have described the stabilization of lysosomes isolated from rat liver, or from other cells from other species. Once again there is a considerable discrepancy in the literature. For example factors as diverse as the pH, temperature and composition of the incubation medium appear to affect substantially the results obtained in this type of assay and in the case of lysosomes isolated from rats which had received aspirin-like drugs there are reports suggesting both that the organelles are protected (see for example Ignarro, 1972) or not protected (Pollock and Brown, 1971). There also seems to be a considerable discrepancy between species in as much as aspirin-like drugs in general have been reported to stabilize lysosomes from guinea-pig peritoneal leucocytes but not those from rabbit (Ignarro and Colombo, 1972).

The salicylates are also found to inhibit many enzymes. For example phosphodiesterases from brain and heart as well as other tissues are sensitive to some aspirin-like drugs although aspirin itself does not appear to be effective in this respect (Stefanovich, 1974). For example many authors have reported inhibition of the catalytic activity of enzymes involved in the metabolism of carbohydrates, amino acids as well as peptides, or proteins (Skidmore and Whitehouse, 1966) as well as mucopolysaccharides. Nucleic acid turnover is also reported to be altered by aspirin-like drugs (cf. Westwick *et al.*, 1972). Once again however the activity of the salicylates, and other non-steroidal anti-inflammatory drugs in these tests does not appear to correlate, at least in any meaningful way, with their anti-inflammatory activity (McCoubrey *et al.*, 1970).

Probably the most widely known 'pre-prostaglandin' hypothesis to explain the activity of the aspirin-like drugs prior to the prostaglandin era was that these drugs interfered in some way with oxidative phosphorylation. This area has been reviewed in detail by the originators of the idea and others (for example Whitehouse and Haslam, 1962; Whitehouse, 1964). Briefly, it has been shown that salicylates (and indeed many other aspirin-like drugs) in 'high therapeutic' doses can uncouple oxidative phosphorylation in isolated mitochondria and that this uncoupling action is also seen in mitochondria taken from aspirin treated animals (Mehlman *et al.*, 1972). The mechanism is not known and once again however there does not appear to be any strict correlation between the anti-inflammatory properties of the salicylates and other aspirin-like drugs and their ability to uncouple oxidative phosphorylation *in vivo* or *in vitro* although, interestingly, the uncoupling potencies correlate well with the ability of these drugs to bind to albumin.

The uncoupling effect is undoubtedly important in understanding the side effects of high therapeutic doses of the drugs.

154

7.3.2 The Prostaglandin Era

Not many of the ideas recounted in the previous section served to provide a satisfying explanation for the activity of the aspirin-like drugs and there were several reasons for this. Firstly, as we have seen, there was generally little or no correlation between the activity of the salicylates or other aspirin-like drugs to inhibit a particular biochemical event and their observed anti-inflammatory profile. Furthermore, there was often little theoretical justification for the alleged mechanism. It was not clear how (for example) inhibition of oxidative phosphorylation, or binding to albumin could provide an anti-inflammatory effect. To complicate matters further, it was not at that time understood how the analgesic, antipyretic and anti-inflammatory activities were linked.

Another objection to many of the earlier ideas was that the concentrations needed to achieve the inhibitory effect under examination were only observed at supra-therapeutic levels: this was a serious objection especially in the light of the fact that salicylates and many other aspirin-like drugs are substantially bound to plasma albumin so that the free concentration of the drug in the plasma following an oral dose is often quite small.

Although many of the early theories did not shed much light on the mechanism of action of the aspirin-like drugs at least one group provided some interesting data which were to be important to the research work which followed. Colliers' solution to the problem of how these drugs worked was both original and significant. He termed aspirin 'an anti-defensive' drug because of its ability to prevent the physiological defence mechanisms of pain, fever and inflammation from functioning normally (Collier, 1969). Together with his group, Collier demonstrated that aspirin blocked bronchoconstriction in guinea-pigs caused by SRS-A and bradykinin injection and also blocked the contraction of the isolated tracheobronchial muscle induced by the same agents.

It was not clear to the group how this bronchoconstrictor response was inhibited. Initially, Collier suggested that 'A-receptors' (i.e. those that could be blocked by aspirin) were involved in the spasmogenic response to these agents, but he later abandoned this concept, writing instead that the drugs acted '. . . rather by inhibiting some underlying cellular mechanism . . .' (Collier, 1969).

Vane tells us that the idea that aspirin blocked prostaglandin synthesis came to him while reviewing some experiments in which he and a colleague had demonstrated that aspirin prevented the release of 'RCS' from guinea-pig and dog lung. At the time, 'RCS' was thought by Vane to be an intermediate in the generation of prostaglandins and since agents that released RCS presumably did so by causing its synthesis then 'a logical corollary was that aspirin might well be blocking the synthesis of prostaglandins' (Vane, 1972).

What followed is now well known. In 1971 three papers appeared in *Nature* demonstrating that aspirin and several other aspirin-like drugs blocked prostaglandin synthesis in a cell-free system (Vane, 1971), in an isolated perfused organ (Ferreira *et al.*, 1971) and in human platelets following oral administration (Smith and Willis, 1971). The importance of this discovery was heightened because of the growing realization that the prostaglandins were involved in the pathogenesis of inflammation, fever and pain.

This discovery initiated a new phase of research into the biochemistry of the aspirin-like drugs and provoked an enormous literature. In the original papers only aspirin, indomethacin and sodium salicylate had been tested as inhibitors but it was soon demonstrated that nearly all the commonly used aspirin-like drugs were inhibitors of the cyclo-oxygenase enzyme and, most important, that this inhibition could be achieved following therapeutic concentrations of these drugs (Flower *et al.*, 1972).

In contrast to many of the other proposed test systems there appeared to be a general correlation between the anti-inflammatory activity of the aspirin-like drugs and their anti-cyclo-oxygenase activity. Indeed, several quite striking correspondences were observed, particularly between some pairs of enantiomers. The observations of Ham and his colleagues (1972) and of Tomlinson and co-workers (1972) are especially noteworthy. The latter group observed that there was a very impressive correlation between the anti-enzyme and anti-inflammatory actions in the case of naproxen and its enantiomer. Naproxen itself was 150 times more potent than aspirin against bovine seminal vesicle cyclo-oxygenase and 200 times more potent against adjuvant-induced arthritis in rats. The enantiomer of naproxen was much less potent against the cyclo-oxygenase (only twice as potent as aspirin) and had almost no activity in the arthritis test. Takeguchi and Sih (1972) also reported similar findings with another series of enantiomeric pairs and indeed took the matter even further using the cyclo-oxygenase test to screen for inhibitors which were subsequently found to have anti-inflammatory properties.

This ability of the cyclo-oxygenase to distinguish between dextro- and laevo-rotatory isomers is lacking in all other *in-vitro* tests of inflammatory drugs and reinforces the idea that this test can be used to pick out candidate compounds for *in-vivo* anti-inflammatory testing.

As with all *in-vitro* tests, not all inhibitors that are discovered will turn out to be effective *in vivo*. The tests cannot predict whether or not the drug will reach its target when given orally and neither can it reveal drugs that must first be metabolized to active compounds. A very interesting case in point is the anti-inflammatory sulindac, which must be oxidized to its sulphone derivative and then reduced to the corresponding sulphide *in vivo* before it becomes active (Van Arman *et al.*, 1976). The biologically active sulphide is more than 500 times more potent that sulindac itself as an inhibitor of the cyclo-oxygenase, again confirming the correlation between the enzyme test and therapeutic activity.

Whilst it is true to say that virtually all the aspirin-like drugs inhibit the cyclo-oxygenase enzyme it seems impossible to generalize about the nature of inhibitory activity; in fact, with one or two exceptions, their mechanism of inhibition is unclear. Appropriately enough however the mechanism of action of aspirin itself is reasonably well established and Roth and Siok (1978) have established that aspirin inactivates the cyclo-oxygenase enzyme by acetylating a serine at the active site.

7.3.3 Anomalies

There is now a great deal of evidence to suggest that the prostaglandins are involved in the pathogenesis of fever, inflammation and pain, and that the principal mechanism of action of the aspirin-like drugs is brought about by interfering with their synthesis. This evidence has been well rehearsed in many reviews and also in this book. It will not be repeated in this chapter. There are however some interesting discrepancies in the literature concerning the activity of these drugs.

Ironically, the chief problem concerns the activity of the archetypal drug, salicylic acid. Even in the early experiments it was evident that the *in-vitro* activity of this drug was extremely low compared with its close relative, aspirin. This was worrying because the two drugs appeared virtually equiactive *in vivo*, not only in terms of their therapeutic effects but also in their ability to block prostaglandin formation in inflammatory exudates (Willis *et al.*, 1972) or in healthy volunteers (Hamberg *et al.*, 1972). The work of the latter author is especially important because it clearly demonstrates that oral salicylate reduces the whole body generation of prostaglandins as estimated by the output of metabolites in the urine. In this interesting study there was a detectable latency in the anti-cyclo-oxygenase action of salicylic acid when compared to aspirin or indomethacin.

How then does salicylic acid produce its effect? Various ideas have been explored, indeed it has been suggested that the therapeutic levels of salicylate in the plasma are sufficient to inhibit prostaglandin synthesis in any case (Higgs in this book). Other authors have suggested that salicylic acid has first to be metabolized to an active inhibitor (Vane,

1972; Willis *et al.*, 1972; Blackwell *et al.*, 1975). With reference to this latter hypothesis, the metabolism of salicylate has been fairly well investigated and several metabolites have been tested as putative inhibitors of the cyclo-oxygenase. Although it is true that certain dihydroxy acid metabolites of salicylic acid were considerably (about 34 times) more potent cyclo-oxygenase inhibitors than the parent compound (Flower, 1974; Blackwell *et al.*, 1975), because of the low conversion to these compounds *in vivo* it seems unlikely that the formation of these substances could account for the full observed activity of salicylic acid. It could be that some hitherto undiscovered metabolite, maybe even aspirin itself, is responsible for the anti-cyclo-oxygenase activity of salicylic acid. It is indeed an irony that the first anti-inflammatory used by man, and the simplest drug from the chemical viewpoint, should have such a complex mode of action.

Another problem of a similar nature arose with the drug, paracetamol. This drug is a potent antipyretic and analgesic agent but did not seem active against cyclo-oxygenase preparations obtained from peripheral tissues such as the spleen. This seems to fit with the idea that the drug displayed low anti-inflammatory activity but sheds no light upon its ability to produce an antipyretic and analgesic effect.

In 1972, Flower and Vane published data suggesting that paracetamol was more active on the brain cyclo-oxygenase than on that of peripheral tissues and that this explained the apparent differences in biological activity. Although this idea was controversial, several papers have lent credence to the general proposition. For example Tolman *et al.*, (1983) have shown quite clearly that when paracetamol is given orally it produces a selective inhibition of brain cyclo-oxygenase although the exact mechanism by which it does this was not settled. More recently, Ferrari and his colleagues (1990) have shown that aspirin, paracetamol and several commonly used aspirin-like drugs inhibited the *ex-vivo* production of prostaglandin E_2 in brains removed from mice which had received the drugs orally. They demonstrated that there was a good correlation with both their potency as inhibitors of mouse brain cyclo-oxygenase *in vitro* as well as their anti-nociceptive action in a mouse abdominal constriction test. Again this lent further support to the concept of selective action of this particular member of the family.

We will conclude this section on potential mechanisms by referring to a totally novel and potentially exciting finding made by Wu and his colleagues (Sanduja *et al.*, 1991) which could shed light upon the salicylate controversy. Wu has found both salicylate itself (as well as some other aspirin-like drugs including paracetamol) active in depressing transcription of cyclo-oxygenase messenger RNA in endothelial cells. This surprising finding could suggest yet another action of these deceptively simple anti-inflammatory agents.

REFERENCES

Binderup, L., Bramm, E. and Arrigoni-Martelli, E. (1982) The effect of some anti-rheumatic drugs *in vivo* on the response of spleen cells to concanavalin A in rats with chronic inflammation. *Int. J. Immunopharm.*, **4**, 57–66.

Blackwell, G., Flower, R.J. and Vane, J.R., (1975) Some characteristics of the prostaglandin synthesizing system in rabbit kidney microsomes. *Biochim. Biophys. Acta*, **398**, 178–90.

Boyer, J., Daniel, D., Akeson, W.H. *et al.* (1977) Effect of salicylate therapy on cartilage destruction in experimental arthrosis. *Clin. Orthop. Rel. Res.*, **126**, 302–4.

Brown, J.H. and Schwartz, N.L. (1969) Interaction of lysosomes and anti-inflammatory drugs. *Proc. Soc. Exp. Biol. Med*, **131**, 614–20.

Brown, J.H., Mackay, H.K., and Rigillo D.A. (1967) A novel *in vitro* assay for anti-inflammatory agents based on stabilization of erythrocytes. *Proc. Soc. Exp. Biol. (NY)*, **125**, 837–43.

Chaplin, M.D., Roszkowski, A.P. and Richards, R.K. (1973) Displacement of thiopental from plasma proteins by non-steroidal anti-inflammatory agents. *Proc. Soc. Exp. Biol. Med*, **143**, 667–71.

Collier, H.O.J. (1969) A pharmacological analysis of aspirin. *Adv. Pharmacol. Chemother.*, **7**, 333–405.

Cordeiro, R.S.B., Silva, P.M.R., Martins, M.A. and Vargaftig, B.B. (1986) Salicylates inhibit PAF-acether-induced rat paw oedema when cyclo-oxygenase inhibitors are ineffective. *Prostaglandins*, **32**, 719–27.

Crawford, J.P. (1988) Pharmacological modulation of localized inflammatory reactions: the non-steroidal anti-inflammatory drug as an adjunct to therapy. *J. Manip. Physiolog. Therapeut.*, **11**, 17–23.

De Clerck, F., Vermylen, J. and Reneman, R. (1975) Effects of suprofen, an inhibitor of prostaglandin biosynthesis, on platelet function, plasma coagulation and fibrinolysis I. *In vitro* experiments. *Arch. Int. Pharmacodyn Ther.*, **216**, 263–79.

Desa, F.M., Chander, C.L., Howat, D.W. *et al.* (1988) Indomethacin and cartilage breakdown. *J. Pharm. Pharmacol*, **40**, 667–70.

Desa, F.M., Moore, A.R., Chander, C.H. *et al.* (1989) Cellular interaction in cartilage degradation. *Int. J. Tiss. React.*, **11**, 213–17.

Desnoyers, P., Labume, J., Conrad J. and Samama, M. (1972) Research on the mechanism of synthetic thrombolytic agents. *Acta Univ. Carol* [med] (Praha). **52**, 33–40.

Dingle, J.T., Page-Thomas, D.P., King, B., and Bard, D.R. (1987) *In vivo* studies of articular damage mediated by catabolin/interleukin 1. *Ann. Rheum. Dis.*, **46**, 527–33.

Di Rosa, M. and Willoughby, D.A. (1971) Screens for anti-inflammatory drugs. *J. Pharm. Pharmac.*, **23**, 297–8.

Di Rosa, M., Papadimitriou, J.M. and Willoughby, D.A. (1971) A histopathological and pharmacological analysis of the mode of action of non-steroidal anti-inflammatory drugs. *J. Pathol.*, **105**, 239–56.

Di Rosa, M., Sorrentino, L. and Parente, L. (1972) Non-steroidal anti-inflammatory drugs and leucocyte emigration. *J. Pharm. Pharmac.*, **24**, 575–77.

Doherty, M. (1989) Chondroprotection by non-steroidal anti-inflammatory drugs. *Ann. Rheum. Dis.*, **48**, 617–19.

Domenjoz, R. (1971) Aspects de la chimiotherapie antirhumatismale. *Bull. Chim. Ther.*, **4**, 284–90.

Famaey, J.P. and Whitehouse, M.W. (1975) Interaction between non-steroidal anti-inflammatory drugs and biological membranes. IV. Effects of non-steroidal anti-inflammatory drugs and various ions on the availability of sulfhydryl groups and lymphoid cells and mitochondrial membranes. *Biochem. Pharmacol.*, **24**, 1609–15.

Ferrari, R.A., Ward, S.J., Zobre, C.M. *et al.* (1990) Estimation of the *in vivo* effect of cyclo-oxygenase inhibitors on protaglandin E_2 levels in mouse brain. *Eur. J. Pharmacol.*, **179**, 25–34.

Ferreira, S.H., Moncada, S. and Vane, J.R. (1971) Indomethacin and aspirin abolish prostaglandin release from the spleen. *Nature*, **231**, 237–9.

Flower, R.J. (1974) Drugs which inhibit prostaglandin synthesis. *Pharmacol. Rev.*, **26**, 33–67.

Flower, R.J. and Vane, J.R. (1972) Inhibition of prostaglandin synthetase in brain explains the anti-pyretic activity of paracetamol (4-acetamidophenol). *Nature*, **240**, 410–11.

Flower, R.J., Gryglewski, R., Herbaczynska-Cedro, K. and Vane, J.R. (1972) The effects of anti-inflammatory drugs on prostaglandin biosynthesis. *Nature*, **238**, 104–6.

Garrett, R., Manthey, B., Vernon-Roberts, B. and Brooks, P.M. (1983) Assessment of non-steroidal anti-inflammatory drug combinations by the polyurethane sponge implantation model in the rat. *Ann. Rheum. Dis.*, **42**, 439–42.

Glenn, E.M. and Bowman, B.J. (1969) *In vitro* effects of non-steroidal anti-inflammatory drugs. *Proc. Soc. Exp. Biol. Med*, **130**, 1327–32.

Goldlust, M.B., Rich, L.C. and Harrity, T.W. (1977) Effects of anti-inflammatory agents on the acute response of immune synovitis in rabbits. *Arthrit. Rheum.*, **20**, 937–46.

Green, A.Y., Green, D., Murray, P.A. and Wilson, A.B. (1971) Factors influencing the inhibitory action of anti-inflammatory drugs on carrageenin induced oedema. *Brit. J. Pharmac.*, **41**, 132–9.

Gryglewski, R.J. (1966) The fibrynolytic activity of anti-inflammatory drugs. *J. Pharm. Pharmacol.*, **18**, 474.

Gryglewski, R.J. (1979) Screening and assessment of the potency of anti-inflammatory drugs *in vitro*. In *Anti-inflammatory Drugs* (eds. J.R. Vane and S.H. Ferreira), Springer-Verlag, Berlin, Heidelberg, New York, pp. 4–43.

Ham, E.A., Cirillo, K.J., Zanetti, M. *et al.* (1972) Studies on the mode of action of non-steroidal, anti-inflammatory agents. In *Prostaglandins in Cell Biology* (eds. P.W. Ramwell and B.B. Phariss), Plenum Press, New York, pp. 345–52.

Hamberg, M. (1972) Inhibition of prostaglandin synthesis in man. *Biochem. Biophys. Res. Commun.*, **49**, 720–6.

Hansch, C. and von Kaulla, K.N. (1970) Fibrinolytic congeners of benzoic and salicylic acid. A mathematical analysis of correlation between structure and activity. *Biochem. Pharmacol.*, **19**, 2193–200.

Harada, Y., Tanaka, K., Uchida, Y. *et al.* (1982) Changes in the levels of prostaglandins and thromboxane and their roles in the accumulation of exudate in rat carrageenin-induced pleurisy – a profile analysis using gas chromatography mass spectrometry. *Prostaglandins*, **23**, 881–95.

Howes, E.L. Jr. and McKay, D.G. (1976) The effects of aspirin and indomethacin on the ocular response to circulating bacterial endotoxin in the rabbit. *Investig. Ophthalmol.*, **15**, 648–51.

Hurley, J.V. and Spector, W.G. (1965) A topographical study of increased vascular permeability in acute turpentine-induced pleurisy. *J. Path. Bact.*, **89**, 245–54.

Ignarro, L.J. (1972) Lysosomal membrane stabilization *in vivo*: effects of steroidal and non-steroidal anti-inflammatory drugs on the integrity of rat liver lysosomes. *J. Pharmacol. Exp. Ther.*, **182**, 179–88.

Ignarro, L.J. and Colombo, C. (1972) Enzyme release from guinea pig polymorphonuclear leukocyte lysosomes inhibited *in vitro* by anti-inflammatory drugs. *Nature (New Biol.)*, **239**, 155–7.

Inglot, A.D. and Wolna, E. (1968) Reactions of non-steroidal anti-inflammatory drugs with the erythrocyte membrane. *Biochem. Pharmacol.*, **17**, 269–79.

Issekutz, A.C. and Bhimji, S. (1982a) The effect of non steroidal anti-inflammatory agents on *Escherichia coli* induced inflammation, *Immunopharmacology*, **4**, 11–12.

Issekutz, A.C. and Bhimji, S. (1982b) Effect of non-steroidal anti-inflammatory agents on immune complex and chemotactic factor-induced inflammation. *Immunopharmacology*, **4**, 253–66.

Jain, P., Khanna, N.K. and Godhwani, J.L. (1988) A possible drug interaction between aspirin and L-glutamine on some experimental inflammatory and analgesic models. *Indian J. Exp. Biol.*, **26**, 368–70.

Keleman, E. (1957a) Local inhibition of the testicular extracts-induced oedema of the rat's hind paw. *Acta Physiol. Acad. Sci. Hungary*, **11**, 121–4.

Keleman, E. (1957b) The inhibition by sodium salicylate of oedema of the hind paw of the rat induced by 5-hydroxytryptamine. *Brit. J. Pharmacol.*, **12**, 28–29.

Korolkiewicz, Z., Hac, E., Gcagalo, I., Gorczyca, P. and Lodzinska, A. (1989) The pharmacologic activity of complexes and mixtures with copper and salicylates or aminopyrine following oral dosing in rats. *Agents Actions*, **26**, 355–9.

Lewis, A.J. (1978) A comparison of the anti-inflammatory effects of copper aspirinate and other copper salts in the rat and guinea pig. *Agents Actions*, **8**, 244–50.

Majno, G. and Palade, G.E. (1961) Studies on inflammation. I. The effect of histamine and serotonin on vascular permeability in acute turpentine-induced pleurisy. *J. Biophys. Biochem. Cytol.*, **11**, 571–605.

Majno, G., Palade, G.E. and Schoeffl, G.I. (1961) Studies on inflammation. II. The site of action of histamine and serotonin along the vascular tree. A topographic study. *J. Biophys. Biochem. Cytol.*, **11**, 607–26.

Marcelon, G., Cros, J. and Guiraud, R. (1975) Activity of anti-inflammatory drugs on an experimental model of osteoarthritis. In *Future Trends*

Pharmacology of aspirin and salicylates

in Inflammation II (eds J.P. Giroud, D.A. Willoughby, and G.P. Velo), Birkhauser Verlag, Basel, pp. 191–4.

Martel, R.R., Klicius, J., Metcalf, G. (1984) Effect of etodolac on articular and bone pathology associated with adjuvant arthritis in rats: a comparison with aspirin and naproxen. *Agents Actions*, **14**, 257–64.

Matsubara, T. and Ziff, M. (1987) Inhibition of human endothelial cell proliferation by gold compounds. *J. Clin Invest.* **79**, 1440–3.

McArthur, J.N. and Dawkins, P.D. (1969) The effect of sodium salicylate on the binding of L-tryptophan to serum proteins. *J. Pharm. Pharmacol.*, **21**, 744–50.

McArthur, J.N., Dawkins, P.D., Smith, M.J.H. and Hamilton, E.B.D. (1971) Mode of action of anti-rheumatic drugs. *Brit. Med. J.*, **ii**, 677–9.

McCoubrey, A., Smith, M.H. and Lane, A.C. (1970) Inhibition of enzymes by alkylsalicylic acids. *J. Pharm. Pharmacol.*, **22**, 333–7.

Meacock, S.C.R. and Kitchen, E.A. (1975) Some effects of non-steroidal anti-inflammatory drugs on leucocyte migration. In *Future Trends in Inflammation II* (eds J.P. Giroud, D.A. Willoughby, and G.P. Velo), Birkhauser Verlag, Basel, pp. 320–5.

Mehlman, M.A., Tobin, R.B. and Sporn, E.M. (1972) Oxidative phosphorylation and respiration by rat liver mitochondria from aspirin-treated rats. *Biochem. Pharmacol.*, **21**, 3279.

Mikikits, S., Mortara, A. and Spector, R.G. (1970) Effect of drugs on red cell fragility. *Nature (Lond.)*, **225**, 1150–1.

Miller, W.S. and Smith, J.G. (1966) Effect of acetylsalicylic acid on lysosomes. *Proc. Soc. Exp. Biol. Med*, **122**, 634–6.

Mizushima, Y., Tsukada, W. and Akimoto, T. (1972) A modification of rat adjuvant arthritis for testing anti-rheumatic drugs. *J. Pharm. Pharmacol.*, **24**, 781–5.

Ono, I., Ohura, T., Azami, K. *et al.* (1989) The effects of drugs on the arachidonate cascade in experimentally burned rabbits. *J. Burn Care Rehabil.*, **10**, 314–20.

Paegelow, I. and Werner, H. (1989) Modulation of the IL-1 content by anti-inflammatory drugs during an acute non-specific inflammation. *Agents Actions*, **26**, 189–90.

Pearson, C.M. and Wood, F.D. (1959) Studies of polyarthritis and other lesions induced in rats by injection of mycobacterial adjuvant. *Arthrit. Rheum.*, **2**, 440–59.

Pollock, S.H. and Brown, J.H. (1971) Studies on the acute inflammatory response. III. Glucocorticoids and vitamin E (*in vivo*) attenuate thermal labilization of isolated hepatic lysosomes. *J. Pharmacol. Exp. Ther.*, **178**, 609–15.

Rao, P.S., Cavanagh, D. and Gaston, L.W. (1981) Endotoxic shock in the primate: effects of aspirin and dipyridamole administration. *Am. J. Obstet. Gynecol.*, **140**, 914–22.

Riesterer, L. and Jaques, R. (1970) The influence of anti-inflammatory drugs on the development of an experimental traumatic paw oedema in the rat. *Pharmacology*, **3**, 243–51.

Rosenthale, M.E. and Nagra, C.L. (1967) Comparative effects of some immuno-suppressive and anti-inflammatory drugs on allergic encephalomyelitis and adjuvant arthritis. *Proc. Soc. Exp. Biol. Med.*, **125**, 149–53.

Roth, G.R. and Siok, C.J. (1978) Acetylation of the NH_2-terminal serine of the prostaglandin synthetase by aspirin. *J. Biol. Chem.*, **253**, 3782–4.

Sancilio, L.F. (1968) Effect of acetylsalicylic acid and hydrocortisone on the pleural response to Evans blue carrageenin. *Proc. Soc. Exp. Biol. Med.*, **127**, 597–600.

Sanduja, R., Loose-Mitchell, D. and Wu, K.K. (1991) Inhibition of de novo synthesis and message expression of prostaglandin H synthase by salicylates. *Adv. Prostaglandin Thromboxane Leukotriene Res.*, **21**, 149–52.

Schaper, U., Lueddeckens, G., Forster, W. and Scheuch, D.W. (1988) Inhibition of lipoxygenase (LOX) or of cyclo-oxygenase (COX) improves survival of rats in endotoxin shock. *Biomed. Biochem. Acta*, **47**, 282–5.

Shea, S.M., Caulfield, J.B. and Burke, J.F. (1973) Microvascular ultrastructure in thermal injury: a reconsideration of the role of mediators. *Microvasc. Res.*, **5**, 87–96.

Skidmore, I.F. and Whitehouse, M.W. (1966) Concerning the regulation of some diverse biochemical reactions under the inflammatory response by salicylic acid, phenylbutazone and other acidic anti-rheumatic drugs. *J. Pharm. Pharmacol.*, **18**, 558–60.

Smith, J.B. and Willis, A.L. (1971) Aspirin selectively inhibits prostaglandin production in human platelets. *Nature*, **231**, 235–7.

Smith, M.J.H. and Dawkins, P.D. (1971) Salicylate and enzymes. *J. Pharm. Pharmacol.*, **23**, 729–44.

Smith, M.J.H., Ford-Hutchinson, A.W. and Elliot, P.N.C. (1975) Prostaglandins and the anti-inflammatory activities of aspirin and sodium salicylate. *J. Pharm. Pharmacol.*, **27**, 473–8.

Sofia, R.D., Vassar, H.B. and Nalepa, S.D. (1973) Correlations between pathological changes in the hind paws of rats with adjuvant arthritis and their response to anti-inflammatory and analgesic drugs. *Eur. J. Pharmacol.*, **24**, 108–12.

Solomon, H.M. and Schrogie, J.J. (1967) The effect of various drugs on the binding of warfarin-^{14}C to human albumin. *Biochem. Pharmacol.*, **16**, 1219–26.

Spector, W.G. and Willoughby, D.A. (1959a) The demonstration of the role of mediators in turpentine pleurisy in rats by experimental suppression of the inflammatory changes. *J. Path. Bact.*, **77**, 1–17.

Spector, W.G. and Willoughby, D.A. (1959b) Experimental suppression of the acute inflammatory changes of thermal injury. *J. Path. Bact.*, **78**, 121–32.

Spector, W.G. and Willoughby, D.A. (1968) The origin of mononuclear cells in chronic inflammation and tuberculin reactions in the rat. *J. Path. Bact.*, **96**, 389–97.

Spector, W.G., Walters, M.N.I. and Willoughby, D.A. (1965) Venular and capillary permeability in thermal injury. *J. Path. Bact.*, **90**, 635–40.

Stefanovich, V. (1974) Inhibition of 3',5'-cyclic AMP phosphodiesterase with anti-inflammatory agents. *Res. Commun. Chem. Pathol. Pharmacol.*, **7**, 573–82.

Stenlake, J.B., Williams, W.D., Davidson, A.G. and Downie, W.W. (1971) The effect of anti-inflammatory drugs on the protein-binding of 1,2-^{3}H cortisol in human plasma *in vitro*. *J. Pharm. Pharmacol.*, **23**, 145–6.

Takeguchi, C. and Sih, C.J. (1972) A rapid spectrophotometric assay for prostaglandin synthetase: Application to the study of non-steroidal, anti-inflammatory agents. *Prostaglandins*, **2**, 169–84.

Tanaka, K., Kobayashi, K. and Kazui, S. (1973) Temperature dependent reaction of flufenamic acid with rat erythrocyte membrane. *Biochem. Pharmacol.*, **22**, 879–86.

Tolman, E.L., Fuller, B.L., Marinan, B.A. *et al*. (1983) Tissue selectivity and variability of effects of acetaminophen on arachidonic acid metabolism. *Prostaglandins Leukotrienes Med.*, **12**, 347–56.

Tomlinson, R.V., Ringold, H.J., Qureshi, M.C. and Forchielli, E. (1972) Relationship between inhibition of prostaglandin synthesis and drug efficacy: Support for theory on mode of action of aspirin-like drugs. *Biochem. Biophys. Res. Commun.*, **46**, 552–9.

Van Arman, C.G., Nuss, G.W. and Risley, G.A. (1973) Interactions of aspirin, indomethacin and other drugs in adjuvant-induced arthritis in the rat. *J. Pharmacol. Exp. Ther.*, **187**, 400–14.

Van Arman, C.G., Risley, E.A., Nuss, G.W., *et al*. (1976) Pharmacology of sulindac. In *Clinoril in the Treatment of Rheumatic Disorders: A New Non-steroidal Anti-inflammatory/Analgesic Agent. Proceedings of a Symposium, VII European Rheumatology Congress* (eds E.C. Huskisson and P. Franchimont), Raven Press, New York, pp. 9–36.

Vane, J.R. (1971) Inhibition of prostaglandin synthesis as a mechanism of action for aspirin-like drugs. *Nature*, **231**, 232–5.

Vane, J.R. (1972) Prostaglandins and the aspirin-like drugs. *Hosp. Pract.* (March), 61–71.

Wagner-Jauregg, T., Burlimann, W. and Fischer, J. (1969) Vergleich anti-phlogistischer Substanzen im Plasmaeiweiß Trubungstest nach Mizushima. *Arzneimittel-Forsch.*, **19**, 1532–6.

Walker, W.R., Beveridge, S.J. and Whitehouse, M.W. (1980) Anti-inflammatory activity of a dermally applied copper salicylate preparation (Alcusal). *Agents Actions*, **10**, 38–47.

Walz, D.T., Di Martino, M.J., Griffin, C.L. and Misher, A. (1970) Investigation of the carrageenin-induced rat paw oedema assay and correlation between anti-inflammatory activity and gastric haemorrhage production in the rat. *Arch. Int. Pharmacodyn. Ther.*, **185**, 337–43.

Walz, D.T., Dolan, M.M., Di Martino, M.J. and Yankell, S.L. (1971) Effects of topical hydrocortisone and acetylsalicylic acid on the primary lesion of adjuvant-induced arthritis. *Proc. Soc. Exp. Biol. Med.*, **137**, 1466–9.

Wax, J., Tersman, D.K., Winder, C.V. and Stephens, M.D. (1975) A sensitive method for the comparative bioassay of non-steroidal anti-inflammatory compounds in adjuvant-induced primary inflammation in the rat. *J. Pharmacol. Exp. Ther.*, **192**, 166–71.

Westwick, W.J., Allsop, J. and Watts, R.W.E. (1972) A study of the effect of some drugs which cause agranulocytosis on the biosynthesis of pyrimidines in human granulocytes. *Biochem. Pharmacol.*, **21**, 1955–66.

White, R.P. and Robertson, J.T. (1983) Comparison of piroxicam, meclofena-mate, ibuprofen, aspirin and prostacyclin in a chronic model of cerebral vasospasm. *Neurosurgery*, **12**, 40–6.

Whitehouse, M.W. (1964) Biochemical properties of anti-inflammatory drugs-III. Uncoupling of oxidative phosphorylation in a connective tissue (cartilage) and liver mitochondria by salicylate analogues: relationship of structure to activity. *Biochem. Pharmacol.*, **13**, 319–36.

Whitehouse, M.W. and Haslam, J.M. (1962) Ability of some anti-rheumatic drugs to uncouple oxidative phosphorylation. *Nature (Lond.)*, **196**, 1323–4.

Whitehouse, M.W., Kippen, I. and Klinenberg, J.R. (1971) Biochemical properties of anti-inflammatory drugs. XII. Inhibition of urate binding to human albumin by salicylate and phenylbutazone analogues and some novel anti-inflammatory drugs. *Biochem. Pharmacol.*, **20**, 3309–20.

Willis, A.L., Davison, P., Ramwell, P.W. *et al.* (1972) Release and actions of prostaglandins in inflammation and fever: Inhibition by anti-inflammatory pyretic drugs. In *Prostaglandins in Cellular Biology* (eds. R.W. Ramwell and B.B. Phariss), Plenum Press, New York, pp. 227–59.

Willoughby, D.A. (1975) Human arthritis applied to animal models: towards a better therapy. Herberden Oration 1974. *Ann. Rheum. Dis.*, **34**, 471–8.

Willoughby, D.A. and Ryan G.B. (1970) Evidence for a possible endogenous antigen in chronic inflammation. *J. Pathol.*, **101**, 233–9.

Willoughby, D.A. and Di Rosa, M. (1972) Studies on the mode of action of non-steroid anti-inflammatory drugs. *Ann. Rheum. Dis.*, **31**, 540–2.

Willoughby, D.A., Polak, L. and Turk, J.L. (1968) Suppression of contact hypersensitivity and acute inflammation by anti-complement serum. *Nature*, **219**, 192–4.

Winter, C.A. and Nuss, G.W. (1966) Treatment of adjuvant arthritis in rats with anti-inflammatory drugs. *Arthrit. Rheum.*, **9**, 394–404.

Winter, C.A., Risley, E.A. and Nuss, G.W. (1962) Carrageenin-induced oedema in hind paw of the rat as an assay for anti-inflammatory drugs. *Proc. Soc. Exp. Biol. Med.*, **111**, 544–7.

8 Analgesic actions of aspirin

J. R. VANE and R. M. BOTTING

Although pain is a protective mechanism, to alert the body to potentially injurious stimuli, it is often excessive and the alleviation of pain has been a focus of human effort since earliest times.

One of the earliest recorded methods of combating headaches was that of trephining the skull with a flat-bladed 'Tumi' knife. This was practised by the early Chimù cultures of Northern Peru in the 13th–15th centuries. One such operation is depicted in the carving on the handle of the trephining knife (Fig. 8.1). The patient is supported by an assistant while the doctor applies the knife blade to the skull. Skeletons from that time have been found with trephining holes in the skulls which have healed or where there were several trephining openings in one cranium. It is difficult to imagine that the method was successful!

However, in Europe and the Near East, treatment of pain with plant products was more widely practised. Babylonian and Assyrian texts from 700 BC mention the use of grains of mustard seed, tamarisk and mandrake for toothache. Mandrake is also mentioned in the Ebers papyrus of Ancient Egypt from around 2000 BC as an ingredient of analgesic preparations, which also contained opium, hyoscyamine or cannabis. Hippocrates used lettuce juice, poppy seed oil and willow bark from which he made infusions, decoctions or extracts for treatment of pain and fever. The pharmacopoeias of Dioscorides and Plinius recommended willow bark for the treatment of mild to moderate pain such as that encountered in rheumatic conditions.

Although a major use of aspirin-like drugs is to treat the pain and inflammation associated with chronic inflammatory states, they are extremely effective in ameliorating pain arising from the traumas of surgery, cancer, childbirth and menstruation. The relief of migraine and other types of headache with aspirin-like drugs is also dealt with in Chapter 14.

166

8.1 MEASUREMENT OF PAIN

Pain is difficult to measure. The most reliable way is to use man's description of the subjective experience of pain under controlled experimental conditions (Lewis, 1942; Beecher, 1957; Keele and Armstrong, 1964). However, the study of reflex reactions in laboratory animals has been widely accepted. Throughout the years, many methods for studying pain and analgesia in laboratory animals have been developed; almost as many as the research workers or laboratories that have been interested in the problem. Extensive reviews on the subject are available (Beecher, 1957; Lim, 1968; Collier, 1969a; Swingle, 1974). As in any other scientific field, the multitude of different techniques has been in part a consequence of the lack of precise definition of the parameters being measured; in this instance, pain and analgesia. This has been especially true in relation to the mechanism of action of the 'mild' analgesics, a term applied to substances of the same order of potency as aspirin, to distinguish them from the 'strong' analgesics such as morphine.

The study of mild analgesics by measuring the type of energy used to induce pain, whether it is mechanical, thermal, electrical or chemical, has not led to an understanding of their mechanism of action, perhaps because the stimuli can vary from mild to severe, short to long lasting or non-damaging to traumatic. Moreover, the integrity of the tissue to which any type of stimulation is applied was not considered as a factor of primary importance. The ability of specific stimuli to induce damage or not, and the nature of the tissue being stimulated, were recognized as basic points of reference in the analysis of pain and analgesia (Randall and Selitto, 1957; Lim, 1968).

There are very few quantitative methods for assessing aspirin-like drugs. In tests which involve short lasting stimulation with any type of energy or in which there is no delay between the stimulus and the response, aspirin-like drugs are either inactive or only active when used in very high concentrations (Collier, 1969a). The most popular assays are those derived from Randall and Selitto's technique (1957) and the stretching assays in rodents (Siegmund et al., 1957). The principles of the tests for mild analgesics introduced by Randall and Selitto have been used subsequently in several animal models (Vinegar et al., 1976b). The original yeast-injected rat hind paw model contributed greatly to the development of mild analgesic drugs. However, due to the chemical heterogeneity of commercial yeast preparations which contain enzymes as well as pyrogens, the results have sometimes been difficult to interpret (Randall, 1963). To try to solve this problem, other irritants such as trypsin or carrageenin were used to induce hyperalgesia in later assays (Vinegar et al., 1976a). Aspirin-like drugs

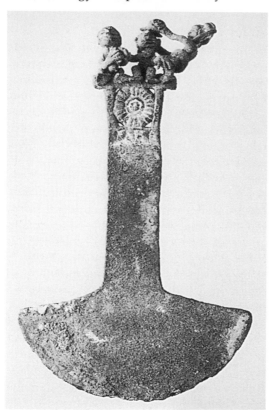

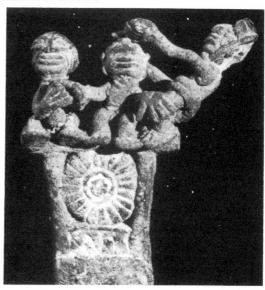

reduced the hyperalgesia which developed between 60 and 180 min after injection of the irritant and raised the threshold of the response to a controlled pressure applied to the inflamed paw (Vinegar et al., 1990). In a recent modification of this test in mice, dilute formalin was used as the inflammatory agent producing two phases of hyperalgesia, 5 min and 20 min, after its injection into a hindpaw (Hunskaar and Hole, 1987; Shibata et al., 1989). Hyperalgesia in the rat hindpaw could be mimicked by injections of PGE_2 or prostacyclin (Ferreira et al., 1978b).

Both mild analgesics and morphine-like drugs inhibit abdominal constriction or the 'stretching' response in the mouse, produced by an intraperitoneal injection of phenylbenzoquinone (Siegmund et al., 1957), acetic acid (Koster et al., 1959) or acetylcholine (Collier et al., 1968). However, these assays are not specific for analgesics (Whittle, 1964; Chernov et al., 1967). Central depressant and stimulant drugs as well as local anaesthetics and amphetamine-like drugs inhibit stretching. In spite of this drawback, the mouse abdominal constriction test is frequently used as a simple and rapid method for the assessment of aspirin-like drugs (Vinegar et al., 1976b; Hunskaar, 1987). Moreover, there is a good correlation between the oral potency of aspirin-like drugs in this test and the human oral dose in clinical practice (Dubinsky et al., 1987). The mechanism responsible for eliciting this complex phenomenon undoubtedly involves the release of prostaglandins (PGs). PGEs, prostacyclin and carbacyclin are all potent inducers of stretching which is not prevented by cyclo-oxygenase inhibitors (Collier and Schneider, 1972; Smith et al., 1985). Moreover, both PGE_2 and 6-keto-$PGF_{1\alpha}$ (the stable product of prostacyclin hydrolysis) have been identified in the pleural cavity during the stretching response to zymosan in mice (Doherty et al., 1987).

Other tests, though not widely used in screening of aspirin-like drugs, include the study of the pseudo-affective response after intra-arterial injection of pain-producing substances described by Guzman et al. (1962) and subsequently developed by Ferreira et al., (1973), the induction of inflammation in the foot joint of the rat (Hesse et al., 1930; Margolin, 1965) or in physiological cavities such as the knee joint of dogs (Pardo and Rodriguez, 1966; Phelps et al., 1966) or pigeons (Brune et al., 1974). Aspirin-like drugs also inhibit the generation of nerve impulses by heat stimulation of the dental receptors of the cat (Scott, 1968), the hypertensive reflex induced by bradykinin (Bk) injections

Figure 8.1 (a) Trepanning knife, Chimú culture (1200–1463), northern Peru (Museum of Ethnology and Prehistory, Hamburg). (b) Handle of trepanning knife with trepanning scene (Museum of Ethnology and Prehistory, Hamburg).

into the knee joint of dogs (Moncada *et al.*, 1975) and the affective response after intra-abdominal injections in humans (Lim *et al.*, 1967).

Woodworth and Sherrington (1904) and Sherrington (1906) described the pseudo-affective response in the decerebrate cat. This response consisted of flexion of the ipsilateral and extension of the contralateral limb after noxious stimulation of the foot. There were also autonomic reflexes such as tachycardia, hypertension, hyperpnoea, and the more complex response of vocalization. These responses were observed after mechanical or electrical stimulation of different cutaneous, muscular or visceral nerves. Moore and Moore (1933), Moore and Singleton (1933) and Moore (1938) observed this response in lightly anaesthetized dogs and cats when irritants were injected intra-arterially in different areas of the body, and showed that they were mediated by afferent pathways entering the medulla via the dorsal roots. Using and developing this technique, Guzman *et al.* (1962) and Lim *et al.* (1964) demonstrated the pain-producing ability of several vasoactive substances released during inflammation; moreover, Lim *et al.* (1964) demonstrated by a cross-circulation experiment in dogs, that the analgesic activity of aspirin-like drugs was a peripheral rather than a central effect. These observations had been made also in man by Keele and Armstrong (1964).

Goetzl *et al.* (1943) stated that theoretically any reflex response could serve as a measure of pain provided that only pain nerve endings are stimulated. The selected standard response should be:

1. Clearly perceptible to the observer;
2. Of such a character as to allow a clear distinction to be made between minimal and sub-minimal stimuli;
3. Constant in its appearance when a stimulus of identical intensity is applied repeatedly;
4. Definite in its onset.

With these criteria in mind and taking into consideration the difficulties of measuring analgesia induced by aspirin-like drugs in laboratory models, two approaches have been used when studying pain and analgesia and its relationship to PG release. First, experiments were carried out on human volunteers using verbal reports as an end point (Ferreira, 1972) and second, measuring the hypertensive reflex induced by pain-producing substances in lightly anaesthetized dogs (Ferreira *et al.*, 1973; Moncada *et al.*, 1974, 1975). These models were chosen because of their comprehensive previous analysis as models for studying pain and because of the clarity with which Lim and co-workers (1964) showed the peripheral effect of aspirin and analgesia.

Due to the developing concept that PGs were involved in the action of algesic substances, vocalization, which many authors agree is the nearest to the human response to pain (Lim, 1968), was not used. This was because this complex response involves higher centres in the central nervous system (CNS), and although clearly observable, it is not as sensitive to slight changes in the intensity of the stimulus and does not allow the study of a 'sensitizing effect' which would need quantitation and a clear difference between minimal and subliminal stimuli (Goetzl et al., 1943). The study of the hypertensive reflex induced by pain-producing substances fulfills the proposed criteria.

With the dog spleen preparation (Ferreira et al., 1973), it has been widely recognized that reflex hypertension induced by injections of Bk is due to the stimulation of pain receptors rather than the mechanical contraction of the spleen (Guzman et al., 1962; Della Bella and Benelli, 1969; Tallarida et al., 1970). Moreover, this response is abolished by dorsal root ganglionectomy or by producing local anaesthesia in the splanchnic nerve.

In the knee joint cavity high concentrations of Bk induce a reflex hypertensive response compatible with that due to the stimulation of pain receptors (Phelps et al., 1966; Melmon et al., 1967). This response is not caused by leakage of the Bk into the general circulation for this would lead to a fall rather than a rise in blood pressure. The hypertension can be blocked by the application of a local anaesthetic such as lignocaine (Moncada et al., 1975); injections of potassium chloride into the synovial cavity, which stimulate pain nerve endings, produce the same reflex hypertension (Moncada et al., 1975). Thus, experiments using two quantitative models for studying pain and analgesia have been instrumental in analysing the mechanisms of analgesia induced by aspirin-like drugs.

8.2 PERIPHERAL MECHANISMS OF PAIN PERCEPTION

8.2.1 Pain Receptors

Two types of skin pain have been recognized since their first description by Lewis and Pochin (1937). One type, characterized by a 'pin prick' or a brisk needle jab into the skin, is well localized, appearing and disappearing quickly, with a low potential for eliciting visceral or somatic reflexes. The second type (the 'ache') consists of a burning pain with a slow onset and a more generalized effect which often persists after the initial stimulus has disappeared. The latter evokes the characteristic cardiovascular and respiratory reflexes which are associated with pain. Available evidence supports the view that these two types of pain are served by two specific sets of peripheral nerve fibres. The pricking pain with its short latency period is transmitted by Aδ fibres; the burning pain with its long latency period is transmitted by polymodal C fibres (Bishop and Landau, 1958; Sinclair and Stokes, 1967; Collins et al., 1966). Pain of a severe and aching quality is evoked by injury to deep structures of the body, such as muscle fascia, joints and tendons. The Aδ and C fibres which occur in the skin are also present in these structures (Gardner, 1950; Paintal, 1960; Iggo, 1962). Lim (1960) proposed that both types of fibres are present in cutaneous as well as visceral or deep areas and that the difference between cutaneous and visceral pain is due to a preponderance of fast 'pricking' pain fibres serving the skin and slow 'aching' pain fibres serving the deep structures. He suggested that this difference would tend to disappear according to the severity or the duration of the injury leading to inflammation.

The identification of pain receptors, as such, has posed many problems. Sherrington (1906) proposed that any type of energy which threatened damage would produce pain. He recognized the lack of stimulus specificity of the nerve endings subserving pain and suggested the use of the word 'nociceptive' to describe stimuli which elicited pain. The finding by Armstrong et al. (1952, 1953) that vasoactive substances, especially kinins, are potent inducers of pain in man and animals (Armstrong et al., 1952, 1953, 1957; Guzman et al., 1962; Keele and Armstrong, 1964) led them to propose that pain receptors in general were chemoreceptors and not nociceptors as suggested by Sherrington (1906).

The only sensory endings with a sufficiently widespread distribution to fulfil the role of pain chemoreceptors are the free terminals of C fibres which have profuse branchings in cutaneous and visceral surfaces extending over all the tegumental areas (Fitzgerald, 1968). These terminals accompany blood vessels (Miller, 1948; Lim et al., 1962) almost everywhere to end in the skin (Weddell et al., 1954), integumental cavities like the joints (Gardner, 1950) or internal viscera (Lim et al., 1962). The stimulation of these pain chemoreceptors may be a complex process and require the development of a sensitized state, as well as a combination of different excitatory substances (reviews by Basbaum and Fields, 1984 and Raja et al., 1988).

Corroborating the idea of multiple mediation of pain, Bk can fail to elicit a pain response but become active in the presence of small amounts of 5-hydroxytryptamine (5-HT) or PGs either exogenously applied or endogenously released (Ferreira et al., 1973; Moncada et al., 1975). In this context, it is important to note the observations of Bishop and Landau (1958) who studied production of pain in subdermal areas and analysed the responses by selective blockade of different nerve fibres. Certain nerve fibres in the subcutaneous tissue of humans responded to ordinary stimuli only under conditions of inflammation. They concluded that such endings register the sequelae of tissue damage rather than the initial injurious incident. They proposed that inflammatory subcutaneous pain is assignable almost entirely to activation of C fibres which seem to be specifically sensitized during the inflammatory process.

Thus, some C fibres are 'silent nociceptors' which do not normally respond to acute noxious, mechanical or thermal stimuli. In joints, such as the knee joints of anaesthetized cats, these fibres are normally unresponsive even to extreme mechanical stimulation. However, injections of inflammatory agents such as kaolin or carrageenin into knee joints caused swelling of the joints and modified the responsiveness of these C fibres. The previously non-responsive afferent fibres developed ongoing activity and began to respond to joint movements that had been previously ineffective. The recruitment of these afferents could be mimicked by close-arterial injections of PGE_2. Thus, PGE_2 induces in articular afferents of normal joints discharges which are similar to those induced by an experimental inflammation (Schaible and Schmidt, 1988a, b). These electrophysiological experiments confirm the behavioural experiments on the dog knee joint in which PGE_2 was detected in inflammatory fluid from the joint and injections of Bk into the joint caused a nociceptive response, which could be prevented with an injection of indomethacin (Rosenthale et al., 1972; Moncada et al., 1975).

After burn injuries, increased responsiveness of afferent nociceptor fibres such as C fibres and myelinated δ fibres results in hyperalgesia of the skin (Bessou and Perl, 1969; LaMotte et al., 1984; Handwerker et al., 1987). In an in-vitro preparation of the rabbit ear, application of noxious levels of heat sensitized C fibre nociceptors and induced ongoing activity in the afferent fibres. This sensitization was blocked by the cyclo-oxygenase inhibitors indomethacin or dipyrone but not by putative substance P antagonists (Cohen and Perl, 1990). These observations provide evidence that increased responsiveness of skin nociceptors after burn injuries may be a result of excessive generation of PGs. Certainly, PGEs have been found in tissue exudates after burn injury (Jonsson et al., 1979) and injections of PGE_2 sensitize some C fibre nociceptors (Handwerker, 1975, 1976; Martin et al., 1987).

The constant stimulation of the CNS resulting from this increased nervous activity can induce central sensitization in which dorsal horn cells of the spinal cord show enhanced ongoing activity and responsiveness to peripheral stimulation (McMahon, 1988; Neugebaeur and

Schaible, 1988; Hoheisel and Mense, 1989). Therefore, changes in excitability of interneurones conducting nociceptive stimuli are initiated by activity in primary afferent C fibres and may result in central hyperalgesia (for review, Woolf, 1989).

8.2.2 Chemical Stimulation of Pain Receptors

Elemental ions and endogenous vasoactive substances are released after almost any kind of damaging stimulation, leading many investigators to search for a chemical which stimulates pain receptors. In pioneering work Lewis (1942) described the development of pain in the forearm of a subject gripping an ergograph once every second during occlusion of the circulation. The time of onset of pain was fairly constant (60–90 s). The pain remained unchanged after the exercise was stopped for as long as the circulation was occluded and disappeared only when the circulation was restored.

Lewis thought that this pain was due to the release of a 'factor P' during muscle exercise which stimulated pain endings but only accumulated during circulatory occlusion in high enough concentrations to produce this effect. This work was extended by Dorpat and Holmes (1955) who demonstrated that 'factor P' could not be just lactic acid or carbon dioxide accumulation or a decrease in pH of the muscle, but thought that it might be potassium released from the muscle cells.

Induction of pain by endogenous vasoactive substances has been studied for many years (Feldberg, 1956), but their pain producing properties were mostly established by Keele and his colleagues (Armstrong et al., 1952, 1953, 1957; Keele and Armstrong, 1964). They applied substances to the denuded base of the cantharidin-induced blister and showed that pain was induced by amines like acetylcholine, 5-HT and histamine; peptides like angiotensin, substance P and Bk; plasma activated by glass; serum, and various inflammatory exudates. Later, Lim and coworkers (Guzman et al., 1962) showed that these substances induced physiological responses indicative of pain when injected into different arteries of lightly anaesthetized dogs. Of all the substances tested, however, only Bk and later, substance P (Potter et al., 1962) produced pain in submicrogram concentrations. All the other substances required concentrations 10–100 times higher. However, claims for one or another substance as a potential mediator of pain were frequently made. Histamine (Rosenthal, 1949, 1950, 1964) has been regarded as a mediator of cutaneous pain and pain of visceral origin referred to the skin. Similarly, it has been proposed that 5-HT is involved in the pain of thrombo-embolic disorders and migraine (Sicuteri, 1968).

The pain-producing actions of the plasma kinins, and later Bk, were first described by Armstrong *et al.* (1952, 1953, 1957). The high potency of Bk in relation to other endogenous vasoactive substances, coupled with the discovery of its formation from kininogens in plasma by a kinin-forming enzyme (Rocha e Silva, 1964), led to the proposal that Bk could be the mediator of inflammatory pain (Lim, 1968). This proposition was supported by the fact that Bk is released during several inflammatory conditions (Rocha e Silva and Garcia Leme, 1972) and that local acidosis characteristic of the acute inflammatory process leads to accumulation of Bk in the inflamed site (Edery and Lewis, 1962).

Bk produces pain when injected intradermally (Cormia and Dougherty, 1960; Lim *et al.*, 1967; Ferreira, 1972), intra-arterially (Burch and De Pasquale, 1962; Coffman, 1966) or intra-abdominally (Lim *et al.*, 1967) in humans and intra-arterially (Guzman *et al.*, 1962; Hashimoto *et al.*, 1964; Ferreira *et al.*, 1973) or intra-articularly (Melmon *et al.*, 1967; Moncada *et al.*, 1975) in dogs. However, not all workers found that Bk induces pain and sometimes a main sensation of warmth is described (Fox *et al.*, 1961). Sicuteri *et al.* (1965) found that Bk induced pain only when the area had been previously sensitized by 5-HT. Moreover, in the blister base, there is tachyphylaxis to the pain-producing property of Bk (Keele and Armstrong, 1964), a phenomenon which is not observed when Bk is injected into a vein previously sensitized by 5-HT (Sicuteri *et al.*, 1965) or when injected intra-arterially in dogs (Guzman *et al.*, 1962).

All these observations, coupled with the facts that levels of recoverable kinins from inflammatory exudates in man and animals are very low (Melmon *et al.*, 1967) and that their concentration does not correlate with the severity of the symptoms in rheumatoid arthritis strongly suggest that Bk is not the sole mediator of pain during inflammation but may be one of the contributors to the pain sensation.

The complexities of the inflammatory response and the nature of the substances involved lead to the conclusion that several mediators, either together or in sequence (Taiwo *et al.*, 1987), contribute to the production of pain. Lipoperoxides, such as 8R,15S diHETE (Ferreira, 1972; Levine *et al.*, 1986b; Taiwo *et al.*, 1987), leukotriene B_4 (Levine *et al.*, 1984), noradrenaline (Ferreira and Nakamura, 1979; Levine *et al.*, 1986a) and platelet-activating factor (Dallob *et al.*, 1987) all cause pain or increased nociception. Interleukin-1β increases nociception in the rat paw by releasing PGs, since the increased pain response can be prevented by indomethacin (Ferreira *et al.*, 1988). The synergism between these substances means that they are not all necessary, nor need they be in any special combination except that Bk has been emphasized as a dominant player (Chapman *et al.*, 1961; Keele and Armstrong, 1964; Rocha e Silva and Garcia Leme, 1972).

A recurrent proposition in the literature is, however, that there is a selective sensitization to pain-producing substances during inflammation because of a background of injury to the tissue (Lewis, 1942; Landau and Bishop, 1953; Guzman *et al.*, 1962). This concept, which is qualitatively different from that postulating the simple interaction of chemical mediators, was developed by Sicuteri *et al.* (1965) and Sicuteri (1968) in relation to 5-HT, as a possible substance responsible for this sensitization, and by Ferreira (1972), Ferreira *et al.* (1973) and Moncada *et al.* (1975) in relation to the sensitizing effects of PGs.

8.2.3 Sensitization of Pain Receptors: Hyperalgesia

Apart from the presence of overt pain during inflammation, there is also a state of hyperalgesia (Lewis and Hess, 1933; Lewis, 1942), defined as a reduced pain threshold to stimuli which are normally non-painful. For example, after sunburn, gentle rubbing of the skin by the clothes can be painful. In fact, Hardy *et al.* (1950) found that after UV light irradiation the skin pain threshold was reduced by 50%. Lewis and Hess (1933) showed that immersing hyperalgesic areas of the body in warm water (40 °C), which is usually not painful, evokes pain within 2–3 s and reaches a peak after 10 s. As the hyperalgesic state increases, lower temperatures provoke pain.

Sensitization of pain receptors to mechanical stimulation has been recognized since the classical description by Lewis *et al.* (1931) of the development of sensitization during muscular exercise in conditions of ischaemia. This type of sensitization has been used by Deneau *et al.* (1953) and Smith *et al.* (1966) to assess pain and analgesia. Sensitization of pain receptors by ischaemia has been described by Sicuteri (1966) who observed in humans the development of pain to a subthreshold dose of Bk injected into the carotid artery after occlusion and by Lim and Guzman (1968) in dogs.

Synergism between chemical substances which activate pain receptors has been observed by several authors. Sensitization of pain receptors to chemical and mechanical stimulation has been described for histamine (Lewis, 1942; Emmelin and Feldberg, 1947), for acetylcholine (Skouby, 1953) and for Bk (Sonina and Khaitin, 1967). Sicuteri *et al.* (1965) showed that 5-HT sensitizes pain receptors in the veins of the dorsal surface of the hand to a previously subthreshold dose of Bk. He proposed that the release of a Bk-like peptide causing vasodilatation in some cranial vessels, and the liberation of 5-HT from blood platelets, may explain headaches related to migraine. Sensitization by 5-HT to the pain induced by Bk was also observed by Ferreira *et al.* (1973) using the dog spleen preparation described by Guzman *et al.* (1962).

By far the most frequently observed sensitization to pain is the one which develops after tissue injuries which lead to inflammation. To quote Lewis (1942): 'The hyperalgesic skin, according to my theory is one which has been brought to this state by the action of certain tissue substances upon the pain nerve endings, the latter being rendered hyperexcitable. It is suggested that these substances are the outcome of processes following at varying intervals according to the nature and severity of tissue injury; the interval is short after cut or burn and long after ultraviolet light'. Lewis thought that the product of the injury that induced the hyperalgesia was a stable pain substance spreading from the injury area through the lymphatic channels. Hardy et al. (1950) agreed with Lewis's concept that after tissue injury, agents were released which excited the terminal nerve endings.

Inflammatory sensitization in man and animals has been used for the study of pain and for assessment of analgesia by several workers. Keele and associates (Keele and Armstrong, 1964) used the denuded base of a cantharadin-induced blister, combining an inflammatory sensitization with the exposure of free nerve endings. Inflammatory sensitization of pain receptors was also used by Hesse et al. (1930) and La Belle and Tislow (1950). However, it was Randall and Selitto (1957) who clearly recognized inflammatory sensitization and successfully used it in animals for the assessment of algesia. Later, several other experimental models were developed (Gilfoil et al., 1963; Margolin, 1965; Winter and Flataker, 1965; Pardo and Rodriguez, 1966).

The concept of hyperalgesia as a state which develops at different intervals after tissue injury and involves the release of chemical mediators has been generally accepted (Lewis, 1942; Hardy et al., 1950; Lim, 1966). Gilfoil and Klavins (1965) made the important observation that in the rat paw hyperalgesia induced by 5-HT, Bk or histamine, given alone or in combination, was somewhat delayed and concluded that the effect was indirect. A delay between the stimulation and the painful response has also been observed in experimental models which do not involve the induction of an inflammatory state.

In 1962, Guzman et al. found that there was delay between injection of a pain-producing substance intra-arterially and the development of the pseudo-affective response in lightly anaesthetized dogs. The delay was much longer than that normally required for somatic reflexes or even the most complicated central pathways and they concluded that changes were necessary at the receptor level before its excitation. Similar delays were observed by Ferreira et al. (1973) using the same experimental model and by Moncada et al. (1975) using the cavity of the knee joint of the dog. Moreover, the latency shortened as the intensity of the stimulus increased and aspirin-like drugs increased the latency, suggesting that they acted on this intermediate step.

Another experimental model in which a lag time occurs between stimulation and effect is the stretching response of mice or rats, after intraperitoneal injection of pain-producing substances (Vander Wende and Margolin, 1956; Siegmund et al., 1957). Some substances such as hypertonic saline induce an early stretch reflex (10–30 s) whereas others like phenylbenzoquinone take about 2 min. Aspirin-type drugs are more effective against the longer latency reflex and Collier (1969a) suggested (as did Winder in 1959) that there might be an intermediate step between the application of the stimulus and the stimulation of pain receptors. Winder called this the development of a pre-inflammatory state and Collier suggested that it was due to the release of a pain producing substance. Later, Collier (1969b) suggested that this could be rabbit aorta contracting substance (RCS; Piper and Vane, 1969), a factor released from the lungs during anaphylaxis and the release of which is inhibited by aspirin-like drugs.

Thus, we may conclude that during inflammation there is a sensitization of pain receptors (hyperalgesia) which develops after the initial trauma and is probably due to the release of inflammatory mediators. There is also a delay period between stimulation and 'pain' response in those tests in which (as in inflammation) weak analgesic agents such as aspirin or paracetamol display an analgesic effect. This delay in response may be due to the noxious stimulus releasing pain mediators or substances which sensitize the pain receptor to normally subthreshold stimulation; weak analgesics possibly act by preventing the generation or release of such mediators. There is strong evidence that the inflammatory mediators which cause hyperalgesia are the PGs.

8.3 PROSTAGLANDIN RELEASE AFTER TISSUE INJURY

8.3.1 Prostaglandins and Pain

Horton (1963) found that PGE_1 did not produce pain when instilled onto a blister base. Similarly, Crunkhorn and Willis (1969, 1971) reported that intradermal injections of microgram doses of PGE_1, PGE_2 or $PGF_{2\alpha}$ did not produce pain. However, Solomon et al. (1968) and Juhlin and Michaelsson (1969) found that the oedematous area caused by intradermal injections of microgram doses of PGE_1 was tender or hypersensitive to touch. In fact, Juhlin and Michaelsson observed hyperalgesia after injections of PGE_1 in doses as low as 10 ng. Moreover, intra-arterial, intravenous or intramuscular injections of PGs of the E series were variously reported to produce pain and headache

(Bevergard and Oro, 1969; Karim, 1971; Collier *et al.*, 1972; Gillespie, 1972). Bk, in contrast, produces systemic and intracranial vasodilatation without pain (Sicuteri *et al.*, 1966). In high concentrations, PGs of the E series produce nociception when injected intra-arterially into the spleen of anaesthetized dogs (Moncada, 1974). In dogs, injections into the knee joint of PGs of the E and F series induced, after a delay, an incapacitation which was untouched by treatment with aspirin-like drugs (Rosenthale *et al.*, 1972). Collier and Schneider (1972) found that PGE_1 or PGE_2 injected into the peritoneal cavity of mice elicited the stretching response and this was not antagonized by aspirin-like drugs. Collier and Schneider (1972) suggested that PGE_1 or PGE_2 could be one of the pain mediators released by noxious stimulation or even the final link between the stimulus and the activation of pain receptors.

Prostacyclin itself (Doherty *et al.*, 1987) or carbacyclin, a stable analogue of prostacyclin, were also potent inducers of the stretching response in mice. A dose-related increase in the number of responses was demonstrated with carbacyclin at 1–100 μg kg^{-1}. Carbacyclin-induced stretching was inhibited by the opiates morphine or dextropropoxyphene, but not by indomethacin (20 mg kg^{-1}; Smith *et al.*, 1985).

Thus, there is general agreement that PGs produce pain only in high concentrations.

8.3.2 Prostaglandins and Hyperalgesia

In 1972, Ferreira observed that subdermal infusions in man of PGE_1 or PGE_2 in low concentrations produced hyperalgesia. Infusions were used to mimic the continuous release of mediators at the site of an injury. The hyperalgesic effect of the PGs was cumulative, since it depended not only on the concentration, but also on the duration of the infusion. Neither Bk nor histamine showed this property.

During separate subdermal infusions of PGE_1, Bk or histamine (or a mixture of Bk and histamine) there was no pain, but when PGE_1 was added to Bk or histamine or a mixture of both, strong pain occurred. Furthermore, in areas made hyperalgesic by an infusion of PGE_1, a second infusion either of histamine or Bk caused pain which gradually increased in intensity. However, at the site where Bk or histamine had been previously infused (without producing hyperalgesia) an infusion of PGE_1 caused little or no pain.

Ferreira concluded that inflammatory mediators such as Bk or histamine had a direct pain-producing action only when the chemical receptors were sensitized by PGs. Another possibility was an indirect action of the mediators on the sensitized receptors due to the oedema they produced.

Pharmacology of aspirin and salicylates

Ferreira also found that histamine, Bk or PGE_1 infusions by themselves did not cause itch. However, when PGE_1 was infused with histamine, itching always preceded pain. PGE_1 infused together with Bk only caused pain. These observations were confirmed by Greaves and McDonald-Gibson (1973) who showed that PGE_1 lowers the threshold of human skin to histamine-evoked itching.

PGE_1 and PGE_2 also sensitize pain nerve endings in the spleen of lightly anaesthetized dogs (Ferreira et al., 1973). In this preparation, sensitization to the reflex hypertension induced by Bk was observed when PGE_1 or PGE_2 was infused in low concentrations into the splenic artery (Fig. 8.2). The response also depended on the depth of the anaesthesia; in deeply anaesthetized dogs, intra-arterial injections of Bk into the spleen induced only a fall in blood pressure similar to that caused by an intravenous injection.

Interestingly, the spleen generates and releases an E_2-like PG continuously into the venous outflow and this release is readily increased by intra-arterial Bk (Ferreira et al., 1973). Thus, it is possible that there is already a background of sensitization and pain-producing substances injected will always find an appropriate environment in which to act. This might be why Lim and co-workers (Lim et al., 1964) found it a suitable model for studying pain and analgesia induced by mild analgesics.

It is important to stress that in this preparation the pain-producing substance must act on a background sensitization caused by spontaneous or induced release of PGs. The released PG is not itself a 'classical' pain mediator, for intra-arterial adrenaline injections do not cause pain but release PGE_2 in similar amounts to Bk injections.

Bk injected in high doses into the knee joint cavity of anaesthetized dogs induces a reflex response compatible with stimulation of pain receptors (Phelps et al., 1966; Melmon et al., 1967). The response depends on the level of anaesthesia and is blocked by a local anaesthetic. Potassium chloride also elicits a similar reflex rise in blood pressure (Moncada et al., 1975). In this preparation, PGE_1 or PGE_2 also have the same sensitizing effect to the pain-producing effects of Bk (Moncada et al., 1974, 1975). In contrast to the spleen, which has a continuous basal release of PGs, normal synovial fluid does not contain PGs (Herman and Moncada, 1975). This correlates well with the observation that the responses to Bk injected into the dog's knee joint were more reproducible after PG release had been induced by a continuous infusion of saline into the joint (Moncada et al., 1975).

Sensitization of pain receptors by PGE_2 has also been described by Kuhn and Willis (1973) and Willis and Cornelsen (1973), who showed the development of hyperalgesia in the rat paw after single

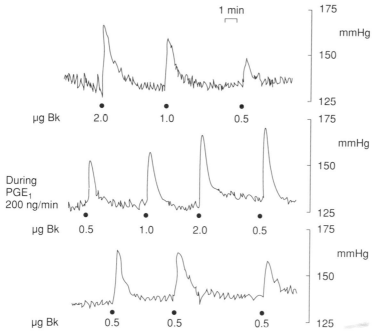

Figure 8.2 Prostaglandin E₁ (PGE₁) potentiates the reflex effect of bradykinin. A continuous tracing of the blood pressure of a dog is shown arranged in three panels. In the upper one, the hypertensive responses to 2.0, 1.0, and 0.5 μg of bradykinin are shown; in the second tracing the same injections are repeated during infusion of prostaglandin E₁ (200 ng min⁻¹). After the infusion (third tracing) the pressor effects of 0.5 μg of bradykinin gradually declined towards pre-treatment levels. Time, 1 min; vertical scales, mm Hg. (Data taken with permission from Ferreira *et al.*, 1973. Copyright 1973, Macmillan Journals Ltd.)

or repeated injections of PGE₂; Juan and Lembeck (1974) observed a similar effect of PGE₁ in the circulation of the rabbit ear, potentiating the pain response induced by several substances. Staszewska-Barczak *et al.* (1976) found that E-type PGs sensitized the surface of the dog's heart to Bk topically applied to the surface (thereby causing a reflex rise in blood pressure) and Handwerker (1975) showed sensitization to thermally-induced discharge of sensory nerves by PGE₂.

The use of infusions (Ferreira, 1972; Ferreira *et al.*, 1973; Moncada *et al.*, 1975) allowed the study of the characteristics of PG-induced hyperalgesia, two important features of which are its cumulative nature and the long duration of the action. The cumulative nature of the PG-induced hyperalgesia was defined by Ferreira (1972) who showed that the hyperalgesic effect of E-type PGs depended not only

181

on the concentration infused but also on the duration of the infusion. Even very small amounts of PGs infused into the knee joint of the dog were able to induce hyperalgesia provided they were maintained for a long enough period (Moncada *et al.*, 1975).

Similar cumulative effects have been described by Willis and Cornelsen (1973) in the rat paw, and by Juan and Lembeck (1974) in the arterial circulation of the rabbit's ear. As a pain-producing substance, Bk does not share this property.

Prostaglandins of the E series cause long-lasting hyperalgesia (Juhlin and Michaelsson, 1969; Ferreira, 1972; Moncada *et al.*, 1975). This may explain why in various pathological conditions such as rheumatoid arthritis or special types of headache there is a delay of several hours before the anti-algesic effect of cyclo-oxygenase inhibitors (such as non-steroidal anti-inflammatory drugs) becomes apparent. However, in many clinical situations and experimental animal models, the analgesic effect of aspirin-like drugs is relatively rapid.

Prostaglandin E_2 hyperalgesia in animals treated with indomethacin (2 mg kg^{-1}) lasts over 5 h, as does carrageenin-induced hyperalgesia. However, when indomethacin is given to rats at the plateau of carrageenin-induced hyperalgesia there is rapid restoration of the pain threshold. Indomethacin partly affects established incapacity induced by endotoxin injected into the dog knee joint, whereas, when given before the challenge, it completely blocks the development of hyperalgesia. These results suggest that in the rat, the stable PGE_2 cannot account for hyperalgesia induced by carrageenin and that in the dog it only contributes in part to the incapacitating effect.

An explanation for this discrepancy was suggested when the unstable prostacyclin was discovered (Moncada *et al.*, 1976). Thus, prostacyclin rather than PGE_2 may be involved for it was more potent than PGE_2 in producing hyperalgesia in both the rat and dog models (Ferreira *et al.*, 1978b). Furthermore, hyperalgesia induced by prostacyclin was immediate and of shorter duration (Fig. 8.3). The presence of 6-keto-$PGF_{1\alpha}$, the non-enzymatic breakdown product of prostacyclin, was demonstrated in inflammatory exudates (Chang *et al.*, 1976). The immediate and short lasting inflammatory effect of prostacyclin was confirmed by Higgs *et al.* (1978).

The difference in the duration of effects of PGE_2 and prostacyclin might explain the effectiveness of cyclo-oxygenase inhibitors in clinical situations. In some headaches, the prompt action of aspirin-like drugs would indicate the participation of prostacyclin, probably generated by the affected vessels. Processes in which the hyperalgesia terminates only after successive administration of the analgesic drug suggest a predominant release of PGE_2 (as in sunburn or back pain, for example).

Both PGE_2 and prostacyclin are released by the irritants injected into the peritoneal cavity of rodents to cause the stretching response and the hyperalgesia. A dilute solution of acetic acid increased the PGE_2 concentration in the peritoneal fluid of rats (Deraedt *et al.*, 1980). SC-19220 and SC-25469, competitive inhibitors of PGE_2 at its receptors (Coleman *et al.*, 1985) prevented stretching induced by acetic acid or an injection of PGE_2 in both mice and rats (Gyires and Torma, 1984; Drower *et al.*, 1987). In mice, prostacyclin is an important mediator of hyperalgesia in zymosan-induced stretching, for a clear parallel was established between the stretching response to this inflammatory agent and the appearance of PGE_2 and 6-keto-$PGF_{1\alpha}$ in the peritoneal fluid. Prostacyclin was found in much larger amounts than PGE_2 and an injection of prostacyclin but not of PGE_2 reversed the analgesia induced by indomethacin (Doherty *et al.*, 1987; Berkenkopf and Weichman, 1988).

In order to examine the hypothesis, that PG hyperalgesia is a metabolic effect, the possibility of mimicking PG hyperalgesia with cyclic adenosine monophosphate (cyclic AMP) analogues and by substances known to increase cyclic AMP formation was investigated (Ferreira and Nakamura, 1979; Taiwo *et al.*, 1989; Ferreira *et al.*,

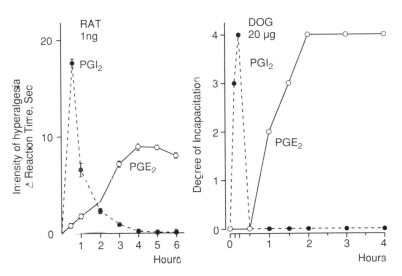

Figure 8.3   Left: Hyperalgesic effect of prostacyclin (PGI_2) and PGE_2 in the rat paw. Rats were treated with indomethacin 2 mg kg^{-1}, i.p., 30 min before the intraplantar injection of prostaglandins. The values indicate the mean and SEM of 6 rats in each group. Right: Incapacitation induced in dogs by intra-articular injection of PGI_2 and PGE_2. The dogs were treated by indomethacin 2 mg kg^{-1}, i.v., just before the intra-articular injection. Each curve was plotted with the median value of three experiments. (Reprinted with permission from Ferreira *et al.*, 1978b. Copyright 1978, Butterworth-Heinemann.)

1990; Taiwo and Levine, 1990). In a modified Randall–Selitto test (Ferreira et al., 1978a), intraplantar injections of PGE_2, prostacyclin, isoprenaline, dopamine, adenosine and dibutyryl or 8-bromo cyclic AMP induced dose-dependent hyperalgesia. The hyperalgesic effects of PGE_2, isoprenaline or dibutyryl cyclic AMP were potentiated after inhibition of phosphodiesterase by local administration of methylxanthines. Caffeine (10 µg), theophylline (20 µg) or isobutylmethylxanthine (1 µg) had no analgesic effect on normal paws. In these experiments, rats were pretreated with indomethacin in order to avoid the release of PGs by the trauma of injection or by the injection of test substances. In this system substances which increased intracellular Ca^{2+} concentrations ($BaCl_2$ or Ca^{2+} ionophore, A23187) also induced hyperalgesia, whereas verapamil and lanthanum (known to block Ca^{2+} influx) were analgesics. These results support the hypothesis that PG-induced hyperalgesia in the rat paw is mediated by a cyclic AMP/Ca^{2+}-dependent process.

While testing the ability of adenylate cyclase stimulators to produce hyperalgesia, it was noticed that noradrenaline, adrenaline or isoprenaline were also able to cause hyperalgesia which could be blocked with propranolol. As a result of this finding, the possible participation of the sympathetic nervous system in the development of inflammatory hyperalgesia in the rat hind paw was investigated (Levine et al., 1986a; Nakamura and Ferreira, 1987). Destruction of peripheral sympathetic neurones or intraperitoneal injections of propranolol reduced inflammatory but not PG-induced hyperalgesia in the paw. When indomethacin only partially inhibited hyperalgesia, an additional reduction could be achieved by removing peripheral sympathetic activity (Nakamura and Ferreira, 1987). Sympathetic postganglionic neurones produce PGE_2 and prostacyclin (measured as 6-keto-$PGF_{1\alpha}$; Gonzales et al., 1989) which could be released in response to stimulation of presynaptic adrenoceptors (Levine et al., 1986a). The pain and hyperalgesia experienced by patients with Raynaud's phenomenon may be caused by an excessive release of these prostanoids (Levine and Taiwo, 1989).

The sympathetic nervous system may be similarly involved in causalgia, the chronic burning pain following nerve injury which is characterized by severe hyperalgesia. The pain is exacerbated by activation of the sympathetic nervous system or by application of noradrenaline (Wiesenfeld-Hallin and Hallin, 1984) and it is often relieved by sympathectomy (Loh and Nathan, 1978).

A state of persistent hyperalgesia can be generated by prolonged periods of pain stimulation, as experienced in the initial stages of chronic pain (Ferreira et al., 1990). Daily injections of PGE_2, dopamine or isoprenaline for 14 days into the foot pad of a rat hind paw caused the development of a persistent hyperalgesic state. In contrast, rats receiving injections of dibutyryl cyclic AMP for 14 days – at doses sufficient to cause an intense, acute and hyperalgesic response – did not show any persistent hyperalgesia. In addition, the duration of the persistent hyperalgesic state depended strongly on the length of the hyperalgesic treatment. Noxious stimulation applied for less than 7 days caused a short-lived hyperalgesic state (1–3 days). However, when the treatment was given for 14 days, the hyperalgesic state was markedly extended (by up to a month). This state of persistent hyperalgesia depends on *de novo* protein synthesis, because two treatments with cycloheximide reduced the intensity of the persistent hyperalgesic state by about 40%. The formation of a regulatory protein, which controls adenylate cyclase activation, might be important in the persistence of chronic pain. When persistent hyperalgesia was blocked, it could be fully restored by a single injection of PGE_2 or dopamine at concentrations which produced a mild and short-lived hyperalgesia in normal paws. It appears therefore, that nociceptor up-regulation can be memorized by nociceptors.

From all these results, it is clear that PGE_2 and prostacyclin, released in almost any form of tissue damage, sensitize the pain receptors to different types of stimulation (chemical, thermal, mechanical). Other mediators released during the inflammatory process interact to stimulate the pain receptors but, at the concentrations present, their activity is probably effective only against a background of sensitization induced by the presence of prostanoids.

8.4 ASPIRIN-LIKE DRUGS AND THEIR MECHANISM OF ANALGESIA

8.4.1 Peripheral Mechanism of Action

Aspirin-like drugs are weak analgesics in contrast to the 'strong' narcotic analgesics like morphine. Several differences separate the groups. Strong analgesics induce tolerance and addiction. They block inhibitory pathways controlling muscle tone, giving rise to the phenomenon described as 'plastic rigidity' or 'Straub tail' in mice and rats. They relieve pain primarily through an effect on the CNS independent of the aetiology of pain. Aspirin-like drugs, on the other hand, do not induce tolerance and addiction. They are selective peripheral analgesics against pain produced in some clinical or experimental conditions, although a central component in the analgesic action of some non-steroidal anti-inflammatory drugs (NSAIDs) has been postulated (section 8.4.2).

Conditions in clinical experience in which aspirin-like drugs are effective as analgesics include pain of low and moderate intensity but not of high intensity (Lim, 1966; Insel, 1990). The pain is usually associated with inflammatory tissue damage, or processes in which the involvement of chemical mediators has been suggested, like post-operative pain, osteo-arthritis, rheumatoid arthritis, ankylosing spondylitis, cancer pain, dysmenorrhea and some forms of headache (Beaver, 1988). Aspirin-like drugs have no measurable activity against pain of high intensity due to muscular spasm, distension of a hollow viscera (DeLeo *et al.*, 1989), acute noxious stimulation of the skin or pain in which nerve trunks are involved.

Aspirin-like drugs are effective in experimental models involving the previous induction of an inflammatory state (Hesse *et al.*, 1930; Randall and Selitto, 1957; Gilfoil *et al.*, 1963; Margolin, 1965; Winter, 1965; Winter and Flataker, 1965; Pardo and Rodriguez, 1966). When there is no previous inflammation, aspirin-like drugs are effective analgesics only when there is a delay between the application of the stimulus and the development of the 'pain response'. For instance there is a delay between the intraperitoneal injection of phenylbenzoquinone and the development of the stretching response (Keith, 1960). Aspirin and other aspirin-type drugs block this delayed stretching response but hardly affect the almost immediate stretching response induced by hypertonic saline (Collier *et al.*, 1968). They have low activity against the early stretching induced by Bk (Collier *et al.*, 1968) but are very active against the delayed response to Bk (Emele and Shanaman, 1963). Aspirin-like drugs are not effective against nociception of short duration induced by pinching or stimulating the tail or toes of mouse, rat or guinea pig (Collier and Chesher, 1956; Winter and Flataker, 1965).

The site of action and the mechanism by which aspirin-like drugs produce analgesia has been the subject of much discussion. An action on the CNS was claimed by Dreser as early as 1899, and for many years since it was maintained as the most plausible explanation, despite increasing evidence for a peripheral mode of action (Woodbury, 1970).

There are several experimental animal models in which inflammation is able to sensitize pain receptors to mechanical and chemical stimulation. Always, hyperalgesia occurs after a latent period, generally when other inflammatory signs or symptoms are developing; but there does not seem to be a strict correlation between oedema and pain (Van Arman *et al.*, 1968; Ferreira *et al.*, 1976). Figure 8.4 illustrates that in the same rat, carrageenin causes greater hyperalgesia than dextran although the oedema produced by the latter was much more intense.

The observation that anti-inflammatory and analgesic activity run parallel in many cases (Randall, 1963) led several authors to believe that at least part of the analgesic activity was peripheral (Randall and Selitto, 1957; Siegmund *et al.*, 1957; Winder, 1959). Some authors suggested that analgesia was an indirect action produced as a consequence of the anti-inflammatory properties (Harris and Fosdick, 1952; Randall and Selitto, 1957; Smith, 1960). This proposition does not explain the results of Guzman *et al.* (1962) in which aspirin-like drugs antagonized pain induced by Bk in conditions in which there is no inflammation. Nor does it explain the fact that in several models aspirin-like drugs are effective as analgesics in doses at which they do not exert anti-inflammatory activity (Gilfoil *et al.*, 1963; Whittle, 1964; Winter, 1965; Winter and Flataker, 1965). Guzman *et al.* (1964) and Lim *et al.* (1964) provided definitive evidence which showed that aspirin-like drugs had a peripheral analgesic activity.

By a cross-circulation experiment in dogs Lim *et al.* (1964) showed that aspirin produced its analgesic action peripherally rather than in the CNS. Bradykinin was injected as the noxious stimulus into the spleen of a dog receiving a splenic circulation from another anaesthetized donor dog. The Bk injection stimulated pain fibres and caused a rise in blood pressure of the recipient animal. Morphine but not aspirin given to the recipient dog prevented this nociceptive response whereas administration of aspirin rather than morphine to the donor dog prevented the rise in blood pressure of the recipient animal. Since aspirin only exerted its analgesic action when its access was limited to the spleen, a peripheral analgesic action of aspirin was strongly indicated (Fig. 8.5). Other authors (Whittle, 1964; Scott, 1968; Takesue *et al.*, 1976; Milne and Twomey, 1980; Rooks *et al.*, 1985; Schweizer and Brom, 1985; Böttcher *et al.*, 1987) using other models have confirmed this concept.

As a mechanism for this peripheral activity Lim *et al.* (1964) and Lim (1968) claimed a direct antagonism at a receptor level between algesic substances and aspirin-like drugs. However, the repeated observation that some sort of inflammation or damage of the tissue needs to be present in order to observe the analgesic effect of aspirin like drugs (Winder, 1959; Randall, 1963; Collier, 1969a) led several authors to suggest that analgesia was produced as a result of an action against pain-producing substances released during inflammation (e.g. Bk, as is inferred from the work of Guzman *et al.*, 1962, and Lim *et al.*, 1964) or against the release of an intermediary substance responsible in the final step for the action of several mediators in inflammation (Collier, 1969a, b) or as Winder (1959) put it, the suppression of some 'pre-inflammatory process' in the course of the reaction by tissues to injury. The same process could lead both to stimulation of pain endings and eventually to frank inflammation.

Three main findings allowed the development of the concept of the mechanism of analgesia induced by aspirin-like drugs. First there was the observation that PG-like activity is released during inflammation

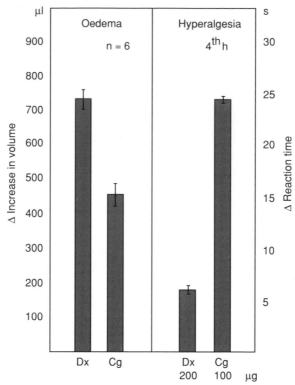

Figure 8.4 Comparison of rat paw oedema and hyperalgesia induced by dextran (Dx) and carrageenin (Cg) in the same animal. Injections of Cg (100 µg) and Dx (200 µg) were made in different paws at 0 and 3 h respectively and measurements of oedema (plethysmography) and hyperalgesia (Randall-Selitto technique) were made at 4 h. Dextran produced a much greater oedema than carrageenin but there was a much smaller hyperalgesia. (Reprinted with permission from Moncada *et al.*, 1978. Copyright 1978, Springer-Verlag, Berlin, Heidelberg.)

(Willis, 1969). Next came the discovery that aspirin-like drugs inhibit the biosynthesis of PGs (Vane, 1971) and third, the finding that PGEs induce hyperalgesia rather than pain in concentrations likely to be present in inflammatory exudates (Ferreira, 1972; Ferreira *et al.*, 1973; Moncada *et al.*, 1975).

It was, therefore, proposed that PGs* sensitize rather than stimulate sensory nerve endings to the pain-producing activity of other stimuli. The pain-producing activity of Bk in the presence of exogenous PGE_2 is unaffected by aspirin-like drugs (Moncada *et al.*, 1975; Fig. 8.6).

The mechanism by which PGs sensitize sensory nerve endings remains unknown; however, electrophysiological techniques have shown an increased response frequency of the receptors to control stimuli, probably by lowering the normally high threshold of polymodal nociceptors associated with C fibres (Chahl and Iggo, 1977; Martin *et al.*, 1987; Cohen and Perl, 1990).

Stimulation of PG receptors generally regulates the synthesis of cyclic AMP by activating or inhibiting adenylate cyclase (Brunton *et al.*, 1976). PGE_2 and prostacyclin stimulate receptors thought to be located on the nociceptive primary afferents (Taiwo and Levine, 1989a), which are linked to adenylate cyclase through a stimulatory guanine nucleotide regulatory protein (G_s; Taiwo and Levine, 1989b). Activation of this system increases intracellular cyclic AMP (Hamprecht and Schultz, 1973; Collier and Roy, 1974a, b; Dismukes and Daly, 1975) and sensitizes the primary afferent nociceptors (Ferreira and Nakamura, 1979). The increased levels of cyclic AMP may be associated with an increased intracellular Ca^{2+} concentration (Greengard, 1979).

The mechanisms of persistent hyperalgesia may be more complex. The sensitizing action of repeated injections of PGE_2 or prostacyclin into rat paws is prevented by pretreatment with a substance P antagonist (Nakamura-Craig and Smith, 1989), indicating that release of substance P mediates their action. Moreover, long lasting hyperalgesia in rat paws can also be induced by multiple injections of substance P, neurokinin A, calcitonin gene-related peptide or 15-hydroperoxyeicosatetraenoic acid (Nakamura-Craig and Gill, 1991; Follenfant *et al.*, 1990). The sustained hyperalgesia with 15-hydroperoxyeicosatetraenoic acid was blocked by the protein kinase inhibitor H-7. Thus, the development of chronic pain may additionally involve release of substance P and stimulation of protein kinase C by the hyperalgesic prostanoids (Negishi *et al.*, 1989).

---

* At the time of the forging of the link between aspirin and the PGs and for several years thereafter, the measurement of PG release in body fluids did not allow clear identification of which PG was involved. For instance, in the early days, relatively high levels of PGE_1 were reported in various tissues but we now know that in mammals (excluding seminal fluid) there is little or no release of PGE_1. It could be that 6-keto PGE_1, the breakdown product of prostacyclin, was the actual culprit in these assays.

In general, we now know that:

1. PGs are not stored, so that concentrations found in tissues or exudates represent new synthesis and release. Since mechanical stimuli in themselves lead to PG synthesis, many of the early observations were confused by extra amounts being formed due to homogenization of tissues, venepuncture, centrifugation of samples, etc.
2. PGE_1 is largely limited in mammals to the seminal fluid.
3. Most tissues release PGE_2 and/or prostacyclin, although $PGF_{2\alpha}$ release is important in the uterus. Formation of PGD_2 is largely limited to mast cells and the brain.

In the following sections, the PGs will be identified wherever the experimental results (with hindsight) allow it; otherwise, when the term 'PGs' is used, it most probably (again with hindsight) refers to PGE_2 and/or prostacyclin.

Pharmacology of aspirin and salicylates

Aspirin-like drugs increase the pain threshold by no more than 50% (Wolff *et al.*, 1941; Winder *et al.*, 1946; Winder, 1947; Deneau *et al.*, 1953) in experimental models, and in clinical conditions they are ineffective against pain of high intensity (see above). This fits with the proposed mechanism of action, for a removal of a sensitization would explain why this analgesic activity can be overcome by increasing the original stimulus and would explain why direct immediate damage of the nerve ending or trunks or, on the other hand, extensive damage leading to massive concentration of pain-producing substances, is unlikely to be affected by aspirin-like drugs.

There are, then, three possibilities. First, as in the spleen model (Guzman *et al.*, 1962; Ferreira *et al.*, 1973), the increased basal release and any stimulated release of PGs is readily blocked by aspirin-like drugs thus allowing an immediate observation of their 'anti-hyperalgesic' effect. Second, there are models in which the stimulus leads to PG release; an example would be the delayed stretching response induced by phenylbenzoquinone or Bk (Keith, 1960; Emele and Shanaman, 1963). Third, in models like the skin or knee joint, an inflammatory state has to develop, leading to PGE_2 release, and only then can the anti-hyperalgesic effects of aspirin-like drugs be observed.

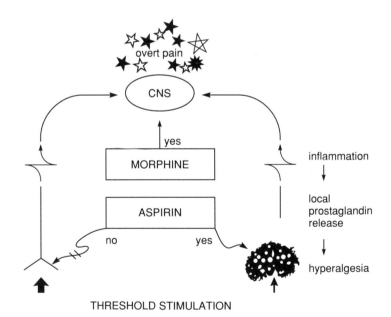

Figure 8.5 An explanation of the analgesic action of aspirin. Details in text. (Reprinted with permission from Ferreira and Vane, 1974. Copyright 1974, Annual Reviews Inc.)

190

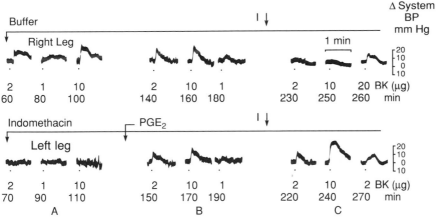

Figure 8.6 Indomethacin fails to antagonize the hypertensive response induced by bradykinin injections in a dog knee joint which is receiving exogenous prostaglandin E_2. The tracings show the changes in systemic blood pressure (mm Hg) of the dog and are arranged in three panels. Panel A (upper part) shows the rise in blood pressure induced by 2, 1, and 10 μg of bradykinin injected into the right knee joint (receiving a Tris-buffer infusion); Panel A (lower part) shows the lack of effect of bradykinin in the left knee joint (receiving an infusion of indomethacin at 1 μg min^{-1}. Panel B shows the responses to the same doses of bradykinin 30 min after adding PGE_2 (50 ng min^{-1}) to the infusion into the left knee joint. This increased the sensitivity so that both joints responded similarly to bradykinin. Panel C shows the responses 30 min after each knee joint received an injection of 1 mg of indomethacin (I). In the right joint (upper part) receiving Tris-buffer, the responses to 2 and 10 μg bradykinin were blocked, and 20 μg only produced an effect similar to that of 2 μg in the left joint, receiving prostaglandin E_2. In this joint, the responses to bradykinin were not inhibited after local indomethacin treatment. The numbers below the doses of bradykinin indicate the time at which each injection was made after the start of the experiment. Time 1 min; vertical scales, variation of blood pressue mm Hg. (Data taken from Moncada *et al.*, 1975, with permission. Copyright 1975, Elsevier BV.)

The knee joint of the dog becomes sensitive to the analgesic effects of aspirin-like drugs when inflammation is induced (Pardo and Rodriguez, 1966; Rosenthale *et al.*, 1966). There is a release of PGE_2 during carrageenin-induced inflammation in this model and a sensitization by PGE_1 or PGE_2 to the pain induced by Bk. Herman and Moncada (1975) observed a close correlation between the concentration of a PGE-like activity and degree of incapacitation during endotoxin-induced inflammation in the knee joint of the dog.

Experimental models in which prostanoids do not seem to be involved like dextran-induced rat paw oedema or passive cutaneous anaphylaxis develop much less hyperalgesia (Van Arman *et al.*, 1968; Moncada *et al.*,

191

1978). Conversely, sunburn hyperalgesia (an example used by Lewis in 1942 to suggest the presence of a factor specifically sensitizing nerve endings) is effectively inhibited by aspirin-like drugs (Hsia et al., 1974) and is a model in which the presence of PGs has been firmly established (Greaves and Sondergaard, 1970).

Patients suffering from chronic headaches are hypersensitive to the pain-producing effects of injections of Bk, and the intracranial pain receptors of rabbits display high sensitivity to Bk (Sicuteri et al., 1966). Interestingly enough, indomethacin is an effective inhibitor of this pain-producing activity of Bk in both man and rabbit. The blockade indicates an involvement of the PG system, probably in the same way as in the dog spleen (Ferreira et al., 1973). Thus, the local release of PGE_2 by injected Bk sensitizes the pain receptors to the pain-producing activity of Bk. Certainly, both in vitro and in vivo, Bk is an effective stimulus for PGE_2 release (Piper and Vane, 1971; McGiff et al., 1972; Moncada et al., 1972; Ferreira et al., 1973).

We can conclude that the aspirin-like drugs do not reduce the effect of prostanoids but reduce only those effects caused by inflammatory substances or stimuli that induce their generation. Such a conclusion depends upon the specific activity of the anti-inflammatory compound on cyclo-oxygenase.

This theory explains the difference between experimental pain and pathological pain (Beecher, 1952; Lim, 1966), explains the specific sensitization described by Landau and Bishop (1953) during inflammation and explains the effectiveness of aspirin-like drugs in experimental models which lead to pathological pain (Winder, 1959; Lim, 1966; Collier, 1969a). As shown in Fig. 8.5 aspirin-like drugs which act mainly peripherally will be active as analgesics only against those forms of pain in which release of prostanoids is involved: however, we suggest that conditions in which a massive release of other mediators is enough to produce a strong stimulation of pain receptors, the presence or absence of modulator prostanoids will not affect the sensation of pain. In these conditions, aspirin-like drugs will not have analgesic activity.

One of the main arguments put forward against the PG theory for explaining analgesia is the existence of aspirin-like drugs which have weak analgesic activity without conspicuous anti-inflammatory activity in man, and paracetamol (acetaminophen) is given as an example. In fact, paracetamol is as effective as aspirin in blocking hyperalgesia in the Randall and Selitto (1958) test, but it should not be overlooked that paracetamol in higher doses also inhibits carrageenin oedema.

It is also possible that analgesia with these drugs is mediated partly through a central site of action (Ferreira et al., 1978a; Ferreira, 1979).

8.4.2 Central Mechanism of Action

Using carrageenin-induced hyperalgesia tests in rats, it was observed that hyperalgesia developed much faster when the contralateral paw had been previously treated with carrageenin (Ferreira et al., 1978a). This was taken as an indication that the local inflammation evoked a central mechanism that facilitated local hyperalgesia. The effects of aspirin, indomethacin, paracetamol and phenacetin injected into the paw and into the cerebral ventricles were also studied. There was a synergistic, anti-algesic effect between central and peripheral administration of these agents. Administration of a specific PG antagonist (SC-19220), either into the cerebral ventricles or into the paw, significantly reduced carrageenin-evoked hyperalgesia. This hyperalgesia in the rat paw could be mimicked only by a combined central and peripheral admin-istration of PGE_2. These results suggest that, in the rat, carrageenin-induced inflammatory hyperalgesia has two components resulting from PG release: a peripheral one due to the local sensitizing action on pain receptors and a central one, possibly due to the participation of central pain circuits. The anti-algesic effect of paracetamol or phenacetin may be partially related to an action on this central component.

The central action of aspirin-like drugs, however, remains controver-sial. In some studies, NSAIDs administered directly into the brain or spinal cord of rats and monkeys increased pain thresholds (Shyu et al., 1984; Shyu and Lin, 1985; Higuchi et al., 1986; Carlsson et al., 1986; Taiwo and Levine, 1988) whereas in others, no analgesic activity could be demonstrated by this route (Nakamura and Shimizu, 1981; Higuchi et al., 1986). Certainly, salicylates injected into the cerebral ventricles of rats and mice reduced peripheral pain and inflammation (Higuchi et al., 1986; Catania et al., 1991). It is interesting that intrathecal injections of low doses of lysine-acetylsalicylate to patients gave relief from chronic pain without at the same time eliciting any centrally-mediated side effects (Devoghel, 1983).

Intravenously injected NSAIDs also reduced the electrical activity evoked in thalamic neurones of rats by stimulation of afferent C fibres in the sural nerve (Carlsson and Jurna, 1987; Groppetti et al., 1988, Carlsson et al., 1988; Jurna and Brune, 1990), and inhibited ex-vivo formation of PGE_2 in rat and mouse brains (Abdel-Halim et al., 1978; Ferrari et al., 1990). These results were taken as evidence for an analgesic action of aspirin-like drugs on the CNS.

The site at which NSAIDs might exert a central analgesic effect is not clear. It may involve activation of descending inhibitory serotoninergic or noradrenergic pathways (Shyu et al., 1984; Shyu and Lin, 1985; Groppetti et al., 1988; Taiwo and Levine, 1988), release of dynorphins

Pharmacology of aspirin and salicylates

(Taiwo and Levine, 1988; Ruda *et al.*, 1988) or antagonism of substance P in the dorsal horns of the spinal cord (Hunskaar *et al.*, 1985). There is also the possibility that PGD_2, as well as PGE_2, may be a mediator of hyperalgesia in the spinal cord (Uda *et al.*, 1990).

In summary, the evidence for a peripheral site of analgesic action of aspirin-like drugs as demonstrated by Lim *et al.* (1964) and extended by Vane and his colleagues (Ferreira *et al.*, 1973; Moncada *et al.*, 1975) has been extensively confirmed (Takesue *et al.*, 1976; Milne and Twomey, 1980; Rooks et al., 1985; Schweizer and Brom, 1985; Böttcher *et al.*, 1987). However, for drugs such as paracetamol, salicylic acid or dipyrone which do not inhibit cyclo-oxygenase at analgesic concentrations (Brune *et al.*, 1981; Brune and Alpermann, 1983; Lanz *et al.*, 1986) or the newer NSAIDs (Attal *et al.*, 1988; Jurna and Brune, 1990), this may not be the complete explanation for their action. Certainly, the analgesic potency of the majority of NSAIDs correlates with their inhibition of cyclo-oxygenase (Table 8.1; Gryglewski, 1978; Ferrari *et al.*, 1990), but with a diverse group of compounds such as the aspirin-like drugs, it is possible that individual members will exhibit additional mechanisms of action unrelated to the main general theme.

8.5 CLINICAL USES OF ASPIRIN-LIKE ANALGESIC DRUGS

Aspirin has been the standard for the peripherally-acting analgesics since 1899. Although paracetamol also came into therapeutic use about that time, it only achieved popularity after 1949 when it was identified as the major active metabolite of phenacetin. An important advance in the treatment of mild to moderate pain has been the development of the newer NSAIDs which are more effective than aspirin or paracetamol and which approach in potency the strong opioid analgesics. They have made a valuable contribution to the relief of various types of non-rheumatic pain such as post-surgical pain, dental pain, post-partum and episiotomy pain, pain of cancer and pain associated with sports injuries. Some provide a much longer duration of pain relief than the standard aspirin-like drugs. Most were introduced in the 1960s and 1970s and Table 8.2 lists some of these newer anti-inflammatory analgesics.

Interest in these drugs as oral analgesics was kindled by studies in the early 1970s, when the use of aspirin was extended to alleviate various types of clinical pain. A randomized double blind crossover study of patients with unresectable cancer found that 650 mg of aspirin was more effective than other commonly used analgesics including 65 mg codeine or 65 mg propoxyphene (Moertel *et al.*, 1972). Similarly, pain resulting from dental surgery has been particularly amenable to aspirin

194

Table 8.1 Comparison of antinociceptive potency of cyclo-oxygenase inhibitors and inhibition of mouse brain microsomal cyclo-oxygenase. Antinociceptive potency was measured as protection against abdominal constriction caused by 3.2 mg kg^{-1} i.p. of acetylchcline. *In-vitro* inhibition of cyclo-oxygenase was measured by incubating each drug with mouse brain microsomes and calculating the percentage decrease in the synthesis of the sum of the four prostaglandins PGE$_2$, PGD$_2$, PGF$_{2\alpha}$ and PGI$_2$ (as 6-keto-PGF$_{1\alpha}$) compared with vehicle control incubations (from Ferrari *et al.*, 1990, with permission. Copyright 1990, Elsevier BV)

Compound	Antinociception ED$_{50}$ (mg kg^{-1})		n^b	Cyclo-oxygenase inhibition in vitro IC$_{50}$		% cyclo-oxygenase inhib. in vitro at ED$_{50}$ of antinociceptive dose[c]
	n^a	(95% c.l.)		µM	(95% c.l.)	
Indomethacin	7	2.2	(0.9–5.6)	4	0.51	(0.47–0.76)	90
Zomepirac Na	5	2.6	(1.3–5.2)	4	0.44	(0.23–0.83)	95
Naproxen Na	4	22	(9–54)	4	6.7	(1.5–30)	90
Ibuprofen	5	17	(8–37)	4	13	(9.6–16)	80
Aspirin[d]	5	20	(60–230)	4	840	(300–2400)	80
Acetaminophen	5	50	(130–180)	4	362	(231–569)	60

[a] n = number of doses with 10 mice per dose. [b] n = number of concentrations tested with three determinations per concentration. [c] The percentage inhibition of *in-vitro* cyclo-oxygenase at the ED$_{50}$ antinociceptive dose. [d] Aspirin has been reported to alkylate the active site of cyclo-oxygenase. Therefore, the value given represents half inactivation of cyclo-oxygenase rather than a true IC$_{50}$ which is based upon competitive binding.

Pharmacology of aspirin and salicylates

Table 8.2. Summary of peripherally-acting analgesic agents

Salicylates	Phenylalkanoic (propionic acids)	Indol-pyrrol acetic acids	p-Amino phenols	Others
Aspirin	Carprofen	Indomethacin	Acetaminophen	Piroxicam
Diflunisal	Fenoprofen	Tolmetin		Mefenamic acid
	Flurbiprofen			Diclofenac
	Ibuprofen			sodium
	Indoprofen			
	Ketoprofen			
	Naproxen			
	Suprofen			

treatment. In a double blind study, aspirin (650 mg) was significantly better than placebo ($P < 0.01$) whereas codeine (30 mg) showed no difference (Cooper and Beaver, 1975). One explanation put forward for the efficacy of aspirin in pain of chronic cancer and post-dental surgery was that it reduced the inflammation which accompanied the pain. The suggestion that aspirin analgesia was a result of its anti-inflammatory activity was proposed by Randall in 1963 and Beaver in 1966. However, for the group of NSAIDs as a whole the anti-rheumatic action does not necessarily parallel their analgesic potency and the anti-rheumatic dose is sometimes much higher than that required for analgesia (Clissold and Beresford, 1987; Todd and Clissold, 1990).

A crucial early study in 1964 showed that a single dose of indomethacin (50 mg) provided comparable analgesia to aspirin (600 mg) in patients with post-operative pain (Sunshine et al., 1964; Fig. 8.7). This important study demonstrated for the first time that indomethacin possessed analgesic activity in a clinical model completely unrelated to rheumatic diseases.

The largest group of NSAIDs and one which comprises the most useful general-purpose analgesics are the propionic acid derivatives (Table 8.2). The prototype of this group is ibuprofen and its major analogues include naproxen, fenoprofen, ketoprofen, suprofen and flurbiprofen. The most sensitive clinical model for the evaluation of the analgesic efficacy of NSAIDs has been that of post-surgical dental pain developed in 1976 by Cooper and Beaver. In a comparison of ibuprofen with aspirin and placebo in this model, ibuprofen 200 mg produced similar analgesia to aspirin 650 mg with ibuprofen 400 mg having a greater peak effect and longer duration of action than this dose of aspirin (Cooper et al., 1977; Fig. 8.8).

196

Whereas ibuprofen has a metabolic half-life of 2 h and is almost completely excreted by 24 h, its analogue naproxen is highly bound to plasma albumen and has a half-life of approximately 13 h. When the usual therapeutic dose of naproxen sodium of 275 mg was compared with aspirin 650 mg and with placebo (Bloomfield *et al.*, 1977), naproxen analgesia was equivalent to and lasted longer than that of aspirin. However, there was a delay of 3 h before the therapeutic activity of naproxen equalled that of aspirin. This delay in onset of analgesic effect is also typical of other NSAIDs which have a long serum half-life and prolonged duration of action such as diflunisal and piroxicam. To speed up the onset of therapeutic effect, the long acting NSAIDs can be administered in an initial loading dose which is twice the subsequent normal dose. Because of their long half-life these drugs can be administered in a single daily dose.

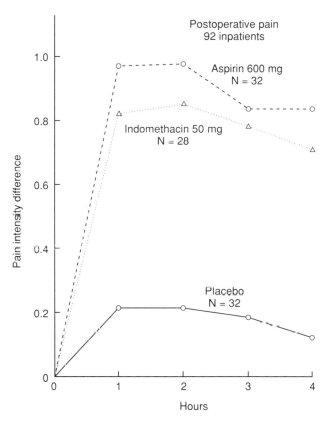

Figure 8.7 Time-effect cuves of indomethacin 50 mg compared with aspirin 600 mg and placebo in 92 patients with postoperative pain. (Adapted from Sunshine *et al.*, 1964, with permission. Copyright 1964, Mosby-Year Book Inc.)

197

Pharmacology of aspirin and salicylates

The analgesia produced by the NSAIDs was related to their inhibition of PG synthesis and to the inhibition of PG-induced hyperalgesia. Prostaglandins of the E and F types have been identified in extracts of menstrual fluid and of the endometrium (Pickles *et al.*, 1965). The concentrations of $PGF_{2\alpha}$ were four times higher in dysmenorrhagic than in non-dysmenorrhagic women and returned to normal levels after treatment with PG synthase inhibitors (Lundstrom *et al.*, 1979). Indomethacin, which is one of the most potent inhibitors of cyclo-oxygenase *in vitro*, as well as ibuprofen, ketoprofen, naproxen and piroxicam have all been evaluated for their effectiveness in the treatment of painful uterine cramps during menstruation. All were shown to be clinically effective and in one double blind comparative study of 68 women, 40 mg piroxicam daily gave equivalent relief from pain to 1600 mg ibuprofen (Pasquale *et al.*, 1988).

The analgesic action of the newer NSAIDs, like that of aspirin, is therefore dependent on their inhibition of peripherally located PG synthesizing enzymes (Flower and Vane, 1974). However, as mentioned earlier in this chapter, animal studies have revealed the possibility of an action of aspirin-like drugs on cyclo-oxygenase in the CNS. More work is needed to evaluate the importance of these observations in practical terms. Perhaps the inhibition of a nociceptive flexion reflex in normal but not in paraplegic patients points to a central component in the analgesic action of ketoprofen (Willer *et al.*, 1989)?

In conclusion, the more recently developed non-steroid anti-inflammatory analgesics are an important advance in the management of clinical pain. They are clearly more potent than aspirin or paracetamol and particularly effective in post-operative pain of various types, post-partum pain, dysmenorrhoea and cancer pain (Dawood, 1988). Some give much longer lasting relief from pain than the standard oral analgesics. Even after two decades of use, the full potential of these new drugs is still being defined in therapeutic practice (Editorial, 1991). Nevertheless, the widespread use of aspirin as an easily available and cheap analgesic will continue in the foreseeable future.

REFERENCES

Abdel-Halim, M.S., Sjöquist, B. and Änggård, E. (1978) Inhibition of prostaglandin synthesis in rat brain. *Acta Pharmacol. Toxicol.*, **43**, 266–72.

Armstrong, D., Day, R.M.L., Keele, C.A. and Markham, J.W. (1952). Pain producing substances in blister fluid and in serum. *J. Physiol. (Lond.)*, **117**, 4P.

Armstrong, D., Day, R.M.L., Keele, C.A. and Markham, J.W. (1953) Observations

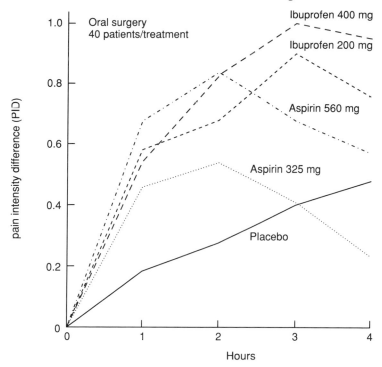

Figure 8.8 Time-effect curves from a dental impaction pain study comparing ibuprofen 200 mg and 400 mg, aspirin 325 mg and 650 mg, and placebo. Time in hours is plotted against pain intensity difference scores. (Adapted from Cooper *et al.*, 1977, with permission. Copyright 1977, W. B. Saunders Company, Philadelphia.)

on chemical excitants of cutaneous pain in man. *J. Physiol. (Lond.)*, **120**, 326–51.

Armstrong, D., Jepson, J.B., Keele, C.A. and Stewart, J.W. (1957) Pain producing substance in human inflammatory exudate and plasma. *J. Physiol. (Lond.)*, **135**, 350–70.

Attal, N., Kayser, V., Eschalier, A. *et al.* (1988) Behavioural and electrophysiological evidence for an analgesic effect of a non-steroidal anti-inflammatory agent, sodium diclofenac. *Pain*, **35**, 341–8.

Basbaum, A.I. and Fields, H.L. (1984) Endogenous pain control systems: Brainstem and spinal pathways and endorphin circuitry. *Ann. Rev. Neurosci.*, **7**, 309–33.

Beaver, W.T. (1966) Mild analgesics, a review of their clinical pharmacology II. *Am. J. Med. Sci.*, **251**, 576–99.

Beaver, W.T. (1988). Impact of non-narcotic oral analgesics on pain management. *Am. J. Med.*, **84**, Suppl. 5A, 3–15.

Beecher, H.K. (1952) Experimental pharmacology and measurements of the subjective response. *Science*, **116**, 157–62.

Pharmacology of aspirin and salicylates

Beecher, H.K. (1957) The measurement of pain. Prototype for the quantitative study of subjective responses. *Pharmacol. Rev.*, **9**, 59–209.

Berkenkopf, J.W. and Weichman, B.M. (1988) Production of prostacyclin in mice following injection of acetic acid, phenylbenzoquinone and zymosan: its role in the writhing response. *Prostaglandins*, **36**, 693–709.

Bessou, P. and Perl, E.R. (1969) Response of cutaneous sensory units with unmyelinated fibers to noxious stimuli. *J. Neurophysiol.*, **3**, 1025–43.

Bevegard, S. and Oro, L. (1969) Effect of prostaglandin E_1 on forearm blood flow. *Scand. J. Clin. Lab. Invest.*, **23**, 347–52.

Bishop, G.H. and Landau, W. (1958) Evidence for a double peripheral pathway for pain. *Science*, **128**, 712–13.

Bloomfield, S.S., Barden, T.P. and Mitchell, J. (1977) Naproxen, aspirin, and codeine in postpartum uterine pain. *Clin. Pharmacol. Ther.*, **21**, 414–21.

Böttcher, I., Schweizer, A., Glatt, M. and Werner, H. (1987) A sulphonamide-indanone derivative CGP 28237 (ZK 34228), a novel non-steroidal anti-inflammatory agent without gastrointestinal ulcerogenicity in rats. *Drugs Exp. Clin. Res.*, **13**, 237–45.

Brune, K. and Alpermann, H. (1983) Non-acidic pyrazoles: inhibition of prostaglandin production, carrageenin oedema and yeast fever. *Agents Actions*, **13**, 360–3.

Brune, K., Bucher, K. and Walz, D. (1974) The avian micro-crystal arthritis. II. Central versus peripheral effects of sodium salicylate, acetaminophen, and colchicine. *Agents Actions*, **4**, 27–33.

Brune, K., Rainsford, K.D., Wagner, K. and Peskar, B.A. (1981) Inhibition by anti-inflammatory drugs of prostaglandin production in cultured macrophages. *Naunyn-Schmiedeberg's Arch. Pharmacol.*, **315**, 269–76.

Brunton, L.L., Wiklund, R.A., Van Arsdale, P.M. and Gilman, A.G. (1976) Binding of (^{3}H) prostaglandin E_1 to putative receptors linked to adenylate cyclase of cultured cell clones. *J. Biol. Chem.*, **251**, 3037–44.

Burch, G.E. and de Pasquale, N.P. (1962) Bradykinin, digital blood flow, and the arteriovenous anastomoses. *Circ. Res.*, **10**, 105–15.

Carlsson, K.H. and Jurna, I. (1987) Central analgesic effect of paracetamol manifested by depression of nociceptive activity in thalamic neurones of the rat. *Neurosci. Lett.*, **77**, 339–43.

Carlsson, K.H., Helmreich, J. and Jurna, I. (1986) Activation of inhibition from the periaqueductal grey matter mediates central analgesic effect of metamizol (Dipyrone). *Pain*, **27**, 373–90.

Carlsson, K-H., Monzel, W. and Ilmar, J. (1988) Depression by morphine and the non-opioid analgesic agents, metamizol (dipyrone), lysine acetylsalicylate, and paracetamol, of activity in rat thalamus neurones evoked by electrical stimulation of nociceptive afferents. *Pain*, **32**, 313–26.

Catania, A., Arnold, J., Macaluso, A. *et al.* (1991) Inhibition of acute inflammation in the periphery by central action of salicylates. *Proc. Natl. Acad. Sci. USA*, **88**, 8544–7.

Chahl, L.A. and Iggo, A. (1977) The effects of bradykinin and prostaglandin E_1 on rat cutaneous afferent nerve activity. *Brit. J. Pharmacol.*, **59**, 343–7.

Chang, W.C., Murota, S. and Tsurufugi, S. (1976) A new prostaglandin transformed from arachidonic acid in carrageenin-induced granuloma. *Biochem. Biophys. Res. Commun.*, **72**, 1259–64.

Chapman, L.F., Ramos, A.O., Goodell, H. and Wolff, H.G. (1961) Neurohumoral features of afferent fibres in man. Their role in vasodilation, inflammation and pain. *Arch. Neurol. (Chic.)*, **4**, 617–50.

Chernov, H.I., Wilson, D.E., Fowler, F. and Plummer, A.J. (1967) Non-specificity of the mouse writhing test. *Arch. Int. Pharmacodyn. Ther.*, **167**, 171–8.

Clissold, S.P. and Beresford, R. (1987) Proquazone. A review of its pharmacodynamic and pharmacokinetic properties and therapeutic efficacy in rheumatic diseases and pain states. *Drugs*, **33**, 478–502.

Coffman, J.D. (1966). The effect of aspirin on pain and hand blood flow responses to intra-arterial injection of bradykinin in man. *Clin. Pharmacol. Ther.*, **7**, 26–37.

Cohen, R.H. and Perl, E.R. (1990) Contributions of arachidonic acid derivatives and substance P to the sensitization of cutaneous nociceptors. *J. Neurophysiol.*, **64**, 457–64.

Coleman, R.A., Humphrey, P.P.A. and Kennedy, I. (1985) Prostanoid receptors in smooth muscle: further evidence for a proposed classification. In *Trends in Autonomic Pharmacology, Vol. 3* (ed. S. Kalsner), Taylor and Francis, Philadelphia, p. 35.

Collier, H.O.J. (1969a) A pharmacological analysis of aspirin. *Adv. Pharmacol. Chemother.*, **7**, 333–405.

Collier, H.O.J. (1969b) New light on how aspirin works. *Nature (Lond.)*, **223**, 35–7.

Collier, H.O.J. and Chesher, G.B. (1956) Antipyretic and analgesic properties of 2 hydroxyisophthalic acids. *Brit. J. Pharmacol.*, **11**, 20–6.

Collier, H.O.J. and Schneider, C. (1972) Nociceptive response to prostaglandins and analgesic actions of aspirin and morphine. *Nature (New Biol.)*, **236**, 141–3.

Collier, H.O.J. and Roy, A.C. (1974a) Morphine-like drugs inhibit the stimulation by E prostaglandins of cyclic AMP formation by rat brain homogenates. *Nature*, **248**, 24–5.

Collier, H.O.J. and Roy, A.C. (1974b). Inhibition of E prostaglandin-sensitive adenyl cyclase as the mechanism of morphine analgesia. *Prostaglandins*, **7**, 361–76.

Collier, H.O.J., Dineen, L.C., Johnson, C.A. and Schneider, C. (1968) The abdominal constriction response and its suppression by analgesic drugs in the mouse. *Brit. J. Pharmacol.*, **32**, 295–310.

Collier, J.G., Karim, S.M.M., Robinson, B. and Somers, K. (1972) Action of prostaglandins A_2, B_1, E_2 and $F_{2\alpha}$ on superficial hand veins of man. *Brit. J. Pharmacol.*, **44**, 374–5.

Collins, W.F., Nulsen. F.E. and Sheally, C.N. (1966) Electrophysiological studies of peripheral and central pathways conducting pain. In *Pain*, (eds. R.S. Knighton and P.R. Dumke) Little Brown & Co., Boston. pp. 33–45.

Cooper, S.A. and Beaver, W.T. (1975) Evaluation of mild analgesics in outpatients. *Clin. Pharmacol. Ther.*, **17**, 231.

Cooper, S.A. and Beaver, W.T. (1976) A model to evaluate mild analgesics in oral surgery outpatients. *Clin. Pharmacol. Ther.*, **20**, 241–50.

Cooper, S.A., Needle, S.E. and Kruger, G.O. (1977) An analgesic relative potency assay comparing aspirin, ibuprofen and placebo. *J. Oral Surg.*, **35**, 898–903.

Pharmacology of aspirin and salicylates

Cormia, F.E. and Dougherty, J.W. (1960) Proteolytic activity in development of pain and itching. Cutaneous reactions to bradykinin and kallikrein. *J. Invest. Dermatol.*, **35**, 21–6.

Crunkhorn, P. and Willis, A.L. (1969) Actions and interactions of prostaglandins administered intradermally in rat and in man. *Brit. J. Pharmacol.*, **36**, 216P–217P.

Crunkhorn, P. and Willis, A.L. (1971) Cutaneous reactions to intradermal prostaglandins. *Brit. J. Pharmacol.*, **41**, 49–56.

Dallob, A., Guindon, Y. and Goldberg, M.M. (1987) Pharmacological evidence for a role of lipoxygenase products in platelet-activating factor (PAF)-induced hyperalgesia. *Biochem. Pharmacol.*, **36**, 3201–4.

Dawood, M.Y. (1988) Nonsteroidal anti-inflammatory drugs and changing attitudes toward dysmenorrhea. *Am. J. Med.*, **84**, Suppl 5A, 23–9.

DeLeo, J.A., Colburn, R.W., Coombs, D.W. and Ellis, M.A. (1989) The differentiation of NSAIDs and prostaglandin action using a mechanical visceral pain model in the rat. *Pharmacol. Biochem. Behav.*, **33**, 253–5.

Della Bella, D. and Bennelli, G. (1969) Bradykinin and the spleen: different reaction *in vivo* and *in vitro*. In *Prostaglandins, Peptides and Amines* (eds P. Mantegazza and E.W. Horton) Academic Press, London, pp. 99–107.

Deneau, G.A., Waud, R.A. and Gowdey, C.W. (1953) A method for the determination of the effects of drugs on the pain threshold of human subjects. *Can. J. Med. Sci.*, **31**, 387–93.

Deraedt, R., Jouquey, S., Delevallee, F. and Flahaut, M. (1980) Release of prostaglandins E and F in an algogenic reaction and its inhibition. *Eur. J. Pharmacol.*, **61**, 17–24.

Devoghel, J.C. (1983) Small intrathecal doses of lysine-acetylsalicylate relieve intractable pain in man. *J. Int. Med. Res.*, **11**, 90–1.

Dismukes, K. and Daly, J.W. (1975) Accumulation of adenosine 3'5'-monophosphate in rat brain slices: effects of prostaglandins. *Life Sci.*, **17**, 199–210.

Doherty, N.S., Beaver, T.H., Chan, K.Y. *et al.* (1987) The role of prostaglandins in the nociceptive response induced by intraperitoneal injection of zymosan in mice. *Brit. J. Pharmacol.*, **91**, 39–47.

Dorpat, T.L. and Holmes, T.H. (1955) Mechanism of skeletal muscle pain and fatigue. *Arch. Neurol. Psychiat (Chic.)*, **77**, 628–40.

Dreser, H. (1899) Pharmakologisches uber Aspirin (Acetylsalicylsäure). *Pfluegers Arch. ges. Physiol.*, **76**, 306–18.

Drower, E.J., Stapelfeld, A., Mueller, R.A. and Hammond, D.L. (1987) The antinociceptive effects of prostaglandin antagonists in the rat. *Eur. J. Pharmacol.*, **133**, 249–56.

Dubinsky, B., Gebre-Mariam, S., Capetola, R.J. and Rosenthale, M.E. (1987) The antialgesic drugs: Human therapeutic correlates of their potency in laboratory animal models of hyperalgesia. *Agents Actions*, **20**, 50–60.

Edery, H. and Lewis, G. P. (1962) Inhibition of plasma kininase activity at slight acid pH. *Brit. J. Pharmacol.*, **19**, 299–305.

Editorial (1991) Postoperative pain relief and non-opioid analgesics. *Lancet*, **337**, 524–6.

Emele, J.F. and Shanaman, J. (1963) Bradykinin writhing: method for measuring analgesia. *Proc. Soc. Exp. Biol. Med. (NY)* **114**, 680–2.

Emmelin, N. and Feldberg, W. (1947) The mechanism of the sting of the common nettle (*Urtica urens*). *J. Physiol. (Lond.)* **106**, 440–55.

Feldberg, W. (1956) The role of mediators in the inflammatory tissue response. *Int. Arch. Allergy*, **8**, 15–31.

Ferrari, R.A., Ward, S.J., Zobre, C.M. *et al.* (1990) Estimation of the *in vivo* effect of cyclooxygenase inhibitors on prostaglandin E_2 levels in mouse brain. *Eur. J. Pharmacol.*, **179**, 25–34.

Ferreira, S.H. (1972) Prostaglandins, aspirin-like drugs and analgesia. *Nature (New Biol.)* **240**, 200–3.

Ferreira, S.H. (1979) Site of analgesic action of aspirin-like drugs and opioids. In *Mechanisms of Pain and Analgesic Compounds* (eds R.F. Beers and E.G. Bassett), Raven Press, New York, pp. 309–21.

Ferreira, S.H. (1980) Peripheral analgesia: mechanism of the analgesic action of aspirin-like drugs and opiate antagonists, *Brit. J. Clin. Pharmacol.*, **10**, 237S–245S.

Ferreira, S.H. and Vane, J.R. (1974) New aspects of the mode of action of non-steroid anti-inflammatory drugs. *Ann. Rev. Pharmacol.*, **14**, 57–73.

Ferreira, S.H. and Nakamura, M. (1979) I-Prostaglandin hyperalgesia. A $cAMP/Ca^{2+}$ dependent process. *Prostaglandins*, **18**, 179–90.

Ferreira, S.H., Moncada, S. and Vane, J.R. (1973) Prostaglandins and the mechanism of analgesia produced by aspirin-like drugs. *Brit. J. Pharmacol.*, **49**, 86–97.

Ferreira, S.H., Harvey, E.A. and Vane, J.R. (1976) Hyperalgesia, inflammatory oedema and prostaglandins. *Proceedings of the VI International Congress of Pharmacology.* Intern Union Pharmacology, p. 426

Ferreira, S.H., Lorenzetti, B.B. and Correa, F.M.A. (1978a) Central and peripheral antialgesic action of aspirin-like drugs. *Eur. J. Pharmacol.*, **53**, 39–48.

Ferreira, S.H., Nakamura, M. and Abreu Castro, M.S. (1978b) The hyperalgesic effects of prostacyclin and PGE_2. *Prostaglandins*, **16**, 31–7.

Ferreira, S.H., Lorenzetti, B.B., Bristow, A.F. and Poole, S. (1988) Interleukin-1β as a potent hyperalgesic agent antagonized by a tripeptide analogue. *Nature*, **334**, 698–700.

Ferreira, S.H., Lorenzetti, B.B. and De Campos, D.I. (1990) Induction, blockade and restoration of a persistent hypersensitive state. *Pain*, **42**, 365–71.

Fitzgerald, M.J.T. (1968) The innervation of the epidermis. In *The Skin Senses* (ed D.R. Kenshalo), Springfield Illinois, pp. 61–83.

Flower, R.J. and Vane, J.R. (1974) Inhibition of prostaglandin biosynthesis. *Biochem. Pharmacol.*, **23**, 1439–50.

Follenfant, R.L., Nakamura-Craig, M. and Garland, L.G. (1990) Sustained hyperalgesia in rats evoked by 15-hydroperoxycicosatetracnoic acid is attenuated by the protein kinase inhibitor H-7. *Brit. J. Pharmacol.*, **99**, 289P.

Fox, R.H., Goldsmith, R., Kidd, D.J. and Lewis, G.P. (1961) Bradykinin as a vasodilator in man. *J. Physiol. (Lond.)*, **157**, 589–602.

Gardner, E. (1950) Physiology of movable joints. *Physiol. Rev.*, **30**, 127–76.

Gilfoil, T.M. and Klavins, I. (1965) 5-hydroxytryptamine, bradykinin, and histamine as mediators of inflammatory hyperesthesia. *Am. J. Physiol.*, **208**, 867–76.

Gilfoil, T.M., Klavins, I. and Grumbach, L. (1963) Effects of acetylsalicylic acid on the oedema and hyperesthesia of the experimentally inflamed rat's paw. *J. Pharmacol. Exp. Ther.*, **142**, 1–5.

Gillespie, A. (1972) Prostaglandin-oxytocin enhancement and potentiation and their clinical applications. *Brit. Med. J.*, **1**, 150–2.

Goetzl, F.R., Burrill, D.Y. and Ivy, A.C. (1943) A critical analysis of algesimetric methods with suggestions for a useful procedure. *Q. Bull. Northwest. Univ. Med. Sch.*, **17**, 280–91.

Gonzales, R., Goldyne, M.E., Taiwo, Y.O. and Levine, J.D. (1989) Production of hyperalgesic prostaglandins by sympathetic postganglionic neurons. *J. Neurochem.*, **53**, 1595–8.

Greaves, M.W. and Sondergaard, J. (1970) Urticaria pigmentosa and factitious urticaria. Direct evidence for release of histamine and other smooth muscle contracting agents in dermographic skin. *Arch. Dermatol.*, **101**, 418–25.

Greaves, M.W. and McDonald-Gibson, W. (1973) Itch: role of prostaglandins. *Brit. Med. J.*, **3**, 608–9.

Greengaard, P. (1979) Some chemical aspects of neurotransmitter action. *Trends Pharmacol. Sci.*, **1**, 27–9.

Groppetti, A., Braga, P.C., Biella, G. *et al.* (1988) Effect of aspirin on serotonin and met-enkephalin in brain: correlation with the antinociceptive activity of the drug. *Neuropharmacology*, **27**, 499–505.

Gryglewski, R.J. (1978) Screening for inhibitors of prostaglandin and thromboxane biosynthesis. *Adv. Lipid Res.*, 327–44.

Guzman, F., Braun, C. and Lim, R.K.S. (1962) Visceral pain and the pseudoaffective response to intraarterial injection of bradykinin and other algesic agents. *Arch. Int. Pharmacodyn. Ther.*, **136**, 353–84.

Guzman, F.m Braun, C., Lim, R.K.S., *et al.* (1964) Narcotic and non-narcotic analgesics which block visceral pain evoked by intra-arterial injections of brady kinin and other algesic agents. *Arch. Int. Pharmacodyn. Ther.* **149**, 571–88.

Gyires, K. and Torma, Z. (1984) The use of the writhing test in mice for screening different types of analgesics. *Arch. Int. Pharmacodyn. Ther.*, **267**, 131–40.

Hamprecht, D. and Schultz, J. (1973) Stimulation by prostaglandin E_1 of adenosine 3'5'-cyclic monophosphate formation in neuroblastoma cells in the presence of phosphodiesterase inhibitors. *Fed. Eur. Biochem. Soc. Lett.*, **34**, 85–9.

Handwerker, H.O. (1975) Influence of prostaglandin E_2 on the discharge of cutaneous nociceptive C-fibres induced by radiant heat. *Pfluegers Arch. Gesamte Physiol. Menschen Tiere*, **355**, Suppl., R 116.

Handwerker, H.O. (1976) Influences of algogenic substances and prostaglandins on the discharges of unmyelinated cutaneous nerve fibers identified as nociceptors. In *Advances in Pain Research and Therapy, Vol. 1* (eds J.J. Bonica, and D. Albe-Fessard), Raven Press, New York, pp. 41–5.

Handwerker, H.O., Anton, F. and Reeh, P.W. (1987) Discharge patterns of afferent cutaneous nerve fibers from the rat's tail during prolonged noxious mechanical stimulation. *Exp. Brain Res.*, **65**, 493–504.

Hardy, J.D., Wolff, H.G. and Goodell, H. (1950) Experimental evidence on the nature of cutaneous hyperalgesia. *J. Clin. Invest.*, **29**, 115–40.

Harris, S.C. and Fosdick, L.S. (1952) Theoretical considerations of the mechanism of antipyretic analgesia. *Bull. Northwest Univ. Dent. Res. Grad. Study*, **53**, 6–9.

Hashimoto, K., Kumakura, S. and Taira, N. (1964) Vascular reflex responses induced by an intra-arterial injection of aza-azepinophenothiazine, andromedotoxin, veratridine, bradykinin, and kallikrein and blocking action of sodium salicylate. *Jap. J. Physiol.*, **14**, 299–308.

Herman, A.G. and Moncada, S. (1975) Release of prostaglandins and incapacitation after injection of endotoxin in the knee joint of the dog. *Brit. J. Pharmacol.*, **53**, 465 P.

Hesse, E., Roesler, G. and Buhler, F. (1930) Zur biologischen Wertbestimmung der Analgetika und ihrer Kombinationen. *Naunyn-Schmiedeberg's Arch. Expt. Pathol. Pharmakol.*, **158**, 247–53.

Higgs, E.A., Moncada, S. and Vane, J.R. (1978) Inflammatory effects of prostacyclin (PGI$_2$) and 6-oxo-PGF$_{1\alpha}$ in the rat paw. *Prostaglandins*, **16**, 153–62.

Higuchi, S., Tanaka, N., Shioiri, Y. *et al.* (1986) Two modes of analgesic action of aspirin, and the site of analgesic action of salicyclic acid. *Int. J. Tissue React.*, **8**, 327–31.

Hoheisel, U. and Mense, S. (1989) Long-term changes in discharge behaviour of cat dorsal horn neurones following noxious stimulation of deep tissues. *Pain*, **36**, 239–47.

Horton, E.W. (1963) Action of prostaglandin E$_1$ on tissues which respond to bradykinin. *Nature (Lond.)*, **200**, 892–3.

Hsia, S.L., Ziboh, V.A. and Snyder, D.S. (1974) Naturally occurring and synthetic inhibitors of prostaglandin synthetase in the skin. In *Prostaglandin Synthetase Inhibitors* (eds H.J. Robinson, and J.R. Vane), Raven Press, New York, pp. 353–61.

Hunskaar, S. (1987) Similar effects of acetylsalicyclic acid and morphine on immediate responses to acute noxious stimulation. *Pharmacol. Toxicol.*, **60**, 167–70.

Hunskaar, S. and Hole, K. (1987) The formalin test in mice: dissociation between inflammatory and non-inflammatory pain. *Pain*, **30**, 103–14.

Hunskaar, S., Fasmer, O.B. and Hole, K. (1985) Acetylsalicyclic acid, paracetamol and morphine inhibit behavioural responses to intrathecally administered substance P or capsaicin. *Life Sci.*, **37**, 1835–41.

Iggo, A. (1962) Non-myelinated visceral muscular and cutaneous afferent fibres and pain. In *The Assessment of Pain in Man and Animals* (eds C.A. Keede and R. Smith), Livingstone, Edinburgh, pp. 74–87.

Insel, P.A. (1990) Analgesic-antipyretics and antiinflammatory agents; drugs employed in the treatment of rheumatoid arthritis and gout. In *The Pharmacological Basis of Therapeutics* (eds A.G. Gilman, T.W. Rall, A.S. Nies and P. Taylor), Pergamon Press, New York, pp. 638–81.

Jonsson, C–E., Shimizu, Y., Fredholm, B. *et al.* (1979) Efflux of cyclic AMP, prostaglandin E$_2$ and F$_{2\alpha}$ and thromboxane B$_2$ in leg lymph of rabbits after scalding injury. *Acta Physiol. Scand.*, **107**, 377–84.

Juan, H. and Lembeck, F. (1974) Action of peptides and other algesic agents on paravascular pain receptors of the isolated perfused rabbit ear. *Naunyn-Schmiedeberg's Arch. Exp. Pathol. Pharmakol.*, **283**, 151–64.

Pharmacology of aspirin and salicylates

Juhlin, L. and Michaelsson, G. (1969) Cutaneous vascular reactions to prostaglandins in healthy subjects and in patients with urticaria and atopic dermatitis. *Acta Dermato-Venereol., (Stockh.)*, **49**, 251–61.

Jurna, I. and Brune, K. (1990) Central effect of the non-steroid anti-inflammatory agents, indomethacin, ibuprofen, and diclofenac, determined in C fibre-evoked activity in single neurones of the rat hypothalamus. *Pain*, **41**, 71–80.

Karim, S. (1971) Action of prostaglandin in the pregnant woman. *Ann. NY Acad. Sci.*, **180**, 483–98.

Keele, C.A. and Armstrong, D. (1964) *Substances Producing Pain and Itch*, Edward Arnold, London.

Keith, E.F. (1960) Evaluation of analgesic substances. *Am. J. Pharm.*, **132**, 202–30.

Koster, R., Anderson, M. and de Beer, E.J. (1959) Acetic acid for analgesic screening. *Fed. Proc.*, **18**, 412.

Kuhn, D.C. and Willis, A.L. (1973) Prostaglandin E_2, inflammation and pain threshold in rat paws. *Brit. J. Pharmacol.*, **49**, 183P–184P.

La Belle, A. and Tislow, R. (1950) A method of evaluating analysis of the antiarthralgic type in the laboratory animal. *J. Pharmacol. Exp. Ther.*, **98**, 19–20.

LaMotte, R.H., Torebjörk, H.E., Robinson, C.J. and Thalhammer, J.G. (1984) Time-intensity profiles of cutaneous pain in normal and hyperalgesic skin: a comparison with C-fiber nociceptor activities in monkey and human. *J. Neurophysiol.*, **51**, 1434–50.

Landau, W. and Bishop, G.H. (1953) Pain from dermal periosteal and fascial endings and from inflammation. *Arch. Neurol. Psychiat. (Chic.)*, **69**, 490–504.

Lanz, R., Peskar, B.A. and Brune, K. (1986) The effects of acidic and non acidic pyrazoles on arachidonic acid metabolism in mouse peritoneal macrophages. *Agents Actions Suppl*, **19**, 125–35.

Levine, J.D. and Taiwo, Y.O. (1989). β-estradiol induced catecholamine-sensitive hyperalgesia: a contribution to pain in Raynaud's phenomenon. *Brain Res.*, **487**, 143–7.

Levine, J.D., Lau, W. and Kwiat, G. (1984) Leukotriene B_4 produces hyperalgesia that is dependent on polymorphonuclear leukocytes. *Science*, **225**, 743–5.

Levine, J.D., Taiwo, Y.O., Collins, S.D. and Tam, J.K. (1986a). Noradrenaline hyperalgesia is mediated through interaction with sympathetic postganglionic neurone terminals rather than activation of primary afferent nociceptors. *Nature*, **323**, 158–60.

Levine, J.D., Lam, D., Taiwo, Y.O. et al. (1986b) Hyperalgesic properties of 15-lipoxygenase products of arachidonic acid. *Proc. Natl. Acad. Sci. USA*, **83**, 5331–4.

Lewis, T. (1942). *Pain*, Macmillan, New York.

Lewis, T. and Hess, W. (1933) Pain derived from the skin and the mechanism of its production. *Clin. Sci.*, **1**, 39–61.

Lewis, T. and Pochin, E.E. (1937) The double pain response of human skin to a single stimulus. *Clin. Sci.*, **3**: 67–76.

Lewis, T., Pickering, G.W. and Rothschild. P. (1931) Observations upon muscular pain in intermittent claudication. *Heart*, 15, 359–83.

Lim, R.K.S. (1960) Visceral receptors and visceral pain. *Ann. NY Acad. Sci.*, **86**, 73–89.

Lim, R.K.S. (1966) Salicylate analgesia. In *The Salicylates* (eds M.J.H. Smith and P.K. Smith), Smith Interscience Publishers, New York, London, Sydney, p. 155.

Lim, R.K.S. (1968) Neuropharmacology of pain and analgesia. In *Pharmacology of Pain* (eds R.K.S. Lim, D. Armstrong and E.G. Pardo), Pergamon Press. Oxford, pp. 169–217.

Lim, R.K.S. and Guzman, F. (1968) Manifestations of pain in analgesic evaluation in animals and man. In *Pain* (eds A. Soulairac, J. Cahn and J. Chartentier), Academic Press, London, New York, pp. 119–52.

Lim, R.K.S., Lin, G.N., Guzman. F. and Braun, C. (1962) Visceral receptors concerned in visceral pain and the pseudoaffective response to intra-arterial injections of bradykinin and other algesic agents. *J. Comp. Neurol.*, **118**, 269–93.

Lim, R.K.S., Guzman, F., Rodgers, D.W. *et al.* (1964) Site of action of narcotic and non-narcotic analgesics determined by blocking bradykinin-evoked visceral pain. *Arch. Int. Pharmacodyn. Ther.*, **152**, 25–58.

Lim, R.K.S., Miller, D.G., Guzman, F. *et al.* (1967) Pain and analgesia evaluated by intraperitoneal bradykinin-evoked pain method in man. *Clin. Pharmacol. Ther.*, **8**, 521–42.

Loh, L. and Nathan, P.W. (1978) Painful peripheral states and sympathetic blocks. *J. Neurol. Neurosurg. Psychiat.*, **41**, 664–71.

Lundstrom, V., Green, K. and Svanborg, K. (1979), Endogenous prostaglandins in dysmenorrhea and the effect of prostaglandin synthetase inhibitors (PGSI) on uterine contractility. *Acta Obstet. Gynecol. Scand. Suppl.*, **87**, 51–6.

McGiff, J.C., Terragno, N.A., Malik, K.U. and Lonigro, A.J. (1972) Release of prostaglandin E like substance from canine kidney by bradykinin. *Circ. Res.*, **31**, 36–43.

McMahon, S.B. (1988) Neuronal and behavioural consequences of chemical inflammation of rat urinary bladder. *Agents Actions*, **25**, 231–3.

Margolin, S. (1965) A simple method for the simultaneous determination of the anti-inflammatory and analgesic properties of drugs. In *Non-Steroidal Antiinflammatory Drugs* (eds S. Garattini and M.N.G. Dukes), Excerpta Medica, Amsterdam, pp. 214–17.

Martin, H.A., Basbaum, A.I., Kwiat, G.C. *et al.* (1987) Leukotriene and prostaglandin sensitization of cutaneous high-threshold C- and A-delta mechanonociceptors in the hairy skin of rat hindlimbs. *Neuroscience*, **22**, 651–9.

Melmon, K.L., Webster, M.E., Goldfiner, S.E. and Seegmiller, J.E. (1967) The presence of a kinin in inflammatory synovial effusion from arthritides of varying etiologies. *Arthritis Rheum.*, **10**, 13–20.

Miller, J.W. (1948) Observations on the innervation of blood vessels. *J. Anat. (Lond.)*, **82**, 68–80.

Milne, G.M. and Twomey, T.M. (1980) The analgesic properties of piroxicam in animals and correlation with experimentally determined plasma levels. *Agents Actions*, **10**, 31–7.

Moertel, C.G., Ahmann, D.L., Taylor, W.F. and Schwartau, N. (1972) A comparative evaluation of marketed analgesics drugs. *N. Engl. J. Med.*, **286**, 813–15.

Pharmacology of aspirin and salicylates

Moncada, S. (1974) Inhibition by aspirin-like drugs of prostaglandin release in the spleen and its effect on the functioning of efferent and afferent nerve fibres. Thesis, University of London.

Moncada, S., Ferreira, S.H. and Vane, J.R. (1972) Does bradykinin produce pain through prostaglandin production? In *Abstracts of the V. International Congress of Pharmacology*, San Francisco, p. 160.

Moncada, S., Ferreira, S.H. and Vane, J.R. (1974) Sensitization of pain receptors of dog knee joint by prostaglandins. In *Prostaglandin Synthetase Inhibitors* (eds H.J. Robinson and J.R. Vane), Raven Press, New York, pp. 189–95.

Moncada, S., Ferreira, S.H. and Vane, J.R. (1975) Inhibition of prostaglandin biosynthesis as the mechanism of analgesia of aspirin-like drugs in the dog knee joint. *Eur. J. Pharmacol.*, **31**, 250–60.

Moncada, S., Gryglewski, R., Bunting, S. and Vane, J.R. (1976) An enzyme isolated from arteries transforms prostaglandin endoperoxides to an unstable substance that inhibits platelet aggregation. *Nature*, **263**, 663–5.

Moncada, S., Ferreira, S.H. and Vane, J.R. (1978) Pain and inflammatory mediators. In *Inflammation* (eds J.R. Vane and S.H. Ferreira), Springer-Verlag, Berlin, Heidelberg, pp. 588–616.

Moore, R.M. (1938) Some experimental observations relating to visceral pain. *Surgery*, **3**, 534–45.

Moore, R.M. and Moore, R.E. (1933) Studies on the pain sensibility of arteries. I. Some observations on the pain sensibility of arteries. *Am. J. Physiol.*, **104**, 259–66.

Moore, R.M. and Singleton, A.O. (1933) Studies on pain sensibility of arteries. II. Peripheral paths of afferent neurones from the arteries of the extremities and of the abdominal viscera. *Am. J. Physiol.*, **104**, 267–75.

Nakamura, H. and Shimizu, M. (1981) Site of analgesic action of a non-steroidal, anti-inflammatory drug, tolmetin sodium, in rats. *Brit. J. Pharmacol.*, **73**, 779–85.

Nakamura, M. and Ferreira, S. H. (1987) A peripheral sympathetic component in inflammatory hyperalgesia. *Eur. J. Pharmacol.*, **135**, 145–53.

Nakamura-Craig, M. and Smith, T.W. (1989) Substance P and peripheral hyperalgesia. *Pain*, **38**, 91–8.

Nakamura-Craig, M. and Gill, B.K. (1991) Effect of neurokinin A, substance P and calcitonin gene related peptide in peripheral hyperalgesia in the rat paw. *Neurosci. Lett.*, **124**, 49–51.

Negishi, M., Ito, S. and Hayaishi, O. (1989) Prostaglandin E receptors in bovine adrenal medulla are coupled to adenylate cyclase via G_i and to phosphoinositide metabolism in a pertussis toxin-insensitive manner. *J. Biol. Med.*, **264**, 3916–23.

Neugebauer, V. and Schaible, H.-G. (1988) Peripheral and spinal components of the sensitization of spinal neurons during an acute experimental arthritis. *Agents Actions*, **25**, 234–6.

Paintal, A.S. (1960) Functional analysis of group III afferent fibres in mammalian muscles. *J. Physiol. (Lond.)*, **52**, 250–70.

Pardo, E.G. and Rodriguez, R. (1966) Reversal by acetylsalicylic acid of pain induced functional impairment. *Life Sci.*, **5**, 775–81.

Pasquale, S.A., Rathauser, R. and Dolese, H.M. (1988) A double-blind, placebo-controlled study comparing three single-dose regimens of piroxicam with ibuprofen in patients with primary dysmenorrhea. *Am. J. Med.*, **84**, Suppl. 5A, 30–4.

Phelps, P., Prockop, D.J. and McCarty, D.J. (1966) Crystal induced inflammation in canine joints. III. Evidence against bradykinin as a mediator of inflammation. *J. Lab. Clin. Med.*, **68**, 433–44.

Pickles, V.R., Hall, W.J., Best, F.A. and Smith, G.N. (1965) Prostaglandins in endometrium and menstrual fluid from normal and dysmenorrhoeic subjects. *J. Obstet. Gynaecol. Brit. Commonw.*, **72**, 185–92.

Piper, P.J. and Vane, J.R. (1969) Release of additional factors in anaphylaxis and its antagonism by anti-inflammatory drugs. *Nature (Lond.)*, **223**, 29–35.

Piper, P.J. and Vane, J.R. (1971) The release of prostaglandins from lung and other tissues. *Ann. NY Acad. Sci.*, **180**, 363–85.

Potter, G.D., Guzman, F. and Lim, R.K.S. (1962) Visceral pain evoked by intra-arterial injection of substance P. *Nature (Lond.)*, **193**, 983–4.

Raja, S.N., Meyer, R.A. and Campbell, J.N. (1988) Peripheral mechanisms of somatic pain. *Anaesthesiology*, **68**, 571–90.

Randall, L.O. (1963) Non-narcotic analgesics. In *Physiological Pharmacology, The Nervous System, Vol. 1, part A* (eds W.S. Root and F.G. Hofmann), Academic Press, New York, pp. 313–16.

Randall, L.O. and Selitto, J.J. (1957) A method for measurement of analgesic activity on inflamed tissue. *Arch. Int. Pharmacodyn. Ther.*, **111**, 409–19.

Randall, L.O. and Selitto, J.J. (1958) Anti-inflammatory effects of Romilar CF. *J. Am. Pharm. Assoc.*, **47**, 313–14.

Rocha e Silva, M. (1964) The participation of substances of low molecular weight in inflammation with special reference to histamine and bradykinin. In *Injury, Inflammation, and Immunity* (eds L. Thomas, J.W. Uhn and L. Grant), Williams & Wilkins, Baltimore, p. 220.

Rocha e Silva, M. and Garcia Leme, J. (1972) *Chemical Mediators of the Acute Inflammatory Reaction*, Pergamon Press, Oxford.

Rooks II, W.H., Maloney, P.J., Shott, L.D. et al. (1985) The analgesic and anti-inflammatory profile of ketorolac and its tromethamine salt. *Drugs Exp. Clin. Res.*, **11**, 479–92.

Rosenthal, S.R. (1949) Histamine as possible chemical mediator of cutaneous pain: painful responses to intradermal injections of perfusates from stimulated human skin. *J. Appl. Physiol.*, **2**, 348–54.

Rosenthal, S.R. (1950) Histamine as possible chemical mediator for cutaneous pain: dual pain response to histamine. *Proc. Soc. Exp. Biol. Med. (NY)* **74**, 167.

Rosenthal, S.R. (1964) Histamine as chemical mediator for cutaneous pain. *Fed. Proc.*, **23**, 1109–11

Rosenthale, M.E., Kassarich, J. and Schneider, F. Jr (1966) Effect of anti-inflammatory agents on acute experimental synovitis. *Proc. Soc. Exp. Biol. Med. (NY)*, **122**, 693–6.

Rosenthale, M.E., Dervinis, A., Massarich, J. and Singer, S. (1972) Prostaglandins and anti-inflammatory drugs in the knee joint. *J. Pharm. Pharmacol*; **24**, 149–50.

Ruda, M.A., Iadarola, M.J., Cohen, L.V. and Young III, W.S. (1988) *In situ* hybridization histochemistry and immunocytochemistry reveal an increase in spinal dynorphin biosynthesis in a rat model of peripheral inflammation and hyperalgesia. *Proc. Natl Acad. Sci. USA*, **85**, 622–6.

Schaible, H.G. and Schmidt, R.F. (1988a) Excitation and sensitization of fine articular afferents from cat's knee joint by prostaglandin E_2. *J. Physiol.*, **43**, 91–104.

Schaible, H.G. and Schmidt, R.F. (1988b) Time course of mechanosensitivity changes in articular afferents during a developing experimental arthritis. *J. Neurophysiol.*, **60**, 2180–95.

Schweizer, A. and Brom, R. (1985) Differentiation of peripheral and central effects of analgesic drugs. *Int. J. Tissue React.*, **7**, 79–83.

Scott, D., Jr (1968) Aspirin action on receptor in the tooth. *Science*, **161**, 180–1.

Sherrington, C.S. (1906) *The Integrative Actions of the Central Nervous System*, Constable, London.

Shibata, M., Ohkubo, T., Takahashi, H. and Inoki, R. (1989) Modified formalin test: characteristic biphasic pain response. *Pain*, **38**, 347–52.

Shyu, K.W. and Lin, M.T. (1985) Hypothalamic monoaminergic mechanisms of aspirin-induced analgesia in monkeys. *J. Neural Transm.*, **62**, 285–93.

Shyu, K.W., Lin, M.T. and Wu, T.C. (1984) Central serotoninergic neurons: their possible role in the development of dental pain and aspirin-induced analgesia in monkeys. *Exp. Neurol.*, **84**, 179–87.

Sicuteri, F. (1966) Vasoneuroactive substances in migraine. *Headache*, **6**, 109–26.

Sicuteri, F. (1968) Sensitization of nociceptors by 5-hydroxytryptamine in man. In *Pharmacology of Pain* (eds R.K.S. Lim, D. Armstrong and E.G. Pardo), Pergamon Press, Oxford pp. 57–86.

Sicuteri, F., Franciullacci, M., Franchi, G. and Del Bianco, P.L. (1965) Serotonin-bradykinin potentiation on the pain receptors in man. *Life Sci.*, **4**, 309–16.

Sicuteri, F., Franchi, P.L. del B. and Franciullacci, M. (1966) Peptides and pain. In *International Symposium on Vasoactive Polypeptides, Bradykinin, and Related Kinins* (eds M. Rocha e Silva and H.A. Rothschild), Edat Sao Paulo, Brazil, pp. 255–61.

Siegmund, E.A., Cadmus, R.A. and Lu, G. (1957). A method for evaluating both non-narcotic and narcotic analgesics. *Proc. Soc. Exp. Biol. Med.* (NY), **95**, 729–31.

Sinclair, D.C. and Stokes, B.A.R. (1967) The production and characterisation of 'Second Pain'. *Brain*, **87**, 609.

Skouby, A.P. (1953) The influence of acetylcholine curarine and related substances on the threshold for chemical pain stimuli. *Acta Physiol. Scand.*, **29**, 340–52.

Smith, P.K. (1960) The pharmacology of salicylates and related compounds. *Ann. NY Acad. Sci*, **86**, 38–63.

Smith, G.M., Egbert, L.D., Markowitz, R.A. *et al.* (1966) An experimental pain method sensitive to morphine in man: the submaximum effort tourniquet technique. *J. Pharmacol. Exp. Ther.*, **154**, 324–32.

Smith, T.W., Follenfant, R.L. and Ferreira, S.H. (1985) Antinociceptive models displaying peripheral opioid activity. *Int. J. Tissue React.*, **7**, 61–7.

Solomon, L.M., Juhlin, L. and Kirschbaum, M.B. (1968) Prostaglandin on cutaneous vasculature. *J. Invest. Dermatol.*, **51**, 280–2.

Sonina, R.S. and Khaitin, V.M. (1967). Increase in the sensitivity of afferent fibres to the stimulating action of potassium ions induced by bradykinin.

Chemoreception and pain-inducing substances. *Fiziol. Zh. SSSR Im. I. M. Sechenova*, **53**, 291–8.

Staszewska-Barczak, J., Ferreira, S.H. and Vane, J.R. (1976) An excitatory nociceptive cardiac reflex elicited by bradykinin and potentiated by prostaglandins and myocardial ischemia. *Cardiovasc. Res.*, **10**, 314–27.

Sunshine, A., Laska, E., Meisner, M. *et al.* (1964) Analgesic studies of indomethacin as analyzed by computer techniques. *Clin. Pharmacol. Ther.*, **5**, 699–707.

Swingle, K.F. (1974) Evaluation for antiinflammatory activity. In *Anti-Inflammatory Agents, Vol. II* (eds R.A. Scherrer and M.W. Whitehouse), Academic Press, New York, pp. 33–122.

Taiwo, Y.O. and Levine, J.D. (1988) Prostaglandins inhibit endogenous pain control mechanisms by blocking transmission at spinal noradrenergic synapses. *J. Neurosci.*, **8**, 1346–9.

Taiwo, Y.O. and Levine, J.D. (1989a) Prostaglandin effects after elimination of indirect hyperalgesic mechanisms in the skin of the rat. *Brain Res.*, **492**, 397–9.

Taiwo, Y.O. and Levine, J.D. (1989b) Contribution of guanine nucleotide regulatory proteins to prostaglandin hyperalgesia in the rat. *Brain Res.*, **492**, 400–3.

Taiwo, Y.O. and Levine, J.D. (1990) Direct cutaneous hyperalgesia induced by adenosine. *Neuroscience*, **38**, 757–62.

Taiwo, Y.O., Goetzl, E.J. and Levine, J.D. (1987) Hyperalgesia onset latency suggests a hierarchy of action. *Brain Res.*, **423**, 333–7.

Taiwo, Y.O., Bjerknes, L.K., Goetzl, E.J. and Levine, J.D. (1989) Mediation of primary afferent peripheral hyperalgesia by the cAMP second messenger system. *Neuroscience*, **32**, 577–80.

Takesue, E.I., Perrine, J.W. and Trapold, J.H. (1976) The anti-inflammatory profile of proquazone. *Arch. Int. Pharmacodyn. Ther.*, **221**, 122–31.

Tallarida, G., Cassone, R., Semprini, A. and Condorelli, M. (1970) Systemic arterial pressure variations induced by the stimulation of bradykinin-sensitive vascular receptors. In *Bradykinin and Related Kinins* (eds F. Sicuteri, M. Rocha e Silva and N. Back), Plenum Press, London, pp. 201–12.

Todd, P.A. and Clissold, S.P. (1990) Naproxen. A reappraisal of its pharmacology and therapeutic use in rheumatic diseases and pain states. *Drugs*, **40**, 91–137.

Uda, R., Horiguchi, S., Ito, S. *et al.* (1990) Nociceptive effects induced by intrathecal administration of prostaglandin D_2, E_2 or $F_{2\alpha}$ to conscious mice. *Brain Res.*, **510**, 26–32.

Van Arman, C.G., Nuss, G.W., Winter, C.A. and Flataker, L. (1968) Proteolytic enzymes as mediators of pain. In *Pharmacology of Pain* (eds R.K.S. Lim D. Armstrong and E.G. Pardo), Pergamon Press, Oxford, pp. 25–32.

Vander Wende, C. and Margolin, S. (1956) Analgesic test based upon experimentally induced acute abdominal pain in rats. *Fed. Proc.*, **15**, 494.

Vane, J.R. (1971) Inhibition of prostaglandin synthesis as a mechanism of action for aspirin-like drugs. *Nature (New Biol.)*, **231**, 232–5.

Vinegar, R., Truax, J.F., Selph, J.L. *et al.* (1976a) Potentiation of the anti-inflammatory and analgesic activity of aspirin by caffeine in the rat. *Proc. Soc. Exp. Biol. Med. (NY)*, **151**, 556–60.

Vinegar, R., Truax, J.F. and Selph, J.L. (1976b) Quantitative comparison of the analgesic and anti-inflammatory activities of aspirin, phenacetin and acetaminophen in rodents. *Eur. J. Pharmacol.*, **37**, 23–30.

Vinegar, R., Truax, J.F., Selph, J.L. and Johnston, P.R. (1990) New analgesic assay utilizing trypsin-induced hyperalgesia in the hind limb of the rat. *J. Pharmacol. Methods*, **23**, 51–61.

Weddell, G., Pallie. W. and Palmer, E. (1954) The morphology of peripheral terminations in the skin. *Q. J. Microsc. Sci.*, **95**, 483–501.

Whittle, B.A. (1964) The use of changes in capillary permeability in mice to distinguish between narcotic and non-narcotic analgesics. *Brit. J. Pharmacol.*, **22**, 246–53.

Wiesenfeld-Hallin, Z. and Hallin, R.G. (1984) The influence of the sympathetic system on mechanoreception and nociception. A review. *Hum. Neurobiol.*, **3**, 41–6.

Willer, J-C., De Broucker, T., Bussel, B. *et al.* (1989) Central analgesic effect of ketoprofen in humans: electrophysiological evidence for a supraspinal mechanism in a double-blind and cross-over study. *Pain*, **38**, 1–7.

Willis, A.L.. (1969) Release of histamine, kinin, and prostaglandins during carrageenin induced inflammation in the rat. In *Prostaglandins, Peptides, and Amines* (eds P. Mantegazza and E.W. Horton), Academic Press, London, pp. 31–8.

Willis, A.L. and Cornelsen, M. (1973) Repeated injection of prostaglandin E_2 in rat paws induces chronic swelling and a marked decrease in pain threshold. *Prostaglandins*, **3**, 353–7.

Winder, C.V. (1947) A preliminary test for analgesic action in guinea-pigs. *Arch. Int. Pharmacodyn. Ther.*, **74**, 176–92.

Winder, C.V. (1959) Aspirin and algesimetry. *Nature (Lond.)*, **184**, 494–7.

Winder, C.V., Pfeiffer, C.C. and Maison, G.L. (1946) The nociceptive contraction of the cutaneous muscle of the guinea pig as elicited by radiant heat, with observations on mode of action of morphine. *Arch. Int. Pharmacodyn. Ther.*, **72**, 329–59.

Winter, C.A. (1965) The physiology and pharmacology of pain and its relief. In *Medicinal Chemistry: Analgesics* (ed. G. Stevens), Academic Press, New York, London, pp. 9–74.

Winter, C.A. and Flataker, L. (1965) Nociceptive thresholds as affected by parenteral administration of irritants and of various anti-nociceptive drugs. *J. Pharmacol. Exp. Ther.*, **148**, 373–9.

Wolff, H.G., Hardy, J.D. and Goodell, H. (1941) Measurement of the effect on the pain threshold of acetylsalicylic acid, acetanilid, acetophenetidin, amino-pyrine, ethylalcohol, trichlorethylene, a barbiturate, quinine, ergotamine tartrate, and caffeine: an analysis of their relation to pain experience. *J. Clin. Invest.*, **20**, 63–80.

Woodbury, D.M. (1970) Analgesic-antipyretics, anti-inflammatory agents, and inhibitors of uric acid synthesis. In *The Pharmacological Basis of Therapeutics* (eds L. S. Goodman and A. Gilman), Collier-Macmillan Ltd, London, pp. 314–47.

Woodworth, R.S. and Sherrington, C.S. (1904) A pseudoaffective reflex and its spinal path. *J. Physiol. (Lond.)*, **31**, 234–43.

Woolf, C.J. (1989) Recent advances in the pathophysiology of acute pain. *Brit. J. Anaesth.*, **63**, 136–46.

9 *Antipyretic actions of aspirin*

A.S. MILTON

9.1 BODY HEAT

If a definition of life were required, it might be most clearly established on that capacity by which the animal preserves its proper
heat under the various degrees of temperature of the medium in
which it lives. The most perfect animals possess this power in a
superior degree, and to the exercise of their vital functions this
is necessary. The inferior animals have it in a lower degree, in a
degree, however, suited to their functions. In vegetables it seems
to exist, but in a degree still lower, according to their more limited
powers, and humbler destination . . .
There is reason to believe that, while the actual temperature of the
human body remains unchanged, its health is not permanently
interrupted by the variation in the temperature of the medium
that surrounds it; but that a few degrees of increase or diminution
of the heat of the system, produces disease and death. A knowledge
therefore of the laws which regulate the vital heat, seems to be the
most important branch of physiology.

James Currie, 1808

So wrote James Currie in his book entitled *Medical Reports on the Effects
of Water as a Remedy in Fever and Other Diseases*. If ever a justification
was needed for research into body temperature regulation and into the
mode of action of drugs affecting body temperature particularly during
fever then it is contained in those two paragraphs.

Of all the symptoms of disease, fever is the one most easily recognized
as being of pathological significance. Even today body temperature is
the first thing that most doctors measure on seeing a sick patient,
and temperature is measured daily in every patient in every hospital
throughout the land; this is because the course of a disease and the
recovery from both disease and surgery can be, in so many cases, most
easily monitored by measuring body temperatures.

Pharmacology of aspirin and salicylates

The symptoms of fever – shivering, cold and clammy extremities, the burning forehead, profuse sweating and the subjective feeling of heat and cold – have been recorded throughout history. The very words we use stem from the classical languages: fever from the Latin *febris*, and pyrexia and pyretic from the Greek *pyretos*. The folklore of fever is vast, with every culture and civilization having its own myths and explanations. The most well known of the early explanations come from the works of Empedocles and Hippocrates. Empedocles of Agrigentum in Sicily (504–443 BC) proposed the doctrine of the four elements, earth, air, fire and water, as the 'four-fold root of all things'. The human body was considered to be composed of these four fundamental elements, with health resulting from a correct balance of all four, and disease an imbalance. Plato and Aristotle introduced the idea of four qualities, 'dry, cold, hot and moist' and combined them with the four elements in the following scheme. Cold and dry represented **earth**, hot and moist represented **air**, hot and dry represented **fire**, and cold and moist represented **water**.

Subsequently, Hippocrates (460–370 BC) put forward the idea of the four humours, blood, phlegm, yellow bile and black bile, in which the scheme of the four elements was modified such that cold and dry represented **black bile**, hot and moist, **blood**, hot and dry, **yellow bile**, and cold and moist, **phlegm**. Hippocrates maintained that illness resulted from an overproduction of one of these four humours and that the body destroyed the excess humours, perhaps by increasing the body's heat (ie. by developing a fever). As Currie says of Hippocrates: 'Perceiving the increase of heat to be the most remarkable symptom in fever, he assumed this for the cause and founded his distinctions of fevers, on the different degrees of the intenseness of this heat. He had not an instrument that could measure this exactly, and necessarily trusted to his sensations'. Hippocrates obviously believed that fever was necessary for the reduction of disease. Galen (AD 131–201), as written in his work *Methodus medendi*, considered that medicines should be classified according to their various humoral contents. Perhaps because of the teachings of Hippocrates and Galen that fever was 'beneficial', the use of drugs as antipyretics does not appear in their writings, or indeed the writings of physicians up until the nineteenth century. Any effect on body temperature was purely accidental to their curing of the disease. In the seventeenth century one of the most eminent medical men of his time, Thomas Sydenham (1624–1689), revised the Hippocratic methods of observation and stated, 'Nature calls in fever as her usual instrument for expelling from the blood any hostile matters that may lurk in it' (Latham, 1848). Again, quoting from Currie, 'It was the postulate of Sydenham that every disease is nothing else but an endeavour of nature to expel morbific matter of one kind or another, by which her healthy operations are impeded'. However, in the late nineteenth and in this century physicians have generally regarded fever as being harmful to the body and have made every effort to reduce it. Surprisingly, in spite of these modern views there are those who believe that except in life-threatening situations fever may indeed be beneficial to the organism (Kluger, 1980).

Modern studies on pyretics and antipyretics and our understanding of fever stem from two important developments. The first was the introduction of the clinical thermometer. The first thermometer is properly attributed to Galileo, who is said to have invented it some time between the years 1593 and 1597. The first clinical thermometer was described by Sanctorius in 1625, but it was not until the second decade of the eighteenth century that the measuring thermometer was described by Fahrenheit.

The importance of thermometry may be best described in the words of Carl Wunderlich as recorded by Seguin (Wunderlich and Seguin, 1871):

> Thermometry has truly discovered, according to the vivid expression of Wunderlich, a new world, the one dreamed of by Currie, the law of the action of external upon human temperature. But his therapeutic application of the two relative terms of caloric to the treatment of disease is only the initial impulse of an immense revolution, whose subsequences, hidden to the view of the far-seeing Currie, are hardly traceable in our horizon; I mean, the calorific and frigorific action of all our medicines, vegetables and their alkaloids, metals, metaloid bodies and gases. This entirely new field of observation, and of therapeutic action, would vanish like a mirage if thermometry could be suppressed. But, far from this impious impossibility, thermometry will find out even the positivism of empiricism in the law of concordance of the apparently most discording treatments; and will reconcile schools which were divided, only because they did not know that their far diverging means converged to the same action and object – the keeping up of normal temperature, that is to say, life; and the suppressing of the sources of pathological temperatures – that is, death, *in propria persona*.

The second important development was the publication by Stone in 1763 of a paper in the *Philosophical Transactions of the Royal Society of London* on the use of an extract of willow bark in the treatment of fever. This is the first scientific paper to describe not only the use of an antipyretic drug, but in particular a salicylate for this purpose

(Fig. 9.1). However, according to Hanzlik (1927) the use of decoctions of willow bark as a 'general febrifuge' goes back to ancient times, and he indicates that this use continued throughout the mediaeval period until the general introduction of salicylates at the end of the nineteenth century. However, according to the teaching of the medical profession based upon the work of Hippocrates and Galen one must assume that somewhere along the line folk medicine and the practice of the medical profession were not as one in the use of drugs to reduce fever. Hanzlik recounts the use of willow bark as a successful substitute for cinchona bark during the Napoleonic Wars (1803–1815) in the treatment of fever. In 1798 Longmore wrote a paper on 14 soldiers who were poisoned in Quebec after consuming a 'decoction of certain plants' in which he states that an extract of gaultheria (which contains methyl salicylate) 'is frequently used by Canadians and is said to be cooling and grateful ptisan in fevers'. Until 1874 quinine was the main antipyretic, its use, of course, being primarily in the treatment of malarial fever.

It is interesting to remember that extracts of plants such as willow, which contain substances which we now refer to as salicylates, had been used for centuries in medical treatment, but that no mention of their antipyretic action is recorded until the paper of Stone in 1763. For example, Hippocrates recommended juice of the poplar tree for eye diseases and the leaves of willow trees in childbirth. Celsus, in the first century AD, used juices of willow trees for removing corns and Discorides recommended their use for earache, skin diseases, and gout. Galen recommended their use for bloody wounds and ulcers. Similarly one can find mention of many plants containing salicylate in the herbals of the Middle Ages and the Renaissance. Neither Currie nor Wunderlich mention antipyretic drugs in their writings. The former regarded direct cooling of the body as the method of treatment of fever, and Wunderlich was primarily concerned with observations made during various fevers and the progress of the disease.

Just as this section began with the words of James Currie, perhaps it is fitting to conclude with the words that he wrote in the Preface to his work and addressed to the Right Honourable Sir Joseph Banks.

> About eighteen years ago when I was at Edinburgh I discovered that the accounts given of the temperature of the human body under disease, even by the most approved authors, are, with a few exceptions, founded, not on any exact measurement of heat, but on the sensations of the patient himself, or his attendants.
>
> Impressed with the belief, that till more accurate information should be obtained respecting the actual temperature in different circumstances of health, and disease, no permanent theory of vital

[195]

XXXII. *An Account of the Success of the Bark of the Willow in the Cure of Agues. In a Letter to the Right Honourable* George Earl of Macclesfield, *President of R. S. from the Rev. Mr.* Edmund Stone, *of* Chipping-Norton *in* Oxfordshire.

My Lord,

Read June 2d, 1763.

AMong the many useful discoveries, which this age hath made, there are very few which, better deserve the attention of the public than what I am going to lay before your Lordship.

There is a bark of an English tree, which I have found by experience to be a powerful astringent, and very efficacious in curing aguish and intermitting disorders.

About six years ago, I accidentally tasted it, and was surprised at its extraordinary bitterness; which immediately raised me a suspicion of its having the properties of the Peruvian bark. As this tree delights in a moist or wet soil, where agues chiefly abound, the general maxim, that many natural maladies carry their cures along with them, or that their remedies lie not far from their causes, was so very apposite to this particular case, that I could not help applying it; and that this might be the intention of Providence here, I must own had some little weight with me.

Figure 9.1 An account of the success of the bark of the willow in the cure of agues. First page of the paper presented to the Royal Society of London on 2 June 1763 by the Reverend Edward Stone. (Note the error in the title, where his name is incorrectly printed as *Edmund* Stone) (courtesy of Aberdeen University Library).

motion could be established, nor any certain progress made in the treatment of those diseases in which the temperature is diminished or increased.

Your faithful and very obedient Servant
James Currie
Liverpool 31st October, 1797

9.2 BODY TEMPERATURE REGULATION

9.2.1 Introduction

Homeothermic animals maintain their deep body temperature within a fairly narrow range despite considerable variations in both their external and internal environments. In order to keep deep body temperature, or perhaps more accurately body heat content, within these limits, body heat production must be in equilibrium with heat loss, otherwise body temperature will either rise or fall depending on which of these two parameters is the larger. Thermoregulation is therefore simply the mechanism by which heat loss and heat production are regulated.

The hypothalamus is generally considered to be the principal thermoregulatory site in the brain. However, it is clear that additional structures such as the medulla oblongata and spinal cord contain thermosensitive neurones. Behavioural thermoregulation is probably under the control of the higher centres of the brain, although the hypothalamus would appear to be the most important. Interpretation of the physiological responses in terms of engineering concepts has created difficulty in understanding the role of the hypothalamus. Engineers and physicists have designed models of thermoregulation which have become so complicated that they are difficult to understand. However, one of the simpler concepts is that of the hypothalamus as a thermostat, with it being set, for example, at approximately 37.5 °C in man, and that any deviation from this temperature is immediately corrected by appropriate changes in either heat gain or heat loss mechanisms. In this concept of a thermostat it is often said, for example, that fever is the result of bacterial pyrogen, resetting the thermostat at a higher temperature.

At its simplest, the hypothalamus may be looked upon as a black box into which afferent impulses from the temperature sensitive nerve endings in the skin, deep body structures, and also from within the central nervous system itself are continually flowing. The efferent impulses which emerge from the hypothalamus are then responsible for changes in physiological processes resulting in either heat gain or heat loss. That is, if the incoming information indicates that the body temperature is too high the efferent signals going out will be concerned with lowering body temperature, whereas if the input to the hypothalamus suggests body temperature is too low then the efferent signals will be concerned with raising deep body temperature. Thus, at thermal neutrality the total sum of input from cold sensors and heat sensors would be zero and there would be zero efferent activity. Another difficulty which arises from earlier experimentation is the idea that the hypothalamus itself is heat sensitive. This is probably a misconception. If one considers the black box hypothesis it would seem unnecessary to regard the hypothalamus itself as being temperature sensitive. In fact, it would probably be at a considerable disadvantage as this is an area concerned solely with the processing of information. This does not exclude the possibility that parts of the hypothalamus or surrounding structures may demonstrate thermosensitivity, and experiments have been performed in which the hypothalamic area has been heated or cooled resulting in changes in deep body temperature irrespective of the thermal state of the animal. When considering various neurotransmitter substances and neuromodulators which are thought to be involved in thermoregulation it is apparent that the large majority produce more than one effect on deep body temperature. They may, for example, cause either a fall or a rise in deep body temperature in the same species, depending on experimental conditions, or they may produce different effects in different species, causing a rise in one species and a fall in deep body temperature in other species. There is only a limited number of neurotransmitters and therefore it is not surprising that the same transmitter should be implicated in more than one pathway. This is in no way different from the fact that acetylcholine is the neurotransmitter at all autonomic ganglia, both sympathetic and parasympathetic, and yet in many cases the parasympathetic and sympathetic responses are working in opposite directions. Confusion also arises following the injection of relatively large amounts of substances directly into the brain which reach more than one part at the same time. The effect seen will depend on the relative sensitivity of these pathways to the substance in question and also variations in experimental techniques, in environmental conditions and anatomical differences between species.

The commonest disturbance of thermoregulation is fever, which is the increase in deep body temperature following infection and inflammation. Fever almost certainly occurs as a result of changes in the central control of deep body temperature brought about by pyrogenic substances released following infection and inflammation. It therefore

219

differs from the hyperthermia associated with, for example, exposure to a hot environment, or following heavy exercise. These hyperthermic events occur as a result of the inability of the body to balance heat loss and heat gain, whereas during fever the balance is maintained but at a higher temperature than normal.

9.2.2 Heat Gain Mechanisms

In order to gain heat homeothermic animals must increase their heat production. This is accomplished in two ways, first, by heat production in brown adipose tissue, and, secondly, by increased muscular effort which is normally manifested as shivering. Poikilothermic animals which do not have the ability to increase their body metabolism increase body temperature by moving into a hotter environment.

9.2.3 Heat Loss Mechanisms

There are two primary mechanisms by which heat loss is accomplished, first, by varying the amount of heat loss by conduction and convection from the skin and this is accomplished by changes in vasomotor tone. As long as air temperature is below skin temperature increasing blood flow through the peripheral areas will increase heat loss, whereas vasoconstriction and decrease of blood through the periphery will decrease heat loss. If ambient temperature is above blood temperature then heat loss cannot be accomplished by changes in vasomotor control. The other main mechanism by which heat is lost from the body is by evaporative heat loss as a result of either sweating or panting.

9.2.4 Behavioural Thermoregulation

Changes in deep body temperature can be affected by changing the environment. Particularly in poikilothermic animals, moving in and out of a hot or cold environment will change body temperature and in higher animals moving into the shade or out into the sun will also have similar affects. Man has in addition the ability to alter his microclimate by the putting on and taking off of clothes.

9.3 MEDIATORS OF FEVER

9.3.1 The Acute Phase Response

The acute phase of the immune response (often abbreviated to the acute phase response) is a term now used to describe the changes which occur in the body following infection, inflammation and tissue damage. The response includes immunological, haemolytic and metabolic changes. The response may take several days to fully implement. However, one of the earliest and most easily identified events that occurs is fever. For almost 50 years investigations have been conducted to determine what sort of mechanisms are involved in the acute phase response and whether the responses are derived from the invading micro-organisms or from the infected animal. It is now generally accepted that it is a two-stage process with molecules collectively known as exogenous pyrogens derived from the invading organisms, for example, endotoxin (lipopolysaccharide) derived from the cell walls of Gram-negative bacteria, and muramyl dipeptide derived from Gram-positive bacteria, which stimulate the release of endogenous substances within the body which then trigger the host response. Various factors have been implicated in the acute phase response, for example, endogenous leucocyte mediator (LEM), lymphocyte activating factor (LAF), mononuclear cell factor (MCF) and endogenous pyrogen (EP). It is now generally accepted that all these factors are either the same molecule or very closely related molecules. It is for this reason that they have now all been grouped together under the term interleukin-1. (For a complete review of interleukin-1, see Dinarello, 1984.)

9.3.2 Interleukin-1

Interleukin-1 (IL-1) is a polypeptide with several biological activities regulating host defence immune responses, for example, stimulation of thymocyte proliferation via the induction of IL-2 release, stimulation of β-lymphocyte maturation and proliferation, fibroblast growth factor activity and induction of acute phase protein synthesis by hepatocytes. It is synthesized by a number of cells, particularly monocytes and macrophages upon stimulation with a variety of agents, including lipopolysaccharide, muramyl dipeptide and phorbol myristate acetate (Dinarello, 1984). It was originally speculated that these activities did not reside in only one protein, but in a family of proteins. Recently, molecular cloning techniques have established that there are two distinct genes in the human genome which encode for two forms of the IL-1 molecule, a form with an isoelectric point (pI) of 5, termed IL-1α and a pI 7 form termed IL-1β (Auron *et al.*, 1985; March *et al*, 1985). Both molecules are synthesized as precursors of 31 000 molecular weight which are post-translationally processed to biologically active proteins of 17 000 molecular weight. Murine, bovine and rabbit IL-1 have all been cloned. IL-1α and murine IL-1 appear to be closely related at the level of the amino acid sequence with 62% homology, whereas IL-1β is only distantly related to either human IL-1α (26%) or murine IL-1 (30% homology). Despite the differences in primary structure, the evidence available indicates that murine IL-1, human IL-1α and human IL-1β all bind to the same receptor (Kilian *et al.*, 1986) and have similar biological activities (Oppenheim *et al.*, 1986).

As far as the pathology of fever is concerned the most important action of IL-1 is its ability to stimulate arachidonic acid metabolism, and the most consistently observed effect is the increased production of prostaglandin E_2 from various cell types including human macrophages (Kunkel *et al.*, 1986) and fibroblasts (Mizel *et al.*, 1981; Newton and Covington, 1987).

In spite of the low homology of human interleukin 1α and interleukin 1β the pyrogenic responses to the two molecules appear to be remarkably similar. Human recombinant IL-1α and IL-1β when injected intravenously into conscious rabbits produced identical fever response curves illustrated by a monophasic fever lasting for approximately 2 h. The dose response curves were also parallel. However, interleukin 1β on a molecular weight for weight basis was found to be approximately five-fold more active than interleukin 1α. Responses to both interleukins were completely inhibited by ketoprofen given 30 min before the injection of the interleukins and ketoprofen produced defervescence when given at the height of the febrile response of either interleukins (Davidson *et al.*, 1989, 1990).

9.4 ANTIPYRESIS

9.4.1 Introduction

From the time that Stone reported on the antipyretic action salicylates in 1763 up until 1970 we had no idea of how infection raised body temperature producing fever, or how antipyretic drugs reduced fever. The general consensus was that during fever the hypothalamic 'thermostat' was set to a higher level and the body regulated its temperature around this new elevated level and that somehow involving a central action salicylates reset the 'thermostat' to its original setting. This view can be seen promulgated in pharmacology textbooks right up until the beginning of the 1970s (Goodman and Gilman, 1970).

One action often claimed for aspirin is that it induces sweating. This represents a misunderstanding of body temperature regulation. Even if one considers the old idea of salicylates 'resetting' the hypothalamic thermostat an elevated temperature can only be reduced by a decrease in heat production and an increase in heat loss. In man the most efficient way for reducing heat is by evaporative heat loss, i.e. sweating. Sweating, therefore, is a consequence of resetting the thermostat with the body having to reduce heat content. It is not due to a direct action of the salicylates. With this in mind a proper understanding of body temperature regulation explains the apparent paradox that there is a feeling of being too hot as the fever 'breaks', and this is due to peripheral vasodilatation, which is another means by which heat is lost from the body. Often a feeling of cold is felt during the onset of fever which is due to peripheral vasoconstriction (and hence clammy extremities) and shivering because these two parameters enhance heat gain and therefore will result in an elevated temperature, i.e. fever.

The modern era of our understanding of fever commenced in 1970 when Milton and Wendlandt injected various prostaglandins into the cerebroventricular system of the conscious cat. The first experiment showed that PGE_1 in microgram quantities produced a marked rise in deep body temperature, accompanied by shivering and vasoconstriction and with the animal adopting a 'curled up' position, symptoms very similar to those observed following the central administration of bacterial endotoxins. A report of this first observation was published by Milton and Wendlandt in 1970. One of the most exciting findings of this early work was the observation that the antipyretic drug 4-acetamidophenol (4-Ac) (paracetamol, acetaminophen), had no effect on the febrile response to PGE_1, in contrast to its actions in suppressing fever produced by the central administration of endotoxins, which Milton and Wendlandt had previously reported in 1968. From their observations of PGE_1 and 4-Ac Milton and Wendlandt put forward the proposal that 'PGE_1 may be acting as a modulator in temperature regulation and that the action of antipyretics may be to interfere with the release of PGE_1 by pyrogen'. At that time there was no experimental evidence to indicate how antipyretic drugs might affect the release of prostaglandins. However, the answer was to come a few months later when Vane (1971) showed that the non-steroidal anti-inflammatory drugs including aspirin inhibited the synthesis of prostaglandins from arachidonic acid by lung homogenate. Vane suggested that since fever could be mimicked by prostaglandins, and because of the

223

Pharmacology of aspirin and salicylates

proposed involvement of prostaglandins in inflammation and pain, the prostaglandins were mediators in all three of these pathological conditions, and the non-steroidal anti-inflammatory drugs produced their antipyretic, anti-inflammatory and analgesic actions by inhibiting the synthesis of the prostaglandins. This proposal of Vane's provided an answer to the question of why aspirin-like drugs should have these three apparently dissimilar therapeutic actions.

9.4.2 Non-steroidal Anti-inflammatory Drugs including Aspirin as Antipyretics

Since first proposed by Vane in 1971 it is now generally accepted that the non-steroidal anti-inflammatory drugs (NSAIDs), including aspirin, all produce their major actions by inhibiting the fatty acid cyclo-oxygenase enzyme. In the majority of recent experiments using NSAIDs as antipyretics and studying the role of the prostaglandins in fever, aspirin itself has been little used and the majority of research work involves the use of other NSAIDs, such as indomethacin, ketoprofen or the rather anomalous 4-Ac (paracetamol). Hence, the results described in this chapter are mainly concerned with the NSAIDs as a group, and not specifically related to aspirin itself. In 1982, Kim *et al.* reviewed the chemistry and structure activity relationship of the NSAIDs with particular reference to their antipyretic action.

9.5 PROSTAGLANDINS AND FEVER

In their paper in 1970 on the effects of the prostaglandins Milton and Wendlandt found that prostaglandin A_1, $F_{1\alpha}$ and $F_{2\alpha}$ were inactive at the same dose levels as PGE_1 with respect to thermoregulation effects. In a more detailed investigation Milton and Wendlandt (1971a) showed that prostaglandin E_2 produced exactly the same thermoregulatory response in the cat as PGE_1 and also that PGE_1 and PGE_2 were equally potent. They also showed that PGE_1 was hyperthermic in the rabbit. In another publication Milton and Wendlandt (1971b) reported on the hyperthermic effects of PGE_1 in the rat. By 1971 Feldberg and Saxena had confirmed the original observations of Milton and Wendlandt on the hyperthermic effects of PGE_1 in the cat and had also shown that this substance was hyperthermic in the rabbit and rat. In addition, they made two important discoveries: first, that when PGE_1 was infused into the cerebroventricular system of the cat, the hyperthermia produced was sustained for only as long as the infusion lasted; thereafter, deep body temperature returned to the pre-infusion level. Secondly, they

224

located the site of action of PGE_1 as the pre-optic area of the anterior hypothalamus (PO/AH). The observations of Milton and Wendlandt and of Feldberg and Saxena indicated that prostaglandins would be an ideal endogenous substance for modulating increases in body temperature, including fever, since it was active in very small amounts, its duration was short, it acted in the area of the brain considered to be the centre of thermoregulation, and it was hyperthermic in all the species to which it had at that time been administered.

In 1970 Milton and Wendlandt reported that a prostaglandin-like substance had been found in cat cerebrospinal fluid (CSF) during pyrogen fever; and in 1973 Feldberg and Gupta obtained CSF from the third cerebral ventricle in the conscious cat and assayed it for contractile activity, using the rat fundus strip preparation of Vane (1957). They found that in afebrile animals activity was very low or absent; whereas during fever produced by injecting pyrogen directly into the third cerebral ventricle, the activity was considerably greater. On administration of the antipyretic 4-Ac, the fever abated, and the contractile activity of the CSF was again low. Feldberg *et al.* (1973) collected CSF from the cisterna magna in the conscious cat and assayed it for PG-like activity. They found that the O-somatic antigen of *Shigella dysenteriae* produced a fever when administered both into the third ventricle and into the cisterna magna, and also when given intravenously. In all cases during the febrile response, the PG-like activity of the CSF increased, and the three antipyretic drugs, acetylsalicylic acid (aspirin), 4-Ac and indomethacin, all abolished fever; and at the same time the PG-like content of the CSF fell (Fig.9.2). Thin-layer chromatography of the CSF samples followed by bioassay and radioimmunoassay indicated that the prostaglandin present in the CSF of the cat during fever was prostaglandin E_2. As previously reported in Milton and Wendlandt in 1971 in the cat, PGE_2 is of equal potency to PGE_1 in producing hyperthermia It was therefore concluded by Feldberg *et al.* that the prostaglandin released during pyrogen fever and responsible for the hyperpyrexia was PGE_2.

As mentioned earlier in this chapter, bacterial endotoxins, tissue damage and other stimuli that produce fever stimulate the synthesis and release of the low-molecular-weight protein now called interleukin-1 and previously known as leucocytic pyrogen or endogenous pyrogen (EP). Harvey and Milton (1975) prepared endogenous pyrogen from cat peritoneal exudate cells and injected this either intravenously in a single dose or infused it intravenously into conscious cats: the CSF was collected and assayed for PGE_2. Doses of EP prepared from 5×10^6 cells produced a mean rise in temperature of 1.5 °C, and PGE_2 increased from less than 1 ng ml^{-1} to a mean of 3.2 ng ml^{-1} at the height of the

Pharmacology of aspirin and salicylates

febrile response. If the EP (4×10^6 cell exudate per ml) was infused at a rate of 0.5 ml min^{-1} for 5 min followed by 0.05 ml min^{-1}, a rapid rise in deep body temperature was produced and was sustained for as long as the infusion was continued; and PGE$_2$ levels rose from less that 1 ng ml^{-1} to between 2.7 and 5 ng ml^{-1} and remained elevated until the infusion was stopped. Harvey and Milton also obtained

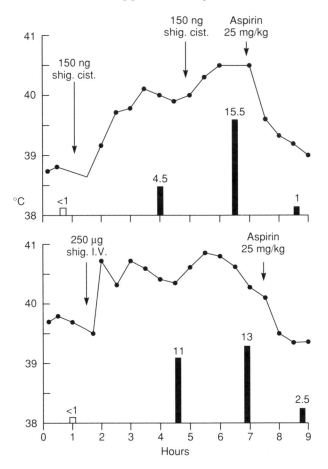

Figure 9.2 Records of rectal temperatuve from two unanaesthetized cats. The height of the columns and the values above refer to PGE$_1$-like activity in ng ml^{-1} of cisternal CSF; the position of the columns refers to the time but not the duration of the CSF collection. In the top record the first and second arrows indicate injections of 150 ng pyrogen into the cisterna magna, and the third arrow indicates an i.p. injection of aspirin 25 mg kg^{-1}. In the bottom record the first arrow indicates an i.v. injection of 250 µg pyrogen and the second arrow an i.p. injection of aspirin 25 mg kg^{-1}. (From Feldberg *et al.*, 1973, with permission.)

226

plasma from cats during fever produced by the administration of O-somatic antigen of *S.dysenteriae* injected either intravenously or into the cerebroventricular system. The plasma was infused into the jugular vein of conscious cats previously made tolerant to *S.dysenteriae*. This was to prevent any possibility of a febrile response to *S.dysenteriae* endotoxin that might still have been circulating in the donor animal, though this was unlikely as endotoxin is very rapidly removed from the circulation by body tissues. When the plasma was taken from cats receiving endotoxin intravenously and infused into the recipient cats, an increase in deep body temperature was observed, and this was associated with an increase in the CSF PGE_2 levels. Plasma obtained from the donor that had received no endotoxin, but 0.9% sodium chloride instead, was found to be non-pyrogenic when infused into recipient cats; and no increase in CSF PGE_2 levels was found. In a cat that developed a post-operative fever, the deep body temperature was found to be 40.5 °C. A sample of CSF was taken and found to contain 7.8 ng ml^{-1} PGE_2. Plasma taken from this animal was infused into a recipient cat and produced a sustained fever, the temperature rising by 1.5 °C; and the PGE content of the CSF of the recipient increased from less than 1 ng to 3.8 ng.

In experiments in which Harvey and Milton injected EP into the conscious cat, they found that the anti-pyretic 4-Ac not only reduced the fever and lowered the elevated prostaglandin levels following central administration of EP, but also did so during intravenous infusion of EP. When the antipyretic agent was given while the EP infusion was maintained, antipyresis occurred in the presence of circulating EP. Similar results were obtained when plasma from a febrile cat was infused into an afebrile recipient animal. Again, 4-Ac reduced the fever.

Saxena *et al.* (1979) measured the prostaglandin-like activity of human CSF obtained from pyrexic patients with bacterial or viral infections. The CSF was obtained by lumbar puncture and tested for biological activity on the rat fundus strip preparation. Biological activity was assayed against a known solution of prostaglandin E_1. PGE-like activity was found in the CSF of patients suffering from high fever (39 °C) of short duration (less than 3 days). From their experimental records it would appear that a 1 ml sample of CSF obtained from a patient with tubercular meningitis contained approximately 1 ng PGE, and a sample from another patient with typhoid fever contained 3 ng PGE ml^{-1}. Prostaglandin-like activity was found in patients suffering from viral encephalitis or pyrogenic meningitis, and also in cases of undiagnosed fever. Prostaglandin-like activity was only occasionally detectable when the fever was of a lower magnitude (less than 39 °C) or of longer duration (5 days or more). No activity was present in the CSF of afebrile patients. The authors suggest that prostaglandins may play some role in the initial stages of pyrexia in man.

9.6 THERMOREGULATORY MECHANISMS BY WHICH PROSTAGLANDINS INCREASE BODY TEMPERATURE

In order to study the way in which prostaglandins raise deep body temperature, Bligh and Milton (1973) observed the effects of infusing PGE_1 into the cerebroventricular system of the conscious Welsh Mountain sheep. The sheep was chosen as the experimental animal for this study because of its ability to maintain a constant deep body temperature when exposed to a wide range of ambient air temperatures, varying from below freezing to above deep body temperature. It does this by regulating both heat loss and heat gain mechanisms. The responses can be regularly monitored. Bligh and Milton used three ambient temperatures, namely 10, 18 and 45 °C and recorded deep body temperature, ear-skin temperature, respiratory rate, and the presence or absence of shivering. The results of their experiments on one particular sheep are shown in Table 9.1. PGE_1 was infused at a rate of 2.5 μg min^{-1}. When the ambient air temperature was cold (10 °C), respiratory rate was low (minimizing evaporative heat loss), and the ear-skin temperature was the same as the air temperature, indicating vasoconstriction. Occasional bursts of electrical activity recorded from a thigh muscle indicated shivering. These measurements showed that the animal was maintaining its deep body temperature by minimizing heat loss and occasionally increasing heat production. When PGE_1 was infused, there was no change in ear-skin temperature, the respiratory rate dropped slightly, and violent shivering was recorded. This results in an immediate rise in deep body temperature. The elevated temperature was maintained so long as the infusion of PGE_1 lasted. However, as soon as the infusion was stopped, the animal began to pant and continued to do so until all the heat gained during the infusion of the PGE_1 had been lost and body temperature had returned to normal. In contrast, when the animal was exposed to an ambient temperature of 45 °C – that is, when the ambient temperature was above deep body temperature – the ear blood vessels were fully dilated, and vigorous panting was observed, with no sign of shivering. The animal was therefore actively preventing deep body temperature rising by evaporative heat loss. Under these conditions, when the PGE_1 infusion was started, the respiratory rate dropped dramatically; but there was no vasoconstriction, and no shivering was observed. Deep body temperature rose rapidly due to the depression of evaporative heat loss with the animal being unable to lose heat.

Table 9.1 PGE₁ infusion into the lateral ventricle of sheep

	Control	Effects of PGE$_1$ infusion	Measurements 1 hour after PGE$_1$ infusion
Ambient temperature 10 °C			
T rec. (°C)	39.3	40.8	40.2
T ear (°C)	10.8	9.9	11.0
Resp. rate/min	35	30	105
EMG	0/+	+++	0
Ambient temperature 45 °C			
T rec. (°C)	39.0	42.5	41.0
T ear (°C)	44.0	44.7	44.6
Resp. rate/min	220	30	324
EMG	0	0	0
Ambient temperature 18 °C			
T rec. (°C)	39.5	41.2	40.5
T ear (°C)	28.0	23.5	28.2
Resp. rate/min	150	30	270
EMG	0	++	0

Note: T rec. = rectal temperature; T ear = ear temperature; EMG = electromyographic recording from thigh muscle.

Immediately the PGE₁ infusion was stopped, panting recommenced, and the respiratory rate rose well above the pre-infusion level. This was maintained until deep body temperature had returned to normal. When the sheep was maintained at 18 °C the ear-skin temperature lay between air temperature and deep body temperature, indicating controlled vaso-motor tone. There was no shivering, but a relatively rapid respiratory rate was recorded, indicating some measure of evaporative heat loss. It should be remembered that, although the animals were at a room temperature of 18 °C, this is considerably greater than that normally experienced during a summer day in the mountains. The PGE₁ infusion produced a fall in respiratory rate, a decrease in ear-skin temperature – indicating vasoconstriction – and an occasional burst of shivering. Deep body temperature rose rapidly. When the PGE₁ infusion was stopped, shivering ceased, ear-skin temperature rose – indicating vasodilatation – and the respiratory rate rose, indicating evaporative heat loss. The deep body temperature soon returned to normal.

These experiments on the Welsh Mountain sheep provide consid-erable insight into our understanding of the thermoregulatory effects of the prostaglandins. They show that PGE₁ increases deep body temperature by inhibiting the heat loss mechanisms through inhibition of evaporative heat loss by panting, and by inhibiting surface heat loss through vasoconstriction. The prostaglandins stimulate heat gain mechanisms by increasing metabolic heat production through shivering.

Using the 1971 model of Bligh et al., these results can be interpreted as indicating an action for PGE_1 somewhere on the pathway between cold sensors and heat production in the effectors before the origin of crossed-inhibitory influences on the pathways between warm sensors and heat loss effect. The predominant pattern of thermoeffector activity depended upon ambient air temperature and therefore on the thermoregulatory pathways being driven at that time. During the infusion of the PGE_1, the maintained elevated temperature reflects a new equilibrium between heat gain and heat loss. There is no need to postulate the archaic view that the prostaglandins and therefore fever produce a resetting of the body thermostat to a higher temperature. Of particular interest were the observations that as soon as the PGE infusion was stopped, the animal rapidly lost the heat gained, and deep body temperature was rapidly restored to normal. This is reminiscent of the effects of antipyretic drugs in reducing fever. Again, it is unnecessary to postulate that antipyretic drugs act by resetting the thermostat back to normal.

Milton et al. reported in 1981 and 1983 that in the endotoxin-resistant MF1 mouse, injection of PGE_2 icv produced a coordinated increase in oxygen consumption, vasoconstriction and rise in deep body temperature.

9.7 PROSTAGLANDINS AND NORMAL BODY TEMPERATURE REGULATION

Though there can be no doubt that prostaglandins are involved in fever, the evidence would point to their not being involved in the control of normal body temperature. Cammock et al. (1976) subjected conscious cats to both heat (45 °C) and cold (0 °C), collected CSF from the cisterna magna, and measured the PGE content by radioimmunoassay. They found that during cold stress lasting for approximately 2 h, the animals assumed a crouched position to conserve body heat and exhibited vigorous and continuous shivering, vasoconstriction, and piloerection. The animals' deep body temperature was maintained during the cold stress. However, the PGE levels of the CSF were unchanged from those measured when the animals were maintained at an ambient temperature of 25 °C. In contrast, when the animals were exposed to heat stress, they stretched out to maximize heat loss, panted, and sweated from the paw pads. However, they were unable to maintain their deep body temperature, which rose steadily. No changes in the PGE levels of the CSF were observed, however. Subsequently, Bernheim, *et al.* (1980) subjected rabbits to cold and heat exposure and also to cooling and heating of the hypothalamus. They collected CSF from the third ventricle and assayed it for PGE activity by radioimmunoassay. Neither exposure to heat or cold nor changes in hypothalamic temperature produced any changes in the PGE levels of the CSF, whereas administration of endogenous pyrogen to the same animals produced marked increases in PGE.

These results indicate that prostaglandins do not appear to be involved in normal body temperature regulation and the results also explain why antipyretic drugs have little effect in the afebrile state. Occasionally it has been reported that the cyclo-oxygenase inhibitors have been observed to lower resting deep body temperature, but only minimally (Milton, 1972). Recent experiments by Rotondo *et al.* (1988) have shown that at rest there are detectable levels of the PGE_2 circulating in the blood and these are reduced to undetectable levels by the cyclo-oxygenase inhibitor ketoprofen and at the same time they observed a slight fall in deep body temperature. Interestingly, they found that heat stress, producing increases in deep body temperature, was without effect on circulating PGE_2 levels.

9.8 DOES ASPIRIN EXERT ITS ANTIPYRETIC ACTION AT A PERIPHERAL OR CENTRAL SITE?

There is no evidence that exogenous pyrogens produce fever directly in the central nervous system but act as previously described in initiating the synthesis of interleukin-1/endogenous pyrogen. Following systemic infection, if indeed either exogenous or endogenous pyrogen were to produce fever by acting directly on the brain, they would have to cross the blood brain barrier. All of the studies using radiolabelled endotoxins have failed to show the penetration of radioactivity into the brain (Dascombe and Milton, 1979). However, since endotoxins produce fever via the intermediate protein, interleukin-1, there indeed is no reason why endotoxins should have to penetrate into the brain. However, this then raises the question as to whether IL-1/EP itself can in fact get into the central nervous system. Again, as with endotoxin there is no convincing evidence that IL-1/EP can actually cross the blood brain barrier and localize in the pre-optic area of the hypothalamus. Dinarello *et al.* (1978) have reported that when human purified ^{125}I-labelled IL-1 is administered to rabbits no radiolabelled pyrogen was detected in either the anterior hypothalamus or the fourth ventricle although its administration produced fever. More recently Stitt (1985) has suggested that endogenous pyrogens cannot enter into neuropile but could act in the area of the *organum vasculosum laminae terminalis* (OVLT) which strictly lies outside the blood brain barrier and may initiate the synthesis and release of neuromodulators for fever at that site. Even more recently, Blatteis *et al.* (1989) have shown that when ^{125}I-interleukin-1α, was given systemically they could find no evidence of any interleukin-1 in the whole brains of the animals, as determined by radioactivity and, also, when they implanted microdialysis probes into the pre-optic area of the hypothalamus there was again no evidence of any radioactivity, in contrast to finding radioactivity in blood, lungs, liver, kidney and urine. Finally, they injected [125]I- IL-1α bilaterally into the pre-optic area of three conscious guinea-pigs. All these animals developed fever and were killed during the rise in body temperature. Two large grainy areas were located bilaterally in the pre-optic area of the hypothalamus at the sites of the injections. There was no evidence that the radioactivity had spread and no obvious disappearance of the [125]I- IL-1α from the PO. In their discussions, Blatteis *et al.* suggest that though pyrogenic doses of circulating IL-1 probably do not enter the brain the IL-1 may interact with receptors in the area of the OVLT and that this interaction may, in turn, introduce cellular signals that transduce the original message and pass it into the brain.

9.9 PYROGENS AND CIRCULATING PROSTAGLANDIN LEVELS

In 1988, Rotondo *et al.* reported that not only bacterial endotoxin but also the interferon-inducer Poly I:C and endogenous pyrogen/interleukin-1 all increase circulating blood levels of PGE_2. The increase was parallel to the increase in body temperature, increasing as fever developed and falling as the fever abated. Prior administration of the non-steroidal anti-inflammatory drug ketoprofen completely abolished the rise in body temperature and the rises in PGE_2 levels (Fig.9.3). Ketoprofen given during the peak of fever produced rapid and complete defervescence; blood PGE_2 levels decreased to undetectable levels.

In a subsequent study Abul and Milton (1989) measured the levels of PGE_2 in CSF in rabbits in which a cannula had previously been implanted into the third cerebral ventricle, using push-pull perfusion. They found that both Poly I:C and IL-1/EP increased the amount of PGE_2 and the increase paralleled the increase in body temperature. Ketoprofen completely inhibited the febrile response and the PGE_2 levels in the perfusate were not detectable.

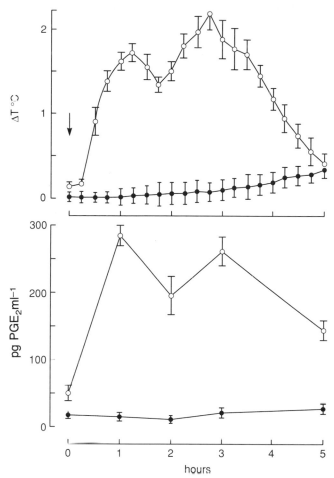

Figure 9.3 The effect of LPS on body temperature and blood PGE$_2$ levels with and without ketoprofen pre-treatment. Ketoprofen (3 mg kg^{-1}, closed circles) or sterile saline (open circles) was given s.c. 15 min before LPS (0.2 µg kg^{-1}) given *i.v.* at the time indicated by the arrow. Rectal temperature was measured continuously and calculated as a change from the basal level. Blood samples were taken at various intervals for the measurement of PGE$_2$ which was estimated by radioimmunoassay. n = 4, ± sd. (From Rotondo *et al.*, 1988, with permission.)

9.9.1 Actions of Pyrogens on Phospholipase A$_2$ Activity

The primary event in the synthesis of the prostaglandins and other eicosanoids is the availability of arachidonic acid. Arachidonic acid does not exist in the free form but only as a constituent of endogenous cell phospholipids. There are two separate pathways involved in making arachidonic acid available from cell constituents – one involving phospholipase A_2 (PLA_2) and the other a diacylglycerol-lipase (Fig. 9.4).

Phospholipase A_2 catalyses the hydrolysis of arachidonic acid from the 2-position of phosphatidyl-choline and other phosphatides present in cell membranes. Diacylglycerol-lipase hydrolyses diacylglycerol (DAG), this substrate having been made available by the action of phospholipase C on phosphatidyl-inositol.

In 1987 Milton and Rotondo investigated the effects of rabbit endogenous pyrogen, recombinant human interleukin-1 (rhIL-1), and tumour necrosis factor (TNF) on PLA_2 activity in purified synaptic plasma membranes and mononuclear leucocyte subcellular fractions from rabbit and purified PLA_2 from snake venom. In addition, they studied the effects of bacterial lipopolysaccharide, Poly I:C, and PGE_2 on the purified PLA_2. PLA_2 activity was estimated by measuring the production of [^{14}C]arachidonic acid from [^{14}C]arachidonyl phosphatidyl-choline after incubation with calcium ions and calmodulin.

They found that rabbit EP increased the PLA_2 activity of both the mononuclear leucocyte fractions and the purified PLA_2 in the order of threefold; rhIL-1 also significantly increased the activity of both preparations, though only 1.3-fold. Preincubation of both EP and rhIL-1 at 80 °C abolished their stimulating activity. In contrast, TNF inhibited the PLA_2 activity of both preparations. LPS inhibited the purified PLA_2 preparation, and Poly I:C and PGE_2 were without effect. The PLA_2 activity of the synaptic membrane was much less than that of the mononuclear leucocyte fractions. None of the pyrogens had any effect.

Milton and Rotondo concluded from their results that endogenous pyrogen and interleukin-1 stimulate PLA_2 activity in mononuclear leucocytes but not in neuronal membranes and that this may be a direct effect on the enzyme itself.

9.9.2 Phospholipase C: Action of Pyrogens on Inositol-Phosphate Accumulation in Cells

Much attention has been paid recently to the role of phosphatidyl-inositol (PI) metabolism in the transduction of extracellular signals into intracellular events. It has been shown that the hydrolysis of membrane phosphatidyl-inositol 4–5 bis-phosphate is an important early event in cell activation in a variety of systems. Hydrolysis of phosphatidyl-inositol 4–5 bis-phosphate catalysed by phospholipase C produces two prospective intracellular messengers: inositol 1–4–5 tris-phosphate (IP_3) and diacylglycerol. IP_3 functions to mobilize calcium ions from intracellular stores, whereas DAG activates protein-kinase C and in addition may be broken down to arachidonic acid by the enzyme DAG lipase. Thus indirectly phospholipase C increases the intracellular availability of arachidonic acid and hence increases eicosanoid biosynthesis (Fig. 9.4). The ability of IP$_3$ to mobilize the intracellular calcium necessary for phospholipase A$_2$ activity in a variety of tissues raises the possibility that bacterial lipopolysaccharide

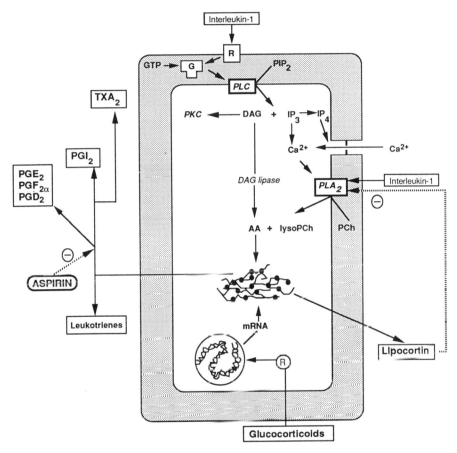

Figure 9.4 Schematic representation of activation of phospholipase A$_2$ by interleukin-1. PLA$_2$ = phospholipase A$_2$; PLC = phospholipase C; R = receptor; G = GTP-binding protein; DAG = diacyglycerol; PIP$_2$ = phosphatidyl-inositol-bis-phosphate; IP$_3$ = inositol-trisphosphate; AA = arachidonic acid; lyso PCh = lysophosphatidyl-choline; PKC = protein kinase C; DAG lipase = diacylglycerol-lipase; PCh = phosphatidyl-choline; mRNA = messenger RNA; TXA$_2$ = thromboxane A$_2$; PGI$_2$ = prostacyclin; PGE$_2$ = prostaglandin E$_2$; PGF$_{2\alpha}$ = prostaglandin F$_{2\alpha}$; PGD$_2$ = prostaglandin D$_2$ (adapted from Milton and Rotondo, 1989).

235

and other pyrogenic immunomodulators may stimulate phosphatidyl-inositol turnover in leucocytes. Kozak *et al.* (1988, 1989) reported on the results of the experiments that they had carried out on the effects of lipopolysaccharide, muramyl-dipeptide (MDP), and Poly I:C on the accumulation of inositol phosphates (IP) in leucocytes. They found that all three pyrogens increased the IP level in monocytes, with the maximum increase occurring when the cells were incubated with the pyrogens for 2 h. If incubations were carried out for less than 1 h, no accumulation occurred. In a separate series of experiments they found that the protein synthesis inhibitor anisomycin reduced the LPS-stimulated IP increase. In contrast to the effects of LPS, Poly I:C and MDP, interleukin-1 increased the IP levels in the monocytes within 10 min, the maximum being reached after 30 min. The action of IL-1 was not inhibited by anisomycin. They conclude that in view of the longer period required by the exogenous immunomodulators before a significant increase in IP level was observed and the inhibition by anisomycin, it would appear that the increase in IP levels in response to LPS in particular requires a protein mediator. A likely candidate for this protein mediator is IL-1, as a rapid increase in the IP levels was observed when this immunomodulator was used. These results suggest that the increase in IP levels in response to the exogenous immunomodulators does not occur directly and that this is not a likely mechanism by which the exogenous immunomodulators trigger the biosynthesis of interleukin-1. It would appear more likely that interleukin-1 exerts its vast array of actions, including possible prostanoid production, by this signal transduction mechanism.

9.9.3 Pyrogen-stimulated Release of Prostaglandin E_2 from Monocytes

In 1989 Abul and Milton reported on their studies into the effects of pyrogens on the release of prostaglandin E_2 from rabbit monocytes. Monocytes were incubated with LPS, Poly-I:C and IL-1/EP at different concentrations and for varying periods of time. During a 24-h period unstimulated monocytes released 160 ± 21 pg of $PGE_2/10^4$ cells. When Poly-I:C was present in a concentration of 1 μg ml^{-1}, 380 ± 25 pg PGE_2 was released. Similar increases were observed with 10 μg ml^{-1} LPS and 50 pg ml^{-1} IL-1/EP. When the monocytes were incubated with any of the three pyrogens in the presence and absence of the non-steroidal anti-inflammatory agent, ketoprofen, not only was the pyrogen-stimulated PGE_2 release abolished but also in unstimulated monocytes the spontaneous release decreased. The release of PGE_2 from monocytes pretreated with the protein synthesis inhibitor, anisomycin, before challenging them with LPS and Poly-I:C, was markedly reduced, whereas in contrast anisomycin had no effect on the release stimulated by IL-1/EP.

From the results of the experiments described in this section it would appear that interleukin-1/EP is stimulating the synthesis and release of prostaglandin E_2 from peripheral sites. It is the PGE_2 and not the bacterial pyrogen or IL-1/EP which crosses the blood brain barrier into the central nervous system to act in the area of the pre-optic anterior hypothalamus to raise deep body temperature. Since the anti-pyretic drugs inhibit the peripheral synthesis of prostaglandin E_2 in the whole animal and also inhibit the stimulation of cells to produce prostaglandin E_2 it would seem most probable that antipyretic agents are indeed acting to prevent fever by a peripheral and not a central action. This would explain why antipyretic drugs such as indomethacin, which are known to penetrate only very slowly into the CNS, are in fact most effective antipyretic drugs when administered peripherally.

That pyrogens can produce fever when injected directly into the CNS is well documented. However, the time course of the action is very different from that when they are given peripherally. One possibility is that the pyrogens have to pass from the central nervous system back into the periphery in order to stimulate IL-1 release and, hence, prostaglandin synthesis, or more likely, as was suggested by Dascombe and Milton (1979) when pyrogens are injected directly into the brain they initiate a local inflammatory response which results in the subsequent production of prostaglandins. This inflammatory response to centrally administered pyrogens can be blocked by antipyretic drugs, including aspirin, which can penetrate into the central nervous system (Milton, 1972).

9.10 FUNCTION OF FEVER

9.10.1 Introduction

One question which needs to be answered is whether fever is beneficial. Is fever part of the mechanism by which the host responds to infection, in which case it should not be treated, or is it a toxic reaction to the invading organism and therefore should be treated? Fever can occur in a large number of animals from such lowly ones as the leech right up to man. In non-mammalian species fever results normally as a consequence of behavioural thermoregulation where the organism, if it can, deliberately moves into a warmer environment. For example, the survival rates of bacteria-infected lizards increase if they are held at a higher ambient temperature than when they are kept at a lower temperature (Kluger *et al.*, 1975) and it has been suggested that fever may have evolved in reptiles as a resistance mechanism to decrease morbidity and mortality (Bernheim and Kluger, 1976). The idea that fever functions as a mechanism of host defence is not new. In clinical practice fever therapy has been used in the treatment of several diseases, for example, persons suffering from paralysis attributed to syphilis were treated by being made febrile with infectious blood of malarial patients (Wagner-Jauregg, 1927), and typhoid vaccine was used to treat resistant forms of gonorrhoea (Knight *et al.*, 1943). The exact mechanism behind reducing diseases by elevating body temperature is not certain. Some studies indicate that there is a direct effect between high temperature and the decreased growth or decreased survival of pathogenic organisms. Gonococcus, the micro-organism responsible for causing gonorrhoea, is killed at a temperature of 40 °C (Speirer, 1931). Carpenter *et al.* in 1933 reported similar results and suggested that fever would be a useful therapeutic agent in the treatment of gonorrhoea. Indeed, the growth of many species of bacteria, for example strains of pneumococci, are inhibited by febrile temperatures, as was discussed by Bennett and Nicastri (1960).

Another direct effect of high temperature on pathogens is believed to be an inhibitory effect on viral ribonucleic acid. Lwoff (1959, 1969) investigated several aspects of the direct effects of temperature on the growth of poliomyelitis virus. The yield of virus growth in tissue culture at 37 °C was 250 times greater than that at 40 °C. He concluded that this effect was not due to destruction of virus by high temperature but rather that the growth was being impaired. However, some viruses, such as herpes simplex, seem to grow better at elevated or febrile temperatures. Fever therapy has also been used in anti-tumour treatment. Overgaard (1977) has reviewed the effects of high temperature on malignant cells and concludes that various types of cells appear to be selectively destroyed when they are heated between 40 and 43 °C. Another mechanism by which fever or elevated body temperature appears to act as a defence mechanism against microbial infection is by indirect action between the pathogens and the immune response. Several of the cytokines have been shown to be increased in elevated body temperatures. These include interferons and interleukin-2 which are thought to participate in various aspects of the immune response (Ho, 1970; Dinarello, 1984; Downing and Taylor, 1987). In addition, Downing and Taylor examined different parameters of the immune response in man by raising body temperature to 39 °C by placing individuals in a warm-water bath. They found that IL-2 and NK cell numbers were increased during elevated body temperature. While lymphocyte transformation was depressed tumour necrosis factor was unchanged. Although the survival rate of rabbits injected with Gram-negative bacteria increases as fever rises to about 1.5 °C above the normal temperature, if the temperature then rises further, the number of surviving animals decreases (Kluger and Vaughn, 1978). Furthermore, fever increases the toxicity of endotoxin in rabbits, mice and rats (Connor and Kass, 1961; Atwood and Kass, 1964). Similar disagreements between the beneficial and deleterious effects in man have been reviewed by Bennett and Nicastri (1960). In general, the magnitude of fever is associated with the severity of the infection and as a result patients with a high fever tend to have the highest mortality rate. Therefore, the beneficial role of fever in man is still obscure. Indeed, in clinical practices fever can be detrimental to humans if it is not treated, especially in children where fever can induce seizures. A child who has had a single febrile convulsion is much more likely to become epileptic (Annegers et la., 1979). Other situations in which fever should be treated have been reviewed by Dinarello (1982).

9.10.2 Endogenous Antipyresis

In recent years the concept that the body produces an endogenous antipyretic has been put forward. In 1979 Cooper et al. reported on the antipyretic action of arginine vasopressin (AVP, antidiuretic hormone). This has led to the view that perhaps AVP has role as a regulator limiting fever and preventing temperature rising to too high a level with consequent danger to the host. As well as AVP other brain peptides, for example, adrenocorticotrophic hormone, (ACTII), and α-melanocyte-stimulating hormone (αMSH), a fragment of ACTH, may also be involved in limitation of fever (Lipton et al., 1981; Abul et al., 1987a). Interestingly, AVP can release ACTH from the anterior pituitary, resulting in corticosteroid release from the adrenal cortex. Corticosteroids, such as dexamethasone, though not strictly antipyretic, can limit the extent of the development of fever (Abul et al., 1987b). The action of corticosteroids is thought to be mediated by stimulating the synthesis of an endogenous phospholipase A_2 inhibitor known as lipocortin which prevents the formation of the eicosanoids. AVP which, of course, is also known as antidiuretic hormone, increases water reabsorption from the kidney tubules and maintains the hydration of the body. It is well known that during fever urine production is often markedly reduced. The interrelationship between the antipyretic action of AVP and its action on water conservation during fever has been discussed by Zeisburger (1985).

9.11 CONCLUSION

Fever is one component of the acute phase of the immune response to invading organisms. It is triggered by exogenous pyrogens, constituents of the invading organism, which in turn stimulate the release of an endogenous pyrogen from various cells of the host and which is called interleukin-1.

Interleukin-1, probably acting on peripheral cells such as monocytes and macrophages, stimulates the synthesis and release of eicosanoids including, in particular, prostaglandin E_2. The site of action of inter-leukin-1 to stimulate eicosanoid synthesis is probably the enzyme phospholipase A_2.

Circulating prostaglandin E_2 enters the CNS and in the pre-optic area of the anterior hypothalamus activates heat gain pathways and inhibits heat loss pathways leading to a rise in body temperature, namely fever.

Aspirin and other non-steroidal anti-inflammatory drugs inhibit the fatty acid cyclo-oxygenase enzyme responsible for the synthesis of prostaglandin E_2 resulting thereby in antipyresis. Since the PGE_2 is probably synthesized from peripheral cells the action of aspirin is a peripheral and not a central action.

Except in life-threatening situations, the use of antipyretic drugs, such as aspirin, is questionable. In fact, antipyretics may prolong infection and therefore their use may be disadvantageous.

REFERENCES

Abul, H.T. and Milton, A.S. (1989). The effects of dexamethasone on prosta-glandin E_2 release into rabbit CSF during fever and on the pyrogen stimulated release of prostaglandin E_2 from rabbit monocytes. *J. Physiol. (Lond.)*, **409**, 60P.

Abul, H.T., Davidson, J., Milton, A.S. and Rotondo, D. (1987a). The effects of peripherally administered ACTH1-24 and α-MSH on normal body temperature during fever in the rabbit. *Brit. J. Pharmacol.*, **91**, 493P.

Abul, H.T., Davidson, J., Milton, A.S. and Rotondo, D. (1987b). Dexamethasone pre-treatment is antipyretic toward polyinosinic:polycytidylic acid, lipo-polysaccharide and interleukin-1/endogenous pyrogen. *NaunynSchmiede-berg's Arch. Pharmacol.*, **335**, 305–9.

Annegers, J.F., Hauser, W.A., Elveback, L.R. and Kurland, L.T. (1979), The risk of epilepsy following febrile convulsions. *Neurology*, **29**, 297–303.

Atwood, R.P. and Kass, E.H. (1964). Relationship of body temperature to the lethal action of bacterial endotoxin. *J. Clin. Invest.*, **43**, 151–9.

Auron, P.E., Rosenwasser, L.J., Matsushima, K. *et al.* (1985) Human and murine interleukin-1 possess sequence and structural similarities. *J. Mol. Cell. Immunol.*, **2**, 169–77.

Bennett, I.L. Jr and Nicastri, A. (1960). Fever as a mechanism of resistance. *Bact. Rev.*, **24**, 16–34.

Bernheim, H.A. and Kluger, H.J. (1976). Fever and antipyresis in the lizard *dipsosaurus dorsalis*. *Am. J. Physiol.*, **231**, 198–203.

Bernheim, H.A., Gilbert, T.M. and Stitt, J.T. (1980). Prostaglandin E levels in the third ventricular cerebrospinal fluid of rabbits during fever and changes in body temperature. *J. Physiol. (Lond.)*, **301**, 69–78.

Blatteis, C.M., Dinarello, C.A., Shibata, M. *et al.* (1989) Does circulating interleukin-1 enter the brain? In *Thermal Physiology 1989*, Excerpta Medica International Congress Series 871 (ed. J.B. Mercer), Elsevier, Amsterdam, pp. 385–90.

Bligh, J. and Milton, A.S. (1973) The thermoregulatory effects of prostaglandin E1 when infused into a lateral cerebral ventricle of the Welsh Mountain sheep at different ambient temperatures. *J. Physiol. (Lond.)*, **229**, 30–31P.

Bligh, J., Cottle, W.H. and Maskrey, M.A. (1971) Influence of ambient temperature on the thermoregulatory responses to 5-hydroxytryptamine, noradrenaline and acetylcholine injected into the lateral cerebral ventricles of sheep, goats and rabbits. *J. Physiol. (Lond.)*, **212**, 377–92.

Cammock, S., Dascombe, M.J. and Milton, A.S. (1976) Prostaglandins in thermoregulation. In *Advances in Prostaglandin and Thromboxane Research*, Vol. 1 (eds B. Samuelsson and R. Paoletti), Raven Press, New York, pp. 375–80.

Carpenter, C.M., Boak, R.A., Mucci, L.A. and Warren, S.L. (1933) Studies on the physiologic effects of fever temperatures. The thermal death time of *Neissseria gonorrhoeae in vitro* with special reference to fever temperatures. *J. Lab. Clin. Med.*, **18**, 981–90.

Connor, D.G. and Kass, E.H. (1961) The effect of artificial fever in increasing susceptibility to bacterial endotoxin. *Nature (Lond.)*, **190**, 453–4.

Cooper, K.E., Kasting, N.W., Lederis, K. and Veale, W.L. (1979) Evidence supporting a role for endogenous vasopressin in natural suppression of fever in the sheep. *J. Physiol. (Lond.)*, **295**, 33–45.

Currie, J. (1808), *Medical Reports on the Effects of Water as a Remedy in Fever and other Diseases*, 4th London edn Philadelphia. Presented for James Humphries and for Benjamin and Thomas Kite.

Dascombe, M.J. and Milton, A.S. (1975) The effects of cyclic adenosine 3′, 5′-monophosphate and other adenine nucleotides on body temperature. *J. Physiol. (Lond.)*, **250**, 143–60.

Dascombe, M.J. and Milton, A.S. (1979) Study on the possible entry of bacterial endotoxin and prostaglandin E2 into the central nervous system from the blood. *Brit. J. Pharmacol.*, **66**, 565–72.

Davidson, J., Milton, A.S. and Rotondo, D. (1989) Effect of dexamethasone and ketoprofen on the pyrogenic response to human recombinant interleukin-1α (IL-1α) and interleukin-1β, (IL-1β), *Brit. J. Pharmacol.*, **97**, 429P.

Davidson, J., Milton, A.S. and Rotondo, D. (1990) A study of the pyrogenic actions of interleukin 1α and interleukin 1β, interactions with a steroidal and a non-steroidal anti-inflammatory agent. *Brit. J. Pharmacol.*, **100**, 542–6.

Dinarello, C.A. (1982) The treatment of fever from a clinical viewpoint. In *Pyretics and Antipyretics. Handbook Exp. Pharm.*, Vol. 60 (ed. A.S. Milton), Springer-Verlag, Berlin, Heidelberg, pp. 529–46.

Pharmacology of aspirin and salicylates

Dinarello, C.A. (1984), Interleukin-1. *Rev. Infect. Dis.*, **6**, 51–95.

Dinarello, C.A., Weiner, P. and Wolff, S.M. (1978) Radiolabelling and disposition in rabbits of purified human leukocytic pyrogen. *Inflammation*, **2**, 179–89.

Downing, J.F. and Taylor, M.W. (1987) The effect of *in vivo* hyperthermia on selected lymphokines in man. *Lymphokine Res.*, **6**, 103–9.

Feldberg, W. and Saxena, P.N. (1971) Further studies on prostaglandin E$_1$ fever in cats. *J. Physiol. (Lond.)*, **219**, 739–45.

Feldberg, W. and Gupta, K.P. (1973) Pyrogen fever and prostaglandin-like activity in cerebrospinal fluid. *J. Physiol. (Lond.)*, **228**, 41–53.

Feldberg, W., Gupta, K.P., Milton, A.S. and Wendlandt, S. (1973). The effect of pyrogen and antipyretics on prostaglandin activity in cisternal CSF of unanaesthetized cats. *J. Physiol. (Lond.)*, **234**, 279–303.

Goodman, L.S. and Gilman, A. (1970) *The Pharmacological Basis of Therapeutics*, 4th edn, The Macmillan Company, New York.

Hanzlik, P.J. (1927) Actions and use of salicylates and cinchophen in medicine. In *Medicine Monographs, vol* **9**, Williams and Wilkins, Baltimore.

Harvey, C.A. and Milton, A.S. (1975) Endogenous pyrogen fever, prostaglandin release and prostaglandin synthetase inhibitors. *J. Physiol. (Lond.)*, **250**, 18–20P.

Ho, M. (1970) Factors influencing the interferon response. *Arch. Intern. Med.*, **126**, 135–46.

Kilian, P.L., Kaffka, K.L., Stern, A.S. *et al.* (1986) Interleukin-1α and interleukin-1β bind to the same receptor on T cells. *J. Immunol.*, **136**, 4509–14.

Kim, D.H., Van Arman, C.G. and Armstrong, D. (1982) The chemistry of non-steroidal antipyretic agents: structure-activity relationships. In *Pyretics and Antipyretics. Handbook Exp. Pharm.*, Vol. 60 (ed. A. S. Milton), Springer-Verlag, Berlin, Heidelberg, pp. 317–75.

Kluger, M.J. (1980) *Fever. Its Biology, Evolution, and Function*, Princeton University Press, Princeton NJ.

Kluger, M.J. and Vaughn, L.K. (1978) Fever and survival in rabbits infected with *Pasteurella multocida*. *J. Physiol. (Lond.)*, **282**, 243–51.

Kluger, M.J., Ringler, D.H. and Anver, M.R. (1975) Fever and survival. *Science*, **188**, 166–8.

Knight, H.C., Emory, M.L. and Flint, L.D. (1943) Method of inducing therapeutic fever with typhoid vaccine using intravenous drip technique. US Public Health Service, *Venereal Dis. Inform.*, **24**, 323–9.

Kozak, W., Milton, A.S. and Rotondo, D. (1988) Pyrogenic immunomodulators increase the accumulation of inositol phosphates in monocytes. *Brit. J. Pharmacol.*, **94**, 337P.

Kozak, W., Milton, A.S., Abul, H.T. *et al.* (1989) Lipopolysaccharide, muramyl dipeptide and polyinosinic:polycytidylic acid induce the accumulation of inositol phosphates in blood monocytes and lymphocytes. *Cellular Signalling*, **1**, 345–56.

Kunkel, S.L., Wiggins, R.C., Chensue, S.W. and Larrick, J. (1986) Regulation of macrophage tumour necrosis factor production by prostaglandin E$_2$. *Biochem. Biophys. Res. Comm.*, **137**, 404–10.

Latham, R.G. (1848) The works of Thomas Sydenham, MD, Vol. II, printed for the Sydenham Society, London, p. 138.

Lipton, J.M., Glyn, J.R. and Zimmer, J.A. (1981) ACTH and α-melanotropin in central temperature control. *Fed. Proc.*, **40**, 2760–4.

Longmore, G. (1798) Account of fourteen men of the Royal Artillery of Quebec who were nearly poisoned by drinking a decoction of certain plants. *Ann. Med. Edin.*, **3**, 364–78.

Lwoff, A. (1959) Factors influencing the evolution of viral diseases at the cellular level and in the organism. *Bact. Rev.*, **23**, 109–24.

Lwoff, A. (1969) Death and transfiguration of a problem. *Bact. Rev.*, **33**, 139–46.

March, C.J., Mosley, B., Larsen, A. *et al.* (1985) Cloning, sequence and expression of two distinct human interleukin-1 complementary DNAs. *Nature*, **315**, 641–47.

Milton, A.S. (1972) Prostaglandin E_1 and endotoxin fever and the effects of aspirin, indomethacin and 4-acetamidophenol. In *Advances in Biosciences, Vol. 9*, Pergamon Press, Oxford and Braunschweig Vieweg, pp. 495–500.

Milton, A.S. and Wendlandt, S. (1968) The effect of 4-acetamidophenol in reducing fever produced by the intracerebral injection of 5-hydroxytryptamine and pyrogen in the conscious cat. *Brit. J. Pharmacol.*, **34**, 215P.

Milton, A.S. and Wendlandt, S. (1970) A possible role for prostaglandin E_1 as a modulator for temperature regulation in the central nervous system of the cat. *J. Physiol. (Lond.)*, **207**, 76–7P.

Milton, A.S. and Wendlandt, S. (1971a) Effects on body temperature of prostaglandins of the A, E and F series on injection into the third ventricle of unanaesthetized cats and rabbits. *J. Physiol. (Lond.)*, **218**, 325–6.

Milton, A.S. and Wendlandt, S. (1971b) The effects of 4-acetamidophenol (paracetamol) on the temperature response of the conscious rat to the intracerebral injection of prostaglandin E_1, adrenaline and pyrogen. *J. Physiol. (Lond.)*, **217**, 33–4P.

Milton, A.S. and Rotondo, D. (1987) The effects of pyrogens on phospholipase A2 (PLA2) activity in the rabbit. *J. Physiol. (Lond.)*, **391**, 95P.

Milton, I.II. and Rotondo, D. (1989) *Thermoregulation: Research and Clinical applications*, Cover illustration. (eds. P. Lomax, and E. Schonbaum), Karger, Basel.

Milton, A.S., Pertwee, R.G. and Todd, M. (1981) The effect of prostaglandin E_2 and pyrogen on thermoregulation in the MF1 mouse. *J. Physiol. (Lond.)*, **322**, 59P.

Milton, A.S., Pertwee, R.G. and Todd, M. (1983). Prostaglandin hyperthermia in mice: effects of ambient temperature. In *Environment, Drugs and Thermoregulation* (eds. P. Lomax, and E. Schönbaum), Karger, Basel, pp. 150–2.

Mizel, S.B., Dayer, J.M , Krane, S.M and Mergenhagen, S.E. (1981) Stimulation of rheumatoid synovial cell collagenase and prostaglandin production by partially purified lymphocyte-activating factor (interleukin-1). *Proc. Natl. Acad Sci. USA*, **78**, 2474–77.

Newton, R.C. and Covington, M. (1987) The activation of human fibroblast prostaglandin E production by interleukin 1. *Cell. Immunol.*, **110**, 338–49.

Oppenheim, J.J., Kovacs, E.J., Matsushima, K. and Durum, S.K. (1986) There is more than one interleukin 1. *Immunology Today*, **7**, 45–56.

Overgaard, J. (1977) The effects of hyperthermia on malignant cells *in vivo*. *Cancer*, **39**, 2637–46.

Pharmacology of aspirin and salicylates

Rotondo, D., Abdul, H.T., Milton, A.S. and Davidson, J. (1988) Pyrogenic immunomodulators increase the level of prostaglandin E_2 in the blood simultaneously with the onset of fever. *Eur. J. Pharmacol.*, **154**, 145–52.

Saxena, P.N., Beg, M.M.A., Singhal, K.C. and Ahmad, M. (1979) Prostaglandin-like activity in the cerebrospinal fluid of febrile patients. *Indian J. Med. Res.*, **70**, 495–8.

Speirer, C. (1931) Die unspezifische behandlung der gonorrhoe mit pyrifer. *Derm-Wschr.*, **92**, 13–17.

Stitt, J.T. (1985) Evidence for the involvement of the *organum vasculosum laminae terminalis* in the febrile response of rabbits and rats. *J. Physiol. (Lond.)*, **368**, 501–11.

Stone, E. (1763) An account of the success of the bark of the willow in the cure of agues. *Phil. Trans.*, **53**,195–200.

Vane, J.R. (1957) A sensitive method for the assay of 5-hydroxytryptamine. *Brit. J. Pharmacol.*, **12**, 344–9.

Vane, J.R. (1971) Inhibition of prostaglandin synthesis as a mechanism of action for aspirin-like drugs. *Nature (New Biol.)*, **231**, 232–5.

Wagner-Jauregg, J. (1927) The treatment of *dimentia paralytica* by malaria innoculation. In *Nobel Lectures: Physiology of Medicine, 1922–1941*, Elsevier Publishing Co., New York, pp. 159–62.

Wunderlich, C.A. and Seguin, E. (1871) *Medical Thermometry and Human Temperature* William Wood, New York.

Zeisburger, E. (1985) Role of vasopressin in fever regulation and suppression. *Trends in Pharmacological Sciences*, **6**, 428–30.

10 *The anti-thrombotic and fibrinolytic actions of aspirin*

R.M. BOTTING, R.J. GRYGLEWSKI and J.R. VANE

When blood vessels are injured, circulating platelets adhere to the damaged vessel walls and aggregate, diminishing or arresting the haemorrhage. This interaction between platelets and vessel walls has an easily demonstrable physiological function. There is conclusive evidence that occlusive thrombi in arteries damaged by atherosclerosis contain platelets as the main component (Davies and Thomas, 1981, 1984). The formation of platelet thrombi appears to be very similar to that of haemostatic plugs of platelets.

The pathology of thrombus formation has been studied by subjecting healthy blood vessels to physical injury and this has formed the experimental basis for the present anti-platelet approaches to the therapy of arterial thrombosis. Clinical thrombosis generally occurs at sites of pathological damage to blood vessels due to the presence of atherosclerotic lesions, necrotic tissue or inflammatory cells. Platelets form the core of a developing thrombus to which are added erythrocytes, neutrophils and monocytes trapped in a fibrin/platelet network (Mustard et al., 1990; Ross et al., 1990; Myler et al., 1990).

Platelets do not accumulate on normal, intact endothelial cells. For the formation of most arterial thrombi, erosion of the endothelial lining with consequent exposure of the thrombogenic subendothelium is considered to be necessary (Mustard et al., 1987) leading to adhesion, activation, aggregation and recruitment of further platelets, together with fibrin formation. However, an intact endothelial lining that has been deprived of cyclo-oxygenase activity is also thrombogenic (Gryglewski, 1990).

10.1 PLATELETS

Platelets, the smallest circulating cell fragments in the blood are anucleate and are formed by the breakdown of megakaryocytes made in the bone marrow. They have a life span of 8–11 days and do not normally

Pharmacology of aspirin and salicylates

adhere to each other or to other blood cells. They contain mitochondria, a complex system of microtubules and three types of granules, namely:

1. α granules, which store fibronectin, von Willebrand's factor (vWF), thrombospondin, fibrinogen, platelet factors IV, V and VIII, various growth factors and albumen.
2. Dense granules, which contain 5-hydroxytryptamine (5-HT), adenosine diphosphate (ADP), adenosine triphosphate (ATP) and calcium.
3. Lysosomes, which contain hydrolase enzymes.

In addition, platelets convert arachidonic acid through the cyclooxygenase pathway to the potent proaggregatory and vasoconstrictor eicosanoid thromboxane A_2 (TXA_2) and through the 12-lipoxygenase pathway to 12-hydroperoxyeicosatetraenoic acid (12-HPETE) and 12-hydroxyeicosatetraenoic acid (12-HETE) (later in this chapter).

10.1.1 Platelets and Thrombosis

The formation of arterial thrombi is initiated at sites of vessel injury or where local blood flow is disturbed (Gertz et al., 1981). Serial sectioning of obstructed coronary arteries has established that the platelet thrombus responsible is invariably associated with recent haemorrhage into an underlying atherosclerotic plaque (Constantinides, 1966; Friedman, 1970; Davies and Thomas, 1981). The haemorrhages occur through fissures or fractures in the plaque; the sudden appearance of such a fissure or fracture may well be a random unpredictable event which affects coronary arteries and accounts for the clinical onset of acute coronary thrombosis (Born, 1979).

The plaque on which a thrombus grows has usually narrowed the arterial lumen. At constant blood pressure, the flow of blood is faster through the constriction than elsewhere in the artery. Therefore, high flow and wall shear rates do not prevent the aggregation of platelets as thrombi (Born, 1977). Indeed, the question arises of whether the activation of platelets that precedes their aggregation depends in some way on such abnormal haemodynamic conditions.

Rupture of an atherosclerotic plaque exposes the subendothelial layers of damaged blood vessel walls which are denuded of endothelium. The vascular subendothelium is probably the most thrombogenic natural surface known and fibrillar collagen in the subendothelium is the most potent stimulus for the adherence of platelets (Baumgartner, 1974).

Platelets adhere to the connective tissue of the subendothelium by interacting with a specific adhesion protein named von Willebrand's factor, which is released both from endothelial cells and from platelets.

246

This adhesion protein binds to both platelets and to subendothelial collagen forming a bridge between the platelets and the subendothelium. Platelet adhesion occurs by an initial attachment of the platelet to the vessel wall by a small area of the membrane or through pseudopodia and subsequent spreading (this could be the shape change observed during in-vitro experiments) in which the platelet is more intimately bound to the subendothelium (Leytin et al., 1984). Platelets can also adhere to artificial surfaces or in vitro to collagen but the mechanisms are different, since platelet adhesion to the subendothelium but not to collagen is prevented by prostacyclin (Lapetina, 1986).

An additional chemical factor contributing to adhesion and aggregation of platelets in whole blood is ADP released from red blood cells (Born et al., 1976). Platelets adhere and aggregate more rapidly in whole blood than in platelet-rich plasma, particularly when some lysis of red blood cells has taken place. This effect of red cells on platelets is prevented by the addition of enzymes capable of specifically utilizing ADP (Harrison and Mitchell, 1966). Free ADP can also be found in blood in concentrations sufficiently high to activate platelets (10^{-7}–10^{-6} M ADP; Schmid-Schönbein et al., 1981).

Adhering platelets become activated, release the contents of their granules (including ADP and 5-HT), and form TXA_2. These substances in turn recruit platelets still suspended in the flowing blood to stick to platelets already adhering to the connective tissue and thus a mass of aggregated platelets is formed (Baumgartner, 1973; Baumgartner et al., 1976; Cazevane et al., 1977).

The mechanism by which platelets adhere to collagen involves the platelet membrane glycoproteins Ia and Ib (GPIa and GPIb) together with adhesive proteins on the subendothelial layers such as vWF and fibronectin (Siess, 1989). Von Willebrand's factor is a large, negatively charged molecule which consists of a series of multimers of identical subunits (220 kDa) with increasing molecular mass. It primarily mediates adhesion of platelets at high shear rates such as those which occur in the arterial and capillary vascular beds (Fressinaud et al., 1988). The platelet receptor involved in the binding of vWF is the GPIb glycoprotein. Patients suffering from the Bernard-Soulier syndrome lack this receptor protein and show decreased platelet adhesion (Weiss et al., 1978; Sixma, 1987). The GPIa glycoprotein is the platelet cytoadhesive receptor mediating the binding of platelets to the extracellular matrix.

The binding of platelet to platelet by means of the glycoprotein IIb–IIIa complex (GPIIb/IIIa) linking with fibrinogen is thought to be responsible for aggregation. The binding of fibrinogen to the GPIIb/IIIa receptor requires the participation of calcium. Thrombospondin, released

247

from the endothelium, stabilizes fibrinogen binding and reinforces the platelet–platelet interactions by binding to a site distinct from the GPIIb/GPIIIa receptor (Gerrard, 1988). The GPIIb/IIIa cyto-adhesive receptor, a member of the integrin superfamily, is found only on platelets and megakaryocytes and represents the final common pathway leading to platelet aggregation. Its expression occurs in response to all pro-aggregatory platelet stimuli (Coller, 1990). Antibodies against the GPIIb/IIIa molecule have an anti-aggregatory effect; however, their *in-vivo* effectiveness in man remains to be evaluated.

Whether exposure of the GPIIb/GPIIIa receptor can be modulated through the phosphorylation of the 47 kDa protein, the major substrate for protein kinase C (PKC), remains to be elucidated. The function of the 47 kDa protein is not known, but, stimulation of phospholipase C releases diacylglycerol (DAG) which in turn activates PKC. Substances which prevent the generation of DAG or the activation of PKC have been reported to inhibit platelet aggregation (Siess, 1989).

As the platelet adheres, it goes through the 'shape change' from a disc to a sphere and then forms long pseudopodia. Spheration is associated with assembly of the contractile mechanism and centralization of the granules (Gerrard, 1988). When the stimulus is weak, shape change can occur without subsequent secretion or aggregation. However, with stronger stimuli, platelets will undergo the release reaction and aggregate.

The shape change is associated with the hydrolysis of inositol phospholipids (as a consequence of the activation of phospholipase C) to form inositol 1,4,5-triphosphate (IP_3). Inositol 1,4,5-triphosphate mobilizes intracellular calcium through a receptor-mediated action on the dense tubular system of the platelets. Calcium can also enter the platelets from the external medium by activation of a receptor-operated channel in the plasma membrane adjacent to the GPIIa/GPIIIb receptor. The increase in intracellular calcium leads to the stimulation of a calcium/calmodulin myosin light chain kinase which phosphorylates the myosin light chain and develops actin-activated ATPase activity. This ATPase enzyme interacts with proteins of the platelet cytoskeleton and a rearrangement of filaments causes their contraction which leads to centralization of cytosolic granules.

Coagulation pathways become activated by the surfaces of platelets that have undergone the release reaction, and by tissue factors from the injured vessel, leading to the formation of thrombin. Thrombin itself causes yet further aggregation, release of platelet granule contents and activation of the arachidonic acid pathway. It also catalyses the conversion of fibrinogen to fibrin, which helps to stabilize the mass of aggregated platelets (Mustard *et al.*, 1987). Thrombi which contain large amounts of fibrin should be particularly susceptible to lysis by fibrinolytic agents, for example, streptokinase and tissue plasminogen activator (tPA).

The extent of stimulation and type of granule released from platelets depends on the nature of the stimulus. For example, whereas all platelet stimuli can release the contents of α granules, agents such as thrombin or collagen (but not ADP) cause lysosomal enzyme release. The platelet release reaction is associated with a further phosphorylation of the proteins of the myosin light chain as well as phosphorylation of the 47 kDa protein. Activation of phospholipase A_2 with the subsequent release of the arachidonic acid metabolites, prostaglandin endoperoxides and TXA_2 provides an amplification mechanism to enhance the extent of the release reaction and increase platelet aggregation (Gerrard, 1988). More than 70% of the arachidonic acid liberated in platelets by phospholipase A_2 originates from membrane phosphatidylcholine and phosphatidylethanolamine (Lapetina, 1986). Thromboxane A_2 is the major cyclo-oxygenase product formed by platelets along with small amounts of prostaglandins E_2 and $F_{2\alpha}$.

Platelets from patients with a previous history of ischaemic heart disease exhibit hyperaggregability *in vitro* to various platelet aggregating agents (Meade *et al.*, 1985; Vilén *et al.*, 1985; Rubenfire *et al.*, 1986; Elwood *et al.*, 1991).

10.1.2 Thromboxane Synthesis

The prostaglandin endoperoxides, PGG_2 and PGH_2, were shown by Hamberg *et al.*, (1974) to induce platelet aggregation. This is accompanied by the formation of an unstable vasoconstrictor substance identified as TXA_2 (Hamberg *et al.*, 1975). Thromboxane A_2 has a chemical half-life at body pH and temperature of 30 s, breaking down to the inactive TXB_2. The activity of the rabbit aorta-contracting substance (RCS) released from sensitized guinea-pig lungs, first described by Piper and Vane (1969), can be accounted for by TXA_2. Thromboxane A_2 constricts large blood vessels, has variable vasoconstrictor activity in the microcirculation and is a potent stimulus for platelet aggregation. The enzyme that synthesizes TXA_2 from prostaglandin endoperoxides was first localized in the high-speed particulate fraction of human and horse blood platelets (Moncada *et al.*, 1976a; Needleman *et al.*, 1976). The enzyme has been solubilized and separated from the cyclo-oxygenase (Diczfalusy *et al.*, 1977; Hammarstrom and Falardeau, 1977; Yoshimoto *et al.*, 1977). Thromboxane synthase (TX-synthase) from human platelet 'microsomes' was isolated and characterized as a cytochrome P-450-containing protein with a molecular mass of 58 800 (Haurand and

Ullrich, 1985). This enzyme promotes conversion of PGH_2 to TXB_2 (derived from TXA_2) and to 12L-hydroxy-5,8,10-heptadecatrienoic acid (HHT; with an unknown biological function) in a 1:1 ratio (later in this chapter).

Using polyclonal and monoclonal antibodies directed against purified human platelet TX-synthase and an enzyme-linked immunosorbent assay (ELISA), the enzyme content of different human cells and tissues has been measured (Nüsing and Ullrich, 1990). After platelets, blood monocytes have the highest content of TX-synthase, whereas lung fibroblasts and promyelocytic cells have only very low levels. Contrary to previous reports, no enzyme was found in purified human polymorphonuclear leukocytes (Goldstein *et al.*, 1978; Conti *et al.*, 1987). Of the tissues examined, lung and liver have the highest content, with low levels of enzyme in spleen, kidney, brain, lymph nodes and gall bladder. However, it may also be in some instances that the production of TXA_2 by tissues is due to the presence of migratory cells such as histiocytes or macrophages. High TXB_2 production by some organs such as the kidney may be the result of an inflammatory reaction with monocytes migrating into the tissue and differentiating into macrophages (Morrison *et al.*, 1978). Certain vascular tissues can also produce TXA_2, including human umbilical artery, rabbit pulmonary artery and cultured bovine endothelial cells (Tuvemo *et al.*, 1976; Salzman *et al.*, 1980; Ingerman-Wojenski *et al.*, 1981).

Thromboxane A_2 has been synthesized and its structure confirmed (Bhagwat *et al.*, 1985). Its potent pro-aggregatory effects are due to receptor-activated phosphoinositide metabolism (Siess *et al.*, 1983). The platelet receptors for TXA_2 can be additionally stimulated by the endoperoxide, PGH_2. Platelet responses to both PGH_2 and TXA_2 are blocked by the same antagonists and the putative receptors have been designated TXA_2/PGH_2 receptors (Burch *et al.*, 1985).

10.2 THE VASCULAR ENDOTHELIUM

Endothelial cells generate prostacyclin and endothelium-derived relaxing factor (now identified as nitric oxide, NO), which contribute to the thromboresistant properties of the vascular endothelium (Fig. 10.1).

10.2.1 Prostacyclin

In 1976, Vane and his colleagues discovered that blood vessels made a previously unknown prostanoid which they called PGX (Moncada *et al.*, 1976b), and later renamed prostacyclin (Johnson *et al.*, 1976). This is a bicyclic eicosanoid with a short chemical half-life at physiological pH of approximately 3 min, and which degrades to the relatively inactive 6-oxo-prostaglandin $F_{1\alpha}$(6-oxo-$PGF_{1\alpha}$). As for TXA_2 in platelets (mentioned earlier), synthesis of prostacyclin begins with the release of arachidonic acid from cell membrane phospholipids by phospholipase A_2 or indirectly by phospholipase C. Arachidonic acid is transformed by prostaglandin H synthase (Markey *et al.*, 1987) to the unstable PGG_2 (cyclo-oxygenase activity) and PGG_2 to the unstable PGH_2 (peroxidase activity). Prostaglandin H_2 is then acted upon by microsomal prostacyclin synthase to form prostacyclin (Gryglewski *et al.*, 1976). The cyclo-oxygenase enzyme is inhibited by aspirin and other aspirin-like drugs (Vane, 1971; Flower *et al.*, 1972; Chapter 3 on the mechanism of action of aspirin) and its activity is modulated by hydroperoxides, including 15-HPETE, H_2O_2 and PGG_2. These peroxides also affect the activity of prostacyclin synthase. For example, the activity of cyclo-oxygenase is stimulated by low (10^{-10}–10^{-7} M) and inhibited by high (>10^{-6} M) concentrations of lipid hydroperoxides (Warso and Lands, 1983). Lipid hydroperoxides, e.g. HPETEs, are always inhibitory for prostacyclin synthase (Gryglewski *et al.*, 1976; De Witt and Smith,

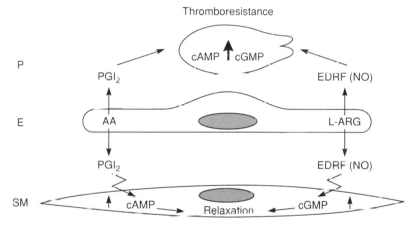

Figure 10.1 Endothelial cells (E) generate prostacyclin (PGI_2) and endothelium-derived relaxing factor/nitric oxide (EDRF/NO). Stimulation of receptors on E by serotonin or adenosine diphosphate released from platelets or thrombin, bradykinin or shear stress leads to release of these vasoactive mediators. Prostacyclin formed from arachidonic acid (AA) relaxes smooth muscle (SM) and inhibits aggregation of platelets (P) by increasing cyclic adenosine monophosphate (cAMP). EDRF/NO formed from L-arginine (L-ARG) also relaxes smooth muscle and inhibits platelet aggregation and adhesion but by increasing cyclic guanosine monophosphate (cGMP). By raising in platelets the levels of cAMP and cGMP simultaneously PGI_2 and EDRF/NO synergize in inhibiting aggregation.

Pharmacology of aspirin and salicylates

1983). This inhibitory action of hydroperoxides may be mediated by oxygen-derived free radicals such as the hydroxyl radical (OH·), which are formed during the reduction of HPETEs to HETEs (Egan *et al.*, 1976; Sagone *et al.*, 1980). Indeed, the inhibition of cyclo-oxygenase from bull seminal vesicles by high concentrations of H_2O_2 is reversed by uric acid or mannitol, which are known OH scavengers (Deby *et al.*, 1984). Hydroperoxides have no effect on thromboxane synthase activity (Ham *et al.*, 1979).

Prostacyclin is the main product of arachidonic acid metabolism by endothelial cells of the larger arteries and veins but it is also formed by endothelial cells of microvessels (Gerritsen, 1987). The ability of the large vessel wall to synthesize prostacyclin is greatest at the intimal surface and progressively decreases toward the adventitia (Moncada *et al.*, 1977). Production of prostacyclin by cultured cells from vessel walls also shows that endothelial cells are the most active producers of prostacyclin (Weksler *et al.*, 1977; MacIntyre *et al.*, 1978). Stripping of the endothelium from a rabbit aorta *in vivo* removed virtually all ability of the luminal surface to produce prostacyclin from exogenously added arachidonic acid. Recovery of prostacyclin production to 60% of that of uninjured vessels took about 35 days and still had not returned completely after 70 days (Weksler *et al.*, 1982).

A number of endogenous substances promote the release of prostacyclin from endothelial cells. These include thrombin, arachidonic acid, PGH_2, adenine nucleotides, trypsin, substance P and bradykinin (for review, Gryglewski *et al.*, 1988). In addition, pulsatile pressure releases prostacyclin from isolated arteries (Quadt *et al.*, 1982; Pohl *et al.*, 1987) which could be an important release mechanism for prostacyclin *in vivo*. However, circulating levels of prostacyclin in plasma are low (3 pg ml^{-1} plasma; Blair *et al.*, 1982) indicating that prostacyclin released by the endothelial cells probably acts as a local mediator on the underlying vascular smooth muscle.

The release of prostacyclin following receptor activation is initiated by a rapid increase in intracellular calcium above a threshold level (>0.8 mM) which then declines but remains above resting levels for several minutes (Pearson *et al.*, 1983). The initial increase in intracellular calcium is due to the release of calcium by IP_3, itself released as a consequence of stimulation of phospholipase C, whereas the sustained elevation of calcium is due to an entry of calcium from extracellular sources. The nature of this influx has not yet been elucidated but it does not occur through voltage operated calcium channels since these do not exist in endothelial cells (Hallam and Pearson, 1986). The increase in intracellular calcium then stimulates phospholipase A_2 and thus the release of arachidonic acid.

252

The release of prostacyclin is dependent on intracellular but not extra-cellular calcium, is transient and decreases upon repeated stimulation with the same agonist (Pearson *et al.*, 1983; Luckhoff and Busse, 1986; White and Martin, 1989). This desensitization does not depend upon a feedback effect of prostacyclin through activation of adenylate cyclase (Czervionke *et al.*, 1979; Brotherton *et al.*, 1982).

Prostacyclin potently inhibits aggregation of platelets, an effect medi-ated by stimulation of platelet adenylate cyclase which results in accu-mulation of cyclic adenosine monophosphate (cAMP; Tateson *et al.*, 1977) and stimulation of protein kinase A. Thus, prostacyclin initiates the phosphorylation of several proteins which are essential for platelet function. These include the 22 000 kDa polypeptide on the dense tubular system, the myosin light chain kinase and the glycoprotein Ib (GPIb) receptor involved in the binding of vWF to the platelet. Furthermore, by inhibiting the activity of the phospholipases A_2 and C, prostacyclin decreases the production of DAG, phosphatidic acid, arachidonic acid and IP_3 (Siess, 1989). Prostacyclin only weakly inhibits adhesion of platelets to thrombogenic surfaces. Its anti-adhesive effi-cacy varies according to the nature of the exposed surface (Adelman *et al.*, 1981). Inhibition by aspirin of endothelial cell cyclo-oxygenase and therefore of prostacyclin release, does not increase the adhesion of platelets to monolayers of endothelial cells (Hoak *et al.*, 1985); however, it does decrease the thromboresistance of rabbit aortic endothelial cells to whole citrated blood (Gryglewski, 1990). The pro-aggregatory effect induced by inhibition of cyclo-oxygenase in endothelial cells is explained by removal of the synergism between prostacyclin and NO, derived either from endothelial or circulating blood cells, which on their own are too low to inhibit platelet aggregation (Radomski *et al.*, 1987a).

Apart from its platelet suppressant and vasodilator actions (for review, Dusting *et al.*, 1986), prostacyclin has other actions which may be protective for the endothelial lining. For example, it promotes the outflow of free cholesterol from endothelial cells, suppresses the accumulation of cholesterol esters by macrophages, inhibits the release of growth factors from endothelial cells, platelets and macrophages (Willis *et al.*, 1986, 1987) and attenuates the release of free radicals and mediators from white blood cells (Kainoh *et al.*, 1990). The fibrinolytic (Dembinska-Kiec *et al.*, 1982; Szczeklik *et al.*, 1983) and cytoprotective actions of prostacyclin are well documented but the mechanisms underlying these effects are poorly understood (Gryglewski *et al.*, 1988). A deficiency in prostacyclin formation by blood vessel walls occurs in atherosclerosis and diabetes, whereas its overproduction is associated with endotoxic shock (Nawroth *et al.*, 1984).

10.2.2 Endothelium-derived Relaxing Factor (Nitric Oxide)

The direct evidence for the obligatory role of the endothelium in certain vascular smooth muscle relaxations was provided by Furchgott and Zawadzki (1980) when they demonstrated that acetylcholine produced relaxation of rings or strips of rabbit aorta only in the presence of an intact endothelium. The factor released from the endothelial cells responsible for the relaxation was called endothelium-derived relaxing factor (EDRF). It is released by a variety of substances including nor-adrenaline, substance P, bradykinin, ATP, ADP, arachidonic acid, 5-HT, histamine, thrombin and the calcium ionophore A23187 (Furchgott, 1984). Endothelium-derived relaxing factor is also released by electrical field stimulation (Frank and Bevan, 1983) and by pulsatile pressure (Rubanyi et al., 1986). Stimuli which activate receptors to release EDRF also largely lead to the release of prostacyclin. This and other evidence suggests that the two mechanisms are coupled (de Nucci et al., 1988).

Endothelium-derived relaxing factor is a labile vasodilator with a half-life of 3–50 s depending upon the experimental system which is being used (Gryglewski et al., 1986). The debate about its identity has lasted from the time of its discovery till the present. Furchgott and Ignarro both proposed at a meeting in 1986 (Khan and Furchgott, 1987; Ignarro et al., 1987) that EDRF was identical to nitric oxide. This was subsequently demonstrated experimentally by Moncada and his co-workers (Palmer et al., 1987) and confirmed by others (Ignarro et al., 1987; Kelm et al., 1988). Cultured endothelial cells stimulated with bradykinin released sufficient quantities of NO to account for the biological actions of EDRF. Further confirmation that EDRF and NO were identical came from studies where their biochemical and pharmacological properties were compared. EDRF and NO exhibit the same stability in buffer solutions and bioassay systems and both are inactivated by superoxide anions and by oxyhaemoglobin (Martin et al., 1985; Gryglewski et al., 1986; Ignarro et al., 1987). Both relax vascular smooth muscle, inhibit platelet function and stimulate soluble guanulate cyclase enzyme (Holzmann, 1982; Rapoport and Murad, 1983). However, some experimenters have suggested that EDRF is not NO but a closely related radical species (Cocks et al., 1985; Long et al., 1987) such as a nitrosothiol (Myers et al., 1990).

In addition to NO release from endothelial cells, NO is also released from human peripheral neutrophils and mononuclear cells (Salvemini et al., 1989). Nitric oxide release from these cells inhibits platelet aggregation, an effect which is markedly potentiated by superoxide dismutase. Furthermore, NO released from human neutrophils synergizes with prostacyclin to inhibit platelet aggregation (Salvemini et al., 1988). Thus, the release of NO from white blood cells can cooperate with release from endothelial cells in maintaining platelets in a quiescent state.

An enzymatic pathway for the conversion of L-arginine to nitrogen oxides was discovered in macrophages by Hibbs *et al.* (1987) and Iyengar *et al.* (1987). They also showed that a substrate analogue, N^G-monomethyl-L-arginine, blocked both the generation of nitrogen oxides and the cytostatic activity of the macrophages. Subsequently, Moncada and co-workers (Palmer *et al.*, 1988) showed a similar pathway in endothelial cells. A cytosolic enzyme in endothelial cells generates NO through the conversion of L-arginine to L-citrulline (Palmer and Moncada, 1989) and NO (Mayer *et al.*, 1989). Its activity is dependent on calcium ($EC_{50} = 60$ μM) and NADPH and is inhibited by L-arginine analogues such as N^G-monomethyl-L-arginine or N^G-nitro-L-arginine (Palmer and Moncada, 1989; Moore *et al.*, 1989; Mayer *et al.*, 1989). These NO synthase inhibitors dramatically raise the blood pressure, confirming that NO must be continuously released (Moncada *et al.*, 1989).

Most agonists which release NO also cause an elevation of intracellular calcium. In contrast to the release of prostacyclin, the release of NO depends primarily on calcium influx into endothelial cells rather than on an intracellular release of calcium (Luckhoff and Busse, 1986; White and Martin, 1989). NO release may be linked to a Na^+/Ca^{2+} exchange mechanism (Schoeffter and Miller, 1986). Unlike prostacyclin release, the generation of NO is sustained and not subject to tachyphylaxis (Kelm *et al.*, 1988; White and Martin, 1989).

The vasodilator and platelet-suppressant properties of NO are mediated through the stimulation of soluble guanylate cyclase enzyme and a subsequent increase in the intracellular levels of cyclic guanosine monophosphate (cGMP). Several *in-vitro* studies have now established that NO released directly from the endothelial cells or applied exogenously in solution inhibits aggregation of platelets in platelet-rich plasma (Azuma *et al.*, 1986) and of washed platelets (Radomski *et al.*, 1987a,b; Furlong *et al.*, 1987; MacDonald *et al.*, 1988; Alheid *et al.*, 1987; Bult *et al.*, 1988). Furthermore, NO inhibits platelet adhesion, as shown in experiments using either intact bovine aortae or monolayers of bovine cultured aortic endothelial cells (Radomski *et al.*, 1987c, Sneddon and Vane, 1988; Venturini *et al.*, 1989). Some studies have also demonstrated a role for NO in the control of platelet function *in vivo*. The concentrations of cGMP in platelets increased after systemic exposure to the EDRF-releasing action of carbachol (Hogan *et al.*, 1988). Methylene blue (an inhibitor of EDRF action) prevented the inhibition by carbachol of ADP-induced accumulation of ^{111}In-labelled platelets in the pulmonary circulation of the rat (Bhardwaj *et al.*, 1988) and cGMP levels in human washed platelets increased after the platelets were injected into a perfused rabbit heart under basal or acetylcholine-stimulated conditions (Pohl and Busse, 1989). It seems likely, therefore, that both basal and stimulated release of NO could be important in the *in-vivo* local regulation of platelet function. Interestingly, prostacyclin and NO synergize to inhibit platelet aggregation but not platelet adhesion (Radomski *et al.*, 1987c).

There is a substantial body of evidence from experimental studies in animals that a deficiency of NO may contribute to the pathogenesis of a number of diseases including hypertension, atherosclerosis and diabetes (review by Gryglewski *et al.*, 1988).

Oxidized low density lipoproteins (LDLs) inhibit endothelium-dependent relaxation (Jacobs *et al.*, 1990) which is also impaired in arteries removed from atherosclerotic or diabetic patients (Bossaller *et al.*, 1987; Andersen *et al.*, 1988) and hypercholesterolaemic rabbits or monkeys (Freiman *et al.*, 1986; Chappell *et al.*, 1987). Patients with atherosclerosis have a high rate of LDL oxidation while the plasma of patients with diabetes contains proteins which enhance adhesion of neutrophils to the vascular endothelium (Andersen *et al.*, 1988). Interestingly, NO and the NO-donor, sodium nitroprusside, inhibit the mitogenesis of fibroblasts and smooth muscle cells (Barrett *et al.*, 1989; Garg and Hassid, 1989). An anti-proliferative action of NO produced by the endothelial cell could prevent the hypertrophy of smooth muscle cells that takes place during the development of atherosclerosis.

10.3 PROSTACYCLIN AND THROMBOXANE BALANCE

As mentioned previously, prostacyclin and TXA_2 are both formed from the endoperoxide PGH_2, derived from arachidonic acid freed from the phospholipids of cell membranes. Thromboxane A_2 is an unstable ($t_{1/2} = 30$ s at 37 °C) powerful vasoconstrictor agent and aggregator of platelets. Prostacyclin is also unstable ($t_{1/2} = 3$ min at 37 °C) but it induces vasodilatation and inhibits platelet aggregation (Vane, 1982; Fig. 10.2).

It was proposed in 1976 that TXA_2 and prostacyclin represent the opposite poles of a homeostatic mechanism for regulation of platelet aggregability *in vivo* (Moncada *et al.*, 1976b). Evidence has been accumulating in recent years that EDRF may additionally be part of this regulating system.

Prostacyclin disperses platelet aggregates *in vitro* (Moncada *et al.*, 1976a; Ubatuba *et al.*, 1979) and in the circulation of man (Szczeklik *et al.*, 1978a). Moreover, it inhibits thrombus formation in models using the carotid artery of the rabbit (Ubatuba *et al.*, 1979) and the coronary artery of the dog (Aiken *et al.*, 1979), protects against sudden death (thought

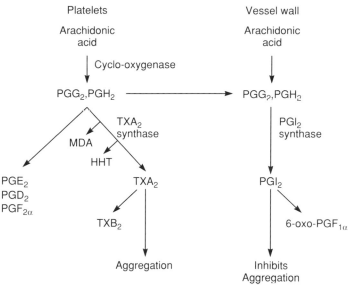

Figure 10.2 Arachidonic acid (AA) metabolism in platelets and blood vessel walls. Prostacyclin (PGI$_2$) and thromboxane A$_2$ (TXA$_2$) are formed from AA by cyclo-oxygenase with the endoperoxides, prostaglandins G$_2$ and H$_2$ (PGG$_2$ and PGH$_2$) as intermediates. They are unstable and break down to the stable and less active 6-oxo-PGF$_{1\alpha}$ and TXB$_2$. Aspirin, by inhibiting cyclo-oxygenase, reduces synthesis of prostacyclin and TXA$_2$. Endoperoxides can be shunted from platelets to the vascular endothelium to increase prostacyclin production. TXA$_2$ synthase metabolizes endoperoxides in platelets to TXB$_2$ and HHT in equal amounts.

to be due to platelet clumping) induced by intravenous arachidonic acid in rabbits (Bayer *et al.*, 1979) and inhibits platelet aggregation in pial venules of the mouse when applied locally (Rosenblum and Sabban, 1979).

As discussed earlier, prostacyclin inhibits platelet aggregation by stimulating adenylate cyclase, leading to an increase in platelet cAMP levels (Tateson *et al.*, 1977). In this respect prostacyclin is much more potent than either PGE$_1$ or PGD$_2$ and its effect is longer-lasting Prostacyclin inhibits platelet aggregation (platelet-platelet interaction) at much lower concentrations than those needed to inhibit adhesion (platelet-collagen interaction) (Higgs *et al.*, 1978). Thus, the loss of NO generation by removed or damaged endothelial cells plus prostacyclin formation by deeper tissues will permit platelets to stick as a monolayer to vascular tissue and to interact with it so allowing platelets to participate in the repair of a damaged vessel wall while at the same time preventing or limiting thrombus formation. In addition, platelets

Pharmacology of aspirin and salicylates

adhering to a site where prostacyclin synthase is present could well feed the enzyme with endoperoxide (Marcus *et al.*, 1980) thereby producing prostacyclin and preventing other platelets from clumping onto the adherent platelets, reinforcing the limitation of the cells to a monolayer.

Shortly after balloon de-endothelialization of the aortae of rabbits there is a closely adherent layer of spread platelets. A small reduction of adherent platelets was observed in animals receiving prostacyclin at 50–100 ng kg^{-1} min^{-1}. Only high infusion rates of 650–850 ng kg^{-1} min^{-1} inhibited this platelet adhesion (Adelman *et al.*, 1981). Eldor *et al.* (1981) have demonstrated that balloon catheter de-endothelialization of the rabbit aorta abolishes the capacity for generation of prostacyclin in the luminal surface which then recovers slowly over a period of 70 days, concomitant with the appearance of neo-intimal cells on the vessel surface. The authors also observed in the de-endothelialized areas a 'carpet of platelets' which slowly disappeared during the process of re-endothelialization. Thus, the loss of NO production from endothelial cells allowed platelet adhesion, but the generation of prostacyclin by the subendothelium prevented platelet aggregates from forming, since prostacyclin potently inhibits aggregation but not adhesion.

All this work suggests that prostacyclin, although not responsible for all the thromboresistant properties of the vascular endothelium, plays a very important part in the limitation of the deposition of platelets to a monolayer, without the formation of aggregates.

The effects of aspirin on the prostacyclin–thromboxane balance in the human have been investigated by FitzGerald and his colleagues and are discussed in Chapter 5 of this book.

10.3.1 Prostacyclin and TXA$_2$ in Disease

A number of cardiovascular, thrombotic diseases have been associated with an imbalance in the prostacyclin–thromboxane system. Platelets from patients with arterial thrombosis, deep venous thrombosis, or recurrent venous thrombosis produce more PG endoperoxides and TXA$_2$ than normal and have a shortened survival time (Lagarde and Dechavanne, 1977). Platelets from rabbits made atherosclerotic by a high fat diet (Shimamoto *et al.*, 1978) or from patients who have survived myocardial infarction (Szczeklik *et al.*, 1978b; Henriksson *et al.*, 1986) or ischaemic stroke (Lee *et al.*, 1989) are abnormally sensitive to aggregating agents and produce more TXA$_2$ than controls. Elevated TXB$_2$ levels have been demonstrated in the blood of patients with Prinzmetal's angina (Lewy *et al.*, 1979) and vasotonic angina (Robertson *et al.*, 1981). Hirsh and colleagues (Hirsh *et al.*, 1981) also studied TXB$_2$

levels in coronary sinus blood of patients with unstable angina. They concluded that local TXA_2 release is associated with recent episodes of angina but were unable to distinguish whether the release was cause or effect. Patients with arteriosclerosis obliterans and diabetes mellitus had more TXB_2 and less 6-oxo-$PGF_{1\alpha}$ in their plasma than control patients without these diseases (Udvardy et al., 1987).

However, measurements of TXA_2 and prostacyclin concentrations in peripheral blood are subject to sampling errors (Fitzgerald et al., 1983a). Assays of the 2,3-dinor metabolites of these eicosanoids in the urine provide a more accurate estimate of their true rate of synthesis (Lawson et al., 1985; Patrono et al., 1986). By measuring urinary 2,3-dinor-thromboxane B_2 and 2,3-dinor-6-oxo-prostaglandin $F_{1\alpha}$, increased synthesis of TXA_2 and prostacyclin was shown in patients during the development of acute myocardial infarction and in unstable angina (FitzGerald et al., 1986; Henriksson et al., 1986). The largest rise in TXA_2 formation occurred in patients with unstable angina indicating a high rate of platelet activation (Fitzgerald et al., 1986). Administration of aspirin only reduced the urinary concentrations of 2,3-dinor-TXB_2 in a proportion of the unstable angina patients, highlighting the problems in assessing the fluctuating TXA_2 production in this disease (Henriksson et al., 1986). The increased prostacyclin synthesis during these cardiovascular disorders may reflect a compensatory response of the vascular endothelium.

In two further studies, the raised blood pressure in patients was associated with an increased ratio of thromboxane A_2 to prostacyclin as measured by the concentrations of their metabolites in the urine. In one study the hypertension was pregnancy-induced (Minuz et al., 1988) whereas in the other it was caused by the administration of cyclosporine A (Förstermann et al., 1989). More recently, an impairment of prostacyclin synthesis was observed in patients with mild essential hypertension which may have contributed to the raised peripheral resistance and increased the incidence of thrombosis characteristic of this disease (Minuz et al., 1990).

In general, it seems that in diseases where there is a tendency for thrombosis to develop, TXA_2 production is elevated whereas prostacyclin production may be either reduced, or elevated. The opposite is found in some diseases associated with an increased bleeding tendency.

10.3.2 Prostacyclin and Atherosclerosis

Lipid peroxides, such as 15-hydroperoxy arachidonic acid (15-HPAA), are potent ($IC_{50} = 0.48$ µg ml^{-1}) and selective inhibitors of prostacyclin generation by vessel wall microsomes or by fresh vascular tissue (Bunting et al., 1976; Gryglewski et al., 1976; Moncada et al., 1976c; Salmon et al., 1978). High concentrations of lipid peroxides have been demonstrated in advanced atherosclerotic lesions (Glavind et al., 1952). Lipid peroxidation induced by free radical formation is known to occur in vitamin E deficiency, the ageing process and perhaps also in hyperlipidaemia accompanying atherosclerosis (Slater, 1972). Accumulation of lipid peroxides in atheromatous plaques could predispose to thrombus formation by inhibiting generation of prostacyclin by the vessel wall without affecting TXA_2 production by platelets. Moreover, platelet aggregation is induced by 15-HPAA and this aggregation is not inhibited by adenosine or PGE_1 (Mickel and Horbar, 1974). D'Angelo and coworkers (D'Angelo et al., 1978) reported that human atheromatous plaques from three patients did not produce prostacyclin. Prostacyclin generation by atherosclerotic arterial tissue has been shown to be significantly lower than from normal arterial tissue but no difference was found between early and advanced atherosclerotic lesions (Sinzinger et al., 1979). This suggests that the early 'fatty streak' may be a biochemically critical stage of the atherosclerotic process. As mentioned earlier, in normal rabbits the production of prostacyclin by the luminal surface of the aorta is abolished by de-endothelialization and slowly recovers with re-endothelialization over a period of about 70 days. However, the recovery of prostacyclin formation did not occur in rabbits made moderately hypercholesterolaemic by diet (Eldor et al., 1982). The same authors have also suggested that the accumulation of cholesteryl esters in the areas of damage of the vessel wall (Falcone et al., 1980) is related to the decrease in prostacyclin synthesis since addition of prostacyclin enhanced acid cholesteryl ester hydrolase activity in cultured vascular smooth muscle (Hajjar et al., 1981) thus suggesting a positive feedback between the prostacyclin system and lipid accumulation in the vessel wall. Bourgain and coworkers (Bourgain et al., 1980), demonstrated that application of 15-HPAA to the outside of mesenteric vessels in vivo in the rat increased the rate of thrombus formation in response to superfusion with ADP. Smooth muscle cells obtained from atherosclerotic lesions and cultured in vitro, consistently produce less prostacyclin than normal vascular smooth muscle cells. This effect persists after subculture (Larrue et al., 1980). In addition, a vitamin E-deficient diet in rats leads to an increase in peroxide levels in the aortae and to a decrease in prostacyclin production in vitro (Okuma et al., 1980). All these results, therefore, suggest that it would be worth exploring whether attempts to reduce lipid peroxide formation by inhibiting peroxidation influence the development of atherosclerosis and arterial thrombosis. Vitamin E acts as an antioxidant and perhaps its empirical use in arterial disease in the past (Marks, 1962; Boyd and Marks, 1963; Haeger, 1968) had, in fact, a biochemical rationale.

Raised concentrations of low density lipoprotein (LDL) are one of the risk factors associated with ischaemic heart disease whereas high density lipoprotein (HDL) is thought to protect against the disease (Medalie et al., 1973; Streja et al., 1978; Kannel et al., 1979). Nordøy and co-workers (Nordøy et al., 1978) were the first to show that LDL reduced the release of a prostacyclin-like substance by human endothelial cells. These observations were extended when it was shown that both LDL (Beitz and Förster, 1980) and oxidized LDL (Gryglewski and Szczeklik, 1981) inhibited, whereas HDL stimulated prostacyclin synthesis. A mixture of low LDL and high HDL also stimulated prostacyclin synthesis. Interestingly, HDL stabilizes prostacyclin and prolongs its half-life in vitro from 5 to 26 min (Morishita et al., 1990). This would enhance the prostacyclin-stimulated hydrolysis of cholesteryl esters (Ho et al., 1980). The half-life of prostacyclin is reduced in patients with myocardial ischaemia due to decreased levels of serum HDL-associated apolipoprotein A-I, which acts as the prostacyclin-stabilizing factor (Aoyama et al., 1990).

Cell proliferation in vitro is inhibited by substances which stimulate cAMP formation (Pastan et al., 1975). Willis et al. (1986, 1987) found that prostacyclin and its analogues suppressed the accumulation of cholesteryl esters by macrophages and also suppressed the release of growth factors from endothelial cells, macrophages and platelets. The latter effect was seen at concentrations that were one tenth of those required to inhibit platelet aggregation. Indeed, prostacyclin inhibited release of platelet-derived growth factor from platelet α granules in preference to β-thromboglobulin and platelet factor IV. In addition, a decrease in the lipid content of vascular wall cells was seen in humans after infusions of prostacyclin. An increased metabolism of cholesteryl esters, under the influence of prostacyclin, could contribute to this effect (Hajjar et al., 1982). Possibly, prostacyclin has a role in the regulation of cell growth in the vascular wall.

10.3.3 Modification of Fatty Acid Precursors

Eicosapentaenoic acid (EPA, C20:5ω3) is a polyunsaturated fatty acid like arachidonic acid (AA, C20:4ω6) but has a higher degree of unsaturation. EPA gives rise to trienoic prostaglandins and when incubated with vascular tissue leads to the release of an anti-aggregating substance (Gryglewski et al., 1979; Fig. 10.3). Synthetic Δ17 prostacyclin or PGI_3 is as potent an anti-aggregating agent as prostacyclin. In contrast, TXA_3 has a weaker pro-aggregatory activity than TXA_2. The fatty

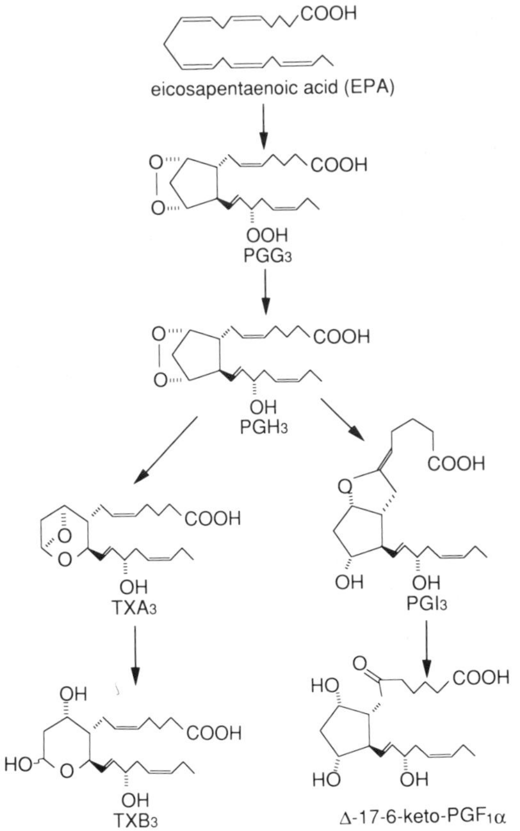

Figure 10.3 Eicosapentaenoic acid is transformed by cyclo-oxygenase into prostaglandin metabolites with three double bonds.

acid available for prostaglandin biosynthesis in Greenland Eskimos is mainly EPA, unlike that in Caucasians which is mainly arachidonic acid (Dyerberg *et al.*, 1978). These differences may explain why Eskimos have a low incidence of acute myocardial infarction, low blood cholesterol levels and an increased tendency to bleed (Dyerberg and Bang, 1979). This prolonged bleeding time is related to a reduction in *ex-vivo* platelet aggregability. The plasma concentrations of cholesterol, triglyceride, low and very low density lipoprotein (VLDL) are low in Eskimos, whereas that of high density lipoprotein is high (Bang and Dyerberg, 1972).

Eicosapentaenoic acid inhibits platelet aggregation in platelet-rich plasma stimulated by ADP, collagen, arachidonic acid, and a synthetic analogue of PGH_2 (Gryglewski *et al.*, 1979). EPA also inhibits aggregation in aspirin- and imidazole-treated platelets and inhibits

262

thrombin-induced aggregation (for review, Moncada, 1982). It is clear, therefore, that both prostaglandin-dependent and -independent pathways of platelet aggregation are inhibited by EPA *in vitro*. *In vivo*, however, EPA is incorporated into platelet phospholipids, to some extent replacing arachidonic acid and exerting an antithrombotic effect either by competing with released arachidonic acid for cyclo-oxygenase and lipoxygenase (Culp et al., 1979; Needleman et al., 1979) or by being converted to the less pro-aggregatory PGH_3 and TXA_3. Studying seven Caucasians who had been on a mackerel diet for 1 week, Siess and colleagues (Siess et al., 1980) showed a reduced sensitivity of platelets to collagen, associated with a reduced ability to produce TXB_2, which was dependent on the ratio of $C20:5\omega3/C20:4\omega6$ in platelet phospholipids. ADP-induced aggregation was significantly reduced in some subjects and platelet aggregation to exogenously added arachidonic acid was unchanged, indicating normal cyclo-oxygenase activity. Similarly, Sanders and co-workers (Sanders et al., 1980, 1981) showed a significant increase in bleeding time of 40% in volunteers who had taken cod liver oil (equivalent to 1.8 g eicosapentaenoic acid) daily for 6 weeks. This was consistent with a decrease in arachidonic acid and an increase in EPA in the platelet phospholipids. This diet also led after 6 weeks to a reduction of anti-thrombin III and blood pressure levels in the volunteers. In accordance with these results Brox and co-workers (Brox et al., 1981) have shown that a supplement of 25 ml of cod liver oil to the diet of normal volunteers leads to a decreased platelet aggregability and a decrease in the formation of TXB_2 during *ex-vivo* platelet aggregation induced by collagen.

A study on volunteers ingesting between 2 and 3 g of EPA daily demonstrated a decrease in platelet aggregability and an increase in bleeding time during the diet period (Thorngren and Gustafson, 1981). Thus, it is clear that EPA feeding leads to a decrease in platelet aggregability and a reduction in TXB_2 formation during *ex-vivo* platelet aggregation.

Metabolites of the trienoic prostaglandins ($\Delta17$–2, 3-dinor-6-keto-prostaglandin $F_{1\alpha}$ and 2,3-dinor-thromboxane B_3; Fig. 10.3) have been identified in the urine of subjects who had ingested EPA or fish oils (Fischer and Weber, 1984; von Schacky et al., 1985a; Knapp et al., 1986) and platelets removed from volunteers taking cod liver oil make TXB_3 from EPA (von Schacky et al., 1985b). While receiving 50 ml of fish oil daily, men with mild essential hypertension initially increased their formation of PGI_3 and prostacyclin. Their diastolic blood pressure simultaneously decreased during the treatment by a mean of 4.4 mm Hg (Knapp and FitzGerald, 1989). Vascular tissues obtained from atherosclerotic patients undergoing coronary bypass surgery, who had been given fish oil for 28 days, produced more prostacyclin than those of similar patients who had not received fish oil (DeCaterina *et al.*, 1990). Analysis of erythrocyte and platelet phospholipids in the atherosclerotic and hypertensive patients and in the human volunteers who had ingested fish oils showed increased incorporation of ω–3 fatty acids into their phospholipids.

In a recent study of more than 2000 patients who had had heart attacks, there was a 30% decrease in recurrence among those who ate at least two meals a week that consisted of fatty fish or who took an equivalent amount of fish oil (Burr *et al.*, 1989). There is also convincing epidemiological evidence that the risk factors for heart disease are decreased by eating fish or taking fish oil (Kromhout *et al.*, 1985). Clearly, a high intake of ω–3 fatty acids in populations with a moderate-to-low consumption of dietary saturated fatty acids is associated with a low incidence of coronary heart disease (Nordøy and Goodnight, 1990).

Overall then, the present evidence suggests that it is well worth while continuing to study the effects of EPA in man. Moreover, concurrent therapy with aspirin should not negate the potentially beneficial effects of ω–3 fatty acid supplementation on the thromboxane–prostacyclin balance (Force *et al.*, 1991).

10.4   ANTI-THROMBOTIC ACTION OF ASPIRIN

10.4.1   Inhibition of Platelet Function

Measurement of *ex-vivo* platelet aggregation and *in vivo* skin bleeding time provide an estimate of *in-vivo* platelet aggregability. Platelet aggregation can be induced in platelet-rich plasma or in suspensions of washed platelets (Radomski and Moncada, 1983) with stimuli such as ADP, adrenaline, collagen or thrombin and estimated photometrically in a Born aggregometer (Born and Cross, 1963, 1964). Substances which activate adenylate cyclase and raise the concentration of cAMP in platelets such as adenosine (Born *et al.*, 1964), PGE_1 or prostacyclin (Moncada and Vane, 1979) prevent aggregation to all stimulating substances. Moreover, platelets from subjects who have ingested aspirin do not aggregate maximally to ADP or collagen, whereas washed platelets from these subjects still respond to the addition of thrombin (Siess, 1989). From this it can be inferred that TXA_2 formation is required for complete aggregation to ADP and for collagen-induced aggregation, but not for that induced by thrombin.

The antiplatelet effect of aspirin is due to its acetylation and irreversible inactivation of platelet cyclo-oxygenase enzyme (Chapter 2), which produces TXA_2 from arachidonic acid. Thromboxane synthesis can be totally prevented by administering one low dose of aspirin (80–100 mg; Weksler *et al.*, 1983) or by as little as 10 mg of aspirin taken daily for 3 weeks (Kallman *et al.*, 1987). Recovery of the ability of platelets to produce TXA_2 depends on the liberation into the circulation of new platelets. Aspirin in moderate doses (325–650 mg) prolongs the average skin bleeding time in normal subjects (Mielke *et al.*, 1969; Deykin *et al.*, 1982; Mielke, 1982; Thorngren *et al.*, 1983) and can lengthen it considerably in patients suffering from haemophilia (Kaneshiro *et al.*, 1969), von Willebrand's disease (Stuart *et al.*, 1979) or chronic renal failure (Gaspari *et al.*, 1987). A single dose of aspirin (5 mg kg^{-1}) increased the bleeding time of normal volunteers by 124% and prevented the appearance of TXB_2 in bleeding time blood (Thorngren *et al.*, 1983), whereas a regular intake of low-dose aspirin (0.43±0.02 mg kg^{-1} day^{-1}) reduced serum TXB_2 levels to almost zero and doubled the bleeding time after 10 days (Gresele *et al.*, 1987; Fig. 10.4).

The consumption of 50 g of ethanol, which alone had no effect on bleeding time, potentiated the increase in bleeding time produced by aspirin (Deykin *et al.*, 1982). Low concentrations of ethanol augment the anti-aggregatory effect of prostacyclin on platelets *ex vivo* and this may be the basis of the *in vivo* synergism between ethanol and aspirin (Jakubowski *et al.*, 1988). Consumption of small amounts of alcohol should, therefore, increase the protective effect of aspirin against sudden coronary death (Hennekens *et al.*, 1979; Marmot, 1984).

10.4.2 Clinical Studies

During the past two decades, numerous randomized clinical trials have taken place assessing the efficacy of aspirin in the prevention of thrombosis. These have covered a wide spectrum of thrombotic conditions encompassing coronary artery and cerebrovascular occlusion, peripheral vascular disease, post-operative deep vein thrombosis, pulmonary embolism and occlusion of physiological or prosthetic vascular grafts (Table 10.1) (for reviews, de Gaetano *et al.*, 1986a; Reilly and FitzGerald, 1988). Although these trials have evaluated aspirin for the prevention of arterial occlusion, a possible fibrinolytic action may contribute to the overall anti-thrombotic effect (later in this chapter).

PRIMARY PREVENTION OF MYOCARDIAL INFARCTION

Most anti-platelet trials have been performed in patients who are already susceptible to vascular occlusive disease (secondary prevention studies). However, two recently reported trials starting with healthy individuals (primary prevention studies), suggest that prophylactic anti-platelet treatment with aspirin can prevent about 30% of all non-fatal myocardial infarctions in apparently healthy male physicians (Peto *et al.*, 1988; Steering Committee of the Physician's Health Study Research Group, 1989). In neither trial was there any reduction in overall vascular mortality and in both there was a slight increase in the incidence of disabling strokes in individuals treated for over 5 years. It is possible, therefore, that the slight benefit derived from aspirin treatment may be outweighed by a small increase in cerebral haemorrhagic disease (Anti-platelet Trialists Collaboration, 1988).

MYOCARDIAL INFARCTION, UNSTABLE ANGINA, TRANSIENT ISCHAEMIC ATTACKS AND STROKE

An overview of 25 randomized trials of anti-platelet treatment in 29 000 patients with a history of transient ischaemic attacks, occlusive stroke, unstable angina or myocardial infarction was published in 1988 by

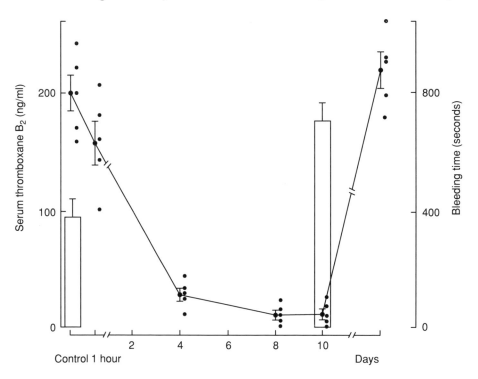

Figure 10.4 Serum thromboxane B_2 (●) and bleeding-time values (columns) during prolonged intake of low-dose aspirin (0.43 ± 0.02 mg kg^{-1} day^{-1}). (Reproduced from Gresele *et al.*, 1987, by permission of The American Society for Clinical Investigation.)

Table 10.1 Major proposed indications for
thrombosis prevention with aspirin

Coronary artery disease
  unstable angina
  myocardial infarction
Aortocoronary bypasses
Coronary angioplasty
Heart valve prosthesis
Transient cerebral ischaemic attacks
Peripheral vascular disease
Lower extremity bypasses
Renal haemodialysis shunts
Extracorporeal circuits
Postoperative deep vein thrombosis
Idiopathic, recurrent venous thrombosis

Peto and his colleagues (Anti-platelet Trialists Collaboration, 1988). In this type of overview, when several different anti-platelet trials are considered, their results may reinforce each other to show a statistically significant effect, whereas the risk reduction in individual trials may not reach significance. The final conclusion was that anti-platelet treatment had no effect on non-vascular mortality, but reduced vascular mortality by 15% and non-fatal stroke or myocardial infarction by 30%.

In addition, there was no significant difference between the effects of medium doses of aspirin (300–325 mg daily) and high doses (900–1500 mg daily). In another study, even lower doses of aspirin (160 mg daily) were administered after suspected acute myocardial infarction and resulted in a 23% reduction of vascular mortality in the 5 weeks following the start of treatment (ISIS–2 Collaborative Group, 1988). A recent study in men with unstable coronary artery disease showed that aspirin (75 mg daily for 3 months) reduced the risk of myocardial infarction and death (RISC Group, 1990). (These trials are discussed in more detail in later chapters of this book.)

GRAFT OCCLUSION

In 1979, Harter *et al.*, described the anti-thrombotic effect of 160 mg of aspirin daily in patients on haemodialysis (Harter *et al.*, 1979). Since that time, a number of trials have reported the beneficial effect of 100–1200 mg aspirin daily in renal haemodialysis shunts, vein graft occlusion after coronary bypass surgery and prosthetic leg artery bypass graft occlusion (Chapter 16).

DEEP VEIN THROMBOSIS AND PULMONARY EMBOLISM

The prophylactic action of aspirin in post-operative deep vein thrombosis and pulmonary embolism has until recently been controversial. Several studies demonstrated a beneficial effect of aspirin in the prevention of deep vein thrombosis either alone (Harris *et al.*, 1977, 1982, 1985; Alfaro *et al.*, 1986), or in combination with dipyridamole (Renney *et al.*, 1976) or sulphinpyrazone (Sauter *et al.*, 1983). Others were unable to confirm this benefit (MRC Steering Committee, 1972; Dechavanne *et al.*, 1975; Stamatakis *et al.*, 1978) possibly due to imperfections in the design of the trials (reviews by Clagett and Reisch, 1988; Hirsh and Levine, 1989).

The Anti-platelet Trialists Collaboration which met in Oxford in March, 1990 (results to be published) resolved this issue in a meta-analysis of all thromboprophylaxis trials of surgical and medical deep vein thrombosis or pulmonary embolism and found a highly significant beneficial effect of aspirin (Chapter 12).

PERIPHERAL VASCULAR DISEASE

The Anti-platelet Trialists Collaboration (1990) also analysed the trials of aspirin in peripheral vascular disease and found a protective effect. This confirmed the results of separate trials of aspirin such as that of Schoop *et al.* (1983) in patients with unilateral femoral artery occlusion. Aspirin significantly reduced occlusion of the contralateral femoral artery in 300 patients already suffering from unilateral femoral artery occlusion.

A subsequent double blind study showed that treatment with aspirin (330 mg three times daily) significantly slowed the development of occlusive arteriosclerosis of the lower limbs (Hess *et al.*, 1985).

10.4.3 Selectivity of Low Doses of Aspirin

Once an inhibition of more than 95% of platelet cyclo-oxygenase has been achieved, a further increase in the dose of aspirin will not produce any increase in anti-thrombotic effect (Patrono, 1989). Daily dosing with 324 mg of aspirin will, therefore, not achieve any more suppression of platelet function than daily administration of 50 mg. Both doses inhibited *ex vivo* thromboxane-dependent platelet aggregation and prolonged *in vivo* bleeding time to the same extent (De Caterina *et al.*, 1985).

However, administration of higher doses of aspirin increases the likelihood of side effects, particularly gastrointestinal toxicity. Evidence from large scale clinical trials indicates that the occurrence of side effects is dose-related in the range of doses between 160 and 1500 mg daily, whereas anti-thrombotic efficacy is not (Anti-platelet Trialists Collaboration, 1988). This separation between anti-thrombotic and gastrointestinal effects is illustrated in Fig. 10.5 (Patrono, 1989).

Likewise, Ritter *et al.*, have shown a clear separation between the inhibition of cyclo-oxygenase of the platelets and that of the blood vessel wall. After treatment with 600 mg of aspirin, the urinary excretion of thromboxane metabolites dropped to zero and did not recover within the experimental period of 6 h. The levels of prostacyclin derivatives also dropped to zero, but recovered completely within 3–5 h (Ritter *et al.*, 1989; Fig 10.6). During daily administration of 20–60 mg of aspirin, measurements of 6-oxo-$PGF_{1\alpha}$ and 2,3-dinor-6-oxo-$PGF_{1\alpha}$ in urine have indicated less than 30% inhibition of prostacyclin production (Patrignani *et al.*, 1982; FitzGerald *et al.*, 1983b; Benigni *et al.*, 1989).

Thus, aspirin potently inhibits thromboxane generation by platelets in doses which largely spare prostacyclin synthesis in the vessel wall. This is attributed to the pharmacokinetics of aspirin after absorption and to the fact that platelets cannot synthesize fresh cyclo-oxygenase enzyme after it has been irreversibly acetylated and inactivated by aspirin (Chapter 2).

10.5 ASPIRIN AND FIBRINOLYSIS

Aspirin-induced suppression of platelet activity (Chapter 5) and salicylate-induced hepatic anti-vitamin K effects (Owens and Cimino 1980) are considered to be responsible for the antithrombotic action of aspirin as well as for the development of a bleeding tendency after ingestion of aspirin. Does activation of fibrinolysis by aspirin contribute to its anti-thrombotic action?

The *in vitro* fibrinolytic activity of aspirin-like drugs was reported as early as 1966 (Gryglewski, 1966). These drugs were shown to interact with the tertiary structure of clot proteins (Gryglewski and Eckstein, 1967) as evidenced by cleavage of protein disulphide bonds (Gryglewski and Panczenko, 1968). This physicochemical phenomenon was claimed to underly the mechanism of fibrinolysis by non-steroidal anti-inflammatory drugs. Indeed, *in vitro* euglobulin clots were dissolved by aspirin, indomethacin, fenamates or ibuprofen only in a narrow range of their millimolar concentrations (Gryglewski, 1970) – a finding which was consistent with a physicochemical concept rather than with an enzymatic activity (von Kaulla, 1974).

These early *in-vitro* studies were followed by reports on increased *ex-vivo* fibrinolytic activity in blood following administration of aspirin to humans (Menon, 1970; Moroz, 1977; Green *et al.*, 1983), rats (Housholder

Pharmacology of aspirin and salicylates

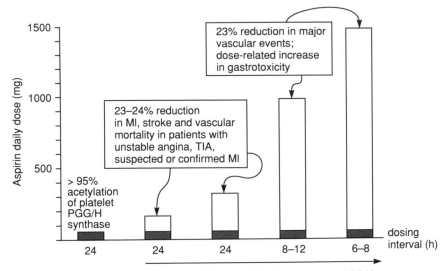

Figure 10.5 Relationship between aspirin daily dosage and biochemical and clinical effects. The shaded area in each column represents the amount of aspirin necessary to achieve >95% suppression of platelet cyclo-oxygenase activity. The open columns depict the doses employed in published clinical trials of secondary prevention. The reduction in major vascular events shows no dose dependence, compatible with almost maximal suppression of TXA$_2$-dependent platelet function in this dose range. There is, however, a dose and dosing interval-dependent increase in gastrointestinal toxicity, consistent with an increase in the extent and duration of extra-platelet cyclo-oxygenase inhibition. GI, gastrointestinal; MI, myocardial infarction; TIA, transient ischaemic attacks. (From Patrono, 1989, with permission. Copyright 1989, Elsevier Science Publishers Ltd, UK.)

et al., 1980) and rabbits (Cattaneo *et al.*, 1983). In patients with coronary heart disease (Jain *et al.*, 1982) and in rats with isoprenaline-induced cardiac micronecrosis (Saxena *et al.*, 1980) plasma fibrinolytic activity was suppressed. Following treatment of these patients with aspirin at a dose of 0.9 g daily for 1–10 days or pretreatment of rats with aspirin at a dose of 30 mg kg^{-1} daily for 7 consecutive days, the low plasma fibrinolytic activity was brought back to control values. In addition, the pretreatment of rats with aspirin protected their myocardium from the damage inflicted by isoprenaline (Saxena *et al.*, 1980).

In healthy volunteers the *ex-vivo* fibrinolytic action of aspirin was attributed either to its hypoglycaemic effect (Menon, 1970) or to activation of the fibrinolytic properties of neutrophils (Moroz, 1977). Indeed, following oral administration of aspirin at a dose of 1.8 g, the fibrinolytic activity of blood increased by 33–150%, while at the same time plasma salicylate levels rose to 0.3–1 mM. *In-vitro* experiments showed that sodium salicylate increased the fibrinolytic activity of both blood and isolated neutrophils to a much greater extent than aspirin did (Moroz, 1977). A biphasic effect of aspirin on fibrinolytic activity of neutrophils was reported in healthy volunteers who were treated

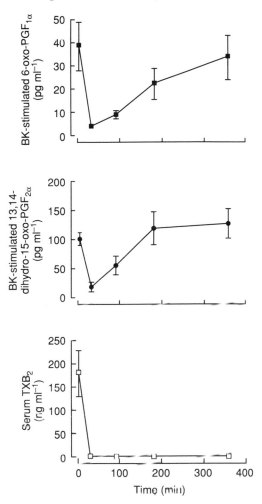

Figure 10.6 Effect of intravenous aspirin on bradykinin-stimulated plasma concentrations of 6-oxo-PGF$_{1\alpha}$ and 13, 14-dihydro-15-oxo-PGF$_{2\alpha}$ and on serum TXB$_2$ concentrations. Nine healthy men (age 23–42 years; weight 72–90 kg), were studied before and at intervals after an intravenous bolus of aspirin (600 mg). Blood for plasma prostaglandin determinations was sampled during the final minute of each of a series of 10 min infusions of bradykinin. Values below detection limit (4 pg ml^{-1}) were taken as at the detection limit. (From Ritter *et al.*, 1989, with permission. Copyright 1989, Macmillan Journals Ltd.)

271

intravenously with lysine acetylsalicylate (LAS) in a dose of 0.9 g. Granulocytes from these volunteers showed an increased fibrinolytic activity 45 min after the administration of LAS, however, 90 min later the fibrinolytic activity of neutrophils decreased well below the control level (Ghezzo *et al.*, 1981a). A similar suppression of the plasminogen-dependent and non-specific fibrinolytic activity of neutrophils was reported in healthy volunteers who received chronic treatment with high (1 g daily for 4 days) but not with low (0.25 g daily for 4 days) doses of aspirin (Ghezzo *et al.*, 1981b).

Thus, in contrast to the platelet-suppressant action of aspirin (Chapter 5) the effect on fibrinolysis does not appear after administration of low doses of aspirin (Ghezzo *et al.*, 1981b; Keber and Keber, 1985; De Gaetano *et al.*, 1986b). An effect of aspirin on fibrinolysis is achieved only at a high range of doses of the drug (Moroz, 1977; Jain *et al.*, 1982; Bjornsson *et al.*, 1989). This effect may present itself either as activation or suppression of particular fibrinolytic parameters (Ghezzo *et al.*, 1981a; Housholder *et al.*, 1980). In other words, aspirin has the potential to act as a pro-fibrinolytic or anti-fibrinolytic agent.

The concept of a dual mechanism of action of aspirin on fibrinolysis also emerged from animal studies. Short-term administration of aspirin (40 mg kg^{-1}) to rats decreased the *ex-vivo* standard fibrin clot lysis time. This would be expected if aspirin decreased the plasma levels of circulating plasminogen activator (Housholder *et al.*, 1980). No matter how refined the methods for measurement of fibrinolysis used, this paper still left us with a message that aspirin can simultaneously evoke two antagonistic actions on the fibrinolytic system.

The pro-fibrinolytic action of aspirin might be due either to inactivation of inhibitors (e.g. PAI-1) (Housholder *et al.*, 1980) or to a change in fibrin structure making it more susceptible to disintegration by plasmin (Bjornsson *et al.*, 1989). In both cases, the acetylating ability of aspirin was proposed as the cause for the change of the structure of the protein in question. One must not forget that apart from aspirin other non-steroidal anti-inflammatory drugs (usually biarylcarboxylic acids) are also capable of dissolving euglobulin clots (Gryglewski, 1966, 1970) and the 'acetylation hypothesis' cannot explain the mechanism of their fibrinolytic action.

The anti-fibrinolytic action of aspirin may result from the inhibition of vascular cyclo-oxygenase by aspirin followed by impaired release of endogenous prostacyclin (Bertele *et al.*, 1989). Prostacyclin is known to exert a moderate fibrinolytic action *in vivo*, most likely through the release of t-PA (Dembinska-Kiec *et al.*, 1982; Musial *et al.*, 1986). Thus the impairment of endogenous prostacyclin release by aspirin is likely to account for the anti-fibrinolytic action of the latter.

Now, let us review the available data for and against the concept of aspirin as a pro- or anti-fibrinolytic agent. In four studies, aspirin, when administered to healthy volunteers in doses of 0.65–1.3 g daily, suppressed the typical responses of the fibrinolytic system to venous occlusion, i.e. aspirin inhibited the venostatic release of t-PA or it diminished an increase of blood fibrinolytic potential as measured by various methods (Levin et al., 1984; De Gaetano et al., 1986b; Keber et al., 1987; Bertele et al., 1989). These findings may support the hypothesis that the anti-fibrinolytic action of aspirin is achieved by breaking a chain of events which lead from the biosynthesis of prostacyclin to the release of t-PA. However, in another study (Bounameaux et al., 1985) aspirin and indomethacin were used as pharmacological tools to disprove the hypothesis that prostacyclin plays a role in the release of t-PA following venous stasis in humans. In this particular study neither indomethacin nor aspirin in doses which inhibited the generation of prostacyclin had any effect on basal or stimulated (by venous stasis) plasma t-PA levels. In two other studies it was demonstrated that aspirin (0.65 g every 12 h for 5 days) neither affected basal plasma t-PA levels (Bjornsson et al., 1989) nor prevented an increase in plasma fibrinolytic activity that was induced by an infusion of 1-desamino-8-D-arginine-vasopressin (DDAVP) into healthy volunteers (Brommer et al., 1984).

The results of the above studies argue against the suppression of the fibrinolytic system by aspirin and more specifically they seem to exclude the participation of prostacyclin and t-PA in the mechanism of anti-fibrinolytic action of aspirin. The next study (Hammouda and Moroz, 1986) takes us a step further. The authors claim 'a modest but significant increase in plasma t-PA response to venous occlusion after aspirin treatment'. Indeed, it means that aspirin acts as a promotor of the release of t-PA in response to venostasis.

The complexity of the issue of anti- and pro-fibrinolytic actions of aspirin has been focused in three recent papers. Bertele et al. (1989) reported that the treatment of healthy subjects with aspirin (0.65 g twice daily) reduced the fibrinolytic response induced by venous occlusion. This anti-fibrinolytic action of aspirin was reversed by iloprost, a stable prostacyclin analogue, however, without a concomitant effect on plasma t-PA and PAI-1 activities. These results may be interpreted as supporting the existence of a link between the anti-fibrinolytic action of aspirin and prostacyclin deficiency, however, involvement of t-PA in this response seems to be dubious.

Bjornsson et al. (1989) have reported that the treatment of healthy volunteers with aspirin (0.65 g every 12 h for 5 days) enhanced the rate of fibrinolysis of plasma clots. This pro-fibrinolytic action of

273

aspirin was associated with a change in plasma levels of neither t-PA nor plasminogen nor fibrinogen. As mentioned earlier the authors suggested N-acetylation of lysyl residues of fibrinogen by aspirin as responsible for its pro-fibrinolytic action. In other words aspirin is thought to weaken the fibrin network of thrombi and thus make them more susceptible to digestion by fibrinolytic enzymes.

Terres *et al.* (1989) have developed a similar idea in their *in-vitro* studies. Combined platelet and fibrin thrombi are susceptible to lysis by urokinase. The thrombolytic effect of urokinase is enhanced by the pretreatment of thrombi with either aspirin or PGE_1. This study pointed to the importance of platelets for building a 'hard' structure of the fibrin clot. Interference with this platelet activity by aspirin or PGE_1 makes the clot more susceptible to lysis by urokinase.

The anti-thrombotic effect of aspirin has generally been ascribed to its inhibitory action on cyclo-oxygenase activity in blood platelets. However, in two different experimental models (Buchanan *et al.*, 1982; Hanson *et al.*, 1985) it has been shown that the anti-thrombotic effect of aspirin may involve mechanisms other than cyclo-oxygenase inhibition. These mechanisms are evident at higher doses than those required for inhibition of cyclo-oxygenase (Bjornsson *et al.*, 1989). One of the possible explanations for this other mechanism of thrombolytic action of aspirin is its fibrinolytic effect which is mediated by making proteins of the clot more susceptible to lysis (Gryglewski and Panczenko, 1968; Gryglewski, 1970; Bjornsson *et al.*, 1989; Terres *et al.*, 1989).

From a practical point of view, one needs to consider the effect of aspirin on the fibrinolytic system only at the high ranges of doses of the drug. It seems that then the pro-fibrinolytic action of aspirin prevails. The anti-fibrinolytic action of aspirin is likely to occur only under particular conditions such as the inhibition of activation of fibrinolysis in response to venous occlusion.

REFERENCES

Adelman, B., Stemerman, M. B., Merrell, D. and Handin, R. (1981) The interaction of platelets with aortic subendothelium: Inhibition of adhesion and secretion by prostaglandin I_2. *Blood*, **58**, 198–205.

Aiken, J.W., Gorman, R.R. and Shebuski, R.J. (1979) Prevention of blockage of partially obstructed coronary arteries with prostacyclin correlates with inhibition of platelet aggregation. *Prostaglandins*, **17**, 483–94.

Alfaro, M.J., Páramo, J.A. and Rocha, E. (1986) Prophylaxis of thromboembolic disease and platelet-related changes following total hip replacement: A comparative study of aspirin and heparin-dihydroergotamine. *Thromb. Haemostasis*, **56**, 53–6.

Alheid, U., Frölich, J.C. and Förstermann, U. (1987) Endothelium-derived relaxing factor from cultured human endothelial cells inhibits aggregation of human platelets. *Thromb. Res.*, **47**, 561–71.

Andersen, B., Goldsmith, G.H. and Spagnuolo, P.J. (1988) Neutrophil adhesive dysfunction in diabetes mellitus: The role of cellular and plasma factors. *J. Lab. Clin. Med.*, **111**, 275–85.

Antiplatelet Trialists Collaboration (1988) Secondary prevention of vascular disease by prolonged antiplatelet treatment. *Brit. Med. J.*, **296**, 320–31.

Aoyama, T., Yui, Y., Morishita, H. and Kawai, C. (1990) Prostaglandin I_2 half-life regulated by high density lipoprotein is decreased in acute myocardial infarction and unstable angina pectoris. *Circulation*, **81**, 1784–91.

Azuma, H., Ishikawa, M. and Sekizaki, S. (1986) Endothelium-dependent inhibition of platelet aggregation. *Brit. J. Pharmacol.*, **88**, 411–15.

Bang, H.O. and Dyerberg, J. (1972) Plasma lipids and lipoproteins in Greenlandic west coast Eskimos. *Acta Med. Scand.*, **192**, 85–94.

Barrett, M.L., Willis, A.L. and Vane, J.R. (1989) Inhibition of platelet-derived mitogen release by nitric oxide (EDRF). *Agents Actions*, **27**, 488–91.

Baumgartner, H.R. (1973) The role of blood flow in platelet adhesion, fibrin deposition, and formation of mural thrombi. *Microvasc. Res.*, **5**, 167–79.

Baumgartner, H.R. (1974) Morphometric quantitation of adherence of platelets to an artificial surface and components of connective tissue. *Thromb. Diath. Haemorrh.*, **60**, 39–49.

Baumgartner, H.R., Muggli, R., Tschopp, T.B. and Turitto, V.T. (1976) Platelet adhesion, release and aggregation in flowing blood: Effects of surface properties and platelet function. *Thromb. Haemostasis*, **35**, 124–38.

Bayer, B-L., Blass, K-E. and Förster, W. (1979) Anti-aggregatory effect of prostacyclin (PGI_2) *in vivo*. *Brit. J. Pharmacol.*, **66**, 10–12.

Beitz, J. and Forster, W. (1980) Influence of human low density and high density lipoprotein cholesterol on the *in vitro* prostaglandin I_2 synthetase activity. *Biochim. Biophys. Acta*, **620**, 352–5.

Benigni, A., Gregorini, G., Frusca, T., *et al.* (1989) Effect of low-dose aspirin on fetal and maternal generation of thromboxane by platelets in women at risk for pregnancy-induced hypertension. *N. Engl. J. Med.*, **321**, 357–62.

Bertele, V., Mussoni, L., Pintucci, G. *et al.* (1989) The inhibitory effect of aspirin on fibrinolysis is reversed by iloprost, a prostacyclin analogue. *Thromb. Haemostasis*, **61**, 286–8.

Bhagwat, S.S., Hamann, P.R., Still, W.C. *et al.* (1985) Synthesis and structure of the platelet aggregation factor thromboxane A_2. *Nature (Lond.)*, **315**, 511–13.

Bhardwaj, R., Page, C.P., May, G.R. and Moore, P.K. (1988) Endothelium-derived relaxing factor inhibits platelet aggregation in human whole blood *in vitro* and in the rat *in vivo*. *Eur. J. Pharmacol.*, **157**, 83–91.

Bjornsson, T.D., Schneider, D.E. and Berger, H. Jr (1989) Aspirin acetylates fibrinogen and enhances fibrinolysis. Fibrinolytic effect is independent of changes in plasminogen activator levels. *J. Pharmacol. Exp. Ther.*, **250**, 159–61.

Blair, I.A., Barrow, S.E., Waddell, K.A. *et al.* (1982) Prostacyclin is not a circulating hormone in man. *Prostaglandins*, **23**, 579–89.

Pharmacology of aspirin and salicylates

Born, G.V.R. (1977) Fluid-mechanical and biochemical interactions in haemostasis. *Brit. Med. Bull.*, **33**, 193–7.

Born, G.V.R. (1979) Arterial thrombosis and its prevention. In *Proc. VIIIth World Congress of Cardiology* (eds. S. Hayase and S. Murao), Excerpta Medica, Amsterdam, pp. 81–91.

Born, G.V.R. and Cross, M.J. (1963) The aggregation of blood platelets. *J. Physiol.*, **168**, 179–95.

Born, G.V.R. and Cross, M.J. (1964) Effects of inorganic ions and of plasma proteins on the aggregation of blood platelets by adenosine diphosphate. *J. Physiol.*, **170**, 397–414.

Born, G.V.R., Honour, A.J. and Mitchell, J.R.A. (1964) Inhibition by adenosine and by 2-chloroadenosine of the formation and embolization of platelet thrombi. *Nature (Lond.)*, **202**, 761–5.

Born, G.V.R., Bergquist, D. and Arfors, K.E. (1976) Evidence for inhibition of platelet activation in blood by a drug effect on erythrocytes. *Nature (Lond.)*, **259**, 233–5.

Bossaller, C., Habib, G. B., Yamamoto, H. *et al.* (1987) Impaired muscarinic endothelium-dependent relaxation and cyclic guanosine 3', 5'-monophosphate formation in atherosclerotic human coronary artery and rabbit aorta. *J. Clin. Invest.*, **9**, 170–4.

Bounameaux, H., Gresele, P., Hanss, M. *et al.* (1985) Aspirin, indomethacin and dasoxiben do not affect the fibrinolytic activation induced by venous occlusion. *Thromb. Res.*, **40**, 161–70.

Bourgain, R.H., Six, F. and Andries, R. (1980) The action of cyclooxygenase and prostacyclin-synthetase inhibitors on platelet-vessel wall interaction. *Artery*, **8**, 96–100.

Boyd, A.M. and Marks, J. (1963) Treatment of intermittent claudication. A reappraisal of the value of α-tocopherol. *Angiology*, **14**, 198–208.

Brommer, E.J.P., Derkx, F.H.M., Barrett-Bergshoeff, M.M. and Schalekamp, M.A.D.H. (1984) The inability of propranolol and aspirin to inhibit the response of fibrinolytic activity and factor VIII-antigen to infusion of DDAVP. *Thromb. Haemostasis*, **51**, 42–4.

Brotherton, A.F.A., MacFarlane, D.E. and Hoak, J.C. (1982) Prostacyclin biosynthesis in vascular endothelium is not inhibited by cyclic AMP. Studies with 3-isobutyl-1-methylxanthine and forskolin. *Thromb. Res.*, **28**, 637–47.

Brox, J.H., Killie, J.E., Gunnes, S. and Nordøy, A. (1981) The effect of cod liver oil and corn oil on platelets and vessel wall in man. *Thromb. Haemostasis*, **46**, 604–11.

Buchanan, M.R., Rischke, J.A. and Hirsh, J. (1982) Aspirin inhibits platelet function independent of the acetylation of cyclooxygenase. *Thromb. Res.*, **25**, 363–73.

Bult, H., Fret, H.R.L., Van der Bossche, R.M. and Herman, A.G. (1988) Platelet inhibition by endothelium-derived relaxing factor from the rabbit perfused aorta. *Brit. J. Pharmacol.*, **95**, 1308–14.

Bunting, S., Gryglewski, R., Moncada, S. and Vane, J. (1976) Arterial walls generate from prostaglandin endoperoxides a substance (prostaglandin X) which relaxes strips of mesenteric and coeliac arteries and inhibits platelet aggregation. *Prostaglandins*, **12**, 897–913.

Burch, R.M., Mais, D.E., Saussy, D.L. Jr and Halushka, P.V. (1985) Solubilization of a thromboxane A_2/prostaglandin H_2 antagonist binding site from human platelets. *Proc. Natl Acad. Sci. USA*, **82**, 7434–8.

Burr, M.L., Fehily, A.M., Gilbert, J.F., *et al.* (1989) Effects of changes in fat, fish, and fibre intakes on death and myocardial reinfarction: Diet and reinfarction trial (DART). *Lancet*, **ii**, 757–61.

Cazevane, J-P., Packham, M.A., Kinlough-Rathbone, R.L. and Mustard, J.F. (1977) Platelet adherence to the vessel wall and to collagen-coated surfaces. In *Thrombosis: Animal and Clinical Models, Vol. 102* (ed. H.J. Day), Plenum Publishing Corp, New York, London, pp. 31–49.

Cattaneo, M., Chahil, A., Somers, D. *et al.* (1983) Effect of aspirin and sodium salicylate on thrombosis, fibrinolysis, prothrombin time and platelet survival in rabbits with indwelling aortic catheters. *Blood*, **61**, 353–61.

Chappell, S.P., Lewis, M.J. and Henderson, A.H. (1987) Effect of lipid feeding on endothelium dependent relaxation in rabbit aortic preparations. *Cardiovasc. Res.*, **21**, 34–8.

Clagett, G.P. and Reisch, J.S. (1988) Prevention of venous thromboembolism in general surgical patients. Results of meta-analysis. *Ann. Surg.*, **208**, 227–40.

Cocks, T. M., Angus, J. A., Campbell, J. H. and Campbell, G. R. (1985) Release and properties of endothelium-derived relaxing factor (EDRF) from endothelial cells in culture. *J. Cell Physiol.*, **123**, 310–20.

Coller, B. S. (1990) Platelets and thrombolytic therapy. *N. Engl. J. Med.*, **322**, 33–42.

Constantinides, P. (1966) Plaque fissures in human coronary thrombosis. *J. Atheroscler. Res.*, **6**, 1–17.

Conti, P., Reale, M., Cancelli, A. and Angeletti, P.U. (1987) Lipoxin A augments release of thromboxane from human polymorphonuclear leukocyte suspensions. *FEBS Lett.*, **225**, 103–8.

Culp, B.R., Titus, B.G. and Lands, W.E.M. (1979) Inhibition of prostaglandin biosynthesis by eicosapentaenoic acid. *Prostaglandins Med.*, **3**, 269–78.

Czervionke, R. L., Smith, J. B., Hoak, J. C. *et al.* (1979) Use of a radioimmunoassay to study thrombin-induced release of PGI_2 from cultured endothelium. *Thromb. Res.*, **14**, 781–6.

D'Angelo, V., Villa, S., Mysliwiec, M., *et al.* (1978) Defective fibrinolytic and prostacyclin-like activity in human atheromatous plaques. *Thromb. Diath. Haemorrh.*, **39**, 535–6.

Davies, M.J. and Thomas, T. (1984) Thrombosis and acute coronary artery lesions in sudden cardiac ischaemic death. *N. Engl. J. Med.*, **310**, 1137–40.

Davis, M.J. and Thomas, T. (1981) The pathological basis and microanatomy of occlusive thrombus formation in human coronary arteries. *Phil. Trans. R. Soc. Lond. B. Biol. Sci.*, **294**, 225–9.

Deby, C., Pincemail, J., Deby-Dupont, G. *et al.* (1984) Secondary chemical reactions mediated by cyclo-oxygenase. In *Icosanoids and Cancer* (eds. H. Thaler-Dao, R. Proletti and P. Gnastes de Paulet), Raven Press, New York, pp. 31–40.

De Caterina, R., Giannessi, D., Boem, A. *et al.* (1985) Equal antiplatelet effects of aspirin 50 or 324 mg/day in patients after acute myocardial infarction. *Thromb. Haemostasis*, **54**, 528–32.

DeCaterina, R., Gianessi, D., Mazzone, A. *et al.* (1990) Vascular prostacyclin is increased in patients ingesting ω–3 polyunsaturated fatty acids before coronary artery bypass graft surgery. *Circulation*, **82**, 428–38.

Dechavanne, M., Ville, D., Viali, J.J. *et al.* (1975) Controlled trial of platelet antiaggregating agents and subcutaneous heparin in prevention of postoperative deep venous thrombosis in high-risk patients. *Haemostasis*, **4**, 94–100.

De Gaetano, G., Cerletti, C., Dejana, E. and Vermylen, J. (1986a) Current issues in thrombosis prevention with antiplatelet drugs. *Drugs*, **31**, 517–49.

De Gaetano, G., Carriero, M.R., Carletti, C. and Mussoui, L. (1986b) Low dose aspirin does not prevent fibrinolytic response to venous occlusion. *Biochem. Pharmacol.*, **35**, 3147–50.

Dembinska-Kiec, A., Kostka-Trabka, E. and Gryglewski, R.J. (1982) Effect of prostacyclin on fibrinolytic activity in patients with arteriosclerosis obliterans. *Thromb. Haemostasis*, **47**, 190.

De Nucci, G., Gryglewski, R., Warner, T.D. and Vane, J.R. (1988) Receptor-mediated release of endothelium-derived relaxing factor and prostacyclin from bovine aortic endothelial cells is coupled. *Proc. Natl Acad. Sci. USA*, **85**, 2334–8.

De Witt, D.L. and Smith, W.L. (1983) Purification of prostacyclin synthase from bovine aorta by immunoaffinity chromatography. Evidence that the enzyme is a hemoprotein. *J. Biol. Chem.*, **258**, 3285–93.

Deykin, D., Janson, P. and McMahon, L. (1982) Ethanol potentiation of aspirin-induced prolongation of the bleeding time. *N. Engl. J. Med.*, **306**, 852–4.

Diczfalusy, U., Falardeau, P. and Hammarstrom, S. (1977) Conversion of prostaglandin endoperoxides to C_{17}-hydroxy acids catalyzed by human platelet thromboxane synthase. *FEBS Lett.*, **84**, 271–4.

Dusting, G.J., Mullane, K.M. and Moncada, S. (1986) Prostacyclin and vascular smooth muscle. In, *Handbook of Hypertension, Vol. 7: Pathophysiology of Hypertension – Cardiovascular Aspects* (eds A. Zanchetti and R.C. Tarazi, Elsevier Science Publishers, BV, Amsterdam pp. 408–26.

Dyerberg, J. and Bang, H.O. (1979) Haemostatic function and platelet polyunsaturated fatty acids in Eskimos. *Lancet*, **ii**, 433–5.

Dyerberg, J., Bang, H.O., Stoffersen, E., Moncada, S. and Vane, J.R. (1978), Eicosapentaenoic acid and prevention of thrombosis and atherosclerosis? *Lancet*, **ii**, 117–19.

Egan, R.W., Paxton, J. and Keuhl, F.A. Jr (1976) Mechanism for irreversible self-deactivation of prostaglandin synthetase. *J. Biol. Chem.*, **251**, 7329–35.

Eldor, A., Falcone, D., Hajjar, D. *et al.* (1981) Recovery of prostacyclin production by de-endothelialized rabbit aorta. Critical role of neointimal smooth muscle cells. *J. Clin. Invest.*, **67**, 735–41.

Eldor, A., Falcone, D.J., Hajjar, D.P. *et al.* (1982) Diet-induced hypercholesterolemia inhibits the recovery of prostacyclin production by injured rabbit aorta. *Am. J. Pathol.*, **107**, 186–90.

Elwood, P.C., Renaud, S., Sharp, D.S. *et al.* (1991) Ischaemic heart disease and platelet aggregation. The Caerphilly Collaborative Heart Disease Study. *Circulation*, **83**, 38–44.

Falcone, D.J., Hajjar, D.P. and Minick, C.R. (1980) Enhancement of cholesterol and cholesteryl ester accumulation in re-endothelialized aorta. *Am. J. Pathol.*, **99**, 81–104.

Fischer, S. and Weber, P.C. (1984) Prostaglandin I$_3$ is formed *in vivo* in man after dietary eicosapentaenoic acid. *Nature*, **307**, 165–8.

Fitzgerald, D.J., Roy, L., Catella, F. and FitzGerald, G.A. (1986) Platelet activation in unstable coronary disease. *N. Engl. J. Med.*, **315**, 983–9.

FitzGerald, G.A., Pedersen, A.K. and Patrono, C. (1983a) Analysis of prostacyclin and thromboxane biosynthesis in cardiovascular disease. *Circulation*, **67**, 1174–7.

FitzGerald, G.A., Oates, J.A., Hawiger, J. *et al.* (1983b) Endogenous biosynthesis of prostacyclin and thromboxane and platelet function during chronic administration of aspirin in man. *J. Clin. Invest.*, **71**, 676–83.

Flower, R., Gryglewski, R., Herbaczynska-Cedro K. and Vane, J.R. (1972) Effects of anti-inflammatory drugs on prostaglandin biosynthesis. *Nature. (Lond.)*, **238**, 104–6.

Force, T., Milani, R., Hibberd, P. *et al.*. (1991) Aspirin-induced decline in prostacyclin production in patients with coronary artery disease is due to decreased endoperoxide shift: analysis of the effects of a combination of aspirin and n-3 fatty acids on the eicosanoid profile. *Circulation*, **84**, 2286–93.

Förstermann, U., Kühn, K., Vesterqvist, O. *et al.* (1989) An increase in the ratio of thromboxane A$_2$ to prostacyclin in association with increased blood pressure in patients on cyclosporine A. *Prostaglandins*, **37**, 567–75.

Frank, G.W. and Bevan, J.A. (1983) Electrical stimulation causes endothelium-dependent relaxation in lung vessels. *Am. J. Physiol.*, **244**, H793-H798.

Freiman, P.C., Mitchell, G.G., Heistad, D.D. *et al.* (1986) Atherosclerosis impairs endothelium-dependent vascular relaxation to acetylcholine and thrombin in primates. *Circ. Res.*, **58**, 783–9.

Fressinaud, E., Baruch, D., Girma, J.P. *et al.* (1988) Von Willebrand factor-mediated platelet adhesion to collagen involves platelet membrane glycoprotein IIb-IIIa as well as glycoprotein Ib. *J. Lab. Clin. Med.*, **112**, 58–67.

Friedman, H. (1970) Pathogenesis of coronary thrombosis, intramural and intraluminal haemorrhage. In *Thrombosis and Coronary Heart Disease, Vol. 4* (ed. L.A. Halonen), Karger, Basel, p. 3.

Furchgott, R. F. (1984) The role of endothelium in the responses of vascular smooth muscle to drugs. *Annu. Rev. Pharmacol. Toxicol.*, **24**, 175–97.

Furchgott, R.F. and Zawadzki, J.V. (1980) The obligatory role of endothelial cells in the relaxation of arterial smooth muscle by acetylcholine. *Nature (Lond.)*, **288**, 373–6.

Furlong, B., Henderson, A.H., Lewis, M.J. and Smith, J.H. (1987) Endothelium-derived relaxing factor inhibits *in vitro* platelet aggregation. *Brit. J. Pharmacol.*, **90**, 687–92.

Garg, U.C. and Hassid, A. (1989) Nitric oxide-generating vasodilators and 8-bromo-cyclic guanosine monophosphate inhibit mitogenesis and proliferation of cultured rat vascular smooth muscle cells. *J. Clin. Invest.*, **83**, 1774–7.

Gaspari, F., Vigano, G., Orisio, S. *et al.* (1987) Aspirin prolongs bleeding time in uremia by a mechanism distinct from platelet cyclooxygenase inhibition. *J. Clin. Invest.*, **79**, 1788–97.

Gerrard, J. M. (1988) Platelet aggregation: Cellular regulation and physiologic role. *Hospital Practice*, 89–108.

Gerritsen, M.E. (1987) Functional heterogeneity of vascular endothelial cells. *Biochem. Pharmacol.*, **35**, 2701–11.

Gertz, S.D., Uretsky, G., Wajnberg, R.S. *et al.* (1981) Endothelial cell damage and thrombus formation after partial arterial constriction: Relevance to the role of coronary artery spasm in the pathogenesis of myocardial infarction. *Circulation*, **63**, 476–86.

Ghezzo, F., Trinchero, P. and Pegoraro, L. (1981a) Changes in granulocyte fibrinolytic activity (FA) induced by *in vivo* treatment with lysine acetylsalicylate (LAS). *Thromb. Haemostasis*, **46**, 761.

Ghezzo, F., Trinchero, P. and Pegoraro, L. (1981b) Effect of aspirin treatment upon fibrinolytic activity of peripheral blood granulocytes. *Acta Haematol.*, **65**, 229–32.

Glavind, J., Hartmann, S., Clemmesen, J. *et al.* (1952) Studies on the role of lipoperoxides in human pathology. II. The presence of peroxidized lipids in the atherosclerotic aorta. *Acta Pathol. Microbiol. Scand.*, **30**, 1–6.

Goldstein, J.M., Mahnsten, C.L., Kindahl, H. *et al.* (1978) Thromboxane generation by human peripheral blood polymorphonuclear leukocytes. *J. Exp. Med.*, **148**, 787–92.

Green, D., Davies, R.O., Holmes, G.I. *et al.* (1983) Fibrinolytic activity after administration of diflunisal and aspirin. *Haemostasis*, **13**, 394–8.

Gresele, P., Arnout, J., Deckmyn, H. *et al.* (1987) Role of proaggregatory and antiaggregatory prostaglandins in hemostasis: Studies with combined thromboxane synthase inhibition and thromboxane receptor antagonism. *J. Clin. Invest.*, **80**, 1435–45.

Gryglewski, R.J. (1966) The fibrinolytic activity of anti-inflammatory drugs. *J. Pharm. Pharmacol.*, **18**, 474.

Gryglewski, R.J. (1970) On the mechanism of fibrinolysis induced by anti-inflammatory drugs. In *Chemical Control of Fibrinolysis – Thrombolysis* (ed. J.M. Schrör), Wiley Interscience, New York, pp. 44–72.

Gryglewski, R.J. (1990) Role of prostacyclin in cardiovascular homeostasis. In *Endogenous Factors of Cardiovascular Regulation and Protection* (eds M. Cantin, R. Paoletti, P. Braquet, and Y. Christen), Excerpta Medica, Amsterdam, pp. 21–59.

Gryglewski, R.J. and Eckstein, M. (1967) Fibrinolytic activity of some biarylcarboxylic acids. *Nature (Lond.)*, **214**, 626.

Gryglewski, R.J. and Panczenko, B. (1968) The influence of sodium flufenacinate on the reaction of protein sulfhydryl groups with β-hydroxyethyl-N-nitrosulfide. *Dissert. Pharm. Pharmacol.*, **20**, 489–96.

Gryglewski, R.J. and Szczeklik, A. (1981) Prostacyclin and atherosclerosis. In *Clinical Pharmacology of Prostacyclin* (eds P.J. Lewis, and J. O'Grady), Raven Press, New York, pp. 89–95.

Gryglewski, R.J., Bunting, S., Moncada, S. *et al.* (1976) Arterial walls are protected against deposition of platelet thrombi by a substance (prostaglandin X) which they make from prostaglandin endoperoxides. *Prostaglandins*, **12**, 685–713.

Gryglewski, R.J., Salmon, J.A., Ubatuba, F.B. *et al.* (1979) Effects of all cis-5, 11, 14, 17 eicosapentaenoic acid and PGH_3 on platelet aggregation. *Prostaglandins*, **18**, 453–78.

Gryglewski, R.J., Palmer, R.M.J. and Moncada, S. (1986) Superoxide anion is involved in the breakdown of endothelium-derived vascular relaxing factor. *Nature (Lond.)*, **320**, 454–6.

Gryglewski, R.J., Botting, R.M. and Vane, J.R. (1988) Mediators produced by the endothelial cell. *Hypertension*, **12**, 530–48.

Haeger, K. (1968) The treatment of peripheral occlusive arterial disease with alpha-tocopherol as compared with vasodilator agents and anti-prothrombin (dicumarol). *Vasc. Dis.*, **5**, 199–213.

Hajjar, D.P., Weksler, B.B., Falcone, D.J. and Minick, C.R. (1981) Prostacyclin alters cholesteryl ester metabolism in cultured aortic smooth muscle cells. *Fed. Proc. Fed. Am. Soc. Exp. Biol.*, **40**, 351 (Abstr.).

Hajjar, D.P., Weksler, B.B., Falcone, D.J. et al. (1982) Prostacyclin modulates cholesteryl ester hydrolytic activity by its effect on cyclic adenosine monophosphate in rabbit aortic smooth muscle cells. *J. Clin. Invest.*, **70**, 479–88.

Hallam, T.J. and Pearson, J.D. (1986) Exogenous ATP raises cytoplasmic free calcium in fura-2 loaded piglet aortic endothelial cells. *FEBS Lett.*, **207**, 95–9.

Ham, E.A., Egan, R.W., Soderman, D.D. et al. (1979) Peroxidase-dependent deactivation of prostacyclin synthetase. *J. Biol. Chem.*, **254**, 2191–4.

Hamberg, M., Svensson, J., Wakabayashi, T. and Samuelsson, B. (1974) Isolation and structure of two prostaglandin endoperoxides that cause platelet aggregation. *Proc. Natl Acad. Sci. USA*, **71**, 345–9.

Hamberg, M., Svensson, J. and Samuelsson, B. (1975) Thromboxanes: a new group of biologically active compounds derived from prostaglandin endoperoxides. *Proc. Natl Acad. Sci. USA*, **72**, 2994–8.

Hammarstrom, S. and Falardeau, P. (1977) Resolution of prostaglandin endo-peroxide synthase and thromboxane synthase of human platelets. *Proc. Natl Acad. Sci. USA*, **74**, 3691–5.

Hammouda, M.W. and Moroz, L.A. (1986) Aspirin and venous occlusion: effects on blood fibrinolytic activity and tissue-type plasminogen activator levels. *Thromb. Res.*, **42**, 73–82.

Hanson, S.R., Harkev, L.A. and Bjornsson, T.D. (1985) Effects of platelet-modifying drugs on arterial thromboembolism in baboons. Aspirin potentiates antithrombotic actions of dipyridamole and sulfipyrazone by mechanism(s) independent of platelet cyclooxygenase inhibition. *J. Clin. Invest.*, **75**, 1591–9.

Harris, W.H., Salzman, E.W., Athanasonlis, C.A. et al. (1977) Aspirin prophylaxis of venous thromboembolism after total hip replacement. *N. Engl. J. Med.*, **297**, 1246–9.

Harris, W.H., Athanasonlis, C.A., Waltman, A.C. and Salzman, E.W. (1982) High and low-dose aspirin prophylaxis against venous thromboembolic disease in total hip replacement. *J. Bone Jt Surg.*, **64A**, 63–6.

Harris, W.H., Athanasonlis, C.A., Waltman, A.C. and Salzman, E.W. (1985) Prophylaxis of deep-vein thrombosis after total hip replacement. *J. Bone Jt Surg.*, **67A**, 58–62.

Harrison, M.J.G. and Mitchell, J.R.A. (1966) The influence of red blood cells on platelet adhesiveness. *Lancet*, **ii**, 1163–4.

Harter, H.R., Burch, J.W., Majerus, P.W. et al. (1979) Prevention of thrombosis in patients on haemodialysis by low-dose aspirin. *N. Engl. J. Med.*, **301**, 577–9.

Haurand, M. and Ullrich, V. (1985) Isolation and characterization of thromboxane synthase from human platelets as a cytochrome P-450 enzyme. *J. Biol. Chem.*, **260**, 15059–67.

Hennekens, C.H., Willett, W., Rosmer, B. *et al.* (1979) Effects of beer, wine, and liquor in coronary deaths. *J. Am. Med. Assoc.*, **242**, 1973–4.

Henriksson, P., Wennmalm, A., Edhag, O. *et al.* (1986) *In vivo* production of prostacyclin and thromboxane in patients with acute myocardial infarction. *Brit. Heart J.*, **55**, 543–8.

Hess, H., Mietaschk, A. and Deichsel, G. (1985) Drug-induced inhibition of platelet function delays progression of peripheral occlusive arterial disease: a prospective double-blind arteriographically controlled trial. *Lancet*, **i**, 415–21.

Hibbs, J.B., Taintor, R.R. and Vavrin, Z. (1987) Macrophage cytotoxicity: role for L-arginine deiminase and imino nitrogen oxidation to nitrite. *Science*, **235**, 473–6.

Higgs, E., Moncada, S., Vane, J. *et al.* (1978) Effect of prostacyclin (PGI_2) on platelet adhesion to rabbit arterial subendothelium. *Prostaglandins*, **16**, 17–22.

Hirsh, J. and Levine, M. (1989) Prevention of venous thrombosis in patients undergoing major orthopaedic surgical procedures. *Brit. J. Clin. Practice*, **65** (Symp. Suppl.), 2–8.

Hirsh, P., Hillis, L., Campbell, W. *et al.* (1981) Release of prostaglandins and thromboxane into the coronary circulation in patients with ischemic heart disease. *N. Engl. J. Med.*, **304**, 685–91.

Ho, Y.K., Brown, M.S. and Goldstein, J.L. (1980) Hydrolysis and excretion of cytoplasmic cholesteryl esters by macrophages: stimulation by high density and other agents. *J. Lipid Res.*, **21**, 391–8.

Hoak, J. C., Brotherton, A. A., Czervionke, R. L. and Fry, G. L. (1985) Role of prostacyclin in inhibiting platelet adherence to cells of the vessel wall. In *Interaction of Platelets with the Vessel Wall* (eds J.A. Oates, J. Hawiger and R. Ross), American Physiological Society, Bethesda, Maryland, pp. 117–24.

Hogan, J.C., Lewis, M.J. and Henderson, A.H. (1988). *In vivo* EDRF activity influences platelet function. *Brit. J. Pharmacol.*, **94**, 1020–2.

Holzmann, S. (1982) Endothelium-induced relaxation by acetylcholine associated with larger rises in cyclic GMP in coronary arterial strips. *J. Cyclic Nucleotide Res.*, **8**, 409–19.

Housholder, G.T., Moorrees, L.L. and Houston, A.A. (1980) Fibrinolysis in the rat after short-term aspirin therapy. *J. Oral Surg.*, **38**, 412–16.

Ignarro, L.J., Buga, G.M., Wood., K.S., *et al.* (1987) Endothelium-derived relaxing factor produced and released from artery and vein is nitric oxide. *Proc. Natl Acad. Sci. USA*, **84**, 9265–9.

Ingerman-Wojenski, C., Silver, M.J., Smith, J.B. and Macarak, E. (1981) Bovine endothelial cells in culture produce thromboxane as well as prostacyclin. *J. Clin. Invest.*, **67**, 1292–6.

ISIS-2 (Second International Study of Infarct Survival) Collaborative Group. (1988) Randomized trial of intravenous streptokinase, oral aspirin, both, or neither among 17,187 cases of suspected acute myocardial infarction: ISIS-2. *Lancet*, **ii**, 349–60.

Iyengar, R., Stuehr, D.J. and Marletta, M.A. (1987) Macrophage synthesis of nitrite, nitrate, and N-nitrosamines: precursors and role of the respiratory burst. *Proc. Natl Acad. Sci. USA*, **84**, 6369–73.

Jacobs, M., Plane, F. and Bruckdorfer, K. R. (1990) Native and oxidized low density lipoproteins have different inhibitory effects on endothelium-derived relaxing factor in the rabbit aorta. *Brit. J. Pharmacol.*, **100**, 21–6.

Jain, A., Mehrotra, T.N., Goel, V.K. *et al.* (1982) Effect of aspirin on plasma fibrinolytic activity in patients of coronary heart disease. *J. Assoc. Physicians India*, **30**, 441–3.

Jakubowski, J.A., Vaillancourt, R. and Deykin, D. (1988) Interaction of ethanol, prostacyclin, and aspirin in determining human platelet reactivity *in vitro*. *Arteriosclerosis*, **8**, 436–41.

Johnson, R.A., Morton, D.R., Kinner, J.H. *et al.* (1976) The chemical structure of prostaglandin X (prostacyclin). *Prostaglandins*, **12**, 915–28.

Kainoh, M., Imai, R., Umetsu, T. *et al.* (1990) Prostacyclin and beraprost sodium as suppressors of activated rat polymorphonuclear leukocytes. *Biochem. Pharmacol.*, **39**, 477–84.

Kallman, R., Nieuwenhuis, H.K., de Groot, P.G. *et al.* (1987) Effects of low doses of aspirin, 10 mg and 30 mg daily, on bleeding time, thromboxane production and 6-keto-PGF$_{1\alpha}$ excretion in healthy subjects. *Thromb. Res.*, **45**, 355–61.

Kaneshiro, M.M., Mielke, C.H. Jr, Kasper, C.K. and Rapaport, S.I. (1969) Bleeding time after aspirin in disorders of intrinsic clotting. *N. Engl. J. Med.*, **281**, 1039–42.

Kannel, W.B., Castelli, W.P. and Gordon, T. (1979) Cholesterol in the prediction of atherosclerotic disease. New perspectives based on the Framingham study. *Ann. Intern. Med.*, **90**, 85–91.

Keber, J. and Keber, D. (1985) No significant effect of chronic aspirin use on fibrinolytic response to venous occlusion in coronary patients. *Thromb. Res.*, **39**, 761–5.

Keber, I., Jercb, M. and Keber, D. (1987) Aspirin decreases fibrinolytic potential during venous occlusion but not during acute physical activity. *Thromb. Res.*, **46**, 205–12.

Kelm, M., Feelisch, M., Spahr, R. *et al.* (1988) Quantitative and kinetic characterization of nitric oxide and EDRF release from cultured endothelial cells. *Biochem. Biophys. Res. Commun.*, **154**, 236–44.

Khan, M.T. and Furchgott, R F. (1987) Additional evidence that endothelium-derived relaxing factor is nitric oxide. In *Pharmacology, Proceedings of the Xth International Congress of Pharmacology (IUPHAR)* (eds. M.J. Rand, and C. Raper), Elsevier Sciences Publishers BV, Amsterdam, pp. 341–44.

Knapp, H.R. and FitzGerald, G.A. (1989) The antihypertensive effects of fish oil. *N. Engl. J. Med.*, **320**, 1037–43.

Knapp, H.R., Reilly, I.A.G., Alessandrini, P. and FitzGerald, G.A. (1986) *In vivo* indexes of platelet and vascular function during fish-oil administration in patients with atherosclerosis. *N. Engl. J. Med.*, **314**, 937–42.

Kromhout, D., Bosschieter, E.B. and de Lezenne Coulander, C. (1985) The inverse relation between fish consumption and 20-year mortality from coronary heart disease. *N. Engl. J. Med.*, **312**, 1205–9.

Lagarde, M. and Dechavanne, M. (1977) Increase of platelet prostaglandin cyclic endoperoxides in thrombosis. *Lancet*, **i**, 88.

Pharmacology of aspirin and salicylates

Lapetina, E. G. (1986). Inositide-dependent and independent mechanisms in platelet activation. In *Phosphoinositides and Receptor Mechanisms* (ed. J.W. Putney, Jr.), Alan R. Liss Inc., New York, pp. 271–86.

Larrue, J., Rigaud, M., Daret, D. *et al.* (1980) Prostacyclin production by cultured smooth muscle cells from atherosclerotic rabbit aorta. *Nature (Lond.)*, **285**, 480–2.

Lawson, J.A., Brash, A.R., Doran, J. and FitzGerald, G.A. (1985) Measurement of urinary 2, 3-dinor-thromboxane B_2 and thromboxane B_2 using bonded-phase phenylboronic acid columns and capillary gas chromatography-negative-ion chemical ionization mass spectrometry. *Anal. Biochem.*, **150**, 463–70.

Lee, T.-K., Chen, Y-C., Kuo, T-L. *et al.* (1989) Effect of low dose acetylsalicylic acid upon plasma thromboxane B_2 levels and platelet aggregation in ischemic stroke patients. *Clin. Chim. Acta*, **184**, 323–8.

Levin, R.I., Harpel, P.C., Weil, D. *et al.* (1984) Aspirin inhibits vascular plasminogen activator activity *in vivo*. *J. Clin. Invest.*, **74**, 571–80.

Lewy, R., Smith, J., Silver, M. *et al.* (1979) Detection of thromboxane B_2 in peripheral blood of patients with Prinzmetal's angina. *Prostaglandins Med.*, **2**, 243–8.

Leytin, V.L., Gorbunova, N.A., Misselwitz, F. *et al.* (1984) Step-by-step analysis of adhesion of human platelets to a collagen-coated surface; defect in initial attachment and spreading of platelets in von Willebrand's disease. *Thromb. Res.*, **34**, 51–63.

Long, C. J., Shikano, K. and Berkowitz, B. A. (1987) Anion exchange resins discriminate between nitric oxide and EDRF. *Eur. J. Pharmacol.*, **142**, 317–18.

Luckhoff, A. and Busse, R. (1986) Increased free calcium in endothelial cells under stimulation with adenine nucleotides. *J. Cell. Physiol.*, **126**, 414–20.

MacDonald, P.S., Read, M.A. and Dusting, G.J. (1988) Synergistic inhibition of platelet aggregation by endothelium-derived relaxing factor and prostacyclin. *Thromb. Res.*, **49**, 437–49.

MacIntyre, D.E., Pearson, J.D. and Gordon, J.L. (1978) Localisation and stimulation of prostacyclin production in vascular cells. *Nature (Lond.)*, **271**, 549–51.

Marcus, A.J., Weksler, B.B., Jaffe, E.A. and Broekman, M.J. (1980) Synthesis of prostacyclin from platelet-derived endoperoxides by cultured human endothelial cells. *J. Clin. Invest.*, **66**, 979–86.

Markey, C.M., Alward, A., Weller, P. E. and Marnett, L. J. (1987) Quantitative studies of hydroperoxide reduction by prostaglandin H synthase. *J. Biol. Chem.*, **262**, 6266–79.

Marks, J. (1962) Critical appraisal of the therapeutic value of α-tocopherol. *Vitamins and Hormones*, **20**, 573–98.

Marmot, M.G. (1984) Alcohol and coronary heart disease. *Int. J. Epidemiol.*, **13**, 160–7.

Martin, W., Villani, G.M., Jothianandan, D. and Furchgott, R.F. (1985) Selective blockade of endothelium-dependent and glyceryl trinitrate-induced relaxation by hemoglobin and by methylene blue in the rabbit aorta. *J. Pharmacol. Exp. Ther.*, **232**, 708–16.

Mayer, B., Schmidt, K., Humbert, P. and Bohme, E. (1989) Biosynthesis of endothelium-derived relaxing factor: A cytosolic enzyme in porcine aortic endothelial cells Ca^{2+}-dependently converts L-arginine into an activator of soluble guanylyl cyclase. *Biochem. Biophys. Res. Commun.*, **164**, 678–85.

Meade, T.W., Vickers, M.V., Thompson, S.G. *et al.* (1985) Epidemiological characteristics of platelet aggregability. *Brit. Med. J.*, **290**, 428–32.

Medalie, J.H., Kahn, H.A., Neufeld, H.N. *et al.* (1973) Myocardial infarction over a five-year period. I. Prevalence, incidence and mortality experience. *J. Chronic Dis.*, **26**, 63–84.

Menon, J.S. (1970) Aspirin and blood fibrinolysis. *Lancet*, **i**, 364.

Mickel, H. and Horbar, J. (1974) The effect of peroxidized arachidonic acid upon human platelet aggregation. *Lipids*, **9**, 68–71.

Mielke, C.H. Jr (1982) Aspirin prolongation of the template bleeding time: influence of venostasis and direction of incision. *Blood*, **60**, 1139–42.

Mielke, C.H. Jr, Kaneshiro, M.M., Maher, I.A. *et al.* (1969) The standardized normal Ivy bleeding time and its prolongation by aspirin. *Blood*, **34**, 204–15.

Minuz, P., Covi, G., Paluani, F. *et al.* (1988) Altered excretion of prostaglandin and thromboxane metabolites in pregnancy-induced hypertension. *Hypertension*, **11**, 550–6.

Minuz, P., Barrow, S.E., Cockcroft, J.R. and Ritter, J.M. (1990) Prostacyclin and thromboxane biosynthesis in mild essential hypertension. *Hypertension*, **15**, 469–74.

Moncada, S. (1982) Biological importance of prostacyclin. *Brit. J. Pharmacol.*, **76**, 3–31.

Moncada, S. and Vane, J.R. (1979) Pharmacology and endogenous roles of prostaglandin endoperoxides, thromboxane A$_2$ and prostacyclin. *Pharmacol. Rev.*, **30**, 293–31.

Moncada, S., Needleman, P., Bunting, S. and Vane, J.R. (1976a) Prostaglandin endoperoxide and thromboxane generating systems and their selective inhibition. *Prostaglandins*, **12**, 323–9.

Moncada, S., Gryglewski, R., Bunting, S. and Vane, J.R. (1976b) An enzyme isolated from arteries transforms prostaglandin endoperoxides to an unstable substance that inhibits platelet aggregation. *Nature (Lond.)*, **263**, 663–5.

Moncada, S., Gryglewski, R.J., Bunting, S. and Vane, J.R. (1976c) A lipid peroxide inhibits the enzyme in blood vessel microsomes that generates from prostaglandin endoperoxides the substance (prostaglandin X) which prevents platelet aggregation. *Prostaglandins*, **12**, 715–37.

Moncada, S., Herman, A.G., Higgs, E.A. and Vane, J.R. (1977) Differential formation of prostacyclin (PGX or PGI$_2$) by layers of the arterial wall. An explanation for the antithrombotic properties of vascular endothelium. *Thromb. Res.*, **11**, 323–44.

Moncada, S., Palmer, R.M.J. and Higgs, E.A. (1989) Biosynthesis of nitric oxide from L-arginine. A pathway for the regulation of cell function and communication. *Biochem. Pharmacol.*, **38**, 1709–15.

Moore, P.K., al-Swayeh, O.A., Chong, N.S.W. *et al.* (1989) L-N^G-nitro arginine (NOARG) inhibits endothelium-dependent vasodilatation in the rabbit aorta and perfused rat mesentery. *Brit. J. Pharmacol.*, **98**, 905P.

Morishita, H., Yui, Y., Hattori, R. *et al.* (1990) Increased hydrolysis of cholesteryl ester with prostacyclin is potentiated by high density lipoprotein through the prostacyclin stabilization. *J. Clin. Invest.*, **86**, 1885–91.

Moroz, L.A. (1977) Increased blood fibrinolytic activity after aspirin ingestion. *N. Engl. J. Med.*, **296**, 525–9.

Morrison, A.R., Nishikawa, K. and Needleman, P. (1978) Thromboxane A_2 biosynthesis in the ureter obstructed isolated perfused kidney of the rabbit. *J. Pharmacol. Exp. Ther.*, **205**, 1–8.

MRC Steering Committee. (1972) Effect of aspirin on postoperative venous thrombosis. *Lancet*, **ii**, 441–5.

Musial, J., Wilczynska, M., Sladek, K. *et al.* (1986) Fibrinolytic activity of prostacyclin and iloprost in patients with peripheral arterial disease. *Prostaglandins*, **31**, 61–70.

Mustard, J.F., Kinlough-Rathbone, R.L. and Packham, M.A. (1987) The vessel wall in thrombosis. In *Hemostasis and Thrombosis* (eds R.W. Colman, J. Hirsh, V.J. Marder and E.W. Salzman), J. Lippincott Co. Philadelphia, PA, pp. 1073–88.

Mustard, J.F., Packham, M.A. and Kinlough-Rathbone, R.L. (1990) Platelets, blood flow and the vessel wall. *Circulation*, **81** (Suppl. 1), I-24–I-27.

Myers, P. R., Minor, R.L. Jr, Guerra, R. Jr *et al.* (1990) Vasorelaxant properties of the endothelium-derived relaxing factor more closely resemble S-nitrosocysteine than nitric oxide. *Nature (Lond.)*, **345**, 161–3.

Myler, R.K., Frink, R.J., Shaw, R.E. *et al.* (1990) The unstable plaque: Pathophysiology and therapeutic implications. *J. Invest. Cardiol.*, **2**, 117.

Nawroth, P. P., Stern, D. M., Kaplan, K. L. and Nossel, H. L. (1984) Prostacyclin production by perturbed bovine aortic endothelial cells in culture. *Blood*, **64**, 801–6.

Needleman, P., Moncada, S., Bunting, S. *et al.* (1976) Identification of an enzyme in platelet microsomes which generates thromboxane A_2 from prostaglandin endoperoxides. *Nature (Lond.)*, **261**, 558–60.

Needleman, P., Raz, A., Minkes, M.S. *et al.* (1979) Triene prostaglandins: Prostacyclin and thromboxane biosynthesis and unique biological properties. *Proc. Natl Acad. Sci. USA*, **76**, 944–8.

Nordøy, A. and Goodnight, S.H. (1990) Dietary lipids and thrombosis: Relationships to atherosclerosis. *Arteriosclerosis*, **10**, 149–63.

Nordøy, A., Svensson, B., Wiebe, D. and Hoak, J.C. (1978) Lipoproteins and the inhibitory effect of human endothelial cells on platelet function. *Circ. Res.*, **43**, 527–34.

Nüsing, R. and Ullrich, V. (1990) Immunoquantitation of thromboxane synthase in human tissues. *Eicosanoids*, **3**, 175–80.

Okuma, M., Takayama, H. and Uchino, H. (1980) Generation of prostacyclin-like substance and lipid peroxidation in vitamin E-deficient rats. *Prostaglandins*, **19**, 527–36.

Owens, M.R. and Cimino, C.D. (1980) The inhibitory effect of sodium salicylate on synthesis of factor VIII by the perfused rat liver. *Thromb. Res.*, **18**, 839–45.

Palmer, R.M. and Moncada, S. (1989) A novel citrulline-forming enzyme implicated in the formation of nitric oxide by vascular endothelial cells. *Biochem. Biophys. Res. Commun.*, **158**, 348–52.

Palmer, R.M.J., Ferrige, A.G. and Moncada, S. (1987) Nitric oxide accounts for the biological activity of endothelium-derived relaxing factor. *Nature (Lond.)*, **88**, 411–15.

Palmer, R. M. J., Ashton, D. S. and Moncada, S. (1988) Vascular endothelial cells synthesize nitric oxide from L-arginine. *Nature (Lond.)*, **33**, 664–6.

Pastan, I.H., Johnson, G.S. and Anderson, W.B. (1975) Role of cyclic nucleotides in growth control. *Annu. Rev. Biochem.*, **44**, 491–522.

Patrignani, P., Filabozzi, P. and Patrono, C. (1982) Selective cumulative inhibition of platelet thromboxane production by low-dose aspirin in healthy subjects. *J. Clin. Invest.*, **69**, 1366–72.

Patrono, C. (1989) Aspirin and human platelets: from clinical trials to acetylation of cyclooxygenase and back. *Trends Pharmacol. Sci.*, **10**, 453–8.

Patrono, C., Ciabattoni, G., Pugliese, F. *et al.* (1986) Estimated rate of thromboxane secretion into the circulation of normal humans. *J. Clin. Invest.*, **77**, 590–4.

Pearson, J.D., Shakey, L.L. and Gordon, J.L. (1983) Stimulation of prostagladin through purinoceptors of cultured porcine endothelial cells. *Biochem. J.*, **214**, 273–6.

Peto, R., Gray, R., Collins, R. *et al.* (1988) Randomized trial of prophylactic daily aspirin in British male doctors. *Brit. Med. J.*, **296**, 313–16.

Piper, P.J. and Vane, J.R. (1969) Release of additional factors in anaphylaxis and its antagonism by anti-inflammatory drugs. *Nature (Lond.)*, **223**, 29–35.

Pohl, U. and Busse, R. (1989) EDRF increases cyclic GMP in platelets during passage through the coronary vascular bed. *Circ. Res.*, **65**, 1798–803.

Pohl, U., Dezsi, L., Simon, B. and Busse, R. (1987) Selective inhibition of endothelium-dependent dilation in resistance-sized vessels *in vivo*. *Am. J. Physiol.*, **253**, H234–H239.

Quadt, J. F. A., Voss, R. and Ten-Hoor, F. (1982) Prostacyclin production of the isolated pulsatingly perfused rat aorta. *J. Pharmacol. Methods*, **7**, 263–70.

Radomski, M.W. and Moncada, S. (1983) An improved method for washing of human platelets with prostacyclin. *Thromb. Res.*, **30**, 383–9.

Radomski, M.W., Palmer, R.M.J. and Moncada, S. (1987a) The anti-aggregating properties of vascular endothelium: interactions between prostacyclin and nitric oxide. *Brit. J. Pharmacol.*, **92**, 639–46.

Radomski, M.W., Palmer, R.M.J. and Moncada, S. (1987b) Comparative pharmacology of endothelium-derived relaxing factor, nitric oxide and prostacyclin in platelets. *Brit. J. Pharmacol.*, **92**, 181–7.

Radomski, M.W., Palmer, R.M.J. and Moncada, S. (1987c) The role of nitric oxide and cGMP in platelet adhesion to vascular endothelium. *Biochem. Biophys. Res. Commun.*, **148**, 1482–9.

Rapoport, R. M. and Murad, F. (1983) Agonist-induced endothelium-dependent relaxation in rat thromboxane aorta may be mediated through cGMP. *Circ. Res.*, **51**, 352–57.

Reilly, I.A.G. and FitzGerald, G.A. (1988) Aspirin in cardiovascular disease. *Drugs*, **35**, 154–76.

Renney, J.T.G., Sullivan, G.F. and Burke, P.F. (1976) Prevention of postoperative vein thrombosis with dipyridamole and aspirin. *Brit. Med. J.*, **1**, 992–4.

RISC Group (1990) Risk of myocardial infarction and death during treatment with low dose aspirin and intravenous heparin in men with unstable coronary artery disease. *Lancet*, **336**, 827–30.

Pharmacology of aspirin and salicylates

Ritter, J.M., Cockcroft, J.R., Doktor, H.S. *et al.* (1989) Differential effect of aspirin on thromboxane and prostaglandin biosynthesis in man. *Brit. J. Clin. Pharmacol.*, **28**, 573–9.

Robertson, R., Robertson, D., Roberts, J. *et al.* (1981) Thromboxane A_2 in vasotonic angina pectoris. Evidence from direct measurements and inhibitor trials. *N. Engl. J. Med.*, **304**, 998–1003.

Rosenblum, W.I. and El Sabban, F. (1979) Topical prostacyclin (PGI_2) inhibits platelet aggregation in pial venules of the mouse. *Stroke*, **10**, 399–401.

Ross, R., Masuda, J., Raines, E.W. *et al.* (1990) Localization of PDGF-B protein in macrophages in all phases of atherogenesis. *Science*, **248**, 1009–12.

Rubanyi, G.M., Romero, J.C. and Vanhoutte, P.M. (1986) Flow-induced release of endothelium-derived relaxing factor. *Am. J. Physiol.*, **250**, H1145–H1149.

Rubenfire, M., Blevins, R.D., Barnhart, M. *et al.* (1986) Platelet hyperaggregability in patients with chest pain and angiographically normal coronary arteries. *Am. J. Cardiol.*, **57**, 657–60.

Sagone, A. L., Wells, R. M. and De Mocko, C. (1980) Evidence that OH production by human PMNs is related to prostaglandin metabolism. *Inflammation*, **4**, 65–71.

Salmon, J.A., Smith, D.R., Flower, R.J. *et al.* (1978) Further studies on the enzymatic conversion of prostaglandin endoperoxide into prostacyclin by porcine aorta microsomes. *Biochim. Biophys. Acta*, **523**, 250–62.

Salvemini, D., Sneddon, J.M., Kondo, K. *et al.* (1988) 'EDRF' released from human neutrophils and prostacyclin acts synergistically to inhibit platelet aggregation. *Brit. J. Pharmacol.*, **95**, 728P.

Salvemini, D., de Nucci, G., Gryglewski, R.J. and Vane, J.R. (1989) Human neutrophils and mononuclear cells inhibit platelet aggregation by releasing a nitric oxide-like factor. *Proc. Natl Acad. Sci. USA*, **86**, 6328–32.

Salzman, P.M., Salmon, J.A. and Moncada, S. (1980) Prostacyclin and thromboxane A_2 synthesis by rabbit pulmonary artery. *J. Pharmacol. Exp. Ther.*, **215**, 240–7.

Sanders, T.A.B., Naismith, D.J., Haines, A.P. and Vickers, M. (1980) Cod-liver oil, platelet fatty acids, and bleeding time. *Lancet*, **i**, 1189.

Sanders, T.A.B., Vickers, M. and Haines, A.P. (1981) Effect on blood lipids and haemostasis of a supplement of cod-liver oil, rich in eicosapentaenoic and docosahexaenoic acids, in healthy young men. *Clin. Sci.*, **61**, 317–24.

Sauter, R.D., Koch, E.L., Myers, W.O. *et al.* (1983) Aspirin-sulfinpyrazone in prophylaxis of deep venous thrombosis in total hip replacement. *J. Am. Med. Assoc.*, **250**, 2649–54.

Saxena, K.K., Gupte, B., Srivastave, R.K. and Prasad, D.N. (1980) Prevention of chemically induced myocardial damage and concomitant changes in fibrinolytic system by acetylsalicylic acid in rats. *Indian J. Exp. Biol.*, **18**, 410–13.

Schmid-Schönbein, H., Born, G.V.R., Richardson, P.D. *et al.* (1981) Rheology of thrombotic processes in flow: the interaction of erythrocytes and thrombocytes subjected to high flow forces. *Biorheology*, **18**, 415–44.

Schoeffter, P. and Miller, R.C. (1986) Role of sodium–calcium exchange and effects of calcium entry blockers on endothelial-mediated responses in rat isolated aorta. *Mol. Pharmacol.*, **30**, 53–7.

Schoop, W., Levy, H., Schoop, B. and Gaentzsch, A. (1983) Experimentelle and klinische Studie zu der sekundären Prevention der periphere Arteriosklerose. In *Thrombocytenfunktionshemmer* (eds. A. Bollinger and K. Rhyner), Thieme Verlag, Stuttgart, pp. 49–58.

Shimamoto, T., Kobayashi, M., Takahashi, T. *et al.* (1978) An observation of thromboxane A_2 in arterial blood after cholesterol feeding in rabbits. *Jpn Heart J.*, **19**, 748–53.

Siess, W. (1989) Molecular mechanisms of platelet activation. *Physiol. Rev.*, **69**, 58–178.

Siess, W., Roth, P., Scherer, B. *et al.* (1980) Platelet-membrane fatty acids, platelet aggregation, and thromboxane formation during a mackerel diet. *Lancet*, **i**, 441–4.

Siess, W., Siegel, F.L. and Lapetina, E.G. (1983) Arachidonic acid stimulates the formation of 1,2-diacylglycerol and phosphatidic acid in human platelets. Degree of phospholipase C activation correlates with protein phosphorylation, platelet shape change, serotonin release and aggregation. *J. Biol. Chem.*, **258**, 11236–42.

Sinzinger, H., Feigl, W. and Silberbauer, K. (1979) Prostacyclin generation in atherosclerotic arteries. *Lancet*, **ii**, 469.

Sixma, J.J. (1987) Platelet adhesion in health and disease. *Thromb. Haemostasis*, **7**, 127–46.

Slater, T.F. (1972) *Free Radical Mechanisms in Tissue Injury*, Pion Ltd, London.

Sneddon, J.M. and Vane, J.R. (1988) Endothelium-derived relaxing factor reduces platelet adhesion to bovine endothelial cells. *Proc. Natl Acad. Sci. USA*, **185**, 2800–4.

Stamatakis, J.D., Kakkar, V.V., Lawrence, D. *et al.* (1978) Failure of aspirin to prevent postoperative deep vein thrombosis in patients undergoing total hip replacement. *Brit. Med. J.*, **1**, 1031.

Steering Committee of the Physicians' Health Study Research Group (1989) Final report on the aspirin component of the ongoing physicians' health study. *N. Engl. J. Med.*, **321**, 129–35.

Streja, D., Steiner, G. and Kwiterovich, P.O. Jr (1978) Plasma high-density lipoproteins and ischaemic heart disease: studies in a large kindred with familial hypercholesterolemia. *Ann. Intern. Med.*, **89**, 871–80.

Stuart, M.J., Miller, M.L., Davey, F.R. and Wolk, J.A. (1979) The post-aspirin bleeding time: a screening test for evaluating hemostatic disorders. *Brit. J. Haematol.*, **43**, 649–59.

Szczeklik, A., Gryglewski, R.J., Nizankowski, R. *et al.* (1978a) Circulatory and anti-platelet effects of intravenous prostacyclin in healthy men. *Pharmacol. Res. Commun.*, **10**, 545–56.

Szczeklik, A., Gryglewski, R., Musial, J. *et al.* (1978b) Thromboxane generation and platelet aggregation in survivals of myocardial infarction. *Thromb. Diath. Haermorrh.*, **40**, 66–74.

Szczeklik, A., Kopec, M. and Slade, K. (1983) Prostacyclin and the fibrinolytic system in ischaemic vascular disease. *Thromb. Res.*, **29**, 655–60.

Tateson, J.E., Moncada, S. and Vane, J.R. (1977) Effects of prostacyclin (PGX) on cyclic AMP concentrations in human platelets. *Prostaglandins*, **13**, 389–97.

Terres, W., Beythien, C., Kupper, W. and Bleifield, W. (1989) Effects of aspirin and prostaglandins on *in vitro* thrombolysis with E_1 urokinase. *Circulation*, **79**, 1309–14.

Pharmacology of aspirin and salicylates

Thorngren, M. and Gustafson, A. (1981) Effects of 11-week increases in dietary eicosapentaenoic acid on bleeding time, lipids and platelet aggregation. *Lancet*, **ii**, 1190–3.

Thorngren, M., Shafi, S. and Born, G.V.R. (1983) Thromboxane A_2 in skin-bleeding-time blood and in clotted venous blood before and after administration of acetylsalicylic acid. *Lancet*, **i**, 1075–8.

Tuvemo, T., Strandberg, K., Hamberg, M. and Samuelsson, B. (1976) Maintenance of the tone of the human umbilical artery by prostaglandin and thromboxane formation. *Adv. Prostaglandin Thromboxane Res.*, **1**, 425–8.

Ubatuba, F.B., Moncada, S. and Vane, J.R. (1979) The effect of prostacyclin (PGI_2) on platelet behaviour, thrombus formation *in vivo* and bleeding time. *Thromb. Haemostasis*, **41**, 425–35.

Udvardy, M., Török, I. and Rak, K. (1987) Plasma thromboxane and prostacyclin metabolite ratio in atherosclerosis and diabetes mellitus. *Thromb. Res.*, **47**, 479–84.

Vane, J. R. (1971) Inhibition of prostaglandins as a mechanism of action for aspirin-like drugs. *Nature (Lond.)*, **231**, 232–5.

Vane, J. (1982) Prostacyclin: a hormone with a therapeutic potential. *J. Endocrinol.*, **95**, 3P–43P.

Venturini, C. M., Del Vecchio, P. J. and Kaplan, J. E. (1989) Thrombin induced platelet adhesion to endothelium is modified by endothelium derived relaxing factor (EDRF). *Biochem. Biophys. Res. Commun.*, **159**, 349–54.

Vilén, L., Johansson, S., Kutti, J. *et al.* (1985) ADP-induced platelet aggregation in young female survivors of acute myocardial infarction and their female controls. *Acta Med. Scand.*, **217**, 9–13.

Von Kaulla, K.N. (1974) Niflumic acid, prototype of a multiaction anti-thrombotic agent. *Experientia*, **30**, 959–61.

Von Schacky, C., Fischer, S. and Weber, P.C. (1985a) Long-term effects of dietary marine ω-3 fatty acids upon plasma and cellular lipids, platelet function and eicosanoid formation in humans. *J. Clin. Invest.*, **76**, 1626–31.

Von Schacky, C., Siess, W., Fischer, S. and Weber, P.C. (1985b) A comparative study of eicosapentaenoic acid metabolism by human platelets *in vivo* and *in vitro*. *J. Lipid Res.*, **26**, 457–64.

Warso, M. A. and Lands, W. E. M. (1983) Lipid peroxidation in relation to prostacyclin and thromboxane physiology and pathophysiology. *Brit. Med. Bull.*, **39**, 277–80.

Weiss, H.J., Turitto, V.T. and Baumgartner, H.R. (1978) Effect of shear rate on platelet interaction with subendothelium in citrated and native blood. I. Shear rate-dependent decrease of adhesion in von Willebrand's disease and the Bernard–Soulier syndrome. *J. Lab. Clin. Med.*, **92**, 750–64.

Weksler, B.B., Marcus, A.J. and Jaffe, E.A. (1977) Synthesis of prostaglandin I_2 (prostacyclin) by cultured human and bovine endothelial cells. *Proc. Natl Acad. Sci. USA*, **74**, 3922–6.

Weksler, B.B., Eldor, A., Falcone, D. *et al.* (1982) Prostaglandins and vascular endothelium. In *Cardiovascular Pharmacology of the Prostaglandins* (eds A.G. Herman, P.M. Vanhoutte, H. Denolin and A. Goossens), Raven Press, New York, pp. 137–48.

Weksler, B.B., Pett, S.B. and Alonso, D. (1983) Differential inhibition by aspirin

290

of vascular and platelet prostaglandin synthesis in atherosclerotic patients. *N. Engl. J. Med.*, **308**, 800–5.

White, D.G. and Martin, W. (1989) Differential control and calcium-dependence of production of endothelium-derived relaxing factor and prostacyclin by pig aortic endothelial cells. *Brit. J. Pharmacol.*, **97**, 683–90.

Willis, A.L., Smith, D.L. and Vigo, C. (1986) Suppression of principal atherosclerotic mechanisms by prostacyclins and other eicosanoids. *Prog. Lipid Res.*, **25**, 645–66.

Willis, A.L., Smith, D.L., Vigo, C. and Kluge, A.F. (1987) Effects of prostacyclin and orally active stable mimetic agent RS-93427–007 on basic mechanisms of atherogenesis. *Lancet*, **ii**, 682–3.

Yoshimoto, T., Yamamoto, S., Okuma. M. and Hayaishi, O. (1977) Solubilization and resolution of thromboxane synthesizing system from microsomes of bovine blood platelets. *J. Biol. Chem.*, **252**, 5871–4.

PART FOUR
Therapeutic applications

11 Use of aspirin in inflammatory diseases

J.M.C. AXON and E.C. HUSKISSON

11.1 INTRODUCTION

Aspirin was for decades the unchallenged first-line treatment for rheumatoid arthritis (RA) and many other inflammatory arthropathies. That it no longer occupies this exalted position is due not to a lack of efficacy, but to the side effects which particularly limit the use of larger doses needed to achieve an anti-inflammatory effect; also to the availability of other drugs with better side effect profiles. Aspirin, combining analgesic, anti-inflammatory and antipyretic actions, is still a useful agent in many clinical situations varying from influenza to Still's Disease. Its price advantage over newer alternatives ensures that it is still held as an anti-inflammatory in poorer countries; newer formulations have increased its acceptability but raised the cost. It has obvious advantages as an analgesic and antipyretic in many rheumatic diseases.

11.2 ANALGESIC ACTION OF ASPIRIN IN ARTHRITIS

It is conventional to supplement regular anti-inflammatory drug therapy for RA with single doses of simple analgesics and aspirin remains a satisfactory agent for this purpose. Huskisson (1974) found that patients tended to obtain their own analgesics without prescription if they were not provided. Huskisson and Hart (1972a) found that patients with RA took an average of 9.2 tablets daily of which 4.2 were simple analgesics taken 'on demand'. The number of tablets taken were related to pain threshold and disease severity.

At the same time, Lee et al. (1974a) looked at the prescribing habits in the Glasgow area, and their results help to explain the discrepancy of why patients buy alternative 'over-the-counter' medication. They looked at 125 patients referred by 75 general practitioners. These all had RA as defined by the criteria of the American Rheumatism Association as written by Ropes *et al.* (1958). Each patient was questioned about the first drug prescribed for his arthritis. The findings were as follows: only 47 of the patients had received salicylates as the first drug and 18 had never had them at all. Sixty-three patients were prescribed soluble aspirin which was the most frequent. Only 60 had been given an adequate dose and only 62 an adequate course of treatment with salicylates. In 28 patients, salicylates had been stopped on account of side effects. About one-third of the patients had been prescribed oral corticosteroids. Regional differences in prescribing are well known, as noted by Dunlop and Inch (1972), but why salicylates were not prescribed more, when at the time they were clearly the drug of first choice, remains a mystery. The fact that a high percentage of patients in this study were treated with corticosteroids is also surprising, particularly in some cases, before a non-steroidal had been prescribed and against the then current recommendations.

Huskisson and Hart (1972b) drew attention to the fact that pain threshold variations led to more or less tablets being taken. They looked at 106 patients with RA, 50 with ankylosing spondylitis, and 50 normal controls. Pain threshold was measured by a slightly modified Keele's method (1954) at the same time of day and by the same observer. They concluded that there was no evidence that pain threshold affected the course of the disease, and that patients with higher pain thresholds showed no tendency to greater disability, more severe radiographical changes or involvement of weight-bearing joints. The pain threshold remained remarkably constant despite in-patient treatment and relapses of the disease. There were striking differences found between patients with RA and those with ankylosing spondylitis (AS) which were not explicable either by the younger age or male sex of the patients with AS. The higher pain threshold in AS may be due to a different attitude transmitted by the physician to the patient with this disease. The overall conclusion was that measures to raise pain threshold can safely form part of the treatment of the disease, and patients should be encouraged to live life to the full. However, pain threshold is clearly unaffected by analgesics.

There have been relatively few comparisons of the efficacy of different analgesics in arthritis, although there are many comparative studies of different anti-inflammatory agents. Huskisson (1974) described a method for making such comparisons and reported three experiments: the first comparing analgesic tablets, the second soluble analgesics in different colours, and the third a new analgesic with a standard and placebo. The trials were designed to take advantage of the consistent polyad method described by Kendal (1963). This method of testing simple analgesics in RA proved to be satisfactory when pain relief scores were used to measure effectiveness. Preference was a less satisfactory method.

Placebo is, of course, strikingly efficacious in arthritis as in other conditions. There was a striking difference between the efficacy of different coloured placebos, red proving to be the most effective. Placebo was more effective when given after an active analgesic than when given before. Single doses of aspirin, codeine and dextropropoxyphene with paracetamol were equally effective when given in single doses in RA. Pentazocine, paracetamol and the new analgesic were intermediate in effectiveness between these agents and placebo.

Huskisson concluded that aspirin and dextropropoxyphene with paracetamol were the first choices for effectiveness, with dextropropoxyphene with paracetamol having a slight advantage due to fewer side effects. Oral pentazocine could not be recommended because of its side effects. Lack of toxicity is a particularly important feature in view of the rather modest effects of these drugs. They produce only slight to moderate pain relief, whereas placebo is not much less effective. Brooks et al. (1982) followed up this study by comparing five analgesics in 12 patients with osteo-arthritis (OA) and 12 with RA. The drugs were dextropropoxyphene, aspirin, dextropropoxyphene and paracetamol, paracetamol, dextropropoxyphene and aspirin, and placebo. No significant difference was found between the analgesics used. They concluded that cost is a major determinant of use, with dextropropoxyphene and its combinations being more expensive than aspirin or paracetamol alone. They also concluded that no ideal interval analgesic has yet been found with regard to pain relief and lack of side effects for each individual patient.

Finally, Dieppe and Huskisson (1978), have shown that the newer drug diflunisal (discussed in greater detail below) at a dose of 500–700 mg a day is more effective than aspirin 2–3 g in the treatment of osteoarthritic pain. The studies performed have been in a double-blind fashion with various physical and laboratory parameters being measured. They concluded that although aspirin is the cheapest analgesic available in osteoarthritis, diflunisal offers advantages in being more potent and somewhat safer than aspirin for the gastrointestinal tract. Its analgesic effect is longer than that of aspirin and lasts for at least 8 h and up to 12 h. It is well absorbed after oral administration, with peak concentrations at about 2 h.

11.3   ANTI-INFLAMMATORY ACTION IN ARTHRITIS

11.3.1   Introduction

The role of aspirin and the salicylates has changed considerably over the last 30 years. Initially, aspirin trials in the 1960s were used to study the anti-inflammatory and analgesic effect in rheumatic conditions. In particular, it was compared to prednisolone and some of the early non-steroidal anti-inflammatories (NSAIDs), and formed the backbone of management in inflammatory conditions. With the many new NSAIDs produced in the 1970s, it became an important standard in the comparative trials. It had a known anti-inflammatory effectiveness with recognized side effects.

In association with these new trials came a realization of a need to measure inflammation by a standard test. Hence aspirin was used to compare various procedures in the hope of finding a simple, quick and cheap method of assessing inflammatory conditions in the clinic.

11.3.2   Methods of Measuring Inflammation

Before discussing the early and important trials of aspirin, a short review of the various methods used will be made. Patients with rheumatoid arthritis have a combination of pain and inflammation. Assessments fall into three groups: objective, subjective and mixed (Hart and Huskisson, 1972). As far back as 1959, Beecher saw the need for the 'properly controlled, quantitative approach' that was needed to evaluate the reversible features of the disease.

In general, the design of clinical therapeutic trials of anti-rheumatic drugs is the short term, double-blind cross over method, with the new drug being tested against an established medication and/or placebo. This was the method used by Deodhar *et al.* in 1973 which will be discussed later. Other objective and semi-objective parameters are also used including digital joint circumference measurement (Boardman and Hart, 1967; Webb *et al.*, 1973), grip strength (Lee *et al.*, 1974a), and radioisotope joint uptake (Dick *et al.*, 1970a, b, 1971; Dick, 1972) with a comparison to clinical methods (Dick *et al.*, 1970b). These tests were found to be relatively insensitive when compared to patients' pain response and an articular index of joint tenderness (Ritchie *et al.*, 1968) and composite indices (Lansbury, 1958, 1968).

The need for faster methods to speed up the clinical therapeutic trial led to the use of the patients' subjective evaluation of pain relief and drug effectiveness as a means of testing and comparing the therapeutic efficacy of new and established anti-rheumatic agents (Lee *et al.*, 1973a, b, 1976). The majority of these methods have been reviewed by Lee *et al.* (1973a, b).

More recent studies have used patient compliance as a measure of efficacy of NSAIDs in the treatment of arthritic conditions. A drug which does not adequately relieve pain or which produces intolerable side effects will be quickly discarded by patients (Capell *et al.*, 1979).

11.3.3 History of Aspirin's Anti-inflammatory Action

Aspirin has been known for many years to have analgesic, anti-inflammatory and antipyretic effects. The evidence for these actions is based largely on clinical studies in acute rheumatic fever. Surprisingly, it was not until 1965 that an anti-inflammatory action was demonstrated in rheumatoid arthritis by Fremont-Smith and Bayles.

There had been earlier studies comparing aspirin to cortisone (MRC and Nuffield Foundation, 1954a) and the use of cortisone as an adjuvant to manipulation compared with tablets of aspirin, codeine and phenacetin (MRC and Nuffield Foundation, 1954b). Neither of these studies showed any striking advantage of cortisone over salicylate medication. They were controlled and measured joint tenderness, range of movement and grip strength, tests of dexterity, haemoglobin level, erythrocyte sedimentation rate (ESR) and overall clinical assessments. These patients were followed initially for 1 year, but were kept on for a longer trial over 4 years (MRC and Nuffield Foundation, 1957). Patients were assessed on a well being scale as well as by haemoglobin and ESR. Therefore, no accurate assessment of inflammation was carried out and the conclusions after 4 years were firstly that the introduction of cortisone had not affected the prognosis in early rheumatoid arthritis and secondly that there was little difference between the therapeutic effect of aspirin and cortisone. The Empire Rheumatism Council in 1955 also studied the effect of aspirin and cortisone over 1 year in 100 patients. Clinical improvement and radiological deterioration were monitored and similar conclusions to the above trials of no significant difference were found

So, although there was plenty of clinical as well as laboratory experience (Dixon *et al.*, 1963) of the anti-inflammatory effect of salicylates, no one had performed a controlled trial using set dosage and answered the question: do salicylates have a clinically significant anti-inflammatory effect in the treatment of rheumatoid arthritis?

Fremont-Smith and Bayles (1965), in one of the most important clinical trials in rheumatoid arthritis, demonstrated the importance of the anti-inflammatory action of aspirin in relieving pain. When aspirin was withdrawn, it was impossible to achieve adequate pain relief, even with narcotic analgesics. These authors studied 12 patients (11 rheumatoid arthritis, 1 systemic lupus erythematosus (SLE)) with early active arthritis using acetylsalicylic acid (ASA), a buffered preparation. The dose was increased until the largest tolerated dose was reached. The final dose ranged from 3.6 to 7.5 g per 24 h with an average of 5.2 g. The trial was not blinded due to the typical side effects of aspirin at this dose level, namely tinnitus, deafness, perspiration and nausea. The patients were studied in a metabolic ward so compliance was assumed. The variables of rest, activity and physiotherapy were kept constant initially but over a week proved impossible. Disease activity was measured by finger-joint size (jeweller's rings), range of joint motion (goniometer), grip strength (sphygmomanometer cuff), finger volume (water displacement), and serial comparative photographs (Polaroid) of selected involved joints. They found that aspirin reduced objective measures of inflammation although there were no statistics. Patients that had their aspirin stopped rebounded after 48 h, as documented by an increasing ring size of every proximal interphalangeal joint, despite adequate analgesia in the form of meperidine hydrochloride. They concluded that intensive administration of ASA led to a clinically significant anti-inflammatory effect and recommended that patients with active RA should receive salicylates regularly in the largest tolerated dose.

A larger study in the same year by Mainland and Sutcliffe used 499 patients in a double-blind parallel group trial. They demonstrated a significant difference in the number of swollen joints, grip strength and walking time but not in duration of morning stiffness between placebo and aspirin 3.9 g daily. There were 51 dropouts and patients continued to use other medications during the 7 day periods. This experience, however, allowed the Co-operating Clinics Committee of the American Rheumatism Association (1965) to draw up reference tables for the use of other workers to help classify patients according to the degree of severity of the signs and symptoms of disease activity.

To achieve an anti-inflammatory action in rheumatoid arthritis, aspirin must be given in large doses. This important phenomenon was elegantly demonstrated by Boardman and Hart in 1967. Their aim was to establish a quantitative method for measuring joint size by a technique based on the use of a standard jeweller's ring under double-blind controlled conditions, and to differentiate reduction in swelling, an index of anti-inflammatory activity, from pain relief or analgesic effect with various doses of salicylates. They made four experiments, comparing a known anti-inflammatory agent in the form of prednisolone 7.5 mg daily and placebo, a known analgesic, paracetamol 6 g daily and placebo, high dose salicylate in its glycinated form at

5.3 g and low dose salicylate 2.6 g, and in the fourth arm of the trial, low dose salicylate and placebo. There were between 13 and 18 patients in each trial with 1 week on the drug and 2 weeks free.

As well as joint size, grip strength was also measured by one observer, with a tablet count but no plasma salicylate levels measured. The results showed a significant difference of prednisolone over placebo, high dose salicylate over low dose salicylate and low dose salicylate over placebo. Side effects were not a problem in the trial. They concluded that joint size, when measured serially, was a good index of specific anti-inflammatory effect, and reduction in this measure was achieved by high doses of salicylate but not by low doses. Patients on the high dose showed an improvement in 48 h, but the rate of response was not clear as it was a 7 day trial.

The initial trials were short, and barely more than 1 week. Calabro and Paulus in 1970 designed a double-blind crossover experiment involving two drugs and a placebo. Eighteen RA patients were followed up over a period of 30 weeks. The patients took either 5.9 g of buffered aspirin, salicylamide or placebo for 8 weeks. In the interval, they took only 2–6 g of aspirin.

By using the Lansbury systemic index, five criteria were evaluated: duration of morning stiffness, time of onset of fatigue, aspirin need, grip strength, and ESR. Using Lansbury's tables (1958), the findings were converted to a percentage difference. The results showed a therapeutic improvement in 14 (78%) of 18 patients while receiving aspirin, 4 (22%) while receiving salicylamide, and 2 (11%) while on placebo. On finishing 5.9 g of aspirin daily, 14 relapsed within 48 h despite maintenance on 2.6 g. Ototoxicity occurred in 10 out of the 18 patients without undue distress. However, these side effects revealed to the doctors and some of the 10 patients, which ones were on aspirin.

They concluded that the anti-inflammatory action of aspirin is dependent upon the largest tolerated or subtinnitus doses. They confirmed the exacerbation of symptoms on withdrawal of high dose aspirin. Although this was not new, they observed that patients with advanced disease had a more favourable response to aspirin and not to analgesic or placebo. Also, those patients with a high Latex fixation titre of 1:2560 or greater failed to respond to any drug. They also found that a reduction in ESR as objective evidence of the efficacy of aspirin depended on a properly individualized dosage. By the early 1970s, it became clear that the anti-inflammatory effects of salicylates were not particularly dramatic, especially in their ability to relieve pain and reduce swelling in chronic inflammatory joint disease. Therefore in 1973, Deodhar *et al.* set up a double-blind, crossover clinical trial to assess the relative merits of different assessment methods, and to document the response of patients to a week's course of sodium salicylate 1 g qds, indomethacin 25 mg qds, ibuprofen 400 mg tds and prednisolone 2.5 mg qds. The same doctor assessed the patient at the end of each week.

The assessments included a pain index (Jasani et al., 1968), articular index (Ritchie et al., 1968), grip strength (MRC and Nuffield Foundation, 1954a; Co-operating Clinics Committee of ARA, 1965), digital joint circumference (Boardman and Hart, 1967; Webb et al., 1973), and ^{99m}Tc knee joint uptake (Dick et al., 1970a, 1971; Dick, 1972). The results showed that all four active drugs produced a response measurably better than placebo, but comparison between the four active drugs showed no conclusive evidence that any one drug was superior to the other three active drugs. Out of the assessment methods, patients' pain score and articular index proved the best. The ^{99m}Tc knee joint uptakes gave similar results to the clinical scores of knee joint inflammation with clear differences between active and placebo drugs. Grip strength was helpful but less sensitive, and digital joint circumference was not discriminating.

Of particular interest in this study was the finding that acetylsalicylic acid produces more pain relief than sodium salicylate. There was no particular reason for this as sodium salicylate has been found to be an effective anti-rheumatic agent (Dick et al., 1969).

The good points with regard to this study were the one physician observer reducing assessment variation. The trial was also an in-patient study so compliance was recorded and the extraneous factors such as daily rest and activity were better controlled. However, hospital care has a beneficial influence on RA so that the in-patient improvement may not indicate future progress as out-patients. Also, some of the patients had been on steroids or cryotherapy which may alter the results.

However, the main conclusion of the study was that no single assessment method can be relied on to measure the change in severity of the disease. The opinion of the patient was mirrored best by the articular index of joint tenderness and the pain score.

In 1974, Multz et al. used a dose of 3.6 g of aspirin to evaluate the duration of placebo substitution required to elicit a relapse in patients with active RA on aspirin. Thirty-three patients with classical or definite RA (Ropes et al., 1958) not on steroids, were given placebo for up to 1 week before changing to aspirin. Lansbury indices were calculated (Lansbury, 1958) and were found to provide a sensitive indicator between drug and placebo.

Overall, 3 days of placebo exposure were required to produce an exacerbation, and when transferred to aspirin a further 3 days to reduce inflammation. The conclusions were important in that they showed short-term placebo administration can provide adequate negative control without prolonged placebo administration. Secondly, aspirin in an intermediate dose of 3.6 g day^{-1} has anti-inflammatory activity which is clinically useful. In previous studies, doses of 5.2 g day^{-1} (average) given by Fremont-Smith and Bayles (1965), 5.3 g day^{-1} (Boardman and Hart, 1967), and 5.9 g day^{-1} (Calabro and Paulus, 1970) were clearly too high and gave rise to unacceptable side effects.

11.3.4 Conclusion

In conclusion, there are many studies reported that show an anti-inflammatory effect of aspirin and the salicylates. However, there is still great debate on the actual long-term effect on the disease process. Most of the problems lie in the procedures that are used to measure the efficacy of drug treatment. They are either subjective such as pain or morning stiffness, or they are semi-objective by measuring articular index and grip strength. They give a good indication of the progress of the disease and response to drugs, but little about the pathogenesis of the condition in the joints or systemic effect. Measuring ESR and acute-phase proteins seem to reflect a secondary change rather than changes fundamental to the disease progress (Wright and Amos, 1980) so they tend to be considered as important indicators. Thermography and uptake of radioisotopes from the circulation give a measure of the signs of joint inflammation. The value of radiological examination depends on interpretation and can be very variable. Therefore a combination of clinical, laboratory and radiological assessments provides the most reliable view of disease progression. This makes comparison of salicylate effectiveness with other drugs very difficult.

Boyle and Buchanan, (1971) concluded that, although aspirin has an anti-inflammatory effect, there is little evidence to show that it influences the downhill course of patients with severe RA. There is more evidence with regard to second-line agents, with corticosteroids producing symptomatic relief and a lower ESR (Wright and Amos, 1980). The role of aspirin and other salicylates must remain an important first time treatment with its influence on progression on rheumatoid disease still open to question depending on a multifactorial analysis of therapeutic responses (Rainsford, 1984).

11.4 ANTIPYRETIC ACTIVITY OF ASPIRIN IN ARTHRITIS

There is very little doubt about the efficacy of the salicylates (ie aspirin, benorylate, diflunisal, salicylate and its derivatives) in clinical states of fever and those induced experimentally. Seed (1965) showed that aspirin is 1–5 times more potent than sodium salicylate in treating the fevers from cancer and low-grade episodes from chronic infections. Aspirin remains the drug of choice in juvenile arthritis complicated by fever and newer non-steroidals have been found to be less effective as antipyretics.

Claims have been made that paracetamol is as effective an antipyretic as aspirin and that the former drug is the safer of the two for children (Jaffe, 1981). However, the toxicity of paracetamol to the liver and kidneys in the underdeveloped state of metabolic detoxification mechanisms in early childhood leaves its safety in question.

11.5 OTHER INDICATIONS FOR USE

The use of aspirin as an anti-inflammatory drug in RA and as an analgesic in osteo-arthritis (OA) have already been discussed in depth. Aspirin is also frequently used in juvenile arthritis, sero-negative arthropathies and most soft tissue lesions. At very high doses, it may be of help in the treatment of acute gout and severe ankylosing spondylitis, but modern drugs have take over the role of salicylates.

11.5.1 Gout

Aspirin or salicylates at doses greater than 3.5 g daily induce uricosuria and hence are considered potentially beneficial in the treatment of gout. Long-term salicylate therapy, however, compares unfavourably with other ways of controlling uric acid levels, mainly because of side effects and the large number of tablets required. At low doses, urate retention is induced by salicylates which are therefore contra-indicated in gout. Salicylates in low doses also antagonize the actions of some of the uricosuric drugs.

Diflunisal in a dose of 250–375 mg daily has been shown to increase uric acid excretion. It has also been shown to antagonize urate retention as seen in thiazide diuretic therapy. The mechanism is uncertain, but the fact that lower doses are required together with the advantage of reduced gastrointestinal irritation suggests a possible role in the treatment of gout.

11.5.2 Juvenile Rheumatoid Arthritis

The role of aspirin has decreased in recent years with the introduction of newer non-steroidal drugs. However, benorylate has recently been used in the treatment as the younger patient prefers the liquid formulation.

The gastric irritant effect is also less than that of aspirin. Ansell (1986) states that aspirin should be reserved for those children who have failed to respond to simple non-steroidals and for those with systemic onset disease. She states that it must be given in a dose of 80–100 mg kg^{-1} over a 24 h period. The liver function tests should be monitored, especially as the systemic form leaves children more vulnerable to aspirin-related dysfunction. Calabro (1983) states that aspirin should always be tried first. He also says that a maximum dose of 130 mg kg^{-1} is indicated in young patients with high spiking fever. Serum levels of salicylates should also be monitored for hepatotoxicity and overdosage.

The possibility of Reye's syndrome should also be considered even though it is extremely rare. Patients should be told to stop aspirin in the event of a viral epidemic, such as influenza or chicken pox. If the child starts to vomit or have a gastric upset, they should be seen straight away to determine the salicylate level and liver function tests.

The hypermobility syndrome is a condition more commonly present than recognized. Symptoms in children seem to occur at night with aspirin providing the best therapy, particularly enteric coated aspirin.

11.5.3 Systemic Lupus Erythematosus (SLE)

Aspirin has been shown to be highly effective in alleviating the manifestations of SLE, such as inflammation, fever and serositis. Results have shown a considerable improvement but this must be weighed against the frequent hepato-nephrotoxic manifestations of aspirin toxicity in this condition (Hughes, 1979).

11.5.4 Rheumatic Fever

This condition is now rare in the UK. However, aspirin is still the preferred drug and starting doses in children and adolescents are about 60 mg kg^{-1} divided into four daily doses. If the symptoms are not suppressed, the dose can be increased to about 180 mg kg^{-1} daily. This is often adequate, but a small number of cases require corticosteroids after the fourth day if there are no signs of remission.

11.5.5 Ankylosing Spondylitis

In rheumatoid arthritis and osteo-arthritis most non-steroidal anti-inflammatory drugs including aspirin are more or less equally efficacious and hundreds of clinical trials demonstrate equivalence of one compound to another. While indomethacin is therefore as effective as aspirin in rheumatoid and osteo-arthritis, it is clearly more effective in ankylosing spondylitis (Godfrey and *et al.*, 1972) and the same is probably true of phenylbutazone. These two drugs have been particularly favoured in the treatment of ankylosing spondylitis which is one of the few indications in which aspirin has little place.

11.6 FORMULATION AND ASPIRIN

Aspirin is the oldest and cheapest non-steroidal anti-inflammatory drug. In low doses (300–600 mg), it is an effective analgesic and remains the drug of choice for many sorts of pain. However, in up to 50% of patients taking the higher anti-inflammatory dose in rheumatoid arthritis (3.6–4.2 g day^{-1}), the side effects of dyspepsia (nausea, vomiting and epigastric pain), tinnitus, and occult blood loss cannot be tolerated (Nuki, 1983).

These side effects of aspirin led manufacturers to produce a range of products that are all similar in the manner in which they are metabolized and eliminated but differ in their rates of disintegration, dissolution and absorption, and the site of their absorption (Dromgoole *et al.*, 1981).

11.6.1 Acetylsalicylic Acid (Aspirin)

(a) LIQUID PREPARATIONS

These are infrequently used due to their instability in solution. They hydrolyse to acetate and salicylate within days (Morgan and Truitt, 1956). A solution can be obtained by dissolving soluble and buffered tablets which will remain stable if used within a short time.

(b) PLAIN TABLETS

These tablets are ingested and disintegrate in the stomach. Plain aspirin tablets are only slightly soluble (1 in 300 in water) and have no buffering capacity. They are easy to take, but cause gastric mucosal injury. Formulation and particle size have been varied to aid absorption and reduce blood loss. Microfined aspirin is absorbed more rapidly than products with coarser particles (Levy *et al.*, 1967). However, there are conflicting data on gastric bleeding. Coarser particles may be associated with an increase (Gyory and Stiel 1968), while other studies (Leonards and Levy, 1967) have found no statistical difference. The aspirin content of standard tablets is usually 300 or 325 mg.

(c) BUFFERED TABLETS

These preparations have been developed to reduce the likelihood of gastric injury which is caused partly by the initial damage to the lining of the gastric mucosa. The 'buffered' tablets contain insoluble calcium and magnesium antacids. These raise the pH locally which enhances solubility, and hence increases absorption. However, when plain and buffered aspirin tablets, as well as solutions of acetylsalicylic acid and sodium acetylsalicylate were measured after administration, the solutions were absorbed more rapidly than buffered aspirin. The plain aspirin was the slowest (Leonards, 1963).

Effervescent buffered aspirin (e.g. Alka-seltzer) containing sodium bicarbonate is available but is undesirable for long-term therapy because of the amount of sodium and bicarbonate and the increase in urinary pH leading to increased excretion of salicylic acid. Aspirin combined with glycine (e.g. Paynocil) does not have these undesirable effects (Anon., 1978).

(d) ENTERIC COATED TABLETS

This form of tablet was designed to bypass gastric fluids and dissolve rapidly in the small intestine and therefore avoid bleeding from the less resistant gastric mucosa. The ideal product resists disintegration at acid pH, disintegrates rapidly at the approximately neutral pH of the small intestine, is completely bioavailable in terms of total salicylate, and achieves significant plasma acetylsalicylic acid concentrations (Champion et al., 1975). However, there are various factors that affect absorption and plasma levels. These include the disintegration characteristics of the tablet, differences in the rate of gastric emptying in humans, food in the stomach, and drugs such as metoclopramide (Dromgoole et al., 1981). The enteric coated tablets have, however, been found to have significantly lower peak plasma salicylate concentration than following aspirin solution (Leonards and Levy, 1965). During chronic usage, these differences are small, but it is recommended that occasional serum salicylate levels are measured. Twice daily dosage has been shown to be well tolerated and will produce the best therapeutic levels without gastrointestinal bleeding (Benson et al., 1976).

(e) TIMED-RELEASE TABLETS

In these tablets, aspirin particles are microencapsulated in matrices of wax, resins, plastics, or polymers giving different rates of disintegration. This allows a delayed absorption with a flatter salicylate

307

level-time curve and will reduce the peak plasma salicylate after one dose. This does not help when aspirin is used in high doses, although there may well be a reduction in gastrointestinal bleeding (Frenkel *et al.*, 1968).

(f) SOLUBLE TABLETS

These are a combination of aspirin, calcium carbonate and citric acid and are taken dissolved in water. The soluble preparation is more rapidly absorbed than standard aspirin and produces half as much occult bleeding (Leonards and Levy, 1969). However, these minor differences in occult bleeding are not usually of clinical significance; and there is no correlation between occult bleeding and gastric side effects.

(g) SUPPOSITORIES

The rectal route has been used to avoid gastrointestinal irritation. However, there is a longer absorption half-life of 3 h compared to 15–30 mins by the oral route. This leads to subtherapeutic levels dependent on the retention time (time between insertion and first defaecation). Maximum absorption occurs after 10 h retention, whereas 2 h gives 20–40% absorption (Gibaldi and Grundhofer, 1975). Generally, the bioavailability of salicylates from suppositories is less than that of oral salicylate preparations, and close monitoring is required to control the amount of drug available.

(h) TABLETS AND CAPSULES

Combinations with other drugs, such as paracetamol, codeine and caffeine, are not recommended for anti-inflammatory use due to the toxic effects of the other drugs.

(i) ALUMINIUM–ASPIRIN COMPOUNDS

Aloxiprin contains 500 mg aspirin in a 600 mg tablet. The rest is made up of a polymeric condensation of aluminium oxide. Liberation of aspirin by hydrolysis is slow in the stomach, but rapid in the small intestine at a higher pH. Faecal occult blood loss is less than with aspirin (Wood *et al.*, 1962).

11.6.2   Other Salicylates

(a) SODIUM SALICYLATE

This salt is soluble in water (1 in 1 of water) and more rapidly absorbed from solution than aspirin. It lacks the acetyl ester radical making it a less potent analgesic and reducing its granulocyte and platelet anti-adhesiveness (Weiss et al., 1968). The sodium content may cause cardiac failure in certain patients, but it is an effective anti-inflammatory in rheumatoid arthritis and induces less gastric bleeding than aspirin (Leonards and Levy, 1973).

(b) MAGNESIUM SALICYLATE

The long-term treatment of rheumatic diseases is contra-indicated due to the possibility of hypermagnesaemia. It would also not be recommended in those with renal failure.

(c) CHOLINE SALICYLATE

This salt has several potential advantages, although it is not used widely. It consists of a relatively benign cation and salicylic acid. It is absorbed rapidly (peak 10 min) with minimal gastric bleeding (Pierson et al., 1961). It is well tolerated and was initially marketed as a liquid. It is claimed to be effective for the treatment of rheumatic diseases (Scully, 1961).

11.6.3   Newer Salicylates

(a) CHOLINE MAGNESIUM TRISALICYLATE (TRILISATE)

Choline salicylate (293 mg) has been combined with magnesium salicylate (362 mg) to provide 500 mg of salicylate and overcome the hygroscopic nature of choline salicylate. This is therefore a non-acetylated salicylate moiety with a long plasma half-life allowing twice daily dosage. When compared with plain aspirin, 975 mg qds and buffered aspirin, 975 mg qds, similar levels of serum salicylate were achieved when 1.5 g were given twice daily (Binus et al., 1982). Gastrointestinal side effects are considerably reduced when compared with aspirin (Sun and Sun, 1971) and the incidence is comparable to that associated with ibuprofen therapy. The risk of tinnitus and deafness with high doses remains. Nevertheless, choline magnesium trisalicylate

309

overcomes many of the disadvantages of plain or soluble aspirin (the number of tablets required and gastric irritation), although in common with other modern anti-inflammatories, it is very expensive.

(b) SALICYLSALICYLIC ACID (SALSALATE)

Salsalate is almost insoluble in the acid pH of the stomach, but soluble in the near neutral pH of the small intestine. After absorption, salsalate is slowly hydrolysed to two molecules of free salicylic acid; 500 mg of salicylsalicylic acid are equivalent to 698 mg of acetylsalicylic acid in salicylic acid content. It has been shown to produce satisfactory blood salicylate levels (Mielants et al., 1981). There are also claims that it causes less gastric bleeding than aspirin (Leonards, 1969), as it is largely absorbed from the small intestine (Aberg and Larsson, 1970). There is significant anti-rheumatic activity when used with aspirin (Denson and Thompson, 1960; Paris and Newfield, 1963) and also when used alone (Deodhar et al., 1977), so that it may prove superior to aspirin in the long-term treatment of rheumatoid arthritis.

(c) BENORYLATE

This is the paracetamol ester of aspirin (Robertson, 1973). After absorption, it is hydrolysed to release both drugs. Four grams of benorylate is equivalent to 2.4 g of aspirin so a 4 g twice daily dosage is effective in adults and around 200 mg kg^{-1} bodyweight per day given morning and evening is usually needed in children (Ansell, 1982). A 2g dose of benorylate has been shown to have potent anti-inflammatory activity (Rosner et al., 1973). The relative freedom from gastric mucosal bleeding (Croft et al., 1972) may be due to its neutral formulation unique among aspirin compounds, with hydrolysis occurring after absorption. However, it is by no means free of gastric irritant effect (Bain and Burt, 1970; Sperryn et al., 1973). Its efficacy has been established (Beales et al., 1972; Franke and Manz, 1972), and hence is a useful addition to the available drugs for the treatment of rheumatic diseases. The twice daily administration of the liquid form is a great advantage for children going to school. It is also available in tablet form.

(d) DIFLUNISAL

Diflunisal is a derivative of aspirin, differing chemically in having an extra ring with two fluorine atoms added, the acetyl group having been removed (Hannah et al., 1977). In contrast to other salicylic acid derivatives, diflunisal is not metabolized to salicylic acid but is excreted in the urine unchanged (Brogden *et al.*, 1980). It has four advantages over conventional aspirin. The simple analgesic action is prolonged, lasting up to 12 h. It can be given twice daily because of its longer plasma half-life. It is more effective than aspirin. It causes fewer side effects than aspirin and does not cause metabolic acidosis in overdosage. Tinnitus and deafness are not a problem either. It is well tolerated in human subjects (Tempero *et al.*, 1977) and causes less gastric irritation than aspirin (Andrew *et al.*, 1977). Its main use is as a long acting analgesic as opposed to a powerful anti-inflammatory agent. It has some value in the treatment of osteo-arthritis (Andrew *et al.*, 1972), chronic low backache (Hickey, 1982), and has an allopurinol-like action (Ambacelli and Fenaccioli, 1982).

11.7 ACETYLSALICYLATE OR SALICYLATE

For much of the century acetylsalicylic acid, ASA or aspirin, has been preferred to sodium salicylate on historical and theoretical grounds. Ferreira and Vane (1974) had shown acetylsalicylate to be superior to salicylate as an analgesic and anti-inflammatory in animal models.

However, with the more recent introduction of non-acetyl group salicylic acid formulations, the role of ASA as the major drug has been doubted. The first trial to be described was by Blechman and Lechner (1979) comparing choline magnesium trisalicylate (CMT) with ASA. One hundred and thirty-one patients were entered into the multicentre double-blind trial over 7 weeks. The results showed that both were highly effective in reducing the severity of the symptoms of RA, with CMT achieving the greater reduction in the number of swollen joints than ASA. The incidence of adverse side effects per patient was significantly less with CMT (ASA, 32.1%, CMT, 16.3%). A larger percentage of ASA patients (50.8%) reported adverse side effects than did CMT patients (28.4%). With the twice daily dosage of CMT as well, this may well prove more desirable for patients.

These results have been repeated by Giuliano and Scharff (1980) on 40 patients with a maximal daily dosage of salicylates of 3000 mg while on gold therapy. Rothwell (1983) reviewed the above trials plus an endoscopic trial by Kilander and Dotevall (1983) and concluded that CMT in an equivalent dose was as or more effective than ASA in the treatment of rheumatoid arthritis. He went on to comment that the acetyl radical did not confer efficacy to salicylate in the treatment of the disease.

Salsalate, in a more recent trial by April *et al.* (1987), has been compared with aspirin in 233 patients with rheumatoid arthritis over 12 weeks. The median dose of salsalate was 3 g daily and aspirin 3.6 g daily. The results showed that both were equally as effective, but there was a higher incidence of serious gastrointestinal effects in the aspirin patients.

Brogden *et al.* reviewed the literature on diflunisal, a difluorophenyl derivative of salicylic acid, and concluded that it is a more potent analgesic, anti-inflammatory agent and antipyretic than aspirin. This has been supported by comparative studies on diflunisal and aspirin. De Silva *et al.* (1980) showed it to be as effective an anti-inflammatory as aspirin in a dose of 500 mg twice daily. Side effects were minor and responded well to reduction of dosage and disappeared on withdrawal of the drug.

Benorylate has also proved a useful addition to the non-acetylated group. Bain and Burt (1970) used a low dose of 4 g versus 2.4 g of aspirin daily, and increased this to 6 g and 3.6 g respectively. This preliminary evaluation showed benorylate to be well tolerated and suggested that it is as effective as aspirin. Sasisekhar *et al.* (1973) used a dose of 8 g daily in a double-blind double-dummy cross-over comparison versus 4.8 g of aspirin. Both preparations were found to be equipotent, causing significant decrease in pain score and morning stiffness. Interestingly, higher salicylate levels were found during aspirin therapy leading to a higher incidence of salicylism while on aspirin.

The supremacy of acetylsalicylic acid, as has been mentioned, was not challenged till the early 1970s. Calabro and Paulus (1970), in a study of 18 RA patients, concluded that aspirin was the superior analgesic and anti-inflammatory agent compared to non-acetylated compounds. Deodhar *et al.* (1973), however, showed sodium salicylate, in clinical therapeutic trials in RA, to be equally efficacious to indomethacin 100 mg daily, ibuprofen 1200 mg daily and prednisolone 10 mg daily. The first study to compare aspirin with sodium salicylate in RA was not until Preston *et al.*'s (1989) trial in 18 patients over 2 weeks. The results showed that 4.8 g daily of sodium salicylate was equipotent to the same dose of aspirin in pain relief, reduction in articular index of joint tenderness, increase in grip strength, decrease in digital joint circumference and patients' assessment. Preston *et al.* strongly concluded that non-acetylated salicylates should be prescribed in preference to acetylated salicylates. This is based on reduced gastrointestinal mucosal damage, and reduced hypersensitivity reactions to sodium salicylate.

11.8 ASPIRIN, SALICYLATE AND THEIR ESTERS COMPARED WITH ACIDIC NSAIDS

Aspirin has been used as a standard in many clinical trials where the efficacy of new NSAIDs has been analysed. These new propionic acid derivatives have challenged and now succeed aspirin's proud place in the anti-inflammatory hierarchy. The side effects are seldom serious and seldom lead to withdrawal of treatment. Huskisson *et al.* (1976) compared four propionic acid derivatives and showed the striking individual variation in response which occurs with drugs of this type. More recently, the older NSAIDs have been used to compare newer formulations of salicylic acid. For example Deodhar *et al.* (1977) compared salsalate as a new anti-rheumatic with indomethacin and placebo.

Many of the initial studies have been conducted by the drug companies, particularly the large multicentre studies, leading to a uniformity in the analysis. However, a number of the early studies used aspirin in a suboptimal dose below 4–6 g daily.

Diamond *et al.* (1975), in a double-blind multicentre trial of 119 patients with RA, used aspirin at 3.6 g daily and naproxen at 500 mg daily which is half of the latter's now current dose. Some of the patients were maintained on corticosteroids and/or gold throughout the study. The results of the study tended to set a trend. Using subjective assessments and measurement of grip strength, walking time, number of clinically affected joints, duration of morning stiffness and time to fatigue, as well as ESR measurements, there was no significant difference between the drugs in the parameters studied. However, the gastrointestinal side effects were fewer in the naproxen group.

As well as straight comparisons of two drugs, there were studies comparing combined therapy. Willkens and Segre (1976) performed an 8 week double-blind crossover trial of naproxen or placebo against a background of constant dose aspirin. Clinical relevance was maintained by administering a dose of aspirin arrived at by prior individualized titration to tolerance. Patient preference was clear cut in that the combination was preferred at a significantly higher level. Interestingly, patients on higher doses of aspirin tended to show less incremental improvement with the addition of naproxen. There was also no increase in adverse effects during combined therapy.

Experience with naproxen led to studies comparing it with new salicylic acid derivatives and other new non-steroidals. Huskisson *et al.* (1982) compared diflunisal, the fluorinated derivative of aspirin, and diclofenac sodium, an acetic acid derivative, with naproxen. The trial was designed to resemble the ideal way of treating patients, demonstrating individual preferences. The incidence of side effects was similar with 750 mg naproxen, 150 mg diclofenac, and 1000 mg diflunisal daily. Each was also chosen by a significant group of patients as continuation therapy at the end of the study.

Devereaux and Douglas (1983) confirmed the similar analgesic and anti-inflammatory effect of 750 mg daily naproxen and diflunisal 1000 mg daily in 47 out-patients for 3 weeks. This study again showed the need for a wide selection, as patient preference revealed definite individual variation.

Huskisson *et al.* (1974) commented on the comparative efficacy of aspirin 6 g daily with fenoprofen 2.4 g daily in 60 patients for 24 weeks. Again, this study proved fenoprofen to be as effective as aspirin in relieving the pain of rheumatoid arthritis but with considerably less side effects. Almost half of the patients failed to continue aspirin therapy for 6 months and the remainder were able to take on average only 4 g daily. Even at this dose, almost half of the patients continued to have tinnitus or deafness.

The other major comparisons have been with ibuprofen and indomethacin. Blechman *et al.* (1975) found up to 1600 mg ibuprofen to be similar to 3.6 g aspirin in both efficacy and tolerance over 1 year. This study showed that many of the early trials used too low a dose of non-steroidal drugs. Even later, studies by Ehrlich *et al.* (1980), when the dose of ibuprofen was increased to 2400 mg daily, failed to compare with an adequate dose of salicylic acid. Here choline magnesium trisalicylate was used in inadequate dosages with 3000 mg salicylate daily as an equivalent.

Indomethacin provided an early useful NSAID to compare initially with acetylsalicylic acid and later with the introduction of aloxiprin, benorylate and salsalate. Pinals and Frank (1967) found no benefit of indomethacin over ASA in 24 patients over a 1 month period using an increasing dose of 50 mg to 200 mg by the fourth week. The dose of ASA was similarly increased from 1.6 g daily to 6.4 g daily.

Huskisson and Hart (1972b) found 100 mg indomethacin at night superior to 3.6 g aloxiprin in a single dose study. They again stated the importance of correct timing and dosage of the drug. Benorylate proved a more impressive anti-inflammatory when compared with 150 mg of indomethacin. Franke and Manz (1972) matched 40 patients and gave a daily dose of 6 g of benorylate. Both drugs produced a significant improvement in the disease as assessed by objective measurements and both drugs were extremely well tolerated. They concluded that benorylate was a useful addition to the therapeutic range for the treatment of rheumatoid disease.

11.9 CONCLUSION

Aspirin is the 'Gold standard' anti-inflammatory drug. At the turn of the century, it was successfully synthesized by Felix Hoffmann of Bayer-Elberfeld expressly as an anti-inflammatory agent to be used in rheumatism. Even with the advent of cortisone in 1949 and its dramatic effect on a number of inflammatory conditions, aspirin still remained the first choice drug in the 1960s.

Aspirin has both central and peripheral actions. Its effects are most useful if it can be tolerated at full doses in rheumatoid athritis and other inflammatory arthropathies and in inflammatory episodes in osteo-arthritis. In contrast, its analgesic action is helpful throughout the whole dosage range and brings quick pain relief of short duration.

Gastrointestinal intolerance, experienced by up to 50% of patients given anti-inflammatory doses of aspirin, has been the main reason for changing to a wide range of other NSAIDs. Initially, the use of enteric coated and soluble aspirin tablets to some degree reduced gastric disturbances. Newer preparations of salicylates, such as diflunisal and choline magnesium trisalicylate with a lower incidence of side effects than aspirin, have maintained their position in the therapy of rheumatoid arthritis. However, the more recently available NSAIDs are effective in lower doses than aspirin and their side effects are seldom serious enough to lead to withdrawal of treatment. Thus, propionic acid derivatives including naproxen, fenoprofen, ibuprofen and other NSAIDs, are being widely prescribed and taking over from the salicylates as drugs of first choice for rheumatoid arthritis.

Therefore, with no single analgesic (non-steroidal) anti-inflammatory drug consistently providing adequate relief for each patient, the salicylates maintain a prominent place among the growing list of useful NSAIDs.

REFERENCES

Aberg, G. and Larsson, R.S. (1970) Pharmacological properties of some anti-rheumatic salicylates. *Acta Pharmacol. Toxicol.* **28**, 249–57.

Ambacelli, U. and Fenaccioli, G.F. (1982) Allopurinol like action of diflunisal. *Arthritis Rheum.*, **25**, 474–5.

Andrew, A., Rodda, B. Verhaest, L. and Van Winzum, C. (1977). Diflunisal: six months experience in osteoarthritis. *Brit. J. Clin. Pharmacol.*, **4**, (Suppl 1), 455–525.

Anon. (1978) Which preparation of aspirin? *Drug Ther. Bull.*, **16**, 13.

Ansell, B.M. (1982) Juvenile chronic arthritis. *Drug Treatment of Rheumatic Diseases*, 2nd Edn (ed. F.D. Hart) ADIS Health Science Press, Sydney, p.186.

Ansell, B.M. (1986) Juvenile arthritis. *Practitioner*, **230**, 343–50.

April, P.A., Curran, M.J., Ekholm, B.P. *et al.* (1987) Multicentre comparative study of salsalate versus aspirin in rheumatoid arthritis. *Arthritis Rheum.*, **30**, 593.

Bain, L.S. and Burt, R.A.P. (1970) The treatment of rheumatic disease, a double-blind trial comparing buttered aspirin with benorylate. *Clin. Trials J.*, **7**, 307–12.

Beales, D.L. Barry, H.C. and Grahame, R. (1972) Comparison of aspirin and benorylate in the treatment of rheumatoid arthritis. *Brit. Med. J.*, **2**, 483–5.

Beecher, H.K. (1959), *Measurement of subjective response*. Oxford University Press, New York.

Bensen, W.G., Laskin, C.A., Paten, T.W. *et al.* (1976) Twice daily dosing of enteric coated aspirin in patients with rheumatoid disease. *J. Rheumatol.*, **6**, 351–6.

Binus, M.A., Lyon, J.A. and Nicholas, J.L. (1982) Comparable serum salicylate concentrations from choline magnesium trisalicylate, aspirin and buffered aspirin in rheumatoid arthritis. *Arthritis Rheum.*, **25**, 464–6.

Blechman, W.J. and Lechner, B.L. (1979) Clinical comparative evaluation of choline magnesium trisalicylate and acetylsalicylic acid in rheumatoid arthritis. *Rheum. Rehab.*, **18**, 119–24.

Blechman, W.J., Schmid, F.R., April, P.A. *et al.* (1975) Ibuprofen or aspirin in rheumatoid arthritis therapy. *JAMA*, **233**, 336–40.

Boardman, P.L. and Hart, F.D. (1967) Clinical measurement of the anti-inflammatory effects of salicylates in rheumatoid arthritis. *Brit. Med. J.*, **4**, 264–8.

Boyle, J.A. and Buchanan, W.W. (1971) *Clinical Rheumatology*, Blackwell Scientific Publications, Oxford, Edinburgh, pp. 169–72.

Brogden, R.N., Heel, R.C., Pakes, G.E. *et al.* (1980) Diflunisal: a review of its pharmacological properties and therapeutic use in pain and musculoskeletal strains and sprains and pain in osteoarthritis. *Drugs*, **19**, 84–106.

Brooks, P.M., Dougan, M.A., Mugford, S. and Meffin, E. (1982) Comparative effectiveness of 5 analgesics in patients with rheumatoid arthritis and osteoarthritis. *J. Rheumatol.*, **9**, 723–6.

Calabro, J.J. (1983) Optimum management of juvenile chronic polyarthritis. *Drugs*, **26**, 530–42.

Calabro, J.J. and Paulus, H.E. (1970) Anti-inflammatory effect of acetyl salicylic acid in rheumatoid arthritis. *Clin. Orthop. Rel. Res.*, **71**, 124–31.

Capell, H.A., Rennie, J.A.N., Rooney, P.J. *et al.* (1979) Patient compliance: a novel method of testing non-steroidal anti-inflammatory analgesics in rheumatoid arthritis. *J. Rheumatol.* **6**, 584–93.

Champion, G.D., Day, R.O., Graham, G.G. and Paull, P.D. (1975) Salicylates in rheumatoid arthritis. *Clin. Rheumat. Dis.*, **1**, 245–65.

Co-operating Clinics Committee of the American Rheumatism Association. (1965) A seven day variability study of 499 patients with peripheral rheumatoid arthritis. *Arthritis Rheum.*, **8** 302–34.

Croft, D.N., Cuddigan, J.H.P. and Sweetland, C. (1972) Gastric bleeding and benorylate, a new aspirin. *Brit. Med. J.*, **iii**, 545–7.

Denson, L.J. Thompson, M.D. (1960) A new salicylate therapy for treatment of arthritic diseases. *J. Med. Soc. New Jersey*, **57**, 314.

Deodhar, S.D., Dick, W.C., Hodgkinson, R. and Buchanan, W.W. (1973) Measurement of clinical response to anti-inflammatory drug therapy in rheumatoid arthritis. *Q. J. Med. NS*, **42**, 387–401.

Deodhar, S.D., McLeod, M.M., Dick, W.C. and Buchanan, W.W. (1977) A short-term comparative trial of salsalate and indomethacin in rheumatoid arthritis. *Curr. Med. Res. Opinion,*, **5**, 185–8.

De Silva, M., Hazleman, B.L. and Dippy, J.E. (1980) Diflunisal and aspirin: a comparative study in rheumatoid arthritis. *Rheum. Rehab.*, **19**, 126–30.

Devereaux, M.D. and Douglas, W.A.C. (1983) A double-blind, comparative study of diflunisal and naproxen in the treatment of rheumatoid arthritis. *Eur.J. Rheum. Inflam.*, **6**, 274–8.

Diamond, H., Alexander, S., Kuzell, W. *et al.* (1975) Naproxen and aspirin in rheumatoid arthritis: a multicentre double-blind crossover comparison study. *J. Clin. Pharmacol.*, **15**, 335–9.

Dick, W.C. (1972) The use of radioisotopes in normal and diseased joints. *Semin Arthritis Rheum.*, **1**, 301–25.

Dick, W.C., Dick, P.H., Nuki, G. *et al.* (1969) Effect of anti-inflammatory drug therapy on clearance of ^{133}Xe from knee joints of patients with rheumatoid arthritis. *Brit. Med.* J., **3**, 278.

Dick, W.C., Neufeld, R.R., Prentice, A.G. *et al.* (1970a) Measurement of joint inflammation: a radioisotopic method. *Ann. Rheum. Dis.*, **29**, 135–7.

Dick, W.C., Grayson, M.F., Woodburn, A. *et al.* (1970b) Indices of inflammatory activity: Relationship between isotope studies and clinical methods. *Ann. Rheum. Dis.* **29**, 643–8.

Dick, W.C. Deodhar, S.D., Provan, C.J. *et al.* (1971) Isotope studies in normal and diseased knee joints: ^{99M}Tc uptake related to clinical assessment and to synovial perfusion measured by the ^{133}Xe clearance technique. *Clin. Sci.*, **40**, 327–36.

Dieppe, P.A. and Huskisson, E.C. (1978) Diflunisal and acetylsalicylic acid: A comparison of efficacy in osteoarthritis; of nephrotoxicity, and of anti-inflammatory activity in the rat. In *Diflusinal in Clinical Practice* (ed K. Miehlke) Futura Publishing Company Inc., New York, pp. 57–61.

Dixon, A.St J., Martin, B.K., Smith, M.J.H. and Wood, P.H.N, (Eds) (1963) *Salicylates; an International Symposium*, Boston, Little Brown & Co., London.

Dromgoole, S.H., Furst, D.E. and Paulus, H.E. (1981) Rational approaches to the use of salicylates in the treatment of rheumatoid arthritis. *Semin. Arthritis Rheum.*, **11**, 257–83.

Dunlop Sir D. and Inch, R.S. (1972) Variations in pharmaceutical and medical practice in Europe. *Brit. Med* J., **3**, 749–52.

Ehrlich, G.E., Miller, S.B., Zeiders, R.S. (1980) Choline magnesium trisalicylate versus ibuprofen in rheumatoid arthritis. *Rheum. Rehab.*, **19**, 30–41.

Empire Rheumatism Council (1955) Multicentre controlled trial comparing cortisone acetate and acetylsalicylic acid in the long-term treatment of rheumatoid arthritis. *Ann. Rheum. Dis.*, **14**, 353–70.

Ferreira, S.H. and Vane, J.R. (1974) New aspects of the mode of action of non-steroidal anti-inflammatory drugs. *Ann. Rev. Pharmacol.*, 14, 57–73.

Franke, M. and Manz, G. (1972) Benorylate and indomethacin in the treatment of rheumatoid arthritis: a double-blind clinical trial. *Curr. Ther. Res.*, **14**, 113–22.

Fremont-Smith, K. and Bayles T.B. (1965) Salicylate therapy in rheumatoid arthritis. *JAMA*, **192**, 1133–6.

Frenkel, E.P., McCall, M.S., Douglas, C.C. *et al.* (1968) Faecal blood loss following aspirin microspherule administration. *J. Clin. Pharmacol* **8**, 347–51.

Therapeutic applications

Gibaldi, M. and Grundhofer, B. (1975) Bioavailability of aspirin from commercial suppositories. *J. Pharm. Sci.* **64**, 1064–6.

Giuliano, V. and Scharff, E.V. (1980) Clinical comparison of two salicylates in rheumatoid arthritis patients on maintenance gold therapy. *Curr. Ther. Res.*, **28**, 61–71.

Godfrey, R.G., Calabro, J.J. Mills, D. and Maltz B.A. (1972) A double blind cross over trial of aspirin, indomethacin and phenylbutazone in ankylosing spondylitis. *Arthritis Rheum.*, **15**, 110.

Gyory, A.Z and Stiel, J.N. (1968) Effect of particle size on aspirin-induced gastrointestinal bleeding. *Lancet*, **ii**, 300–2.

Hannah, W.V., Ruyle H., Jones, A.R. *et al.* (1977) Discovery of diflunisal. *Brit. J. Clin. Pharmacol.*, **4**, 75–135.

Hart, F.D. and Huskisson, E.C. (1972) Measurement in rheumatoid arthritis. *Lancet*, **i**, 28–30.

Hickey, R.F. (1982) Chronic low back pain: a comparison of diflunisal and paracetamol. *New Zealand Med. J.*, **95**, 312–4.

Hughes, G.R.V. (1979) The treatment of SLE: the case for conservative treatment. *Clin. Rheum. Dis.*, **5**, 641–55.

Huskisson, E.C. (1974) Simple analgesics for arthritis. *Brit. Med. J.*, **4**, 196–200.

Huskisson, E.C. and Hart, F.D. (1972a), The use of indomethacin and aloxiprin at night. *The Practitioner*, **208**, 248–51.

Huskisson E.C. and Hart, F.D. (1972b) Pain threshold and arthritis. *Brit. Med. J.* **4**, 193–5.

Huskisson, E.C., Wojtulewski, J.A., Berry, H. *et al.* (1974) Treatment of rheumatoid arthritis with fenprofen: comparison with aspirin. *Brit. Med. J.* **1**, 176–80.

Huskisson, E.C., Woolf, D.L., Balme, H.W. *et al.* (1976) Four new anti-inflammatory drugs: responses and variations. *Brit. Med. J.*, **1**, 1048–9.

Huskisson, E.C. Dieppe, P.A., Scott, J. and Jones, H. (1982) Diclofenac sodium, diflunisal, and naproxen: patient preferences for anti-inflammatory drugs in rheumatoid arthritis. *Rheum. Rehab.*, **21**, 238–42.

Jaffe, S.Y. (1981) *Arch. Intern. Med.*, **141**, 286–92.

Jasani, M.K., Downie, W.W., Sammels, B.M. and Buchanan, W.W. (1968) Ibuprofen in rheumatoid arthritis. Clinical study of analgesic and anti-inflammatory activity. *Ann. Rheum. Dis.*, 27, 457–62.

Keele, K.D. (1954) Pain sensitivity tests. The pressure algameter. *Lancet*, **i**, 636–9.

Kendal, M.G. (1963) *Rank Correlation Methods*, 3rd edn, Griffin, London.

Kilander, A. and Dotevall, G. (1983) Endoscopic evaluation of the comparative effects of acetylsalicylic acid and choline magnesium trisalicylate on human gastric and duodenal mucosa. *Brit. J. Rheumatol.*, **22**, 36.

Lansbury, J. (1958) Report of a three year study on the systemic and articular indexes in rheumatoid arthritis. *Arthritis Rheum.*, **1**, 505–22.

Lansbury, J. (1968) Clinical appraisal of the activity index as a measure of rheumatoid activity. *Arthritis Rheum.*, **11**, 599.

Lee, P., Sturrock, R.D., Kennedy, A. and Dick,W.C. (1973a) The evaluation of anti-rheumatic drugs. *Curr. Med. Res. Opinion*, **11**, 427–43.

Lee, P., Webb, J., Anderson J. and Buchanan, W.W. (1973b) Method for

318

assessing therapeutic potential of anti-inflammatory anti-rheumatic drugs in rheumatoid arthritis. *Brit. Med. J.*, **2**, 685–8.

Lee, P. Ahola, S.J., Grenan, D., *et al.* (1974a) Observations on drug prescribing in rheumatoid arthritis. *Brit. Med. J.*, **1**, 424–6.

Lee, P., Baxter, A., Dick, W.C. and Webb, J. (1974b) An assessment of grip strength measurement in rheumatoid arthritis. *Scand. J. Rheumatol.*, **3**, 17–23.

Lee, P., Anderson, J.A., Miller. J., Webb, J. and Buchanan, W.W. (1976) Evaluation of analgesic action and efficacy of anti-rheumatic drugs: study of 10 drugs in 684 patients with rheumatoid arthritis. *J. Rheumatol.*, **3**, 283–94.

Leonards, J.R. (1963) The influence of solubility on the rate of gastrointestinal absorption of aspirin. *Clin. Pharmacol. Ther.*, **4**, 476–9.

Leonards, J.R. (1969) Absence of gastrointestinal bleeding following administration of salicylsalicylic acid. *J. Lab. Clin. Med.*, **74**, 911.

Leonards, J.R. and Levy, G. (1965) Absorption and metabolism of aspirin administered in enteric coated tablets. *JAMA*, **193**, 99–104.

Leonards, J.R. and Levy, G. (1967) The role of dosage form in aspirin-induced gastrointestinal bleeding. *Clin. Pharmacol. Ther.*, **8**, 400–8.

Leonards, J.R. and Levy, G. (1969) Reduction or prevention of aspirin-induced occult blood loss in man. *Clin. Pharmacol. Ther.*, **10**, 571–5.

Leonards, J.R. and Levy, G. (1973) Gastrointestinal blood loss from aspirin and sodium salicylate tablets in man. *Clin. Pharmacol. Ther.*, **14**, 62–6.

Levy, G., Leonards, J.R. and Procknal, J.A. (1967) Interpretation of in vitro dissolution data relative to the gastrointestinal absorption characteristics of drugs and tablets. *J. Pharm. Sci.*, **56**, 1365–7.

Mainland, D. and Sutcliffe, M.J. (1965) Aspirin in rheumatoid arthritis, a seven day double-blind trial preliminary report. *Bull. Rheum. Dis.*, **16**, 388–91.

Mielants, H., Veys, E.M., Verbruggen, G. and Schelstraete K. (1981) Comparison of serum salicylate and gastrointestinal blood loss between salsalate and other forms of salicylates. *Scand. J. Rheumatol*, **10**, 169–73.

Morgan, A.M. and Truitt, E.B. (1956) Evaluation of acetylsalicylic acid esterase in aspirin metabolism. *J. Pharm. Sci.*, **54**, 1640–5.

MRC and Nuffield Foundation (1954a) A comparison of cortisone and aspirin in the treatment of early cases of rheumatoid arthritis. *Brit. Med. J.*, **1**, 1224–7.

MRC and Nuffield Foundation (1954b) Joint report on cortisone and codeine. *Brit. Med. J.*, **1**, 233–5.

MRC and Nuffield Foundation (1957) Long-term results in early cases of rheumatoid arthritis treated with either cortisone or aspirin. *Brit. Med. J.*, **1**, 847–50.

Multz, C.V., Bernhard, G.C., Blechman, W.C. *et al.* (1974) A comparison of intermediate-dose aspirin and placebo in rheumatoid arthritis. *Clin. Pharmacol. Ther.*, **15**, 310–15.

Nuki, G. (1983) Non-steroidal analgesia and anti-inflammatory agents. *Brit. Med. J.*, **287**, 39–43.

Paris, L. and Newfield, H. (1963) Morning stiffness in arthritis. *Clin. Med.*, **70**, 2029.

Therapeutic applications

Pierson, R.N., Holt, P.R., Watson, R.M. *et al.* (1961) Aspirin and gastrointestinal bleeding. *Am. J. Med.*, **31**, 259–65.

Pinals, R.S. and Frank, S. (1967) Relative efficacy of indomethacin and acetylsalicylic acid in rheumatoid arthritis. *N Engl. J. Med.*, **276**, 512–14.

Preston, S.J., Arnold, M.H., Beller, E.M. *et al.* (1989) Comparative analgesic and anti-inflammatory properties of sodium salicylate and acetylsalicylic acid (aspirin) in rheumatoid arthritis. *Brit. J. Clin. Pharmacol.*, **27**, 607–11.

Rainsford, D. (1984) *Aspirin and the Salcylates*, Butterworths, London, Boston.

Ritchie, D.M., Boyle, J.A., McInnes, J.M. *et al.* (1968) Clinical studies with an articular index for the assessment of joint tenderness in patients with rheumatoid arthritis. *Q. J. Med. NS*, **37**, 393–406.

Robertson, A. (1973) Benorylate – the rationale: a symposium on benorylate. *Rheum. Rehab.*, **12**, 7–16 (Suppl. issue).

Ropes, M.W., Bennett, G.A., Cobb, S. *et al.* (1958) 1958 Revision of diagnostic criteria for rheumatoid arthritis. *Bull. Rheum. Dis.*, **9**, 175–6.

Rosner, I., Mottot, G., Khalil, V. and Legros, J. (1973). Experimental data on benorylate and their clinical relevance. *Rheum. Rehab.*, Suppl., 59–65.

Rothwell, K.G. (1983) Efficacy and safety of a non-acetylated salicylate, choline magnesium trisalicylate, in the treatment of rheumatoid arthritis. *J. Int. Med. Res.*, **11**, 343–8.

Sasisekhar, P.R., Penn, R.G., Haslock, I. and Wright, V. (1973) A comparison of benorylate and aspirin in the treatment of rheumatoid arthritis. *Rheum. Rehab.*, Suppl., Symposium on Benorylate, 31–8.

Scully, F.J. (1961) Choline salicylate: an effective well tolerated drug for treatment of rheumatic diseases. *South. Med. J.*, **53**, 12–6.

Seed, J.C. (1965) A clinical comparison of the antipyretic potency of aspirin and sodium salicylate. *Clin. Pharmacol. Ther.*, **6**, 354–8.

Sperryn, M.M., Hamilton, E.B.D. and Parsons, V. (1973) Double-blind comparison of aspirin and benorylate in rheumatoid arthritis. *Ann. Rheum. Dis.*, **32**, 157–61.

Sun, D.H. and Sun, S. (1971) Salicylate therapy. *Fla. Fam. Physician*, **28**, 33–41.

Tempero, K.F., Cirillo, V.J. and Steelman, S.L. (1977) Diflunisal: a review of pharmacodynamic properties, drug interactions, and special tolerability studies in humans. *Brit. J. Clin. Pharmcol.*, **4**, 315–65.

Webb, J., Downie, W.W., Dick, W.C. and Lee, P. (1973) Evaluation of digital joint circumference measurements in rheumatoid arthritis. *Scand. J. Rheumatol.*, **2**, 127–31.

Weiss, H.J., Aledorf, L.M. and Kochwas, S. (1968) The effect of salicylates on the haemostatic properties of platelets in man. *J. Clin. Invest.*, **217**, 2169–80.

Willkens, R.F. and Segre. E.J. (1976) Combination therapy with naproxen and aspirin in rheumatoid arthritis. *Arthritis Rheum.*, **19**, (4) 677–82.

Wood, P.H.N., Harvey-Smith, E.A. and Dixon, A. St. J. (1962) Salicylates and gastrointestinal bleeding. Acetylsalicylic acid and aspirin derivatives. *Brit. Med. J.*, i, 669–75.

Wright, V. and Amos, R. (1980) Do drugs change the course of rheumatoid arthritis? *Brit. Med. J.*, **280**, 964–6.

12 Aspirin and myocardial infarction with an annotation on venous thrombosis

T.W. MEADE

12.1 INTRODUCTION

Aspirin now plays a central part in preventing the recurrence of myocardial infarction (MI) and may well have a place in preventing first episodes as well. Before considering the evidence for these conclusions it is, however, worth summarizing quite recent changes in views on the pathogenesis of MI not just for their historical interest but because they set the scene for what aspirin may or may not be able to achieve and also because of their possible implications for the future.

The term 'coronary thrombosis' was first used many years ago and clearly implies recognition of a thrombotic component in ischaemic heart disease (IHD). The increasing volume of research after 1945, stimulated by the growing epidemic of IHD, was however largely directed towards the role of lipids. The thrombotic contribution was largely overlooked. The topic only re-emerged comparatively recently and, when it did, was characterized by two major controversies. The first was whether thrombosis precedes or follows transmural MI. In the former case, anti-thrombotic agents might be expected to prevent recurrences or first events. In the latter, they would not prevent onset although they might modify the subsequent course. To begin with, the issue was settled, as far as it then could be, by a consensus view of the evidence, which concluded that thrombosis does precede and probably causes transmural infarction (Chandler et al., 1974). With the advent of thrombolytic therapy and the need to establish the rationale for its use and its effects, coronary angiography clearly demonstrated the high frequency of total coronary occlusion during MI (DeWood et al., 1980) and there is now no doubt about the significance of thrombosis in transmural MI (Davies, 1987). The place of thrombosis in subendocardial infarction is less clear (Davies, 1987), though probably real. The second controversy – again, settled only quite recently – was the place of thrombosis in sudden coronary death. In the 1970s, reports of platelet thrombi and microemboli in the coronary vessels of those dying sudden vascular deaths (Haerem, 1974) were often viewed, wrongly, with scepticism. It was not until the results of a series of particularly careful autopsy studies became available in the 1980s (Davies and Thomas, 1984; Dantzig and Becker, 1986; El Fawal *et al.*, 1987; Frink *et al.*, 1988) that the almost universal occurrence of thrombosis in sudden coronary death was recognized and accepted as directly contributing to these events. Most though not all sudden coronary deaths are the result of a ruptured atheromatous plaque in which thrombosis either contributes to the intramural pathology or to luminal occlusion, or both. The minority of events in which thrombosis is not apparently associated with plaque rupture – between 2% (Davies and Thomas, 1984) and about 25% (El Fawal *et al.*, 1987) – are interesting in suggesting that characteristics of the circulating blood, such as the degree of intrinsic platelet aggregability or of coagulability, play a part in initiating some arterial thrombi as well as contributing to the development of those initiated by plaque rupture or leakage. The observation that thrombi associated with sudden coronary death do not totally occlude the arterial lumen as often as those causing transmural MI may be due to the intense fibrinolytic activity accompanying sudden death with the consequence that thrombi initially responsible for the episode are at least partially lysed by the time of autopsy (Meade *et al.*, 1984; Davies, 1987). The underlying pathology of MI and sudden coronary death is probably the same, or at least very similar. The clinical outcome of thrombosis in the coronary circulation may largely depend on whether or not conducting tissue is involved (Davies and Thomas, 1984).

In summary, most pathologists who have studied the pathogenesis of IHD now agree that thrombosis is causally involved in MI, in most sudden coronary deaths and also in unstable angina pectoris (Davies and Thomas, 1985; Falk, 1987). The probable role of thrombosis in atherosclerosis as well should also be remembered (Duguid, 1970).

As interest in thrombosis and IHD mounted, most attention was directed towards the contribution of platelets. Their very rapid adhesion to damaged endothelium and then to each other is central to arterial thrombosis. The formation and incorporation of fibrin is a slower event but it is fibrin which gives many developing thrombi their ultimate stability and volume. There are many platelet agonists, of which thrombin is one. It may therefore be that activation of the coagulation system contributes to platelet aggregation as well as to fibrin formation. Coronary artery thrombi may vary from predominantly platelet bodies in the vessel wall to mainly fibrin accumulations in the lumen. A recent biochemical (as distinct from morphological) study concluded that fibrin formation and platelet activation are probably equally important in the early hours of MI (Rapold *et al.*, 1989). If so, this is added reason for recognizing that the mechanical obstruction of the coronary artery is due to two main processes and that the most effective approach to anti-thrombotic therapy may involve platelet-active agents and anticoagulants simultaneously, a topic discussed in more detail in a later section.

12.2 OBSERVATIONAL AND EXPERIMENTAL STUDIES

Much of the early evidence that aspirin might confer some protection against MI came from observational studies. These provided a powerful stimulus for the randomized controlled trials (RCT) that then followed. Since there is still a good deal of uncertainty about the rationale for randomized treatment allocation, it is worth briefly summarizing.

Randomization ensures that treatment allocation in any individual participant in an RCT is, indeed, made at random so that this allocation has not been influenced by characteristics of the patient that might affect outcome. For example, a clinician might tend, consciously or not, to avoid anticoagulants after MI in patients with heart failure. Since heart failure is associated with a poor prognosis, any tendency of this kind will obviously favour anticoagulants, which will have been used more frequently in those without heart failure and therefore with a better prognosis anyway. The correct procedure is either to exclude all patients with heart failure from the trial in the first place or to ensure that those with and without this complication all stand the same chance of drawing active or placebo treatment – that is, by randomization. Provided the trial is large enough, randomization will ensure that the treated and placebo groups are, as groups, identical in all respects other than the trial treatment. Under these circumstances, differences in outcome can only be due to treatment. The very small minority of those who still advocate the use of historical controls, or other methods for establishing a control series not based on randomization, often claim that differences between the two groups can be allowed for in the analysis by adjusting for imbalances in characteristics other than the treatment under investigation – for example, age differences, differences in proportions with heart failure and in other features known to be associated with outcome. But no adjustment whatever can be made for imbalances in characteristics that have not been measured or whose existence and association with outcome the investigators may not even be aware of. Randomization ensures identical groups, not only in terms of characteristics known to influence outcome, but also of those not measured or not even identified.

Therapeutic applications

That these considerations are not just theoretical is well exemplified by randomized and non-randomized comparisons of the effects of oral anticoagulants on mortality following MI. In an illuminating review of six RCTs and 20 non-randomized comparisons, Armitage (1980) showed that the benefit in the former was about 20%, compared with about 50% in the latter. Almost certainly, the explanation for the contrast lies in the inability of non-randomized comparisons to allow fully for imbalances in characteristics other than treatment that are associated with a greater or lesser risk of dying during the study period. The biases so introduced may be as large as or even larger than the effect of the agent under study.

12.2.1 Analysing Randomized Controlled Trials (RCTs)

An important recent development has been the introduction of over-views or meta-analyses for simultaneously assessing the results and implications of all the trials of a particular treatment, rather than relying on the results of separate trials. The main argument for this approach (which has now been used for aspirin, β-blockers and thrombolytic therapy, for example) is that most trials are too small to give clear indications on their own, and that more precise estimates and therefore greater practical utility will be available from analyses based on the results of all the available trials. Details of the technique are available in the report from the Antiplatelet Trialists' Collaboration (1988). The contribution that each trial makes to the meta-analysis depends on its size, particularly the number of events – the larger the trial the greater its contribution. Results depend on the sum of the separate within-trial contributions. The method makes no comparisons between individual trials. It is not assumed that treatment effects are the same in different trials or that the patients or subjects on which they are based are necessarily comparable. Another leading principle of meta-analysis, and a compelling argument for its use, is the importance of obtaining the results of all the trials of a particular agent, including those that may not have been published as well as those that have. This approach ensures an unbiased as well as a more precise assessment of the effects of the drug in question, since it avoids the potential or actual biases which may undoubtedly occur in reviews based on selected trials and on the subjective opinions of those carrying out these reviews as to which trials to include or specially emphasize. Against meta-analysis, it is argued that some trials are of higher quality than others and this is obviously true. Provided, however, that the results of a poorer quality trial are not biased in the sense (in this context) that treatment was not allocated at random or that the assessment of outcome was somehow influenced by knowledge of the treatment group, the results of the trial nevertheless make a contribution to the data as a whole and its results can therefore justifiably be included. Another argument advanced against some meta-analyses is that an agent such as aspirin has been included in trials in different groups of patients – after MI, after transient ischaemic attacks (TIAs) and stroke, in unstable angina and in the primary prevention of IHD – and, in addition, with the intention of preventing different clinical manifestations in these different groups of patients. Is it therefore justifiable to consider the results of these different sorts of trials together? Resolving this objection depends on the use to which results are to be put. Combining data from trials in patients with a range of clinical conditions may be inappropriate if the objective is to test a scientific hypothesis about aspirin, platelet aggregability and thrombogenesis in a particular condition such as unstable angina. In clinical practice, on the other hand, doctors are often confronted by patients with more than one indication for aspirin – for example, unstable angina and a past history of TIA – who are at risk from several different clinical manifestations of arterial disease – for example, MI and a major stroke. In these circumstances, the indications of a meta-analysis are obviously helpful. Until there is clear evidence that different doses of aspirin may confer different benefits, it is also reasonable to include in meta-analyses all the trials based on what is a wide range of doses (though it would be misleading to press the principle so far that possible dose-dependent effects were overlooked) and also, again in the absence of clear differences, to include the results of trials using other anti-aggregating agents. Provided the qualifications that have been discussed are borne in mind, however, the use of meta-analysis undoubtedly represents a substantial advance in the evaluation of results from clinical trials.

Another question is the appropriate definition of end-points. Some argue that since vascular disease is the leading cause of death in developed countries, trials of anti-thrombotic agents (and of other drugs for the prevention of arterial disease) should be able to demonstrate a significant reduction in deaths, from whatever cause, and that doctors and their patients are unlikely to be impressed by results that do not show this. Another view is that a trial initiated, on scientific grounds, to test a drug's ability to prevent IHD should place the main emphasis on these results, including non-fatal as well as fatal episodes. Yet another approach is to include all vascular deaths and non-fatal episodes of both IHD and stroke in one category of major vascular events. Obviously, the larger the number of end-points and the ways in which they are considered in combinations, the greater the chance of observing what may in fact be a spurious result. There is no absolutely right or wrong approach. Again, much depends on the context in which the results are being considered.

12.3 ASPIRIN AND MI

The *in vitro* inhibition of platelet aggregation by aspirin was recognized in the late 1960s (e.g. Weiss and Aledort, 1967). The demonstration of this effect was followed in 1974 by two consecutive publications in the *British Medical Journal*, the first a randomized controlled trial from Cardiff and the second a case-comparison study from Boston in the USA. Both are well worth reading partly for historical reasons but also because they contrast the undoubted value of a case-comparison study in suggesting an effect with the need for randomized comparisons to provide firm evidence. The Cardiff trial appeared under the Journal's 'For Debate' heading (Elwood *et al.*, 1974). It had been carried out in 1239 men under the age of 65 discharged from hospital with a confirmed diagnosis of MI. Treatment consisted either of 300 mg powdered aspirin daily or an inert placebo. While the trial was in progress, the investigators were contacted by the group carrying out the case-comparison study, the Boston Collaborative Drug Surveillance Programme, who presented preliminary data suggesting a substantial protective effect of aspirin. The Boston findings were, however, also consistent with the possibility of increased early mortality from MI in those who had taken aspirin recently. The results of the Cardiff trial at that time were disclosed to the Boston group – 6 deaths in those on aspirin, 11 among those in the control group. There was therefore no difficulty about the decision to continue the trial, whose recruitment rate was increased in order to obtain more certain results as quickly as possible. The trial's original design was modified first by the removal of the age restriction and secondly by the inclusion of patients who had been discharged during the previous 6 months as well as those more recently discharged. Recruitment ended in July 1973. The results are summarized in Fig. 12.1. Although mortality was lower in the actively treated group, the difference was not statistically significant at a conventional level. The authors considered the results 'inconclusive' which, in the light of the evidence then available they were, while clearly providing a major stimulus for further trials. In an interesting comment about the appropriate dose of aspirin, the authors favoured a higher dose, a conclusion implemented in the second Cardiff trial (Elwood and Sweetnam, 1979).

The Boston case-comparison study (Boston Collaborative Drug Surveillance Group, 1974) was based on data routinely collected on medicines taken before admission and on discharge diagnoses from a

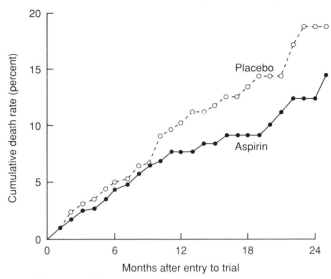

Figure 12.1 First Cardiff trial in 1239 men taking 300 mg aspirin daily or placebo after myocardial infarction; cumulative death rates. (Reproduced from Elwood *et al.*, 1974, with permission of authors and *British Medical Journal.*)

number of hospitals in four countries. When a strong negative association between regular aspirin intake and MI had been established, a second, separate study was undertaken in about 25 000 consecutive admissions to the wards of 24 hospitals in the Boston area. In the first study, three (0.9%) of 325 patients with acute MI gave a history of regular aspirin use before admission, compared with 188 (4.9%) among 3807 controls. The summary risk ratio (SRR) was about 0.2, suggesting a very marked protective effect attributable to aspirin. In the second study, 16 (3.5%) of 451 patients with acute MI gave a history of regular aspirin use before admission compared with 702 (7.0%) among 10 091 controls. The SRR was 0.53, still suggesting a protective effect though less marked than that observed in the first study. Since both studies were based on those who had survived infarction long enough to be admitted to hospital, the associations observed could have been due to high early mortality of patients experiencing infarction who were regular aspirin users. The Boston Group up-dated the findings of their first study in 1976 (Jick and Miettinen, 1976), the results being little altered.

In 1975, Hammond and Garfinkel (1975) reported on findings from the American Cancer Society study which had enrolled over a million men and women most of whom were over the age of 45 in a long-term study principally (as its title suggests) concerned with cancer. At recruitment,

327

each participant had answered a questionnaire that included items on the use of aspirin as 'never', 'seldom' or 'often'. Mortality ratios for deaths from coronary heart disease were almost the same in the three groups, suggesting no association between recent aspirin consumption and mortality from coronary heart disease. At about the same time, the results of the Coronary Drug Project Research Group trial (1976) in 1529 patients with a previous history of MI reported a mortality of 5.8% in those given 972 mg aspirin daily compared with 8.3% in the placebo group, a difference of 30% suggestive of a beneficial effect but not statistically significant at a conventional level. In 1978, another American case-control study suggested no protective effect (Hennekens *et al.*, 1978).

Recently, a further American observational study concluded that the daily use of aspirin increases the risk of kidney cancer and ischaemic heart disease (Paganini-Hill *et al.*, 1989). Given the volume of evidence now available from randomized controlled trials that aspirin reduces the recurrence of MI and probably its incidence as well it is hard to understand the justification for further studies of this kind. Ascertainment of aspirin use was at best approximate, and little if any attempt was made to see whether usage was for reasons that might have been associated with increased risks of cancer or IHD. The possibility that aspirin unmasked pre-existing renal cancer by causing early bleeding was not considered. At least, at an important point in the history of aspirin in cardiovascular disease, it re-emphasized the need to rely on evidence from trials rather than observational studies.

12.3.1 Secondary Prevention

It is worth repeating that more events in trials based on neurological patients (those who have had strokes or transient ischaemic attacks) are due to ischaemic heart disease than to cerebrovascular disease, so that simultaneous consideration of results from trials based on patients who have survived MI, who have had strokes and/or TIAs and those with unstable angina is justified for this reason alone. The frequent occurrence in clinical practice of more than one possible indication for aspirin has already been referred to as another reason.

Clinical decisions about the use of aspirin have to take account of the full range of potential benefits and hazards. So while this chapter is mainly concerned with aspirin in the prevention of MI, brief references are also made to its effect on cerebrovascular disease, where any benefits in cerebral infarction have to be balanced against the possibility of an increase in episodes of cerebral haemorrhage, and to bleeding at various non-cerebral sites.

Further sections on secondary prevention are largely based on the indications of two overviews of all the available evidence from 25 trials (Antiplatelet Trialists' Collaboration, 1988; Hennekens *et al.*, 1989), for reasons considered in the Introduction. In much of what follows, details from both overviews are cited but not always separately referenced in summarizing the findings on particular topics. The original publications should be consulted for details about the individual trials. Here, the only feature of any particular trial to which special attention needs to be drawn is the imbalance between the two groups in the Aspirin Myocardial Infarction Study Research Group trial (1980). In several respects, the actively treated group (1000 mg aspirin daily) was characterized by a significantly higher prevalence of features associated with an increased risk of death, including heart failure and angina pectoris. This imbalance would have the effect of reducing any real benefit attributable to aspirin. However, as the overviews showed (below), corrections for the imbalances make only a marginal difference to their results because the AMIS group of patients is small relative to the total numbers considered.

The Antiplatelet Trialist's Collaboration (1988), or ATC review, placed the main emphasis on 'one important vascular event' as an outcome, i.e. first stroke, MI or vascular death during the scheduled treatment period. Table 12.1 summarizes the 25 trials considered in the ATC review, sub-divided according to the types of patients recruited – those with cerebrovascular disease, those who had survived MI and those with unstable angina. Of the 25 trials, aspirin was used in 19, mostly on its own though in combination with dipyridamole or combined or compared with sulphinpyrazone in others. About 80% of the patients were compliant with treatment at 1 year. Some 17% of the 29 073 patients considered suffered at least one new vascular event.

Figure 12.2, from the ATC review, summarizes the main results, i.e. according to occurrence of first stroke, MI or vascular death. The odds reduction for 'important vascular events' so defined was 25% and highly significant ($P < 0.0001$). There was no convincing evidence of heterogeneity between groups defined according to prior disease, thus justifying their inclusion in one analysis. The possibility that aspirin conferred more benefit in unstable angina than in those with the other two conditions was neither confirmed nor excluded.

Turning now to different measure of outcome, Table 12.2 summarizes the percentage reductions in non-fatal MI and in other outcomes according to the three groups of prior disease already referred to (Hennekens *et al.*, 1989). There was a suggestion that the reduction in strokes might have been somewhat greater for disabling than non-disabling stroke, though this effect was not statistically significant. For vascular death,

Table 12.1 Summary of trials included in ATC review (Antiplatelet Trialists Collaboration, 1988)

First principal investigator and/or title, acronym or centre	Active regime(s)*	No. entered	No. events	Duration, (years, approx)
Patients with cerebrovascular disorders†				
Lowenthal, ESPS	A 975+D225	2500	446	2
Warlow, UK-TIA	A1200 or 300	2435	552	4
Bousser, AICLA	A 990+D225 or A 990	604	109	3
Barnett, CCSG	A1300 or S 800 } or both	585	131	2
Britton, Sweden	A1500	505	115	2
Gent, McMaster	Su 600	447	106	2
Guiraud-Chaumeil, Toulouse	A 900 + D150 or A 900	440	41	3
Fields, AITIA	A1300	303	61	1
Blakely, Toronto	S 800	290	67	3
Sorensen, Denmark DCS	A1000	203	49	2
Acheson, Stoke	D 400–800	169	43	2
Robertson, Tennessee	S 800	148	46	6
Reuther, German TIA	A1500	60	5	2
Patients with MI				
AMIS, Aspirin Myocardial Infarction Study	A1000	4524	874	3
PARIS-II, Persantin-Aspirin Reinfarction Study	A 972 + D225	3128	438	2
PARIS-I	A 972 + D225 A 972	2026	380	3–4
Elwood, Cardiff-II	A 900	1682	314	1
Sherry, ART	S 800	1620	270	1
CDP, Coronary Drug Project	A 972	1529	179	2
Vogel, GDR	A1500	1340	150	2
Elwood, Cardiff-I	A 300	1239	136	1
Cortellaro, ARIS	S 800	727	101	2
Breddin, GAMIS	A1500	626	96	2
Patients with unstable angina				
Lewis, Veterans Administration, VA	A 324	1388	125	0.25
Cairns, McMaster	A1300	555	75	2

A= aspirin; D= dipyridamole; S= sulphinpyrazone; Su= suloctidil; doses in mg daily. TIA= transient ischaemic attack.
* Each active regime compared with no active drug regime.
† Events leading to entry: AITIA, DCS, German trials: TIA; ESPS, AICIA, Acheson trials: TIA or stroke; UK-TIA, CCSG, Toulouse, Tennessee trials: TIA or minor stroke; Swedish, McMaster, Toronto trials: infarct or thrombosis.

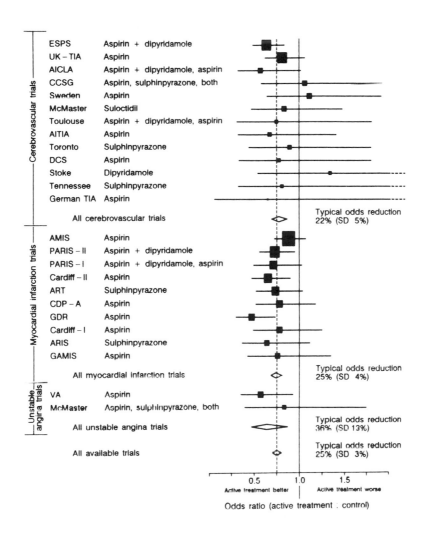

Figure 12.2 Odds ratios (active treatment: control) for first stroke, myocardial infarction, or vascular death during scheduled treatment period in completed antiplatelet trials. Solid symbols and lines show individual trial results and 99% confidence intervals (area of symbol proportional to amount of information contributed). Unfilled symbols show overview results and 95% confidence intervals. Dashed vertical line represents odds ratio of 0.75 suggested by overview of all trial results. Solid vertical line represents odds ratio of unity (no treatment effect). (Reproduced from Antiplatelet Trialists Collaboration, 1988, with permission of authors and *British Medical Journal*.)

331

Therapeutic applications

Table 12.2 Percentage reductions (standard deviations) in odds of specified end-points in different groups of patients (Antiplatelet Trialists Collaboration, 1988)

End-point	Prior cerebro-vascular disease (13 trials)	Prior MI (10 trials)	Recent unstable angina (2 trials)	Any history (25 trials)
Non-fatal MI	35 (12)	31 (5)	35 (17)	32 (5)
Non-fatal stroke	22 (7)	42 (11)	-	27 (6)
All vascular deaths	15 (7)	13 (5)	37 (19)	15 (4)
Any vascular event	22 (5)	22 (4)	36 (13)	25 (3)

For details of aspirin doses, Table 12.1.

the overall reduction was 15%, and highly significant ($P<0.0003$) though apparently smaller than the effect for non-fatal events. Adjustment for the imbalances in AMIS (already referred to) suggests a reduction of 17% rather than 15%. The reason for the quantitative difference between the reductions for non-fatal events and vascular deaths is uncertain. A possible explanation is that some patients in the trials covered by the reviews were taken off aspirin shortly before they died, while others, in the placebo groups, may nevertheless have been given aspirin for one reason or another. Either or both of these effects would result in an under-estimate of the true benefits attributable to aspirin and, on this basis, the ATC review suggested that the reduction in vascular deaths that is really due to aspirin may be about 20%.

There was no clear effect of aspirin on mortality from non-vascular causes, there being 280 such deaths observed compared with 287.3 expected. There was a reduction attributable to aspirin in mortality from all causes, bearing in mind that there were 2431 vascular deaths compared with only 497 non-vascular deaths. While significant ($P<0.0001$), this reduction is not quantified in the reviews, which emphasized the importance of concentrating on clinical events whose course might be modified by aspirin, having first established that there is no evidence of a harmful effect on other disease processes. Because there were relatively few non-vascular deaths, the reduction in mortality from all causes will have been only a little less than the 15% reduction in vascular deaths.

Figure 12.3, also from the ATC review, summarizes the findings on aspirin dose and on the other platelet-active agents considered. The direct comparisons are those where aspirin on its own was compared with either sulphinpyrazone or aspirin and dipyridamole within the same trials. The indirect comparisons do involve comparing effects in

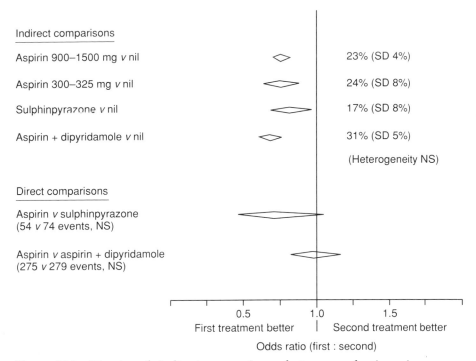

Figure 12.3 Direct and indirect comparisons between reductions in new vascular event rates (first stroke, myocardial infarction, or vascular death) with different antiplatelet agents. Unfilled symbols show 95% confidence intervals for typical odds ratios. (Reproduced from Antiplatelet Trialists Collaboration, 1988, with permission of authors and *British Medical Journal*.)

different trials using different doses or different agents. The direct comparisons, in particular, are based on relatively small numbers of events and neither is statistically significant at a conventional level. It is possible that aspirin is more effective than sulphinpyrazone. There is no reason to believe that aspirin combined with dipyridamole is more effective than aspirin. From the indirect comparisons, there is no evidence that higher aspirin doses are more or less effective than lower doses or that sulphinpyrazone or the combination of aspirin and dipyridamole are more effective than aspirin alone.

How long treatment (for practical purposes, aspirin in a dose of not more than 325 mg daily) should be used is, the review pointed out, still an open question.

The ATC review presented estimates, summarized in Table 12.3, of the absolute numbers of vascular events that might be avoided by platelet active agents used by a hundred people for 2 years. As the review pointed out, 'what matters most is not whether the proportional reduction is 15 or 20% but whether the absolute risk is high (for example, 25% dead within 2 years) or low (5% dead within 2 years)'. For this reason, the number of events saved in primary prevention (i.e. those with no previous history of vascular disease), who are at relatively low absolute risk, is considerably smaller than the number of events avoided in those who have already had events such as MI whose absolute risk of recurrence is very much higher. This consideration emphasizes the importance of trying to identify those at particularly high risk in primary prevention trials, a point covered in further detail later on.

Finally, returning briefly to pathological considerations, a very recent angiographic study (Chesebro et al., 1989) has shown that the combination of aspirin (975 mg daily) and dipyridamole (225 mg daily) reduces the rate of formation of new coronary artery lesions but not the progression of established lesions.

12.3.2 Acute MI

Patients in the secondary prevention trials already reviewed were recruited at varying intervals after acute MI. These trials therefore provide no evidence about aspirin in the acute phase. One trial (Elwood and Williams, 1979) involving a single aspirin tablet at the onset of symptoms of possible infarction was too small to clarify the value or otherwise of aspirin at a very early stage. The second International Study in Infarct Survival, ISIS-2 (ISIS-2 Collaborative

Table 12.3 Approximate numbers of vascular events avoidable by treatment of 100 people for 2 years with aspirin (Antiplatelet Trialists Collaboration, 1988)

Circumstances	Events avoided	
	Fatal	*Other*
History of TIA, minor stroke or unstable angina	1	2
Recent myocardial infarction	2	3
No history of vascular disease (primary prevention)		
At ages 55 – 64	0.1	0.2
65 – 74	0.2	0.4

For details of doses of aspirin, Table 12.1.

Group, 1988), recruited 17 187 patients thought to be within 24 h of the onset of symptoms of suspected MI who had no clear indication for or against streptokinase or aspirin. In fact, 98% of the patients showed some electrocardiographic abnormality. The trial's design was factorial, i.e. there were four treatment groups, one receiving active streptokinase and placebo aspirin, another receiving active aspirin and placebo streptokinase, one receiving both active treatments and one receiving both placebo streptokinase and placebo aspirin. The dose of streptokinase was 1.5 MU given in an infusion over about an hour. Aspirin was given as an enteric-coated preparation in a dose of 162.5 mg, the first tablet being crushed, sucked or chewed to ensure a rapid effect. It is likely that compliance with aspirin was between 90 and 95%. (For reasons explained in more detail later on, it should also be noted that anticoagulants were planned as part of standard care for over 11 000 patients.) The main results were based on vascular deaths occurring during the first 5 weeks, although estimates of survival at 12 and 24 months were also given and showed only marginal convergence or divergence of the trends established at 5 weeks.

The main results of ISIS-2 are summarized in Fig. 12.4. They represent a reduction of 23% ($P<0.0001$) in the odds of death attributable to aspirin, the 95% confidence interval ranging from 15% to 30%. (To be precise, the figure of 23% is based on mortality in all those treated with aspirin, whether or not they also received streptokinase, compared with all those not receiving aspirin, whether they received streptokinase or not. By comparison with Fig. 12.4, the inclusion in the analyses of those receiving streptokinase gave percentages of 11.8% and 9.4% in those on active and placebo aspirin, respectively.) There were 25 non-vascular deaths in those receiving aspirin compared with 39 such deaths in those on placebo aspirin, the consequent reduction in mortality from all causes being significant ($P<0.001$). By contrast with streptokinase, whose beneficial effect was greater the sooner it was used, aspirin conferred a similar benefit among those starting treatment early and late – for example, the odds reduction in those starting treatment within 4 h of the onset of symptoms was 25%, compared with 21% in those starting treatment between 13 and 24 h after the onset of symptoms. In 1000 patients, aspirin probably prevented 25 deaths and between 10 and 15 non-fatal episodes of reinfarction or stroke during the first month and is likely to have prevented a further 20 fatal and 30 non-fatal episodes within 2 or 3 years.

Serious side effects in ISIS-2, principally bleeding, were mostly due to streptokinase. There was no difference in the proportion of patients, 0.4% in both those receiving active and placebo aspirin, who needed transfusion after episodes of bleeding, although minor episodes, i.e.

335

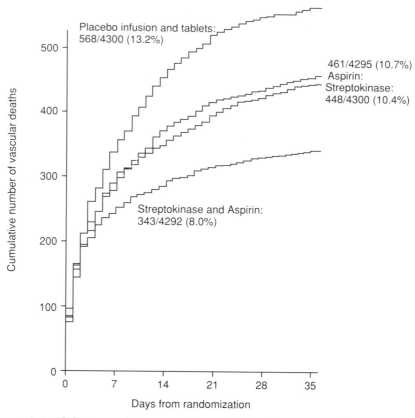

Figure 12.4 ISIS-2; cumulative vascular mortality after suspected acute myocardial infarction. (Reproduced from ISIS-2, 1988, with permission of authors and *Lancet*.)

those not requiring transfusion, did occur significantly more frequently ($P<0.01$) in those on active aspirin. Table 12.4 summarizes the ISIS-2 findings on stroke. There was no evidence of a significant excess of cerebral haemorrhage in those receiving aspirin (by contrast with a definite increase in haemorrhagic strokes due to streptokinase), a point of some importance in considering the results of the primary prevention trials (see below). There were significant reductions in reinfarction ($P<0.00001$) and in cardiac arrest ($P<0.01$) attributable to aspirin.

Figure 12.4 also makes clear the additive effects of aspirin and streptokinase, very strongly suggesting that modification of both platelet activity and of coagulability is more effective in preventing thrombosis than either modification on its own. This finding provides an important starting point for one of the primary prevention trials discussed later.

Table 12.4 Numbers of strokes in ISIS-2 (1988)

	Aspirin (162.5 mg daily)	
	Active N:8587	Placebo N:8600
By aetiology		
Confirmed haemorrhage*	5	2
Other, day 0-1	11	22
Other, after day 1	31	57
Total†	47	81
By outcome		
Died	20	30
Disabled	17	23
Not disabled	10	28
Total†	47	81

*All 7 events probably due to streptokinase.
†$P<0.01$

Another recent trial (not included in the ATC overview) recruited 796 men with unstable coronary artery disease into a factorial trial of 75 mg aspirin daily and intermittent intravenous heparin (RISC Group, 1990). The effect (if any) of heparin was marginal. Aspirin reduced the risk of MI and death by some 60%. This trial clearly supports the value of aspirin in unstable coronary disease demonstrated by the two trials in the ATC overview (Tables 12.1 and 12.2; Fig. 12.2). More generally, the trial's results do again raise the question of whether low doses may indeed be particularly effective because of their beneficial effect on the balance between thromboxane and prostacyclin.

The third international study in Infarct Survival, ISIS-3 (ISIS-3, 1992) on 41,299 patients demonstrated no extra benefit on 35 day or 6 month survival by the addition of heparin to 162 mg day [1] aspirin.

12.3.3 Primary Prevention

Two trials have now reported on aspirin in primary prevention, i.e. the prevention of clinical episodes in those who have not so far experienced these. Both were carried out on male doctors, British or American.

The British trial (Peto *et al.*, 1988) recruited healthy male doctors. Some 20 000 doctors were initially approached. Most were willing to take part but many were ineligible because they were already taking aspirin for one reason or another or gave histories of peptic ulceration, stroke or MI in the past. Nearly half the 5139 doctors eventually entered were under the age of 60. Two thirds were randomly allocated to take 500 mg ordinary, soluble or effervescent aspirin, whichever they preferred, or, if they later asked for it, 300 mg enteric-coated aspirin daily, while the remaining third were randomly allocated to avoid aspirin unless some specific indication for it developed. Treatment was therefore not blind.

In the first year, 661 (19%) of the 3429 doctors allocated to aspirin treatment stopped taking it and during the subsequent 5 years a further 5% stopped each year. In the group allocated to avoid aspirin, about 2% began using it in each year of the study. 'Effectively, therefore, the study assessed the effects of about two-thirds more of the treated than control group taking aspirin regularly.'

During the six or so years of follow up, there were 137 deaths from heart disease and 121 confirmed non-fatal MIs. The main results are summarized in Table 12.5. Death and incidence rates for MI were very similar, suggesting no obvious benefit attributable to aspirin. However, the 95% confidence interval for the effect of aspirin on MI (fatal and non-fatal combined) ranged from 24% more to about 27% fewer events associated with treatment. Aspirin approximately halved the frequency of transient cerebral ischaemic attacks but there was a small, non-significant excess of strokes in those allocated aspirin, with similar patterns for fatal and non-fatal events. The 95% confidence interval for the difference in stroke rates was also wide, ranging from a 25% reduction to a 50% increase. There may have been slightly more disabling strokes in those allocated aspirin, possibly due to haemorrhage. It is, however, important to bear in mind that the lack of a placebo controlled group may have introduced biases into the assessment of the occurrence and consequences of the non-fatal events. There were 15% fewer non-vascular deaths in the aspirin than in the control group, though this difference was not significant at a conventional level. Overall vascular death rates (including sudden death from unknown causes and bleeding from peptic ulcer) were 6% lower in the aspirin treated group.

The Physicians' Health Study in the USA was based on male doctors aged between 40 and 84 in 1982. It evaluated two agents in a factorial design – aspirin in a dose of 325 mg on alternate days for its effects on cardiovascular disease and β-carotene for the prevention of cancer. Thus, there were four treatment groups – one on active aspirin and placebo carotene, one on placebo aspirin and active carotene, one taking both active agents and one taking both placebos. The aspirin component of the trial includes all those recruited, whether or not they were taking carotene, since in both those on active aspirin and on placebo aspirin, half were taking active and half placebo carotene. To begin with, invitations were sent to over a quarter of a million doctors, of whom just over 112 000 responded. Nearly 60 000 were willing to participate in the trial. These doctors were then excluded if they had previously had an MI or cerebrovascular disease and for a variety of other reasons, including current use of aspirin. A total of 33 223 doctors

Table 12.5 Main results of primary prevention trial in British doctors: death and non-fatal event rates per 10000 man-years (Peto *et al.*, 1988)

	Aspirin group (usually 500 mg daily)	Control group
Death rates		
Myocardial infarction	47.3	49.6
Stroke		
haemorrhagic	5.3	4.2
occlusive	4.3	3.2
aetiology unknown	6.4	5.3
Other vascular causes	15.4	21.2
Non-vascular causes	64.8	76.0
Total	143.5	159.5
Non-fatal event rates		
Myocardial infarction		
confirmed	42.5	43.3
possible	11.7	4.2
*Stroke, confirmed	32.4	28.5
probably haemorrhagic	1.6	2.1
probably occlusive	6.9	4.2
aetiology unkown	23.9	22.2
Stroke, possible	3.2	3.2
Transient ischaemic attack		
confirmed†	15.9	27.5
possible†	5.3	14.8
Non-cerebral bleeding	10.6	7.4
Peptic ulcer†	46.8	29.6
Malignant neoplasm	63.2	61.2
Migraine‡	197.1	276.7
Musculo-skeletal disorders‡	544.1	639.9

*Rates of confirmed strokes that were disabling were 19.1 and 7.4 ($p<0.05$) in aspirin and control groups respectively.
†$P < 0.05$.
‡$P < 0.01$

Table 12.6 Main results of primary prevention trial in American doctors: numbers of events (Physicians Health Study Research group, 1989)

	Aspirin (325 mg on alternate days)	
	Active	Placebo
Myocardial infarction		
Fatal*	10	26
Non-fatal†	129	213
Total†	139	239
Stroke		
Fatal	9	6
Non-fatal	110	92
Total	119	98

*$p = 0.007$.
†$p < 0.00001$.
There were 55 500 (approx) person-years of observation in each of the two treatment groups.

were eligible according to the criteria and were enrolled in a preliminary study, during which they were all given active aspirin (and the carotene placebo). After about 18 weeks, those who had changed their minds about participation or shown inadequate compliance were excluded. As a result, 22 071 doctors entered the trial. Clearly, they formed a highly selected group. Instead of the 733 cardiovascular deaths expected, only 88 were confirmed during first 4.8 years of the scheduled 8 years follow-up.

The trial's Data Monitoring Board recommended an early end to the aspirin component of the trial because of the clearly beneficial effects on MI and because the very low cardiovascular risk status of the trial group meant that definitive results on the main end-point, cardiovascular mortality, could not be established until well beyond the scheduled date of termination of the trial. The Steering Committee accepted the Board's recommendation.

The preliminary findings were published in 1988 (Physicians' Health Study Research Group, 1988). The final results were published in 1989 (Physicians' Health Study Research Group, 1989). In between these two publications, representatives of the British and American doctors' trial groups presented an overview of the combined results of both trials (Hennekens et al., 1988), using data from the first of the two American reports. They presented an updated overview (Hennekens et al., 1989) after the final results from the American trial.

The main results of the American trial are summarized in Table 12.6. Aspirin reduced the incidence of both fatal and non-fatal MI, the reduction in risk for both combined being 44%. There were in fact more strokes in those receiving aspirin than placebo, though the difference was not statistically significant.

There was no difference between the actively treated and placebo groups in total cardiovascular mortality, the benefit for MI being offset by somewhat higher numbers in the actively treated group of sudden deaths not obviously due to MI and due to other cardiovascular causes. The addition of sudden death (ICD 798) to fatal events coded as ischaemic heart disease (ICD 410–414) gave 56 deaths in the aspirin group (22 sudden) and 65 in the placebo group (12 sudden), a difference that was not statistically significant. Combining non-fatal MI, non-fatal stroke and death from any cardiovascular cause to indicate 'important vascular events', there were 307 events in those on aspirin compared with 370 in those on placebo, a statistically significant reduction of 18% ($P=0.01$). There were 217 deaths from all causes in the actively treated group compared with 227 in the placebo group.

Two risk factors, age and the blood cholesterol level, appeared to modify the effects of aspirin. Thus, the benefit attributable to aspirin was mainly seen in those aged over 50 and, while benefit was apparent at all cholesterol levels, it appeared greatest at lower levels.

The obvious difference between the British and American trials is the apparent ineffectiveness of aspirin against MI in the former contrasting with the very clear effect in the latter. The overviews (Hennekens et al., 1988, 1989) considered the higher dose of aspirin, the absence of placebo tablets and lower compliance (and other contrasts) in the British trial as possible explanations. Since aspirin doses of 300 mg or more are clearly effective in secondary prevention, it seems unlikely that the dose (500 mg in most cases) used in the British doctors' trial would be ineffective unless there is some unidentified pathological difference between first and recurrent episodes of MI and/or in the way aspirin acts in these two situations. While compliance was indeed lower in the British trial, there was still a very substantial difference between the proportions taking aspirin in the two groups. The overview therefore considered the possibility that the discrepancy between the two results was due to chance and the results were combined (Fig. 12.5). This suggests a 32% reduction in the odds of non-fatal MI attributable to aspirin, an increase (if anything) of 18% in non-fatal stroke and very little if any effect on vascular death. For MI, there was significant heterogeneity between the two trials, raising the possibility that their separate findings do indicate effectiveness in the American study, and ineffectiveness in the British, for whatever reasons. However, the test

Therapeutic applications

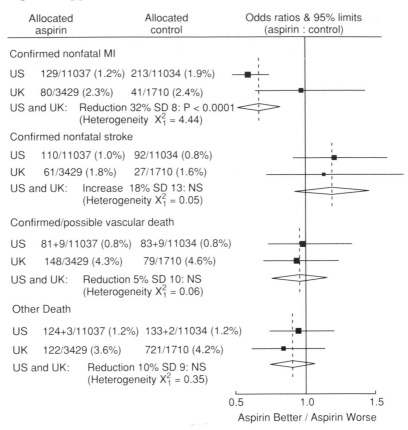

Figure 12.5 Overview of US and UK primary prevention trial results for four end points, odd ratios (aspirin versus control), overall risk reductions, and heterogeneity tests (sum of four heterogeneity X^2 tests = 4.9, NS). For further details, original publication (Hennekens *et al.*, 1989). Symbols, etc, as in Fig. 12.2. (Reproduced with permission of authors and *Circulation* and American Heart Association, Inc.)

for heterogeneity in all four of the outcomes in Fig. 12.5 was not significant.

The absence of any obvious effect of aspirin on the incidence of stroke in the primary prevention trials (if anything, as already indicated, the effect was adverse) compared with the obvious benefit due to aspirin in the secondary prevention trials (already discussed) is also puzzling. It is true that the numbers of strokes in the primary prevention trials are less than those available for the ATC overview but they are by no means trivial. There is no obvious explanation for any differential effect of aspirin on stroke in the settings of secondary and primary prevention. Thrombosis is a frequent occurrence in those who have already had a clinically manifest episode of arterial disease but since a substantial majority of strokes in those so far free of arterial disease are also thrombotic, it is surprising that aspirin appears to confer no protection in this setting. The point must be kept under review for obvious clinical reasons and also for any unexpected indications about different pathogenetic pathways in the onset of stroke.

12.4 BLEEDING

Any benefits attributable to aspirin must, of course, be considered along with potential hazards, principally bleeding.

Cerebral haemorrhage is the most serious type of bleeding that may be due to aspirin. Evidence from the secondary prevention trials is fragmentary. Even in the United Kingdom Transient Ischaemic Attack aspirin trial (UK-TIA Study Group, 1988), few patients who had strokes after entry to the trial came to necropsy or had brain scans early enough to distinguish with certainty between infarction and primary intracerebral haemorrhage. Definite intracerebral haemorrhages occurred in three patients (one of whom died) in the placebo group compared with 13 (nine of whom died) in the combined aspirin treatment groups (the trial having compared 300 and 1200 mg aspirin with placebo treatment). This difference represents a two-fold increase in the odds of haemorrhage attributable to aspirin but it was not statistically significant ($P=0.2$) at a conventional level. The number of episodes in each group almost certainly under-represent the true situation since there may have been other cerebral haemorrhages causing strokes whose underlying pathology was not determined. While this uncertainty clearly influences the absolute incidence of cerebral haemorrhage possibly due to aspirin, it is unlikely to affect the relative risk. Tentatively, therefore, the 'worst case' assumption in secondary prevention is that aspirin may double the risk of cerebral haemorrhage. Since, however, the incidence of haemorrhage is substantially lower than that of cerebral infarction, the absolute as distinct from relative risk of cerebral haemorrhage has to be set against the undoubted reduction in secondary prevention in the risk of stroke as a whole and of MI and will usually be sufficiently low to justify the use of aspirin for the prevention of these much commoner events.

Tables 12.5 and 12.7 show results on possible cerebral haemorrhage from the two primary prevention trials. In the British trial, there may have been about one more fatal haemorrhagic stroke per 10 000 man-years in those taking aspirin. For non-fatal strokes, there was, at face value a slightly lower incidence of 'probably haemorrhagic' stroke in those taking aspirin. There was, however, a significant excess of 'disabling' stroke in those taking aspirin, though, as the trial report itself points out, the difference may be due to bias in assessing the extent of residual disability after stroke. In the subgroup experiencing haemorrhagic stroke in the American trial, there was an increased risk associated with aspirin that was of borderline statistical significance. There were about 55 000 person-years of observation in each of the aspirin treated and placebo groups. There may, therefore, have been about two haemorrhagic strokes induced by aspirin per 10 000 person-years of observation (with the reservation, once again, that the difference for haemorrhagic stroke between those receiving aspirin or placebo treatment was of only borderline statistical significance). This potential hazard is considerably less than the benefit due to the reduction in MI though if only fatal MI is considered, the balance is more even. Against the possibility that aspirin increases the risk of cerebral haemorrhage in the primary prevention of MI is the lack of clear evidence that it does so in secondary prevention. As with the apparent difference between the two contexts for the effects of aspirin on strokes of whatever kind, it

Table 12.7 Incidence and outcome of different types of stroke in trial in American doctors: numbers of events (Physicians Health Study Research group, 1989)

| | Aspirin (325 mg on alternate days) | |
	Active	Placebo
Ischaemic		
Mild	69	91
Moderate, severe or fatal	21	20
Total	91	82
Haemorrhagic		
Mild	10	6
Moderate, severe or fatal	13	6
Total*	23	12
Unknown cause		
Mild	2	1
Moderate, severe or fatal	1	2
Total	5	4
Total	119	98

*$P = 0.06$.
Grand totals and sub-totals include 5 events of unknown severity.
There were 55 500 (approx.) person-years of observation in each of the two treatment groups.

seems implausible that its effects on cerebral haemorrhage would differ according to whether there has been a previous event. The uncertainty can really only be resolved by further data.

Though generally less serious than cerebral haemorrhage, gastrointestinal bleeding is another potential hazard the extent of which needs to be borne in mind. In the UK-TIA trial (UK-TIA Study Group, 1988) the proportions of patients requiring admission to hospital because of gastrointestinal bleeding were 0.9%, 1.5% and 2.3% respectively in those receiving placebo treatment, 300 mg and 1200 mg aspirin daily. Corresponding figures for any gastrointestinal bleeding (i.e. requiring hospital admission or not) were 1.6%, 2.6% and 4.7%. Table 12.8 shows the findings from the US American primary prevention trial for a range of potential side effects, including gastrointestinal bleeding. There was a clear excess of melaena in those receiving aspirin. Apart from (perhaps even including) this finding, the results may not be unduly worrying although the relatively low dose of aspirin used and the highly selected nature of the trial participants should be remembered.

12.5 CONCLUSION: PRESENT AND FUTURE IMPLICATIONS

With the convincing demonstration that aspirin substantially lowers the recurrence rate in those who have survived at least one MI, its use is rapidly becoming part of routine clinical practice. For example, more than 85% of those in the American primary prevention trial who sustained an MI during the trial decided to take aspirin to reduce the risk of further events. The same trend is occurring in the UK (Collins and Julian, 1991) and in other countries. This development raises two related questions. One concerns the appropriate dose of aspirin, the other the avoidance of bleeding. There is no evidence that more than 325 mg aspirin daily confers greater benefit that this dose, i.e. one conventional tablet a day. The indications of the US Physicians' Health Study and of the ISIS-2 trial are that 160 mg daily is adequate. It is likely that 75 mg or less is effective (RISC Group, 1990; SALT Collaborative Group, 1991; Dutch TIA Trial Study Group, 1991). The lower the dose, the smaller the risk of bleeding, certainly from the gastrointestinal tract. An obvious danger is that the use of aspirin in routine clinical practice will be less closely monitored than in trials, not only for evidence of bleeding and other unwanted effects but also over the selection of patients in the first place. Aspirin can be purchased without a prescription. The publicity surrounding its use for the prevention of arterial disease has already encouraged some patients to take aspirin on their own initiative, a tendency that is almost certain to increase. But the understandable and justified enthusiasm for aspirin that now exists must not be allowed to

Therapeutic applications

Table 12.8 Unwanted events in trial in American doctors: numbers of events (and % experiencing events) (Physicians Health Study Research Group, 1989)

| | Aspirin (325 mg on alternate days) | |
	Active	Placebo
Gastrointestinal symptoms		
Discomfort	2882(26.1)	2823(256)
Other non-infectious disorders*	345(3.1)	288(2.6)
Ulcers		
Gastric	25(0.2)	15(0.1)
Duodenal*	46(0.4)	27(0.2)
Peptic	156(1.4)	129(1.2)
Bleeding		
Easy bruising†	1587(14.4)	1027(9.3)
Haematemesis	38(0.3)	28(0.3)
Melaena†	364(3.3)	246(2.2)
Epistaxis†	862(7.8)	640(5.8)
Other§‡	724(6.6)	596(5.4)

*$P = 0.03$.
†$P < 0.0001$.
‡$P = 0.0004$.
§ Including haematuria and related to shaving or brushing teeth.

obscure its potential hazards. The further use of aspirin in secondary prevention should, therefore, be accompanied by increasing awareness of the need to identify those for whom it may be contraindicated and, in those who do take it, watchfulness for changing circumstances calling for a review of its use.

Turning to primary prevention, the low risk of MI in the two primary prevention trials, particularly in the American trial, has already been referred to. The aspirin doses in both trials were larger than the substantially lower doses, of between about 40 and 80 mg daily, needed for near maximal inhibition of thromboxane production. We do not, therefore, yet know what the benefits and hazards would be of low dose aspirin in men at particularly high risk of MI, and what the balance between benefits and hazards in this group is, including, among the latter, effects of low doses on cerebral haemorrhage. It is important to settle these points before aspirin for primary prevention passes into routine practice. Another question, identified at the beginning of this chapter and whose relevance is reinforced by the results of the ISIS-2 trial, is the extent to which the simultaneous modification of platelet function and fibrin formation may reduce the risk of MI, bearing in mind that many coronary artery thrombi are a mixture of platelet aggregates and fibrin. (If anything (EPSIM Research Group, 1982), anticoagulants on their own may be more effective than aspirin alone). These points – the value of low dose aspirin in high risk men and of simultaneously modifying platelet function and fibrin formation – are under study in the Thrombosis Prevention Trial (TPT) (Meade et al., 1992). This is being carried out through about 100 general practices in the UK in 6000 men so far free of clinically manifest IHD but at substantially increased risk, calculated from information on family history, smoking history, body mass index, blood pressure and blood cholesterol, factor VII activity and fibrinogen levels. Those in the top 20% of the risk score distribution are entered into the trial provided there are no contraindications to aspirin or warfarin. The design of the trial is factorial and double-blind. One group receives active warfarin and placebo aspirin, one active aspirin and placebo warfarin, one both active aspirin and active warfarin and one placebo aspirin and placebo warfarin. The dose of aspirin is 75 mg in a controlled release formulation. The level of oral anticoagulation aimed for is an International Normalized Ratio (INR) of about 1.5. At the low aspirin dose and low INR being used, it may be possible to secure any benefits of combined treatment without an unacceptable incidence of serious bleeding. There is some evidence to support this view. In the ISIS-2 trial, for example, anticoagulation was planned and in most cases implemented for over 11 000 of the 17 187 patients recruited, either as heparin alone, or as heparin and oral anticoagulation or as oral anticoagulation on its own. Among this group, half received active aspirin and half received placebo aspirin. (Active and placebo streptokinase were equally distributed between those on active and placebo aspirin, so the effects of streptokinase can be disregarded.) Major episodes of bleeding, i.e. those requiring transfusion, occurred in 0.4% of those receiving aspirin and also 0.4% of those on placebo aspirin. Major and/or minor episodes occurred in 3.3% of those on aspirin, compared with 2.5% of those on placebo aspirin (ISIS-2 Collaborative Group: personal communication). While there was, therefore, an excess of minor bleeding episodes in those receiving anticoagulants and aspirin compared with those on anticoagulants only, there was no difference in the case of major episodes. In a special study designed to investigate the effects on gastric bleeding of the proposed TPT treatments, warfarin (in doses sufficient to raise the INR to about 1.5) caused no detectable excess, aspirin (75 mg daily) caused a small increase though, as expected, very much less than conventional doses, while the combination caused no more bleeding than could be attributed to the aspirin component on its own (Prichard et al., 1989).

Therapeutic applications

In summary, there is little doubt that in the immediate management of suspected or confirmed MI, patients should take half a tablet (160 mg) of aspirin at once, preferably sucked or chewed, followed by half a tablet (swallowed) daily for at least 5 weeks. For the subsequent, i.e. secondary, prevention of MI, one tablet of aspirin should be taken daily, probably indefinitely. It is difficult to give unequivocal advice about the use of aspirin for the primary prevention of MI, in the light of the rather different indications of the two primary prevention trials and the more even balance between any reduction in the risk of MI due to aspirin, on the one hand, and the possibility of an increased risk of cerebral haemorrhage, on the other. At least one commentator has concluded that there is at present no case for the generalized use of aspirin for primary prevention in apparently healthy people (de Gaetano, 1988). Whether clearer guidance can eventually be given depends on the effects of low dose aspirin, both on MI and on different types of stroke, in high risk men among whom the clinical benefit–hazard balance may differ substantially from the less certain picture emerging from the trials in low risk men.

12.6 ANNOTATION ON VENOUS THROMBOSIS

It is generally considered that aspirin is largely ineffective for the prevention of venous thrombosis, one reason being the less extensive involvement of platelets in venous than arterial thrombi. A recent review (Hirsh and Levine, 1989) suggested that aspirin may achieve a reduction of about 13% in the risk of venous thrombosis after hip surgery, a setting in which many consider aspirin is likely to have its most obvious effect on venous thrombosis. By implication, therefore, it would have less effect in other contexts. Even in hip surgery, however, the use of aspirin has not been widely adopted because of the much greater benefits – so it has been assumed – attributable to heparin and oral anticoagulants. (In British practice, the use of anti-thrombotic agents of any kind for the prevention of post-operative venous thrombosis is at a low level.)

Very recently, the position has changed dramatically as the result of further work from the Antiplatelet Trialists Collaboration (ATC) which now includes an overview of aspirin for the prevention of venous thrombosis based on the results of 51 trials covering 7945 patients. In summary, aspirin reduces the incidence of deep vein thrombosis by between 30% and 40% and of pulmonary embolism by between 60% and 70%. The magnitude of this effect is similar in the different settings of general surgery, trauma surgery, orthopaedic surgery and of medical conditions.

348

Apart from its convincing demonstration of the value of the overview approach, this particular ATC analysis has revealed what may be a major misconception in medical practice and has now started its correction. Because aspirin is easier to administer and manage than heparin or oral anticoagulants, it is likely to replace these agents for the prevention of venous thrombosis where they are currently used and to encourage its adoption and use as effective prophylaxis in countries such as the UK where, as already indicated, the prevention of venous thrombosis by anti-thrombotic measures is not widely practised anyway.

The full results of the most recent ATC overview will probably be published in 1992. Meanwhile, I am grateful to the Collaboration for permission to use this summary of the results in this chapter.

REFERENCES

Acheson, J., Danta, G. and Hutchison, E.C. (1969) Controlled trial of dipyrida-mole in cerebral vascular disease (abstract). *Brit. Med. J.*, **1**, 614–15.

Antiplatelet Trialists Collaboration (1988) Secondary prevention of vascular disease by prolonged antiplatelet treatment. *Brit. Med. J.*, **296**, 320–31.

Armitage, P. (1980) Clinical trials in the secondary prevention of myocardial infarction and stroke. *Thromb. Haemostasis*, **43**, 90–4.

Aspirin Myocardial Infarction Study Research Group (1980) A randomized, controlled trial of aspirin in persons recovered from myocardial infarction. *JAMA*, **243**, 661–9.

Barnett, H.J.M., Gent, M. and Sackett, D.L. and the Canadian Cooperative Study Group (1978) A randomized trial of aspirin and sulfinpyrazone in threatened stroke. *N. Engl. J. Med.*, **299**, 53–9.

Blakely, J.A. (1979) A prospective trial of sulphinpyrazone and survival after thrombotic stroke (abstract). *Thromb. Diathesis Haemorrhag.*, **42**, 161.

Boston Collaborative Drug Surveillance Group (1974) Regular aspirin intake and acute myocardial infarction. *Brit. Med. J.*, **1**, 440–3.

Bousser, M.G., Eschwege, E., Haguenau, M. *et al* (1981) Essai cooperatif controle 'AICLA': Prevention secondaire des accidents ischemiques cerebraux lies a l'atherosclerose par l'aspirine et le dipyridamole. *Rev. Neurol. (Paris)*, **5**, 333–41.

Bousser, M.G., Eschwege, E. and Haguenau, M. (1983) 'AICLA' controlled trial of aspirin and dypridamole in the secondary prevention of atherothrom-botic cerebral ischemia. *Stroke*, **14**, 5 14.

Breddin, K., Loew, D., Lechner, K. *et al.* (1980) Secondary prevention of myocardial infarction: A comparison of acetylsalicylic acid, placebo and phenprocoumon. *Haemostasis*, **9**, 325–44.

Britton, M., Helmers, C. and Samuelsson, K. (1986) High dose salicylic acid after cerebral infarction (abstract). *Stroke*, **17**, 132.

Britton, M., Helmers, C. and Samuelsson, K. (1987) High dose acetylsalicylic acid after cerebral infarction: A Swedish co-operative study. *Stroke*, **18**, 325–34.

Therapeutic applications

Cairns, J.A., Gent, M., Singer, J. et al. (1985) Aspirin, sulfinpyrazone or both in unstable angina. N. Engl. J. Med., 313, 1369–75.

Chandler, A.B., Chapman, I., Erhardt, L.R. et al. (1974) Coronary thrombosis in myocardial infarction. Am. J. Cardiol., 34, 823–33.

Chesebro, J.H., Webster, M.W.I., Smith, H.C. et al. (1989) Antiplatelet therapy in coronary disease progression, reduced infarction and new lesion formation. Circulation, Suppl. II, 80, 1060.

Collins, R. and Julian, D.J. (1991) British Heart Foundation Surveys (1987 and 1989) of United Kingdom treatment policies for acute myocardial infarction. Brit. Heart J., 66, 250–5.

Coronary Drug Project Research Group (1976) Aspirin in coronary heart disease. J. Chron. Dis., 29, 625–42.

Dantzig, J.M. van and Becker, A.E. (1986) Sudden cardiac death and acute pathology of coronary arteries. Eur. Heart J., 7, 987–91.

Davies, M.J. (1987) Thrombosis in acute myocardial infarction and sudden death. In Thrombosis and Platelets in Myocardial Ischemia (eds J.L. Mehta, C.R. Conti and A.N. Brest), F.A. Davis Company, Philadelphia, pp. 151–9.

Davies, M.J. and Thomas, A. (1984) Thrombosis and acute coronary-artery lesions in sudden cardiac ischemic death. N. Engl. J. Med., 310, 1137–40.

Davies, M.J. and Thomas, A.C. (1985) Plaque fissuring – the cause of acute myocardial infarction, sudden ischaemic death, and crescendo angina. Brit. Heart J., 53, 363–73.

de Gaetano, G.D. (1988) Primary prevention of vascular disease by aspirin. Lancet, i, 1093–4.

DeWood, M.A., Spores, J., Notske, R. et al. (1980) Prevalence of total coronary occlusion during the early hours of transmural myocardial infarction. N. Engl. J. Med., 303, 897–902.

Duguid, J.B. (1970) Thrombosis as a factor in the pathogenesis of coronary atherosclerosis. J. Pathol., 58, 202–12.

Dutch TIA Trial Study Group (1991) A comparison of two doses of aspirin (30 mg vs. 283 mg a day) in patients after a transient ischemic attack or minor ischemic stroke. New Engl. J. Med., 325, 1261–6.

El Fawal, M.A., Berg, G.A., Wheatley, D.J. and Harland, W.A. (1987) Sudden coronary death in Glasgow: nature and frequency of acute coronary lesions. Brit. Heart J., 57, 329–35.

Elwood, P.C. (1981) Trial of acetylsalicylic acid in the secondary prevention of mortality from myocardial infarction. Brit. Med. J., 282, 481.

Elwood, P.C. and Sweetnam, P.M. (1979) Aspirin and secondary mortality after myocardial infarction. Lancet, ii, 1313–15.

Elwood, P.C. and Williams, W.O. (1979) A randomized controlled trial of aspirin in the prevention of early mortality in myocardial infarction. J.R. Coll. Gen. Practit., 29, 413–16.

Elwood, P.C., Cochrane, A.L., Burr, M.L. et al. (1974) A randomized controlled trial of acetylsalicylic acid in the secondary prevention of mortality from myocardial infarction. Brit. Med. J., 1, 436–40.

EPSIM Research Group (1982) A controlled comparison of aspirin and oral anticoagulants in prevention of death after myocardial infarction. N. Engl. J. Med., 12, 701–8.

Falk, E. (1987) Thrombosis in unstable angina: pathologic aspect. In Thrombosis *and Platelets in Myocardial Ischemia* (eds J.L. Mehta C.R. Conti A.N. Brest), F.A. Davis Company, Philadelphia, pp. 137–49.

Fields, W.S., Lemak, N.A., Frankowski, R.F. and Hardy, R.J. (1977) Controlled trial of aspirin in cerebral ischemia. *Stroke*, **8**, 301–16.

Fields, W.S., Lemak, N.A., Frankowski, R.F. and Hardy, R.J. (1978) Controlled trial of aspirin in cerebral ischemia. *Stroke*, **9**, 309–18.

Frink, R.J., Rooney, P.A. Jr, Trowbridge, J.O. and Rose, J. (1988) Coronary thrombosis and platelet/fibrin microemboli in death associated with acute myocardial infarction. *Brit. Heart J.*, **59**, 196–200.

Gent, M., Blakely, J.A., Hachinski, V. *et al.* (1985) A secondary prevention, randomized trial of suloctidil in patients with a recent history of thromboembolic stroke. *Stroke*, **16**, 416–23.

Guiraud-Chaumeil, B., Rascol, A., David, J. *et al.* (1982) Prevention des recidives des accidents vasculaires cerebraux ischemiques par les anti-aggregants plaquettaires. *Rev. Neurol. (Paris)*, **138**, 367–85.

Haerem, J.W. (1974) Mural platelet microthrombi and major acute lesions of main epicardial arteries in sudden coronary death. *Atherosclerosis*, **19**, 529–41.

Hammond, E.C. and Garfinkel, L. (1975) Aspirin and coronary heart disease: findings of a prospective study. *Brit. Med. J.*, **2**, 269–71.

Hennekens, C.H., Karlson, L.K. and Rosner, B. (1978) A case-control study of regular aspirin use and coronary deaths. *Circulation*, **58**, 35–8.

Hennekens, C.H., Peto, R., Hutchison, G.B. and Doll, R. (1988) An overview of the British and American aspirin studies. *N. Engl. J. Med.*, **318**, 923–6.

Hennekens, C.H., Buring, J.E., Sandercock, P. *et al.* (1989) Aspirin and other antiplatelet agents in the secondary and primary prevention of cardiovascular disease. *Circulation*, **80**, 749–56.

Hirsh, J. and Levine, M. (1989) Prevention of venous thrombosis in patients undergoing major orthopaedic surgical procedures. *Brit. J. Clin. Pract.*, Symposium Suppl., **65**, 2–8.

ISIS-2 (Second International Study of Infarct Survival) Collaborative Group (1988) Randomized trial of intravenous streptokinase, oral aspirin, both, or neither among 17 187 cases of suspected acute myocardial infarction *Lancet*, **ii**, 349–60.

ISIS-3 (Third International Study of Infarct Survival) Collaborative Group (1992) ISIS-3: a randomised comparison of streptokinase vs tissue plasminogen activator vs anistreplase and of aspirin plus heparin vs aspirin alone among 4/299 cases of suspected acute myocardial infarction. *Lancet*, **339**, 753–70.

Jick, H. and Miettinen, O.S. (1976) Regular aspirin use and myocardial infarction. *Brit. Med. J.*, **1**, 1057.

Klimt, C.R., Knatterud, G.L., Stamler, J. and Meier, P. (1986) Persantine-aspirin reinfarction study, part II: Secondary prevention with persantine and aspirin. *J. Am. Coll. Cardiol.*, **7**, 251–69.

Krol, W.F. and the Persantine-Aspirin Reinfarction Study Research Group (1980) Persantine and aspirin in coronary heart disease. *Circulation*, **62**, 449–61.

Krol, W.F., Klimt, C.R., Morledge, J. *et al.* (1980) Persantine-aspirin reinfarction study: Design, methods and baseline results. *Circulation*, **62** (suppl. II), II-1-II-22.

Therapeutic applications

Lewis, H.D. Jr, Davis, J.W., Archibald, D.G. *et al*. (1983) Protective effects of aspirin against myocardial infarction and death in men with unstable angina: Results of a Veterans Administration cooperative study. *N. Engl. J. Med.*, **309**, 396–403.

Lowenthal, A., Dom. L., Moens, E. and the European Stroke Prevention Study Group (1987) European stroke prevention study: Principal end points. *Lancet*, **ii**, 1351–4.

Meade, T.W., Howarth, D.J., Stirling, Y. *et al*. (1984) Fibrinopeptide A and sudden coronary death. *Lancet*, **ii**, 607–9.

Meade, T.W., Roderick, P.J., Brennan, P.J. *et al*. (1992) Extra-cranial bleeding and other symptoms due to low dose aspirin and low intensity oral anticoagulation. *Thromb. Haemostasis* (in press).

Paganini-Hill, A., Chao, A., Ross, R.K. and Henderson, B.E. (1989) Aspirin use and chronic diseases: a cohort study of the elderly. *Brit. Med. J.*, **299**, 1247–50.

Peto, R., Gray, R., Collins, R. *et al*. (1988) Randomized trial of prophylactic daily aspirin in British male doctors. *Brit. Med. J.*, **296**, 313–16.

Physicians' Health Study Research Group (1988) Preliminary report: findings from the aspirin component of the ongoing Physicians' Health Study. *New Engl. J. Med.*, **318**, 262–4.

Physicians' Health Study Research Group (1989) Final report on the aspirin component of the ongoing Physicians' Health Study. *N. Engl. J. Med.*, **321**, 129–35.

Polli, E.E. and Cortellaro, M. (1983) The Auturan Reinfarction Study. In *Secondary Prevention of Ischaemic Cardiac Events: Present Status and New Perspectives* (eds E.E. Polli and M. Cortellaro), Hans Huber, Berne, pp. 51–60.

Polli, E., Cortellaro, M., Baroni, L. *et al*. (1982) Auturan Reinfarction Italian Study: Sulphinpyrazone in post-myocardial infarction. *Lancet*, **i**, 237–42.

Prichard, P.J., Kitchingman, G.K., Walt, R.P. *et al*. (1989) Human gastric mucosal bleeding induced by low dose aspirin, but not warfarin. *Brit. Med. J.*, **298**, 493–6.

Rapold, H.J., Haeberli, A., Kuemmerli, H. *et al*. (1989) Fibrin formation and platelet activation in patients with myocardial infarction and normal coronary arteries. *Eur. Heart J.*, **10**, 323–33.

Reuther, R. and Dorndorf, W. (1978) Aspirin in patients with cerebral ischaemia and normal angiograms: The results of a double blind trial. In *Acetylsalicylic Acid in Cerebral Ischaemia and Coronary Heart Disease* (eds K. Breddin, W. Dorndorf, D. Loew and R. Marx), Schattauer Verlag, Stuttgart, pp. 97–106.

RISC group (1990) Risk of myocardial infarction and death during treatment with low dose aspirin and intravenous heparin in men with unstable coronary artery disease. *Lancet*, **336**, 827–30.

Robertson, J.T., Dugdale, M., Salky, N. and Robinson, H. (1975) The effect of a platelet inhibiting drug in the therapy of patients with transient ischaemic attacks and strokes. *Thromb. Diathesis Haemorrhag.*, **34**, 598.

SALT Collaborative Group (1991) Swedish Aspirin Low-dose Trial (SALT) of 75 mg aspirin as secondary prophylaxis after cerebrovascular ischaemic events. *Lancet*, **338**, 1345–9.

Sherry, S., Gent, M., Lilienfeld, A. *et al*. (1980) Sulfinpyrazone in the prevention of sudden death after myocardial infarction. *N. Engl. J. Med.*, **302**, 250–6.

Sorensen, P.S., Pedersen, H. Marquardsen, J. *et al.* (1983) Acetyl-salicylic acid in the prevention of stroke in patients with reversible cerebral ischaemic attacks: A Danish cooperative study. *Stroke*, **14**, 15–22.

UK-TIA Study Group (1988) United Kingdom transient ischaemic attack (UK-TIA) aspirin trial: interim results. *Brit. Med. J.*, **296**, 316–20.

Vogel, G., Fischer, C, and Huyke, R. (1981) Prevention of reinfarction with acetylsalicylic acid. In *Prophylaxis of Venous, Peripheral, Cardiac and Cerebral Vascular Diseases with Acetylsalicylic Acid* (eds K. Breddin, D. Loew, K. Ueberla, W. Dorndorf, and R. Marx), Schattauer Verlag, Stuttgart, pp. 123–8.

Weiss, H.J. and Aledort, L.M. (1967) Impaired platelet/connective-tissue reaction in man after aspirin ingestion. *Lancet*, **ii**, 495–7.

13 *Aspirin in ischaemic stroke*

W.S. FIELDS and F. CLIFFORD ROSE

13.1 AETIOLOGY OF ISCHAEMIC STROKE

In order to understand the role which aspirin plays in the prevention of ischaemic stroke, it is essential to have an understanding of the pathogenetic mechanisms underlying this disorder. Chiari (1905) was the first to note that the distal end of the common carotid artery and proximal internal carotid artery were frequently the sites of severe atheromatous plaques. He noted that the internal carotid artery is a frequent site for thrombosis superimposed upon these plaques and, even more significantly, as a source for cerebral embolism, pointing out that in his autopsied cases the intracranial vessels were not diseased. This important concept escaped attention for the most part except for an article by Ramsay Hunt (1914) in which the syndrome of internal carotid artery occlusion was described. The object of his study was the importance of lesions in the main neck arteries in the causation of brain softening. He pointed out that the neck arteries should be checked for 'a possible diminution of sense of pulsation', and added, 'I would also particularly emphasize the occurrence of unilateral vascular changes, pallor, or atrophy of the disc with contralateral hemiplegia in obstruction of the carotid artery'. Regrettably, the findings of Chiari and Hunt received little attention for nearly 40 years, largely because the extracranial arteries were seldom examined *post mortem*. It was only the advent of angiography (Moniz, 1927) that allowed the condition of these arteries to be ascertained in the living patient and brought attention once again to obstructive lesions in the cervical region.

Once the importance of these lesions in the aetiology of ischaemic stroke became more widely recognized (Hutchinson and Yates, 1957), the warning symptoms of a threatened stroke came under scrutiny. Initially, these symptoms, to which the name 'transient ischaemic attacks' (TIA) was given, were thought to be a consequence of narrowing of the extracranial arteries and of haemodynamic origin, but the fact that they responded favourably to anticoagulant therapy made this hypothesis untenable and led to a better understanding of their arterial origin and presumed embolic nature (Barnett, 1975).

Prospective studies which clearly delineate the natural history of TIAs soon led to an appreciation of their seriousness. Millikan (1970) suggested that 4–10% of patients per year who have suffered TIAs will have a stroke or that in 5 years 25–40% will have had a catastrophic cerebral infarction. In another study Baker *et al.* (1962) indicated that 4% of patients suffering TIAs will die each year, mostly from vascular causes, about one-third of which will be stroke. A third study by Friedman *et al.* (1969) undertaken as a population survey in a California retirement community, indicated that 18% of those who developed TIAs would have a stroke within a follow-up period averaging 27 months.

Marshall and Wilkinson (1971) reported that, even with normal angiograms of the carotid artery on the side appropriate to the symptoms in TIA patients, the prognosis was still grave. This also applied when the transient episodes were confined to the retinal circulation in cases of *amaurosis fugax*.

Fisher (1951) was the first to establish a firm link between transient monocular blindness, ipsilateral hemispheric symptoms, and the condition of the carotid artery appropriate to those symptoms. He was also the first to suggest, after he had observed a patient with 'white bodies' passing through the retinal arterioles during an episode of *amaurosis fugax*, that cerebral microemboli might be of platelet origin. Nearly ten years later, Ross (1961) made a similar observation and determined that, following thrombo-endarterectomy of the appropriate carotid artery, the material adherent to the surface of the atherosclerotic plaque was made up of agglutinated platelets and that pliable material shed by the clot had gone downstream and produced transient cerebral and retinal attacks.

Gunning *et al.* (1964) reported a series of patients with cerebral and retinal lesions associated with athcromatous carotid lesions in the extracranial vessels, and demonstrated platelet-fibrin emboli in both the retinal and cerebral arteries. Two of their patients were noted to have the whitish material passing through the retinal arteries during attacks of monocular blindness.

Lougheed *et al.* (1966) studied specimens removed at endarterectomy and found collections of amorphous and presumably platelet-containing material on the surface of ulcerated lesions. Moore and Hall (1968) demonstrated similar material in irregular or ulcerated plaques in specimens removed at operation, including those without significant stenosis but with recurrent episodes of transient cerebral ischaemia which ceased after operation.

Of three cases of *amaurosis fugax* (Levine and Swanson, 1968; Singer,

1969; Mundall *et al.*, 1972) in which there was an association between idiopathic thrombocythaemia and clinical symptoms, there was cessation of the attacks following administration of aspirin in one (Mundall *et al.*, 1972). The dull yellow bodies, which had previously been observed passing through the retinal arterioles during attacks of monocular blindness, were no longer evident. Moreover, the spontaneous aggregation of platelets *in vitro*, even without the addition of a stimulus such as collagen, also ceased with aspirin therapy.

At the beginning of the 1970s, when arteriography became more frequently used in the diagnostic evaluation of patients with cerebrovascular symptoms, it became apparent that there was a clear-cut relationship between TIAs and stroke and ulcerated lesions in the extracranial vessels, particularly at the bifurcation of the common carotid artery (Gomensoro *et al.*, 1973). Ehrenfeld *et al.* (1966) reported 32 cases operated on for carotid lesions in the neck where the presenting complaint had been *amaurosis fugax*; in 18 of these, the internal surface of the carotid bulb was ulcerated and irregular. Kishore *et al.* (1971) undertook a radiographic assessment of the carotid and subclavian-vertebrobasilar arteries in 71 randomly selected patients whom they had seen during their participation in the Joint Study of Extracranial Arterial Occlusion; in 133 carotid arteries examined, there were 24 ulcers (16%) and 21 were completely occluded at the origin of the internal carotid artery.

Surgical experience during the past two decades has indicated that ulcers in carotid bifurcation lesions are far more common than can be demonstrated radiographically or by non-invasive ultrasonic methods (Harrison *et al.*, 1971). From specimens examined following thrombo-endarterectomy or at *post mortem* it is clear that these ulcers may be shallow and virtually undetectable pre-operatively (Moore and Hall, 1968).

It was these facts and clinical assumptions that led to the clinical trials of drugs known to affect platelet activity, either *in vitro* and/or *in vivo*. The rationale for undertaking such studies of antiplatelet drugs was based on the following factors (Barnett, 1975):

1. Cerebro-vascular disease is the third leading cause of death.
2. Cerebral infarction accounts for almost two-thirds of the fatalities from vascular diseases of the brain.
3. Cerebral infarction is frequently preceded by warning TIAs.
4. Once TIAs have occurred, there is a 4–10% risk of stroke each year thereafter.
5. Ulcerated atheromatous lesions in the extracranial arteries and platelet emboli which form on them, have aetiologic importance for TIAs.

356

6. Drugs having an effect on platelet function should be tested to determine their efficacy in the prevention of TIAs and reduction of subsequent stroke and mortality following the onset of TIAs.
7. Pre-thrombotic lesions produced experimentally in the femoral arteries of dogs (Weiss *et al.*, 1968) demonstrated the prophylactic efficacy of aspirin. Moreover, case reports by Mundall *et al.* (1972) and Harrison *et al.* (1971) clearly demonstrated the cessation of multiple attacks of *amaurosis fugax* following treatment with aspirin.

13.2 ASPIRIN AS AN ANTITHROMBOTIC AGENT

Aspirin, the drug which at present seems to be the best suited for use as an antithrombotic agent, has been available for nearly 100 years but it is only within the last 15 years that there has been any understanding of how it works. The story of aspirin begins with Felix Hoffmann, a German research chemist who set out in 1893 to find relief for his father's rheumatoid arthritis. Hoffmann's father found that he could not tolerate the stronger remedies of that day, all of which were dependent on salicylic acid, a chemical relative of 'salicin', an agent originally extracted from willow bark and later shown to be effective in reducing fever. Hoffmann explored contemporary pharmaceuticals looking for other salicin-related agents and finally came upon acetylsalicylic acid, which had been synthesized by another German chemist in 1853 but unappreciated at that time. He found a simpler and less expensive way to make acetylsalicylic acid which he then gave to his father who experienced relief for the first time in 10 years. Hoffmann suggested that his new drug be called 'A-salicin', but his employers at the pharmaceutical firm overruled him and the drug was christened 'Aspirin' when first put on the market in 1899. The name 'Aspirin' is today, with the exception of the USA and Canada, the trademark of the German company, Bayer AG. After the assets of the German company had been seized by the Alien Property Administration during World War I, the names 'Bayer' and 'Aspirin' were bought at a US Government auction in 1918 by the predecessor of Sterling Drug Inc. Sterling lost the rights to 'Aspirin' as a trademark in a court battle in 1921, but it still manufactures Bayer Aspirin in the USA and holds the name 'Aspirin' as a trademark in Canada.

In 1950, Dr Lawrence Craven, a general practitioner in Glendale, California, wrote an article in which he suggested that aspirin, because of its tendency to cause bleeding, might be useful as an antithrombotic agent. He reported that he had stumbled on this idea because he noted a connection between nose bleeds and reports of haemorrhage following tonsillectomy in children chewing too much 'Aspergum', which had been prescribed in small doses for its analgesic effect. They liked the gum so much that they were chewing twenty sticks (4.5 g of acetylsalicylic acid) a day and when denied any more gum, the bleeding stopped. This confirmed his suspicion that there was a relationship between bleeding and aspirin.

Craven also reported that he had been able to induce nose bleeds in himself by taking large doses of aspirin, thereby satisfying his personal belief that it really did affect bleeding. He then related that conclusion to the more accepted idea that anticoagulants are the best therapy for cardiac patients and with this in mind, prescribed either 5 grains (325 mg) or 10 grains (650 mg) daily to his high-risk patients, many of whom were obese, inactive males over the age of 45. In a later article (Craven, 1956) he wrote that approximately 8000 men who had been under his care had adopted a regimen calling for this daily dose of aspirin and mentioned in boldface type what he called a 'surprising result – not a single case of detectable coronary or cerebral thrombosis has occurred among patients who have faithfully adhered to this regimen'. He went on to say that 'the mechanism which brings about occlusion of the coronary arteries also is responsible for thrombosis of cerebral arteries – a much more common finding than blockage of the coronary vessels, albeit less spectacular or catastrophic in nature', and continued 'although patients who have faithfully taken daily doses of aspirin may have suffered minor strokes, which have gone undetected, no major stroke has occurred in roughly 8000 patients who have followed this regimen'. He stated further that no untoward reactions had developed in the normal patients who had adhered to this oral administration of aspirin over a period as long as 6 or 7 years. He felt that 5–10 grains (325–650 mg) of aspirin daily carried practically no hazard and that it might be life saving.

Craven's work was regarded by his colleagues as unscientific and, unfortunately, it appeared in an obscure and not widely disseminated medical journal. Twenty years passed before interest in aspirin for the prevention of thrombosis was revived.

Born (1962a) described a photometric method for the quantification of platelet aggregation, a development that led to further study of the mechanisms underlying aggregation and the subsequent discovery of inhibitors (Born, 1962b) which eventually led to their clinical testing as antithrombotic agents.

In the late 1960s aspirin was shown to have marked effects on platelet function in animals (Evans *et al.*, 1968). Aspirin ingestion suppresses the second phase of aggregation which is induced either by epinephrine (O'Brien, 1968; Sahud and Aggeler, 1969) or a critical concentration of adenosine diphosphate (Born, 1967; Zuker and Peterson 1968). It was also demonstrated that the effects of a single oral dose of aspirin may last for as long as 7 days (Weiss *et al.*, 1968). A further study in patients with rheumatic disease showed that the inhibitory effects of aspirin persist during long-term administration (Atac *et al.*, 1970). These investigators suggested that aspirin held promise as an anti-thrombotic agent. Shortly thereafter, Weiss *et al.* (1970) reported the prevention of experimentally induced arterial thrombosis in dogs by the administration of aspirin. Their report prompted the convening of a meeting in Houston, Texas to develop plans for undertaking a controlled clinical trial of aspirin in patients with transient ischaemic attacks (Fields and Hass, 1971).

13.3 CLINICAL TRIALS OF ANTIPLATELET AGENTS

By 1970, physicians had become more aware of the value of controlled (randomized) clinical trials in determining the efficacy of a drug or other treatment modalities such as surgical intervention and it was then that the first controlled clinical trials of aspirin and other potential antithrombotic drugs were organized.

13.3.1 The Aspirin in Transient Ischaemic Attack Study (AITIA)

This randomized clinical trial, begun in 1972, involved two groups of patients: (1) those who had attacks of monocular blindness (*amaurosis fugax*), hemispheric TIAs, or minor strokes (Fields *et al.*, 1977) and (2) those patients with similar histories in whom a carotid endarterectomy had been performed before they entered the trial (Fields *et al.*, 1978). Subjects were randomly allocated to either aspirin, 650 mg twice daily, or placebo, and followed to determine the incidence of TIAs, cerebral infarction, retinal infarction, or death from any cause. Unfortunately, the number of patients recruited in both arms of this study was small but the analysis published in 1977 demonstrated that in the medically treated group of 178 patients, there was a significance in favour of aspirin when subsequent TIAs were included as end-points. This significance was most apparent in patients with a history of multiple TIAs prior to entry and those with carotid artery lesions on the side appropriate to their TIA symptoms. All subjects entered had arteriograms to verify the location and character of extra- or intra-cranial atherosclerotic lesions.

13.3.2 Canadian Cooperative Study Group

At approximately the same time that the American trial was getting under way, a trial was begun in Canada (Canadian Cooperative

Study Group, 1978) recruiting patients suffering from TIA or minor stroke, who were then randomly allocated to one of four regimens: (1) sulfinpyrazone, 250 mg four times daily; (2) aspirin, 325 mg four times daily; (3) both drugs in the aforementioned dose; or (4) placebo. The final report published in 1978 showed that among the total patient population aspirin reduced the risk of stroke or death by 31%, but this prophylactic benefit appeared to be confined to males. Among women there were more strokes and death for the aspirin takers than for those not receiving the drug. The number of women entered was proportionately low so there was considerable speculation as to whether the sex difference in response might be a statistical artifact. Sulfinpyrazone was shown to be ineffective.

13.3.3 Accidents Ischémiques Cérébraux Liés à L'athèrosclérose (AICLA)

The AICLA Study (Bousser *et al.*, 1983) began in 1975 to determine whether aspirin (1 g daily) or aspirin (1 g) plus dipyridamole (225 mg daily) would produce a significant reduction in the occurrence of fatal and non-fatal cerebral infarction during a 3-year period of follow-up. The authors reported at the end of this trial in 1983 that aspirin had a significant beneficial effect which did not appear to be enhanced by dipyridamole, and noted no difference in response to aspirin between males and females.

13.3.4 Danish TIA-Aspirin Study

Sørenson *et al.* (1983) reported, at the same time as the French study a comparison of patients on either aspirin, 1000 mg daily, or placebo. After an average follow-up period of 25 months, the authors concluded that there was no significant difference between the treatment groups for either stroke or death, and occurrence of TIAs was not reduced by aspirin. Patients referred for carotid surgery were excluded from the trial. If one accepts the conclusion of the American trial that the patients most likely to benefit were those who had carotid lesions appropriate to their cerebral symptoms, then it would appear that many individuals who would have been expected to benefit from aspirin were considered ineligible for inclusion in the trial.

Of the three aforementioned clinical trials, the AITIA study was the only one in which all the patients were subjected to arteriography as a prerequisite for entry. Consequently, the presence or absence of carotid lesions was known in only one-quarter to one-third of the study population.

13.3.5 European Stroke Prevention Study

A total of 2500 patients with a clinical diagnosis of transient ischaemic attack, reversible ischaemic neurologic deficit, or stroke were entered in a multi-centred, double-blind trial. The subjects were randomized to receive either dipyridamole, 75 mg, plus acetylsalicylic acid, 325 mg, or placebo three times daily. There was no group which received dipyridamole only. Follow-up was carried out over a period of 24 months. After an intention to treat analysis, it was reported (ESPS Study Group, 1987) that 473 patients had reached an end-point (stroke or death from any cause), 190 on the active therapeutic agents and 283 on placebo. From this it was concluded that a 33% benefit in favour of the active treatment group had been demonstrated.

13.3.6 United Kingdom-TIA Aspirin Trial

Between 1979 and 1985, 2435 patients considered to have had a transient ischaemic attack or minor ischaemic stroke were randomly allocated to long-term control treatment with either aspirin, 600 mg twice daily (n = 815), aspirin, 300 mg once daily (n = 806), or placebo (n = 814). The treatment was continued with about 85% compliance for another year. This large group of collaborators reported (UK-TIA Study Group, 1988) that the likelihood of suffering one or more of the four categories of events, namely, non-fatal myocardial infarction, non-fatal major stroke, vascular death or non-vascular death, was 18% less in the two groups allocated to receive aspirin than in the group allocated to placebo. No definite difference was noted between responses to the 300 mg and 1200 mg daily doses except that the lower dose produced significantly fewer gastrointestinal symptoms.

13.3.7 The Persantine-Aspirin Trial in Cerebral Ischaemia

Clinical trials in which aspirin was used for medical management of patients with a history of TIA have clearly shown that many patients do not benefit from aspirin therapy. Physicians worldwide had been using aspirin together with dipyridamole on an empirical basis but no controlled trial in patients with stroke symptoms had tested whether that combination of drugs was more effective than aspirin alone. The Persantine-Aspirin Trial started in 1978 was designed to answer that question. During the recruitment period which lasted through 1984, 890 individuals were entered into the trial and allocated randomly to either aspirin 325 mg plus placebo, or aspirin in a similar dose plus Persantine 75 mg four times daily. The results reported in 1985

Therapeutic applications

(American-Canadian Co-operative Study Group, 1985) clearly demonstrated that dipyrimadole contributed no additional benefit when prescribed with aspirin.

13.3.8 The Antiplatelet Trialists Collaboration

A so-called meta-analysis of 25 completed randomized trials employing antiplatelet treatment for patients with a history of transient ischaemic attacks, occlusive stroke, unstable angina, or myocardial infarction were reported in 1988 (Antiplatelet Trialists Collaboration, 1988). These trials included a total of 29 000 patients, 3000 of whom had died. In the aggregate, it appeared that allocation to antiplatelet treatment had no effect on non-vascular mortality but significantly reduced vascular mortality by 15% and non-fatal events (stroke and myocardial infarction) by 30%. Aspirin was at least as effective as any other antiplatelet agent or combinations of such agents.

13.3.9 Dipyridamole as an Antithrombotic Agent

Dipyridamole (Persantine) is still prescribed worldwide as an antiplatelet drug in the management of thrombo-embolic disorders. There is abundant evidence, however, beginning with Acheson *et al.* (1969) and including the French trial of aspirin and dipyridamole (Bousser *et al.*, 1983), the European Stroke Prevention Study (ESPS Study Group, 1987) and the Persantine-Aspirin Trial (American-Canadian Co-operative Study Group, 1985) that this drug contributes nothing to the treatment of transient ischaemic attacks or stroke (Loeliger, 1985). The accumulated data for and against dipyridamole as an antithrombotic agent has been reviewed in depth in an article by FitzGerald (1987). He concludes that, 'Dipyridamole is widely prescribed as an antithrombotic drug – commonly in combination with aspirin. Despite its apparent efficacy at high concentrations in certain animal models involving repeated injury to a previously normal vasculature, an antithrombotic action of dipyridamole in humans remains to be established. In the majority of prospective clinical trials designed to assess the efficacy of dipyridamole, it has been combined with aspirin rather than compared directly with placebo therapy. . . . the emerging consensus does not support its use as an antiplatelet drug'.

13.3.10 The Dutch TIA Study Group

The Dutch TIA Study Group reported the results of trials comparing two doses of aspirin in patients who had had a TIA or minor ischaemic stroke (Dutch TIA Trial Study Group, 1991). The effects of a water soluble preparation of acetylsalicyclic acid of either 30 mg or 283 mg daily were tested in a double blind randomized controlled clinical trial in 3131 patients for an average of 2.6 years. In the group receiving 30 mg aspirin, 14.7% of patients suffered death from vascular causes, non-fatal stroke or non-fatal myocardial infarction, compared to 15.2% in the group receiving 283 mg. In addition, fewer patients in the 30 mg group experienced adverse effects such as bleeding complications or gastrointestinal symptoms. The authors concluded that 30 mg aspirin daily was as effective in preventing vascular events as 283 mg and had fewer adverse effects. Prior to this, a dose of 300 mg aspirin daily had been established as an efficacious dose (UK-TIA Study Group 1988) for the secondary prevention of transient ischaemic attacks or minor ischaemic stroke.

13.4 LOW-DOSE ASPIRIN

What is the correct dose of aspirin for clinical trials? Controversy about the correct dose of aspirin for use as an antithrombotic agent is based largely on evidence that has been accumulated from laboratory studies rather than from clinical trials. As early as 1967, prostaglandin E_1 was found to be the most powerful inhibitor of *in-vitro* aggregation of platelets known at that time (Emmons *et al.*, 1967; Kloeze, 1967) and of the formation of platelet thrombi with embolization in animal models (Emmons *et al.*, 1967). The aspirin effect on bleeding time and on platelet test systems *in vitro* was already known (Miekle *et al.*, 1969) but shortly thereafter, Vane (1971) and colleagues (Needleman *et al.*, 1976) were investigating the anti-inflammatory action of aspirin and concluded that one mechanism of action was the inhibition of prostaglandin synthesis. Their investigations provided the first clue to an understanding of the mechanisms by which prostaglandins and their derivatives influence the interaction between platelets and the vessel wall.

Samuelsson (1972) demonstrated that platelets generated endoperoxides from arachidonic acid within the platelet and that these substances then produced the most powerful known aggregating substance, the unstable thromboxane A_2 (TXA$_2$), which could only be measured after it broke down to stable thromboxane B_2 (TXB$_2$). They noted that a particularly crucial step in this chain was mediated by the enzyme, cyclo-oxygenase, and that this enzyme was irreversibly acetylated and inhibited by aspirin. It was further demonstrated that thromboxanes are not only powerful platelet aggregators but are also vasoconstrictors (Hamberg *et al.*, 1975). This lent support to the idea

363

that aspirin as an inhibitor of TXA_2 synthesis might well be a valuable antithrombotic drug.

Moncada *et al.* (1976) reported that a similar system existed which produced a diametrically opposed end product in the vessel wall. Beginning with arachidonic acid in endothelial cells, cyclo-oxygenase was shown to be able to generate a new series of intermediate endoperoxides which produced an extremely powerful anti-aggregatory, vasodilator substance called 'prostacyclin' (PGI_2).

Aspirin inhibits cyclo-oxygenase by acetylation (Al-Mondhiry *et al.*, 1969; Roth *et al.*, 1975) a process which is irreversible in platelets and results in an enzymatic defect which is permanent on the platelet during its lifetime in the blood. A platelet population which functions in a completely normal fashion will not reappear until 10–14 days after stopping ingestion of aspirin and allowing the bone marrow to generate new platelets. The irreversible nature of the aspirin effect may be explained by the fact that the platelet is a non-nucleated cell, whereas the nucleated cells of the vessel wall can produce new cyclo-oxygenase and prostacyclin production will rapidly recover (Jaffe and Weksler, 1979).

It has been suggested that a dose of aspirin that selectively inhibits TXA_2, while sparing PGI_2 generation in the vascular wall, would enhance the efficacy of aspirin as an antithrombotic agent (Korbut and Moncada, 1978; Patrignani *et al.*, 1982), but the evidence against this being possible is accumulating (Preston *et al.*, 1981; Weksler *et al.*, 1983; Herd *et al.*, 1987; Kyrle *et al.*, 1987; Zaragoza and Le Breton, 1987). Many investigators have become overly enthusiastic about this concept of selective inhibition of the important interacting systems in the platelet and vessel wall, but it seems quite likely that these hypotheses, developed largely on the basis of laboratory evidence, may have nothing whatsoever to do with the prevention of pathologic thrombotic events. Furthermore, not all platelet behaviour is dependent solely on prostaglandin pathways.

Preston *et al.* (1981) gave aspirin to volunteers in a dose of 300 mg which is known to produce prolongation of the bleeding time. A comparison was then made in these subjects of the inhibitory effects of aspirin on prostaglandin synthesis by platelets and by the vessel wall. Two hours after aspirin ingestion, platelet production of TXB_2 was totally inhibited. The bleeding time was prolonged in spite of the fact that there was also a nearly complete inhibition of prostacyclin production. In another study, Jaffe and Weksler (1979), using cultured human endothelial cells, showed that both platelet and endothelial cell cyclo-oxygenase were about equally responsive to the inhibitory effect of low-dose aspirin.

The literature is also confused and controversial with respect to the effect of aspirin on the bleeding time. Treacher *et al.* (1978) estimated the bleeding time after a 1-week regimen of aspirin, 300 mg once daily or 600 mg twice daily. The bleeding time was determined 2 h after the first dose and 2 h after the last dose. The anticipated prolongation of the bleeding time after 2 h was confirmed. Although the bleeding times after 1 week were still prolonged, the prolongation was not quite as marked as at the 2-h reading after the initial dose.

According to Godal *et al.* (1979) the dose of aspirin necessary to produce maximal prolongation of the bleeding time varies from one individual to another (between 1 mg kg^{-1} and 3.5 mg kg^{-1}). They also reported that the bleeding times after aspirin, 425 mg and 3.8 g, were equally prolonged; Rajah *et al.* (1978) obtained maximal prolongation with 1000 mg, and doses of over 2 g were reported by them to produce paradoxical shortening of bleeding time, as had been observed previously by O'Grady and Moncada (1978) using 3.9 g. Girolami *et al.* (1979) also found a paradoxical effect after larger doses. Jørgensen *et al.* (1979), in an attempt to reconcile these differences, showed that paradoxical shortening was present to some extent in individuals under the age of 32 but not in older individuals between ages 66 and 70. They reported further that the bleeding time decreases with age, which raises a serious question regarding the clinical relevance of studies into which young adults have been recruited as subjects (Praga *et al.*, 1973).

In the controversy of the paradoxical effect of aspirin on bleeding time, it should be stressed that the vessels studied were arterioles, which are not affected by atheroma. Consequently, if a large dose of aspirin produces paradoxical shortening of the bleeding time as claimed, it does not necessarily follow that one can extrapolate this observation to the larger arteries of either the coronary or cerebral circulation. Moreover, atheromatous areas in the walls of larger arteries may not have the capacity to produce prostacyclin, and therefore further inhibition by aspirin does not occur.

There may be little clinical relevance in this entire problem of aspirin dosage other than with respect to side effects (Hirsh, 1985). There continues to be controversy over whether the paradoxical shortening of the bleeding time really occurs with large doses of aspirin. The dose necessary to produce such a paradoxical, and perhaps thrombogenic, effect is considerably higher than those doses used for an antithrombotic effect in recently reported and current major clinical trials. It is not even clear whether atheromatous plaques are capable of synthesizing prostacyclin, and patients over 60 years of age with widespread atheroma may produce so little prostacyclin that any further reduction by aspirin is insignificant. Moreover, it is not known whether the endothelium of arteries in older humans generates as much prostacyclin as the endothelium in younger adults, who have been the ones most commonly serving as volunteers for testing these effects.

The only clinical trial thus far in which two different doses of aspirin were compared in a double-blind fashion with placebo is the recently completed UK-TIA Aspirin Trial (1988). As previously stated, the efficacy of the lower dose was equal to that of the larger dose.

Large doses of aspirin have been used for many years by physicians treating rheumatic disease. Such large doses not only totally inhibit the cyclo-oxygenase in platelets but more than likely also affect in a similar manner the cyclo-oxygenase in the vessel wall. In spite of this, rheumatic patients treated with aspirin do not develop severe thrombotic complications. It is also unlikely that cyclo-oxygenase is of absolutely critical importance because its congenital absence in platelets and the vessel wall fails to lead to severe thrombotic disease but instead produces a mild haemorrhagic defect (Pareti *et al.*, 1980).

Unfortunately, the relevance of *in-vitro* tests to clinical antithrombotic activity remains uncertain. Cerletti *et al.* (1985) showed that doses of aspirin which completely inhibit aggregation, induced by arachidonic acid, platelet activating factor and/or epinephrine, are counteracted *in vitro* by combinations of threshold concentrations of these same antagonists. This combination of antagonists in all likelihood approximates more precisely the *in-vivo* situation. Aspirin also appears to have complex reactions with the products of lipoxygenase in both platelets and endothelial cells. Moreover, there is substantial evidence that aspirin influences other aspects of haemostasis (Moroz, 1977), including the release of tissue plasminogen activator (Levin *et al.*, 1984) and at higher doses, the synthesis of vitamin K-dependent coagulation factors (Roncaglioni *et al.*, 1986).

In an editorial published in 1987, Parkin suggests that, 'It is not entirely unexpected that the results of clinical trials of aspirin have not been universally encouraging. It may be that the ideal antithrombotic, platelet-inhibitory regimen should influence multiple pathways of platelet activation and not simply platelet eicosanoids'. He then goes on to point out that 'The candidates for combination testing are legion if we consider the proliferation of new antiplatelet drugs. Furthermore, both adrenergic and calcium blocking agents, drugs which are commonly used in patients with cardiovascular disease, have platelet inhibitory activity which may be synergistic with aspirin' (Greer *et al.*, 1985).

366

13.5 DIFFERENCE IN RESPONSE BETWEEN MALES AND FEMALES

Several of the trials of aspirin as an antithrombotic agent have suggested that aspirin might not be protective for females in circumstances where there was proven benefit for males (Canadian Co-operative Study Group, 1978; Candelise, 1982). It was thought by other investigators that this observation might be due to differences between the sexes in tests of primary haemostasis, as well as in the response of these tests to aspirin, and sex differences in aspirin metabolism. More recent reports (Johnson *et al.*, 1975; Buchanan *et al.*, 1983; Philp and Paul, 1986; Lee *et al.*, 1987), however, have not supported these observations which may simply have been the results of statistical analysis and stem from the fact that anywhere from two to three times as many males as females have been included in the trials to date.

In the future the design for clinical trials of antiplatelet agents will undoubtedly continue to follow the results of further laboratory investigations into haemostatic physiology (De Gaetano *et al.*, 1982). In the laboratory setting the variables can be more easily controlled, the models made less complex, and the time course less protracted.

13.6 CONCLUSIONS

Transient ischaemic attacks are caused by temporary occlusion of either cerebral or retinal blood vessels by circulating platelet thrombi. These thrombi form on atheromatous plaques in the carotid arteries from which they become detached leaving ulcerated lesions. The appearance of TIAs is invariably followed sooner or later by a cerebral ischaemic stroke.

Aspirin has been known since the 1950s to increase bleeding and in uncontrolled trials was thought to prevent TIAs and cerebrovascular strokes. Controlled clinical trials to test aspirin either alone or combined with other anti-platelet drugs in ischaemic stroke were started in 1972 and are still continuing. In a meta-analysis published in 1988, the Antiplatelet Trialists Collaboration reported a significant reduction in vascular mortality and in non-fatal vascular events with aspirin treatment.

Administration of low doses of aspirin which inhibit thromboxane formation in platelets without reducing prostacyclin synthesis in the blood vessel wall has been advocated as the most satisfactory method of treatment. However, experimental evidence suggests that atheromatous vessels make much less prostacyclin than normal ones and that prostacyclin does not play a significant part in preventing the formation of platelet thrombi in atherosclerotic arteries. The most significant effect

Therapeutic applications

of aspirin must therefore be to reduce synthesis of thromboxane by platelets.

Clinical trials of low dose aspirin treatment for secondary prevention of ischaemic stroke are in progress. In one such study (SALT Collaborative Group, 1991), 676 patients received low dose aspirin (75 mg day^{-1}) and 684 were allocated to placebo. The aspirin-treated group showed a reduction of 18% in the risk of stroke or death.

REFERENCES

Acheson, J., Danta, G. and Hutchinson, E.C. (1969) Controlled trial of dipyridamole in cerebral vascular disease. *Brit. Med. J.*, **i**, 614–15.

Al-Mondhiry, H., Marcus, A.J. and Spaet, T.H. (1969) Acetylation of human platelets by aspirin. *Fed. Proc.*, **28**, 576.

American-Canadian Co-operative Study Group (1985) Persantine-aspirin trial in cerebral ischemia, Part II: Endpoint results. *Stroke*, **16**, 406–15.

Antiplatelet Trialists Collaboration (1988) Secondary prevention of vascular disease by prolonged antiplatelet treatment. *Brit. Med.J.*, **296**, 320–31.

Atac, A., Spagunolo, M. and Zucker, M.B. (1970) Long-term inhibition of platelet functions by aspirin. *Proc. Soc. Exp. Biol.*, **133**, 1331–3.

Baker, R.N., Broussard, J.A., Fang, H.C. *et al.* (1962) Anticoagulant therapy in cerebral infarction. *Neurology*, **12**, 823–35.

Barnett, H.J.M. (1975) Platelets, drugs and cerebral ischemia. In *Platelets, Drugs and Thrombosis*, Symp. Hamilton, 1972, Basel, Karger, pp. 233–52.

Born, G.V.R. (1962a) Quantitative investigation into the aggregation of blood platelets. *J. Physiol.*, **162**, 67–8.

Born, G.V.R. (1962b) Aggregation of blood platelets by adenosine diphosphate and its reversal. Nature 194: 927–9.

Born, G.V.R. (1967) Mechanism of platelet aggregation and of its inhibition by adenosine derivatives. *Fed. Proc.*, **26**, 115–17.

Bousser, M.G., Eschwege, E., Hagenau, M. *et al.* (1983) 'AICLA' controlled trial of aspirin and dipyridamole in the secondary prevention of atherothrombotic cerebral ischemia. *Stroke*, **14**, 5–14.

Buchanan, M.R., Rischke, J.A., Butt, R. *et al.* (1983) The sex-related differences in aspirin pharmacokinetics in rabbits and man and its relationship to antiplatelet effects. *Thromb. Res.*, **29**, 125–39.

Canadian Co-operative Study Group (1978) A randomized trial of aspirin and sulfinpyrazone in threatened stroke. *N. Engl. J. Med.*, **299**, 53–9.

Candelise, L., Landi, G., Perrone, P. *et al.* (1982) A randomized trial of aspirin and sulfinpyrazone in patients with TIA. *Stroke*, **13**, 175–9.

Cerletti, C., Latini, R., Del Maschio, A. *et al.* (1985) Aspirin kinetics and inhibition of platelet thromboxane generation – relevance for a solution as to the 'aspirin dilemma'. *Thromb. Haemost.*, **53**, 415–18.

Chiari, H. (1905) Über das Verhalten des Teilungswinkels der Carotis communis bei der Endarteriitis chronica deformans. *Verh. Dtsch. Ges. Path.*, **9**, 326–330.

Craven, L.L. (1950) Acetylsalicylic acid, possible preventive of coronary thrombosis. *Ann. West. Med. Surg.*, **4**, 95–6.

Craven, L.L. (1956) Prevention of coronary and cerebral thrombosis. *Miss. Valley Med. J. (Quincy, IL)*, **78**, 213–15.

De Gaetano, G., Cerletti, C. and Bertelè, V. (1982) Pharmacology of antiplatelet drugs and clinical trials on thrombosis prevention: a difficult link. *Lancet*, **ii**, 974–7.

Dutch TIA Trial Study Group (1991) A comparison of two doses of aspirin (30 mg vs. 283 mg a day) in patients after a transient ischemic attack or minor ischemic stroke. *N. Engl. J. Med.*, **325**, 1261–6.

Ehrenfeld, W.K., Hoyt, W.F. and Wylie, E.J. (1966) Embolization and transient blindness from carotid atheroma. *Arch. Surg.*, **93**, 787–94.

Emmons, P.R., Hampton, J.R., Harrison, M.J.G. *et al.* (1967) Effect of prostaglandin E_1 on platelet behaviour *in vitro* and *in vivo*. *Brit. Med. J.*, **ii**, 468–72.

ESPS Study Group (1987) The European stroke prevention study (ESPS): principal end points, *Lancet*, **ii**, 1351–4.

Evans, G., Packham, M.A., Nishizawa, E.E. *et al.* (1968) Effect of acetylsalicylic acid on platelet function. *J. Exper. Med.*, **128**, 877–94.

Fields, W.S. and Hass, W.K. (1971) *Aspirin, Platelets and Stroke. Background for a Clinical Trial*, Warren H. Green, St Louis.

Fields, W.S., Lemak, N.A., Frankowski, R.F. and Hardy, R.J. (1977) Controlled trial of aspirin in cerebral ischemia. *Stroke*, **8**, 301–16.

Fields, W.S., Lemak, N.A., Frankowski, R.F. and Hardy, R.J. (1978) Controlled trial of aspirin in cerebral ischemia. Part II: Surgical group. *Stroke*, **9**, 309–19.

Fisher, C.M. (1951) Occlusion of the internal carotid artery. *Arch. Neurol. Psychiat.*, **65**, 346–77.

FitzGerald, G.A. (1987) Dipyridamole. *N. Engl. J. Med.*, **316**, 1247–57.

Friedman, G.D., Wilson, S., Mosier, J.M. *et al.* (1969) Transient ischemic attacks in a community. *JAMA*, **210**, 1428–34.

Girolami, A. Cella, G., Zanon, R.D.B. *et al.* (1979) Aspirin and the bleeding time. *Lancet*, **ii**, 205–6.

Godal, H.C., Eika, C., Dybdale, J.M. *et al.* (1979) Aspirin and bleeding time. *Lancet*, **i**, 1236.

Gomensoro, J.B., Maslenikov, V., Azambuja, N. *et al.* (1973) Joint study of extracranial vascular occlusion. VIII. Clinical-radiographic correlation of carotid bifurcation lesions in 177 patients with transient cerebral ischemic attacks. *JAMA*, **224**, 985–91.

Greer, I.A., Walker, J.J., Calder, A.A. and Forbes, C.D. (1985) Aspirin with an adrenergic or a calcium-channel-blocking agent as a new combination therapy for arterial thrombosis. *Lancet*, **i**, 351–2.

Gunning, A.J., Pickering, G.W., Robb-Smith, A.H.T. and Ross Russell, R.W. (1964) Mural thrombosis of the internal carotid artery and subsequent embolism. *Quart. J. Med.*, **33**, 155–95.

Hamberg, M., Svensson, J. and Samuelsson, B. (1975) Thromboxanes: a new group of biologically active compounds derived from prostaglandin endoperoxides. *Proc. Natl Acad. Sci. USA*, **72**, 2994–8.

Harrison, M.G.J., Marshall, J., Meadows, J.C. and Ross Russell, R.W. (1971) Effect of aspirin in amaurosis fugax. *Lancet*, **ii**, 743–4.

Herd, C.M., Rodgers, S.E., Lloyd, J.V. *et al.* (1987) A dose ranging study of the

Therapeutic applications

antiplatelet effect of enteric coated aspirin in man. *Aust. NZ J. Med.*, **17**, 195–200.

Hirsh, J. (1985) Progress review: the relationship between dose of aspirin, side effects and antithrombotic effectiveness. *Stroke*, **16**, 1–4.

Hunt, J.R. (1914) The role of the carotid arteries in the causation of vascular lesions of the brain. *Am. J. Med. Sci.*, **147**, 704–13.

Hutchinson, E.C. and Yates, P.O. (1957) Caratico-vertebral stenosis. *Lancet*, **i**, 2–8.

Jaffe, E.A. and Weksler, B.B. (1979) Recovery of endothelial cell prostacyclin production after inhibition by low doses of aspirin. *J. Clin. Invest.*, **63**, 532–5.

Johnson, M., Ramey, E. and Ramwell, P.W. (1975) Sex and age differences in human platelet aggregation. *Nature (New Biol.)*, **253**, 355–7.

Jørgensen, K.A., Olesen, A.S., Dyerberg, J. and Stoffersen, E. (1979) Aspirin and bleeding time: dependency on age. *Lancet*, **ii**, 302.

Kishore, P.R.S., Chase, N.E. and Kricheff, I.I. (1971) Ulcerated atheroma of carotid artery and cerebral embolism. In *Aspirin, Platelets and Stroke*, (eds W.S. Fields and W.K. Hass), Warren H. Green, St Louis, p 13.

Kloeze, J. (1967) Influence of prostaglandins on platelet aggregation. In *Prostaglandins; Proceedings 2nd Nobel Symposium*, (eds S. Bergstrom and B. Samuelsson,) Interscience, New York, p. 241.

Korbut, R. and Moncada, S. (1978) Prostacyclin (PGI_2) and thromboxane A_2 interaction *in vivo*. Regulation by aspirin and relationship with antithrombotic therapy. *Thromb. Res.*, **13**, 489–500.

Kyrle, P.A., Eichner, H.G., Jäger, U. and Lechner, K. (1987) Inhibition of prostacyclin and thromboxane A_2 generation by low-dose aspirin at the site of plug formation in man *in vivo*. *Circulation*, **75**, 1025–9.

Lee, T-K., Chen, Y-C. and Kuo, T-L. (1987) Comparison of the effect of acetylsalicylic acid on platelet function in male and female patients with ischemic stroke. *Thromb. Res.*, **47**, 295–304.

Levin, R.I., Harpel, P.C., Weil, D. *et al.* (1984) Aspirin inhibits vascular plasminogen activator activity *in vivo*. *J. Clin. Invest*, **74**, 571–80.

Levine, J. and Swanson, P.D. (1968) Idiopathic thrombocytosis. A treatable cause of transient ischemic attacks. *Neurology*, **18**, 711–13.

Loeliger, E.A. (1985) Does dipyridamole have antithrombotic potential? *Thromb. Haem.*, **53**, 437.

Lougheed, W.M., Elgie, R.G. and Barnett, H.J.M. (1966) The results of surgical management of extracranial internal carotid occlusion and stenosis. *Can. Med. Assoc. J.*, **95**, 1279–93.

Marshall, J. and Wilkinson, I.M.S. (1971) The prognosis of carotid ischemic attacks in patients with normal angiograms. *Brain*, **94**, 395–402.

Miekle, C.H., Kaneshiro, M.M., Maher, I.A. *et al.* (1969) The standardized normal Ivy bleeding time and its prolongation by aspirin. *Blood*, **34**, 204–15.

Millikan, C.H. (1970) Anticoagulant therapy in cerebrovascular disease. In *Cerebrovascular Survey Report*, Subcommittee on Cerebrovascular Disease, NINDS, p. 218.

Moncada, S., Gryglewski, R., Bunting, S and Vane, J.R. (1976) An enzyme isolated from arteries transforms prostaglandin endoperoxides to an unstable substance that inhibits platelet aggregation. *Nature*, **263**, 663–5.

Moniz, E. (1927) L'encéphalographie arterielle, son importance dans la locali-sation des tumeurs cérébrales. *Rev. Neurol.*, **2**, 72–90.

Moore, W.S. and Hall, A.D. (1968) Ulcerated atheromata of the carotid artery, a major cause of transient cerebral ischemia. *Am. J. Surg.*, **116**, 237–42.

Moroz, L.A. (1977) Increased blood fibrinolytic activity after aspirin ingestion. *N. Engl. J. Med.*, **296**, 525–9.

Mundall, J., Quintero, P., von Kaulla, K.N. *et al.* (1972) Transient monocular blindness and increased platelet aggregability treated with aspirin. *Neurology*, **22**, 280–95.

Needleman, P., Moncada, S., Bunting, S. *et al.* (1976) Identification of an enzyme in platelet microsomes which generates thromboxane A_2 from prostaglandin endoperoxides. *Nature*, **261**, 558–60.

O'Brien, J.R. (1968) Effects of salicylates on human platelets. *Lancet*, **i**, 779–83.

O'Grady, J. and Moncada, S. (1978) Aspirin: a paradoxical effect on bleeding time. *Lancet*, **ii**, 780.

Pareti, F.I., Maunucci, P.M., D'Angelo, A. *et al.* (1980) Congenital deficiency of thromboxane and prostacyclin. *Lancet*, **i**, 898–901.

Parkin, J.D. (1987) The enigma of aspirin (editorial). *Aust. NZ J. Med.*, **17**, 192–4.

Patrignani, P., Filabozzi, P. and Patrono, C. (1982) Selective cumulative inhibition of platelet thromboxane production by low-dose aspirin in healthy subjects. *J. Clin. Invest.*, **69**, 1366–72.

Philp, R.B. and Paul, M.L. (1986) Salicylate antagonism of acetylsalicylic acid inhibition of platelet aggregation in male and female subjects: Influence of citrate concentration. *Haemostasis*, **16**, 369–77.

Praga, C., Malisardi, P., Pollini, C. *et al.* (1973) Bleeding time and antiaggregating drugs: a controlled study in elderly patients. *Thromb. Res.*, **3**, 13–22.

Preston, F.E., Shipps, S., Jackson, C.A. *et al.* (1981) Inhibition of prostacyclin and platelet thromboxane A_2 after low dose aspirin. *N. Engl. J. Med.*, **304**, 76–9.

Rajah, S.M., Penny, A. and Kester, R. (1978) Aspirin and bleeding time. *Lancet*, **ii**, 1104.

Roncaglioni, M.C., Ulrich, M.M.W., Muller, A.D. *et al.* (1986) The vitamin K antagonism of salicylate and warfarin. *Thromb. Res.*, **42**, 727–36.

Ross, R.W. (1961) Observations on the retinal vessels in monocular blindness. *Lancet*, **ii**, 1422–8.

Roth, G.J., Stanford, N. and Majerus, P.W. (1975) Acetylation of prostaglandin synthase by aspirin. *Proc. Natl. Acad. Sci., USA*, **72**, 3073–6.

Sahud, M.A. and Aggeler, P.M. (1969) Platelet dysfunction – differentiation of a newly recognized primary type from that produced by aspirin. *N. Engl. J. Med.*, **280**, 453–9.

SALT Collaborative Group (1991) Swedish Aspirin Low-dose Trial (SALT) of 75 mg aspirin as secondary prophylaxis after cerebrovascular ischaemic events. *Lancet*, **338**, 1345–9.

Samuelsson, B. (1972) The synthesis and biological role of prostaglandins. *Biochem. J.*, **128**, 4P.

Singer, G. (1969) Migrating emboli of retinal arteries in thrombocythaemia. *Brit. J. Ophthalmol.*, **53**, 279–83.

Therapeutic applications

Sørenson, P.S., Pedersen, H., Marquardsen, J. *et al.* (1983) Acetylsalicylic acid in the prevention of stroke in patients with reversible cerebral ischemic attacks. A Danish Study. *Stroke*, **14**, 15–22.

Treacher, D., Warlow, C.P. and McPherson, K. (1978) Aspirin and bleeding time. *Lancet*, **ii**, 1378–9.

UK-TIA Study Group (1988) United Kingdom transient ischemic attack (UK-TIA) aspirin trial: interim results. *Brit. Med. J.*, **296**, 316–20.

Vane, J.R. (1971) Inhibition of prostaglandin synthesis as a mechanism of action for aspirin-like drugs. *Nature*, **231**, 232–5.

Weiss, H.J., Aledort, L.M. and Kochwa, S. (1968) The effects of salicylates on the hemostatic properties of platelets in man. *J. Clin. Invest.*, **47**, 2169–80.

Weiss, H.J., Danese, C.A. and Voleti, C.D. (1970) Prevention of experimentally induced arterial thrombosis by aspirin (Abstr.). *Fed. Proc.*, **29**, 381.

Weksler, B.B., Pett, S.B., Alonso, D. *et al.* (1983) Differential inhibition by aspirin of vascular and platelet prostaglandin synthesis in atherosclerotic patients. *N. Engl. J. Med.*, **308**, 800–5.

Zaragoza, R. and Le Breton, G.C. (1987) Effect of single dose aspirin on TXA_2 and PGI_2 cyclo-oxygenases *in vivo*. *Hemostasis*, **7**, 40–8.

Zucker, M.B. and Peterson, J. (1968) Inhibition of adenosine diphosphate-induced secondary aggregation and other platelet functions by acetylsalicylic acid ingestion. *Proc. Soc. Exp. Biol. Med.*, **127**, 547–51.

14 The effect of aspirin in headaches and migraine

P.T.G. DAVIES and F. CLIFFORD ROSE

Although migraine and other common headache syndromes have been treated for thousands of years, their scientific study has been active only in the last 50 years. During this period there has been an evolution in diagnostic criteria and classification, concomitant with increased understanding of pathophysiological mechanisms. Headache syndromes can be categorized into primary headaches arising from disturbed physiological mechanisms and secondary headaches where there is an identifiable pathological process (Table 14.1 and 14.2). A more detailed classification, which gives criteria for establishing the diagnosis, has recently been proposed by the Headache Classification Committee of the International Headache Society (1988).

14.1 THE SCOPE OF THE PROBLEM

More than 50 medical conditions may present with headache as the sole or major symptom but only a few of these are commonly seen – tension headache, migraine, and head pain for which a firm diagnosis is never established (Table 14.3). Referral rates to neurology clinics from general practice are about 20 times more frequent for headache than for multiple sclerosis, one of the most common of neurological diseases. Those referred to hospital are only a tiny fraction of headache sufferers in the community. In a population of 100 000, between 79 000 and 83 000 had a headache within the past year, 24 000 in the previous 14 days sufficiently severe to require an analgesic but only 1600 consult their family doctor about headaches each year (Hopkins and Ziegler, 1988).

Primary headache syndromes (tension headache, migraine and cluster headache) far outnumber other types of headache, whether seen in general practice or hospital, and consequently have been the focus of most headache research, but particularly migraine.

373

Table 14.1 Classification of primary headache

Migraine
  Common

  Classical, with focal neurological features (ophthalmic – scintillating scotoma, hemianopic; hemiparaesthetic – cheiro-oral; aphasic; basilar; hemiparetic)

  Migraine variants (ophthalmoplegic; retinal; familial hemiplegic; childhood alternating hemiplegia; equivalents, e.g. aura without headache, abdominal migraine)

Muscle contraction (tension) headache
  Depression
  Anxiety
  Psychogenic (delusional, conversion)

Cluster headache
  Episodic
  Chronic
  Chronic paraxysmal hemicrania
  Atypical variants

14.2 PROBLEMS IN ASSESSMENT OF TREATMENT

Although it has been recognized for many years that the majority of headaches respond to aspirin, the scientific study of this response became significant only when the mechanism of action of aspirin was appreciated. The many formal clinical trials concerning its efficacy in migraine attacks, several studies of prophylactic treatment and a few in tension headache form the basis for this chapter, but there are formidable problems in attempting to quantify therapeutic responses (for review, Steiner and Clifford Rose, 1988).

Although migraine attacks are easily recognized by their characteristic pattern of symptoms, there is no biological marker and no universally accepted definition, with a variety of often widely differing criteria for diagnosis. During the 24 h before the onset of the actual attack there may be non-focal neurological symptoms such as elation, depression or hunger. This is followed by the focal neurological symptoms of the aura, usually visual but may include disturbance of speech, hemianaesthesia or rarely hemiparesis (classical migraine). The headache, often the most severe symptom, is usually unilateral, throbbing and follows the aura, and is associated with nausea and vomiting, photophobia, phonophobia and osmophobia. Without focal symptoms the attack is

Table 14.2 Classification of secondary (symptomatic headache)

Extracranial	Intracranial
Temporal arteritis Carotidynia Periosteal disease	Meningeal (meningitis, encephalitis, subarachnoid haemorrhage, post-lumbar puncture)
	Space-occupying (tumour, haematoma, abscess)
Cranial nerve	Acute raised pressure (cough, exertional, orgasmic, phaeochromocytoma)
Neuralgias (trigeminal, post-herpetic, atypical facial)	Raised venous pressure (otic hydrocephalus, emphysema)
Compression (tumour, aneurysm)	Cerebral oedema (benign intracranial hypertension; malignant hypertension; post convulsive)
Inflammatory (Tolosa–Hunt syndrome) Reflex (ice-cream headache)	*Toxic*
Referred	Fevers
Eyes (glaucoma)	Drugs (alcohol, nitrites, nitrates)
Ear, nose and throat (sinuses, ears)	Drug withdrawal ('hangover', caffeine, analgesics)
Dental (apicitis)	
Cervical	

termed common migraine but the distinction is not always easy and both types may occur in the same patient. In spite of the complex and varied symptomatology, drug efficacy has usually been assessed by its effects on headache, nausea and vomiting, and daily activities.

Besides problems of definition, evaluation in clinical trials is beset by a large number of variables: patient selection, drug dosage, length of treatment and follow-up periods, high placebo response in headache sufferers, a tendency for headaches to remit with time, the subjective nature of headache, and methods of evaluation.

Table 14.3 The differential diagnosis in 906 patients, from a total of 4000 new patients, who presented to the General Neurology Clinic of Charing Cross hospital with headache or facial pain as the major or sole symptom. (Courtesy of Ellis Horwood Ltd, Chichester)

Diagnosis	Number	% of total
Tension headache	296	32.6
Migraine	241	26.6
Headache (cause unknown)	139	15.3
Post-traumatic syndrome	71	7.8
Facial pain (cause unknown)	38	4.1
Depression	29	3.2
Trigeminal neuralgia	29	3.2
Cluster headache	19	2
Malignant intracranial tumour	14	1.5
Benign intracranial tumour	9	1
Temporal arteritis	6	
Post-herpetic neuralgia	5	
Benign intracranial hypertension	4	
Cough headache	3	
Subdural haematoma	2	
Sinus infection	1	

Migraine sufferers commonly experience other types of headache, e.g. tension headache. Those with frequent headaches commonly take too many analgesics which can lead to analgesic rebound headaches. During a migraine attack there is impaired drug absorption by the oral route due to gastric stasis so that other routes of administration, or a combination with an anti-emetic, should be considered.

14.3 ASPIRIN IN THE TREATMENT OF MIGRAINE

With any effective treatment for acute attacks or for prophylaxis of migraine, the question of how the drug is working has implications for hypotheses on pathogenesis.

14.3.1 Pain

The precise location of the headache in migraine is unknown but the most widely accepted view is that it originates from cranial blood vessels which are involved in a sterile inflammatory process. The headache resembles an inflammatory pain because any movement aggravates the headache; this is typical of pain arising in inflamed tissue from the release of mediators, e.g. prostaglandins, serotonin or bradykinin, which lower the threshold of primary afferent fibres, viz the trigeminal nociceptive neurones. The primary afferents are sensitized and stimuli which normally do not generate impulses are now able to do so, producing headache.

There is experimental evidence to support this view. Biopsies from superficial temporal arteries clinically involved in the headache have revealed changes compatible with oedema but without cellular infiltration (Ostfeld et al., 1957). They described changes 'in tissue turgor and a gross appearance of slight to moderate oedema . . . in the area of the headache'. A nociceptive, vasoactive substance termed 'neurokinin' has been isolated from perivascular tissue during a migraine attack (Chapman et al., 1960) while more recent work in animal models has shown that ergotamine and sumatriptan (a newly developed 5-HT$_1$ agonist), both effective in acute treatment, may act by inhibiting neurogenically produced inflammation instead of constricting blood vessels per se (Saito et al., 1988; Buzzi and Moskowitz, 1990). The mechanism by which blood vessels become inflamed is unclear but the simplistic view that vasoconstriction leads to the migrainous aura on an ischaemic basis with subsequent vasodilatation to cause the headache is no longer generally accepted.

A neurogenic origin for the headache based on the trigeminovascular system has been described (Moskowitz et al., 1989), whereby nociceptive fibres from blood vessels may be modulated or even activated at various points from the blood vessel to the brain stem trigeminal complex. Following depolarization, substance P is released from peripheral nerve endings where it can modulate its own nerve terminals, dilate blood vessels, increase vascular permeability, and activate mast cells participating in the inflammatory response. In this system, other modulators affecting the vessel wall–sensory nerve terminal could be biochemical, e.g. prostaglandins, hormones, platelet contents; mechanical, e.g. vessel wall dilatation; ionic, e.g. spreading depression, as well as neural, e.g. sympathetic or parasympathetic.

The concept of inflammatory pain, albeit based largely on circumstantial evidence, is central to current ideas on the mechanism of migraine headache and forms a rational basis for its acute treatment. Aspirin and other non-steroidal anti-inflammatory drugs are often effective in acute therapy, but not universally so, suggesting that other pain transmitters, not involved in the cyclo-oxygenase pathway, may be important, e.g. products of the lipoxygenase pathway or central pain pathways. In the spinal cord there are descending as well as ascending pain modulating pathways and such neurotransmitters as serotonin, enkephalins and prostaglandins could act at various levels to control pain transmission. Aspirin may well have a central action in pain modulation in migraine.

14.3.2 Aspirin and NSAIDs in Acute Migraine Treatment

NON-STEROIDAL ANTI-INFLAMMATORY DRUGS AND ACUTE MIGRAINE TREATMENT

Aspirin can be considered within the family of non-steroidal anti-inflammatory drugs (NSAIDs) and what is found for one member of the group may apply to others. The first studies of a NSAID in acute migraine date back to the 1960s using indomethacin (Sicuteri et al., 1964; Anthony and Lance, 1968) but it was not until the 1970s, with the studies of Vane concerning the inhibition of prostaglandin synthesis by aspirin, that this group of drugs was more fully evaluated for therapeutic efficacy in migraine. Interestingly, indomethacin is not effective for acute treatment and headache is a common side effect.

There is evidence from double-blind, placebo-controlled studies for the efficacy of tolfenamic acid (Hakkarainen et al., 1979), flurbiprofen (Awidi, 1982), naproxen (Johnson et al., 1985; Nestvold et al., 1985) and flufenamic acid (Carasso et al., 1985). The largest study (Johnson et al., 1985) included 110 patients in a parallel trial involving 10 migraine attacks, both common and classical. Twenty-four patients completed the full 10-attack period, 18 had between five and nine attacks, and 28 had less than five attacks. At the onset of an attack, either three 275 mg tablets of sodium naproxen or placebo were taken with a further two tablets 1 h later if needed. Diaries kept by patients indicated changes in symptoms, their duration and any adverse effects, and a significant difference was noted between active drug and placebo in both headache duration and severity, and in the number of additional tablets needed. When the effect between the two treatments was compared in each type of migraine, a significant benefit over placebo was seen only in the common migraine group (16 on active drug, 23 on placebo). The smaller number of classical migraine sufferers (19 on active treatment, 10 on placebo), or the shorter mean duration of symptoms in classical compared to common migraine, may explain this difference.

At the Princess Margaret Migraine Clinic we have found that sodium diclofenac (75 mg) intramuscularly is one of the most effective acute migraine treatments. It is the only non-steroidal anti-inflammatory drug that can be administered parenterally.

Various trials have compared NSAIDs with a reference drug (for review, Pradalier *et al.*, 1988) but only those involving aspirin will be discussed.

ASPIRIN AND ACUTE MIGRAINE TREATMENT

Clinical observations

Ross-Lee *et al.*, (1982a) described a retrospective study of the use of oral aspirin in acute migraine attacks. In a series of 200 consecutive patients drawn from the records of a neurological practice, 87 patients had been advised to take soluble aspirin for their migraine attacks, 93 to take ergotamine (in various forms) and in 20 no drug therapy had been offered. The patients taking aspirin tended to be younger than those taking ergotamine but in other respects the groups were similar. By personal and postal follow-up it was possible to ascertain what had happened to 61 of the original 87 taking aspirin. Twenty-seven (44%) reported that aspirin was usually or always effective for their attacks, whilst another 15 (25%) indicated that the drug was sometimes effective, i.e. aspirin was useful in 69% of cases. The response to aspirin was unrelated to the patient's age, sex or duration of migraine history, nor was the response related to severity or the occurrence of nausea and vomiting. The presence of an aura improved the chance of a good response to aspirin, presumably because attacks were treated at an earlier stage when absorption was greater. Adverse effects reported in 16% were mainly nausea and vomiting, presumably due to the attack itself.

Pharmacokinetic and efficacy studies of aspirin absorption in migraine, different preparations and routes of administration

Volans (1974) studied plasma salicylate levels in 42 patients treated with 900 mg of effervescent aspirin during migraine attacks and in 20 controls. Nineteen of the patients showed significant impairment of aspirin absorption which correlated with severity of headache and with gastrointestinal symptoms at the time of treatment, but not with the duration of the attack or migraine type.

Nausea and/or vomiting are almost universal in migraine attacks and we know from barium meal studies that gastric dilatation occurs at this time. Volans (1975) therefore proceeded to look at the effect of metoclopramide (an anti-nauseant which increases gut motility) on absorption of effervescent aspirin in acute and asymptomatic migraine sufferers and in normal controls. One group of migraineurs was given 900 mg effervescent aspirin only, and a second group then received

10 mg intramuscular metoclopramide, 10 min before the same dose of aspirin. During a migraine attack, and after aspirin alone, there was a significant impairment in the rate of aspirin absorption compared to headache free migraineurs or normal volunteers. With intramuscular metoclopramide treatment, absorption became similar to headache-free migraineurs and normal volunteers; it was concluded that poor aspirin absorption during a migraine attack was due to impaired gastro-intestinal motility with delayed gastric emptying. Both studies can be criticized because, in each, plasma salicylate and not aspirin levels were measured.

Ross-Lee *et al.* (1982b), measured plasma aspirin and salicylate levels at intervals over a 2-h period during migraine attacks in 10 subjects given 900 mg soluble aspirin alone, in 10 subjects given 900 mg soluble aspirin plus 10 mg oral metoclopramide, and in 10 subjects given 900 mg soluble aspirin plus an intramuscular injection of 10 mg metoclopramide. Higher peak aspirin and salicylate levels occurred with the addition of oral or intramuscular metoclopramide. Aspirin appeared earlier in the plasma in those taking oral metoclopramide and there was better early pain relief. By 1 h from dosing, intramuscular metoclopramide was also associated with better pain relief than aspirin alone.

Tfelt-Hansen and Olesen (1984) compared metoclopramide (10 mg) and aspirin (650 mg) in effervescent formulation (Migravess®), with effervescent aspirin (650 mg, Alka-Seltzer®) or placebo in a double-blind crossover study of 118 common migraine sufferers. Eighty five patients completed all three forms of treatment, 11 completed two and six only one. After each form of treatment for a migraine attack, they mailed a report form to the investigators. Additional medication was allowed after 2 h and was taken for 79/95 placebo-treated attacks, 63/92 Migravess-treated attacks, and 51/86 aspirin-treated attacks. Aspirin was significantly better than placebo for pain relief, but not quite significant for nausea relief, whereas Migravess was significantly better than placebo for pain and nausea relief; there was no significant difference between aspirin and the combination with regard to analgesic or antiemetic effects. They concluded that the dose of metoclopramide was probably too low in this preparation.

Brandon *et al.* (1986) looked at a new, pleasant-tasting formulation of aspirin, glycinated aspirin, in normal healthy volunteers and assessed the bioavailability of this preparation when given in a variety of ways; swallowed with 200 ml of water, dissolved sublingually and retained in the mouth, or dispersed on the tongue and swallowed without water. There was no detectable absorption of aspirin when retained in the mouth but equal absorption when swallowed with or without water.

They found no difference in efficacy when the glycinated aspirin was swallowed with or without water during an acute migraine attack and suggested this preparation may be useful in treating attacks when water was not available.

Intravenous aspirin (DL-lysine-acetylsalicylate, Venoprin®) has been available in Japan since 1983, one vial containing 497 mg of aspirin, and it has been used for pain relief in a variety of conditions. About 15 min after its injection in three patients with severe acute migraine attacks 'the headache disappeared completely without any side-effect' (Noda *et al.*, 1985).

Aspirin versus other acute treatments for migraine

Aspirin treatment of acute migraine attacks has been compared with several other acute treatments.

Aspirin versus paracetamol In 1980 the standard treatment for acute migraine attacks at the Copenhagen migraine clinic was metoclopramide 10 mg i.m., diazepam 5 mg orally and then aspirin 1 g orally or paracetamol 1 g orally. Tfelt-Hansen and Olesen compared aspirin with paracetamol in a double blind trial; 435 patients received aspirin and 254 paracetamol. The two groups were not statistically significantly different, and they concluded that aspirin and paracetamol were of equal efficacy in acute migraine.

Aspirin compared to ergotamine and a dextropropoxyphene–aspirin–phenazone combination A double-blind crossover protocol lasting for seven attacks per drug was used (Hakkarainen *et al.*, 1980), and 25 patients (10 classical, 15 common migraine) participated. Doses used were 500 mg of aspirin, 100 mg of dextropropoxyphene and 1 mg of ergotamine tartrate. One repeat dosage of the same medication could be taken after 30 min if required. The percentage of attacks prevented totally by medication was 47% (ergotamine), 41% (dextropropoxyphene compound) but only 18% for aspirin. There was no significant difference between the first two drugs but there was a significant difference with aspirin. The severity of attacks which occurred despite treatment was less in 50% of cases with dextropropoxyphene, 39% of cases with ergotamine and 30% with aspirin (no significant difference between aspirin and ergotamine). Patients had a significantly stronger preference for ergotamine and dextropropoxyphene than for aspirin, but then efficacy was similar in both common and classical migraine.

Aspirin compared to ergotamine and tolfenamic acid Aspirin has been compared against ergotamine tartrate, tolfenamic acid and placebo in 20 patients (8 classical, 12 common migraine) in a crossover study using alternately for every two attacks either aspirin (500 mg), tolfenamic acid (200 mg), ergotamine tartrate (1 mg) or placebo, for a total of 160 attacks (Hakkarainen *et al.*, 1979). The duration of attacks was significantly shortened by all three active drugs when compared with placebo. There was no significant difference between tolfenamic acid and ergotamine either in common or classical attacks but aspirin was not effective in classical attacks when compared with placebo, the explanation given being poor absorption due to gastric stasis.

14.3.3 Aspirin and NSAIDs in migraine prophylaxis

Aspirin is useful in prophylactic treatment of migraine but its mode of action is not clear, although inhibition of prostaglandin production might prevent migraine (for a review of prostaglandins and leukotrienes in migraine, Parantainen *et al.*, 1986).

A variety of prostaglandins have been infused into migraineurs and controls but, with the possible exception of two cases, a migraine attack has never been precipitated (for review, Pradalier *et al.*, 1988).

In 1965, Bergstrom *et al.* infused prostaglandin E_1 (PGE_1), a hyperalgetic vasodilator, intravenously in three healthy volunteers. After 15 min one subject experienced bitemporal headache associated with a visual disturbance consisting of flashing lights and brightly coloured images, and another developed a mild headache. Three years later, Carlson repeated these experiments and infused increasing doses of PGE_1 into eight normal volunteers and found that he could produce headache in all, nausea in three, vomiting in one and photopsia in one. At higher doses the headache was more severe and accompanied by nausea. When prostacyclin (PGI_2) was infused in six healthy males in a double-blind, crossover trial (FitzGerald *et al.*, 1979) three developed headache and one nausea and abdominal pain. Peatfield *et al.* (1981) infused PGI_2 into migraine patients, cluster headache sufferers and controls, but were unable to induce migraine in migraine sufferers: although some experienced headache, this was no greater in migraine subjects that in controls. There is no single hyperalgetic or inflammatory mediator which reliably induces migraine attacks when infused intravenously in migraine sufferers.

The involvement of platelets in migraine attacks is well established but their precise role is controversial (for review, Davies *et al.*, 1988). In one theory (Hanington, 1978), the platelet is primarily involved in migraine and is, at all times, different in migraineurs compared to controls. Trigger factors would physiologically activate these 'abnormal' platelets to produce a gradual but significant increase in serotonin release, causing pathological activation of other platelets at the onset of the attack. This platelet release reaction would lead to vasoconstriction, and the following serotonin depletion to subsequent vasodilatation. This theory stimulated many studies attempting to correlate measurements of platelet aggregation with clinical effects during migraine prophylactic treatment.

Aspirin, and other NSAIDs, are well known for their inhibitory action on platelet aggregation by inhibiting the production of pro-aggregatory prostanoids. Platelet aggregation before and during treatment was studied in 46 patients, each taking aspirin 250 mg daily for 2 months, and in 10 controls (Smith et al., 1984). As other investigators had found, it was noted that platelets are hyperaggregable in migraine patients compared to controls, that aspirin treatment reduced aggregation but this was not associated with any significant clinical improvement. The hypothesis that migraine is primarily a platelet aggregation disorder is no longer tenable (Steiner et al., 1985).

The effects of aspirin 160 mg daily for 3 months was studied in 27 migraine patients in a double-blind, placebo-controlled crossover study (Hosman-Benjaminse and Bolhuis, 1986). No correlation was found between frequency or severity of migraine attacks and the inhibition of ADP-induced platelet aggregation by aspirin, nor was there any difference in efficacy between aspirin and placebo.

The effect of aspirin and flunarizine on platelet activation was studied in two groups of migraine sufferers (common/classic and classic/complicated migraine) and in one group suffering from transient ischaemic attacks (TIAs) (D'Andrea et al., 1985). Plasma levels of beta-thromboglobulin (beta-TG) and platelet factor 4 (PF4), indices of in-vivo platelet activation, were determined before and during treatment with aspirin (50 mg day^{-1}) or flunarizine (10 mg day^{-1}). Before and during treatment, patients with classic and complicated migraine attacks showed a high incidence of in-vivo platelet activation (as did those in the TIA group) whereas common migraine sufferers did not. Administration of aspirin was more effective than flunarizine in reducing beta-TG and PF4 levels in migraine sufferers but aspirin had no effect on these markers in TIA patients. It was concluded that the classic/complicated migraine group differed from the common/classic group in terms of platelet activation which was aspirin-sensitive, while in the TIA group platelet activation occurred through other, non-aspirin sensitive pathways. In a similarly designed study (D'Andrea et al., 1984) basal plasma levels of beta-TG and PF4 were significantly higher in those with classical migraine compared to controls whereas in common migraineurs only beta-TG levels were elevated. The authors suggested that platelet activation occurs *in vivo* in migraineurs during headache-free periods. Aspirin (50 mg day^{-1}) decreased plasma beta-TG and PF4 in both types of migraineurs, so this treatment may prove helpful in 'diminishing the vascular side-effects known to occur in migraine sufferers'.

Further evidence that the inhibition of platelet aggregation is unimportant for migraine prophylaxis comes from studies with dipyridamole. It may be useful in low dosage (100 mg day^{-1}) but higher doses may actually provoke migraine (Hawkes, 1978).

STUDIES OF MIGRAINE PROPHYLAXIS WITH NSAIDS

Placebo-controlled studies

Several studies on NSAID efficacy in migraine prophylaxis have shown the statistically significant superiority of a NSAID over placebo for one of the criteria studied. Ketoprofen (Stensrud and Sjaastad, 1974), tolfenamic acid (Mikkelsen and Viggo Falk, 1982), sodium naproxen (Lindegaard *et al.*, 1980; Welch *et al.*, 1985) and fenoprofen (Diamond *et al.*, 1987) are better than placebo while indomethacin (Sicuteri *et al.*, 1964; Anthony and Lance, 1968) is not.

Studies against a reference drug

Mefenamic acid (500 mg tds) was similar to propranolol (80 mg tds) in a placebo controlled crossover study involving 3-month treatment periods for each of the three substances (Johnson *et al.*, 1986).

STUDIES OF MIGRAINE PROPHYLAXIS WITH ASPIRIN

Placebo-controlled studies

A double-blind crossover study of aspirin, 650 mg twice a day, was carried out against placebo in 12 patients (O'Neill and Mann, 1978), but criteria for the diagnosis of migraine were not exactly stated. Treatment was for 3 months with each agent and in seven patients platelet aggregation to epinephrine and adenosine diphosphate was studied during the trial. In nine patients on aspirin a highly significant reduction in headache frequency was seen, all responders having classical migraine: all the females in the study responded and those with hyperaggregable platelets seemed to respond best of all. Following the idea that platelet aggregation inhibition was an important mechanism in migraine prophylaxis, Masel *et al.* (1980), in a double-blind crossover study, compared aspirin 325 mg twice a day, combined with dipyridamole 25 mg three times a day against placebo in 25 patients. The active treatment was significantly better than placebo with 68% of patients reporting subjective improvement while on active treatment.

In a double-blind parallel group study with 40 patients in each of four groups, one group received dipyridamole 75 mg four times a day, another aspirin 325 mg four times a day, another group dipyridamole 75 mg plus aspirin 325 mg four times a day while the fourth group received placebo (Ryan and Ryan, 1981). The best reduction in attack frequency and severity was with aspirin and dipyridamole combined but both aspirin alone and dipyridamole alone were better than placebo.

The optimum dose of aspirin for migraine prophylaxis is uncertain but there is some evidence in favour of as low a dose as 60–80 mg day^{-1} (Wind and Punt, 1982, 1989).

Perhaps the strongest evidence for the efficacy of aspirin in migraine prophylaxis comes from a 6-year study conducted among 5139 apparently healthy British male doctors to ascertain whether 500 mg of aspirin daily would reduce the incidence of mortality from stroke, myocardial infarction, or other vascular conditions (Peto et al., 1988). Two thirds of the subjects were allocated effervescent or soluble aspirin 500 mg each day (or 300 mg enteric coated aspirin if subsequently requested) while one third were asked to avoid aspirin (there being no placebo group). There was a highly significant decrease in the reporting of migraine attacks in the aspirin-treated group, but it was suggested that more studies were needed to assess the efficacy of aspirin in migraine prophylaxis.

Studies against a reference drug

In a study comparing aspirin with propranolol, 12 patients completed a double-blind, crossover study comparing propranolol 1.8±0.1 mg kg^{-1} day^{-1} and aspirin 13.5±1.2 mg kg^{-1} day^{-1} for 3-month periods (Baldrati et al., 1983). Both drugs resulted in a decrease in migraine indices (product of severity and duration) of 65% on average in comparison with the run-in period, but no difference was found between the drugs in terms of severity, frequency or duration of migraine attacks, suggesting that aspirin was equally as effective as propranolol.

Other studies

The efficacy of a combination of dihydroergotamine (10 mg) with low dose aspirin (80 mg) and placebo in the prophylactic treatment of migraine was studied in a double-blind crossover trial, each arm being of 2 months duration (Bousser *et al.*, 1988). Thirty eight patients completed the study from the 45 starters. The number of attacks was significantly reduced by active treatment but the mean duration, mean severity and the mean score for amount of medication for attacks did not differ significantly. The results were interpreted as showing a modest beneficial effect of the combination in migraine prophylaxis. While the contribution of aspirin to the beneficial effects seen in this study is unclear, the scale of the overall response argues against the marked efficacy of low dose aspirin in migraine prophylaxis which has been suggested by others (Wind and Punt, 1982, 1989).

14.4 ASPIRIN IN THE TREATMENT OF TENSION HEADACHE

It is unfortunate that the most commonly recognized headache of all, tension headache, is the least well understood in pathophysiological terms and, in general, responds poorly to analgesics.

Tension headache is an ill-defined syndrome, the name itself being much disputed and not occurring in the classification of headache by the Ad Hoc Committee of the National Institute of Health (1962), which preferred the term muscle contraction headache. Patients commonly consider that the adjective 'tension' refers to emotional tension when it is really meant as muscle tension. The terms muscle contraction headache, chronic daily headache or benign headache have been used interchangeably. For these reasons such headaches are now classified as tension-type headaches by the Headache Classification Committee of the International Headache Society (1988) since neither muscle contraction nor psychological tension need be the mechanism of headache production.

Tension-type headaches may be episodic or chronic. Mild episodic tension-type headaches are familiar to all and it is easy to determine their provoking factors. Usually lasting less than 12 h, they can last for one or several days. They are usually bilateral, variable in location, dull, aching and non-pulsatile in nature. In most cases, pain is the only symptom, but occasionally increased sensitivity to light, irritability and dizziness may occur. Treatment is commonly a mild analgesic such as aspirin.

In chronic tension-type headache the pain can be constant for days, weeks or years and is generally scored as being more severe than the episodic form but less so than migraine. This group forms the major load in specialist practices and in hospitals and there is a tendency for overuse or abuse of drugs. Prophylactic treatment, for example with amitriptyline, is often effective.

Many mechanisms may be operating, e.g. increased muscle tone, disturbances of endogenous pain controlling pathways, and emotional influences, speculation being made more difficult because patients with tension-type headache do not form a homogeneous group.

While aspirin is an effective agent in episodic tension-type headache (Murray, 1964), so too is ibuprofen (Ryan, 1977). Aspirin (650 mg) has been compared against ibuprofen (400 mg or 800 mg) and placebo in a double-blind, randomized, parallel trial in which patients took the same medication for four successive headaches (Diamond, 1983). Paracetamol was allowed as a rescue medication. Intensity of headache (intense = 4, none = 1), and other symptoms, were recorded before treatment and 3 h post-treatment, and it was found that ibuprofen, at either dose, was significantly more effective than placebo and at least as effective as aspirin but with fewer side effects.

In 269 otherwise healthy subjects with moderately severe headaches which had previously responded to non-prescription medication, a randomized, parallel, double-blind study was done comparing 650 mg aspirin and 1000 mg of paracetamol with each other, and with an identical placebo (Peters et al., 1983). The three groups were demographically similar. Headache intensity and relief scores were obtained over the 6 h following treatment and assessed by analyses of sums of pain intensity differences and values of pain relief scores. Responses for the groups on active medication were significantly better than placebo but not different between active treatments, nor was there any difference in side effects between the three treatments. A subgroup with tension headache (107 persons) responded significantly better to either active medication than to placebo. In subjects with tension-vascular headaches (162) only aspirin at 2 h was superior to placebo, but a direct comparison with paracetamol suggested no real difference. It was concluded that aspirin (650 mg) and paracetamol (1000 mg) are clinically similar in the treatment of headaches.

The time course of pain relief in tension headache after taking 684 mg solid aspirin or 648 mg effervescent aspirin, or matching placebos was studied in 47 patients with 33 patients taking all four trial drugs (Langemark and Olesen, 1987). There was no statistically significant difference between solid and effervescent aspirin but either aspirin was significantly better than placebo for pain relief.

In a study without placebo the efficacy of Micrainin® (meprobamate-acetylsalicylic acid) was compared with aspirin and, not surprisingly, it was found that the addition of an anti-anxiety agent, meprobamate, made Micrainin significantly more effective than aspirin alone (Glassman et al., 1982). The improved response over aspirin paralleled the improved relief in anxiety.

Therapeutic applications

Non-migrainous headache has been claimed to be a useful model for the evaluation of the acute efficacy of oral analgesics (Graffenried and Nuesch, 1980) and a dose relationship for pain relief with aspirin was found to be in the range of 250–1000 mg.

14.5 THE EFFECT OF CAFFEINE AS AN ANALGESIC ADJUVANT

Caffeine is commonly blamed as a migraine precipitant yet is frequently found in over-the-counter analgesic preparations. Of 30 clinical studies involving more than 10 000 patients conducted over the last 20 years the value of caffeine as an analgesic adjuvant was assessed (Laska *et al.*, 1984). Most studies included patients with pain of pelvic origin (dysmenorrhoea, episiotomy pain) but some involved headache and pain following oral surgery. The overall pooled relative potency estimate of an analgesic with caffeine to one without caffeine was 1.41, with 95% confidence limits of 1.23–1.63. It was concluded that to obtain the same amount of response from an analgesic without caffeine would require a dose that is approximately 40% greater than the one with caffeine.

14.6 OTHER TYPES OF HEADACHE

There are a few reports on the use of aspirin in other headache types.

14.6.1 Cluster Headache

This condition, previously called migrainous neuralgia, is much more common in men than women and frequently starts in the 3rd and 4th decades of life. The pain can be extremely severe, lasting from 30 min to 3 h. It is always on the same side of the head, usually centred around the eye which is usually red, watering and has a small pupil (partial Horner's syndrome). The headaches commonly wake the sufferer at night and may occur daily or several times a day during a 6–12-week cluster period, which gives this headache syndrome its name.

Although there have been no formal studies of the use of aspirin in this condition, clinical experience indicates that aspirin is ineffective as an acute treatment.

14.6.2 Chronic Paroxysmal Hemicrania

This type of headache resembles cluster headache with regard to pain localization, intensity and character, but differs in being more common in women, the attacks are more frequent but shorter in duration and are abolished completely by prophylactic indomethacin treatment. The

388

first case in which complete control of chronic paroxysmal hemicrania was achieved using small doses of aspirin has recently been reported in a 9-year old child (Kudrow and Kudrow, 1989).

14.6.3 Alternating Hemiplegia of Childhood

This is a rare syndrome of childhood where recurrent alternating hemiplegia occurs leading to a delay in motor and mental development. In a single case report, improvement in severity, duration and frequency of the attacks on prophylactic treatment was reported with a combination of flunarizine, acetazolamide and aspirin, but the contributing effect of aspirin is difficult to assess (Siemes and Casaer, 1988).

14.6.4 'Intractable Headache and Facial Pain'

In a mixed group of headache and facial pain sufferers the effects of intravenous aspirin was investigated (Fukuda and Izumikawa, 1988). The diagnoses included combined headache (6), common migraine (5), symptomatic trigeminal neuralgia (2), effort migraine (1) and non-migrainous vascular headache (1). One vial containing 497 mg aspirin (DL-lysine-acetylsalicylate; Venoprin) was injected intravenously over 3–5 min. The efficacy was judged as excellent (producing complete relief) in four (common migraine two, effort migraine one, and non-migrainous vascular headache one), good (almost complete relief) in seven (symptomatic trigeminal neuralgia two, common migraine three, combined headache two), and fair (incomplete relief) in four (all combined headache). No serious adverse effects were seen and no comment was made on lesser side effects, but there was no placebo in this small study.

14.6.5 Analgesic Rebound Headaches

Analgesic rebound headache is an often unrecognized clinical syndrome seen in chronic headache sufferers where frequent and excessive use of analgesics (more than 14 tablets per week) such as aspirin and paracetamol perpetuate and worsen pain rather than relieve it. This paradoxical effect of analgesics is termed rebound headache (Rapoport, 1988) and such sufferers are commonly seen in specialist migraine clinics. Most sufferers are aged 30–50 years and have a history of mild, subacute or chronic headache. As the frequency and/or the duration of pain slowly increases, patients gradually use larger and more frequent doses of analgesics. Withdrawing analgesics then improves headache but the washout period can be several weeks. Analgesic rebound headache is more common in headache sufferers than non-sufferers who take similar quantities of analgesics for non-headache pain (Lance *et al.*, 1988)

The long term prognosis of analgesic withdrawal in patients with drug-induced headaches has been studied by admission to hospital for 2 weeks, then follow-up (mean follow-up period = 16.8±13.6 months), of 54 patients, with 38 patients completing the study (Baumgartner *et al.*, 1989). The duration of headache history was 21.9±12.8 years and each patient took an average of 38.8±22.8 tablets or suppositories a week and an average of 2.5 different drugs. All patients had taken at least one drug containing caffeine, 80% of drugs contained ergotamine, 77.1% pyrazolon derivatives, 62.9% barbiturates, 48.6% para-aminophenol derivatives, 42.9% aspirin, 25.7% codeine and 25.7% minor tranquillizers. Analgesics were discontinued abruptly on admission and withdrawal symptoms alleviated by neuroleptics and neurotropics. During the second week of admission varied migraine and tension-type headache prophylactic treatments were instituted as necessary. At the end of the study 76.3% of patients had significantly reduced their analgesic intake, 60.5% had experienced a significant relief of headache both in intensity and frequency while 23.7% were regarded as therapeutic failures. The first 6 months after hospitalization appeared critical for determining long term success. The variables tested for prognostic relevance (age, sex, number of tablets a week, type of drug taken, type of initial headache) were not statistically significant.

14.7 CONCLUSIONS

Most people (80% in any one year) suffer from headache at some stage in their lives and find adequate relief from over-the-counter analgesics. A small proportion of headache sufferers (only about 1.5% per year) seek medical advice and a fraction of these are referred to hospital. At all levels migraine and tension-type headache are by far the most common headaches but neither is sufficiently well understood to explain the beneficial action of aspirin in acute or prophylactic migraine treatment, or in episodic tension-type headache.

In the acute treatment of migraine, benefit is related to drug absorption which is enhanced by drugs that overcome gastric stasis; soluble drug preparations do not show the advantages over solid medication that theory might suggest. Of other routes of aspirin administration studied, intravenous aspirin appears to be that in which further research may prove useful. There is little to choose between aspirin and paracetamol in the acute treatment of migraine.

Further studies are needed to investigate the efficacy of aspirin in migraine prophylaxis, as small doses (80 mg day^{-1}) do not appear to be effective. Aspirin at high dose (650 mg day^{-1}) is effective but benefit is unrelated to an inhibition of platelet aggregation.

In chronic tension-type headache there is a tendency to drug abuse and analgesic rebound headaches are commonly seen in specialist clinics. With appropriate treatment the prognosis is generally good. There are few data on the effect of aspirin in other types of headache syndromes.

Interest in the treatment of headache by the pharmaceutical industry has surged with the recent development of specific serotonin agonists and antagonists. While new and exciting treatments for migraine continue to appear it would be as well to remember the words of Professor Matthews in his book on *Practical Neurology* (1963):

> 'It is a frequent and rather humiliating experience to be told that after all the most recently introduced ergotamine preparations have failed, that a couple of aspirins seem to do the trick.'

REFERENCES

Ad Hoc Committee of National Institutes of Health (1962) Classification of headache. J. Am. Med. Assoc., **179**, 717–18.

Anthony, M. and Lance, J.W. (1968) Indomethacin in migraine. *Med. J. Aust*, **1**, 56–7.

Awidi, A.S. (1982) Efficacy of flurbiprofen in the treatment of acute migraine attacks: a double-blind cross-over study. *Curr. Therap. Res.*, **32**, 492–7.

Baldrati, A., Cortelli, P., Procaccianti, G. *et al.* (1983) Propranolol and acetylsalicylic acid in migraine prophylaxis. Double-blind cross over study. *Acta Neurol. Scand.*, **67**, 181–6.

Baumgartner, C., Wessely, P., Bingol, C. *et al.* (1989) Longterm prognosis of analgesic withdrawal in patients with drug-induced headaches. *Headache*, **29**, 510–14.

Bergstrom, S., Carlson, L.A., Erelund, L.G. and Oro, L. (1965) Cardiovascular and metabolic response to infusions of prostaglandin E_1 and to simultaneous infusions of noradrenaline and PGE_1 in man. *Acta Physiol. Scand.*, **641**, 332.

Bousser, M.G., Chick, J., Fuseau, E. *et al.* (1988) Combined low-dose acetylsalicylic acid and dihydroergotamine in migraine prophylaxis. A double-blind, placebo-controlled crossover study. *Cephalalgia*, **8**, 187–92.

Brandon, R.A., Eadie, M.J., Curran, A.C.W. *et al.* (1986) A new formulation of aspirin: bioavailability and analgesic efficacy in migraine attacks. *Cephalalgia*, **6**, 19–27.

Buzzi, M.G. and Moskowitz, M.A. (1990) The antimigraine drug, sumatriptan (GR43175), selectively blocks neurogenic plasma extravasation from blood vessels in dura mater. *Brit. J. Pharmacol.*, **99**, 202–6.

Therapeutic applications

Carasso, R.L., Odead, P. and Shlomo, Y. (1985) Flufenamic acid in migraine. *Int. J. Neurosci.*, **27**, 67–71.

Carlson, L.A., Eklund, L.G. and Oro, L. (1968) Clinical and metabolic effects of different doses of PGE_1 in man. *Acta Med. Scand.*, **183**, 423–30.

Chapman, L.F., Ramos, A.O., Goodell, H. *et al.* (1960) A humoral agent implicated in vascular headache of the migraine type. *Arch. Neurol.*, **3**, 223.

D'Andrea, G., Toldo, M., Canazi, A. and Ferro-Milone, F. (1984) Study of platelet activation in migraine: control by low doses of aspirin. *Stroke*, **15**, 271–5.

D'Andrea, G., Canazi, A., Toldo, M. and Ferro-Milone, F. (1985) Drugs and platelet activation in migraine and transient ischaemic attacks. *Cephalalgia*, **5** (suppl 2), 103–8.

Davies, P.T.G., Steiner, T.J. and Clifford-Rose, F. (1988) Headache: Part XV – Disturbances of platelet behaviour associated with migraine. *Int. Med. Specialist*, **9**, 83–92.

Diamond, S. (1983) Ibuprofen versus aspirin and placebo in the treatment of muscle contraction headache. *Headache*, **23**, 206–10.

Diamond, S., Soloman, G., Freitag, F. and Mehta, N. (1987) Fenoprofen in the prophylaxis of migraine: a double-blind placebo-controlled study. *Headache*, **27**, 246–9.

FitzGerald, G.A., Friedman, L.A., Mori, M. *et al.* (1979) A double-blind, placebo-controlled crossover study of prostacyclin in man. *Life Sci.*, **25**, 665–72.

Fukuda, Y. and Izumikawa, K. (1988) Intravenous aspirin for intractable headache and facial pain. *Headache*, **28**, 47–50.

Glassman, J.M., Joseph, P., Soyka, M.D. and Pollack, M. (1982) Treatment of muscle contraction headache: Micrainin versus aspirin. *Headache*, **22**, 101–9.

Graffenreid, B. and Nuesch, E. (1980) Non-migrainous headache for the evaluation of oral analgesics. *Brit. J. Clin. Pharmacol.*, **10**, 225S–231S.

Hakkarainen, H., Vapaatalo, H., Gothoni, G. and Parantainen, J. (1979) Tolfenamic acid is as effective as ergotamine during migraine attacks. *Lancet*, **ii**, 326–8.

Hakkarainen, H., Quiding, H. and Stockman, O. (1980) Mild analgesic as an alternative to ergotamine in migraine. A comparative study with acetylsalicyclic acid, ergotamine tartrate and dextropropoxyphene compound. *J. Clin. Pharmacol.*, **20**, 590–5.

Hanington, E. (1978) Migraine: A blood disorder? *Lancet*, **ii**, 501–3.

Hawkes, C.H. (1978) Dipyridamole in migraine. *Lancet*, **ii**, 153.

Headache Classification Committee of the International Headache Society (1988) Classification and diagnostic criteria for headache disorders, cranial neuralgias and facial pain. *Cephalalgia*, **8** (suppl. 7), 1–96.

Hopkins, A. and Ziegler, D.K. (1988) Headache – the size of the problem. In *Headache: Problems in Diagnosis and Management*, (ed. A. Hopkins), W.B. Saunders, London, pp. 1–7.

Hosman-Benjaminse, S.L. and Bolhuis, P.A. (1986) Migraine and platelet aggregation in patients treated with low dose ASA. *Headache*, **26**, 282–4.

Johnson, E.S., Ratcliffe, D.M. and Wilkinson, M. (1985) Naproxen sodium in the treatment of migraine. *Cephalalgia*, **5**, 5–10.

Johnson, R.H., Hornabrook, R.W. and Lambie, D.G. (1986) Comparison of mefenamic acid and propranolol with placebo in migraine prophylaxis. *Acta Neurol. Scand.*, **73**, 490–2.

Kudrow, D.B. and Kudrow, L. (1989) Successful aspirin prophylaxis in a child with chronic paroxysmal hemicrania. *Headache*, **29**, 280–1.

Lance, F., Wilkinson, M. and Parkes, C. (1988) Does analgesic abuse cause headaches de novo (letter). *Headache*, **28**, 61–2.

Langemark, M. and Olesen, J. (1987) Effervescent ASA versus solid ASA in the treatment of tension headache. A double-blind, placebo controlled study. *Headache*, **27**, 90–5.

Laska, E.M., Sunshine, A., Mueller, F. *et al.* (1984) Caffeine as an analgesic adjuvant. *J.Am. Med. Assoc*, **251**, 1711–18.

Lindegaard, K.F., Ovrelio, L. and Sjaastad, O. (1980) Naproxen in the prevention of migraine attacks. A double-blind placebo-controlled crossover study. *Headache*, **20**, 96–8.

Masel, B.E., Chesson, A.L., Peters, B.H. *et al* (1980) Platelet antagonists in migraine prophylaxis. A clinical trial using aspirin and dipyridamole. *Headache*, **20**, 13–18.

Matthews, W.B. (1963) *Practical Neurology*, Blackwell, Oxford.

Mikkelsen, B.M. and Viggo Falk, J. (1982) Prophylactic treatment of migraine with tolfenamic acid. *Acta Neurol*, **66**, 105–11.

Moskowitz, M.A., Buzzi, M.G., Sakas, D.E. and Linnik, M.D. (1989) Pain mechanisms underlying vascular headaches. *Rev. Neurol. (Paris)*, **145**, 181–93.

Murray, W.J. (1964) Evaluation of aspirin in treatment of headache. *Clin. Pharmacol. Ther.*, **5**, 21–5.

Nestvold, K., Kloster, R., Partinen, M. and Sulkava, R. (1985) Treatment of acute migraine attack: Naproxen and placebo compared. *Cephalalgia*, **5**, 115–19.

Noda, S., Itoh, H. and Umezaki, H. (1985) Successful treatment of migraine attacks with intravenous injection of aspirin. *J. Neurol. Neurosurg. Psychiat.* **48**, 1187.

O'Neil, B.P. and Mann, J.D. (1978) Aspirin prophylaxis in migraine. *Lancet*, **ii**, 1179–81.

Ostfeld, A.M., Chapman, L.F., Goodell, H. and Wolff, H.G. (1957) A summary of evidence concerning a noxious agent active locally during migraine. *Arch. Intern. Med.*, **96**, 142.

Parantainen, J., Vapaatalo, H. and Hokkanen, E. (1986) Clinical aspects of prostaglandins and leukotrienes in migraine. *Cephalalgia*, **6** (suppl. 4), 95–101.

Peatfield, R.C., Gawel, M.J. and Clifford Rose, F. (1981) The effect of infused prostacyclin in migraine and cluster headache. *Headache*, **21**, 190–5.

Peters, B.H., Fraim, C.J. and Masel, B.E. (1983) Comparison of 650 mg aspirin and 1000 mg paracetamol with each other, and with placebo in moderately severe headaches. *Am.J.Med.*, **74**, 36–42.

Peto, R., Gray, R., Collins, R. *et al.* (1988) Randomised trial of prophylactic daily aspirin in British male doctors. *Brit. Med. J.*, **296**, 313–16.

Pradalier, A., Clapin, A. and Dry, J. (1988) Treatment review: Non steroid anti-inflammatory drugs in the treatment and long-term prevention of migraine attacks. *Headache*, **28**, 550–7.

Rapoport, A.M, (1988) Analgesic rebound headache. *Headache*, **28**, 662–5.

Therapeutic applications

Ross-Lee, L., Eadie, M.J. and Tyrer, J.H. (1982a) Aspirin treatment of migraine attacks: clinical observations. *Cephalalgia*, **2**, 71–6.

Ross-Lee, L.M., Heazlewood, V., Tyrer, J.H. and Eadie, M.J. (1982b) Aspirin treatment of migraine attacks: plasma drug level data. *Cephalalgia*, **2**, 9–14.

Ryan, R.E. (1977) Motrin – a new agent for the symptomatic treatment of muscle contraction headache. *Headache*, **16**, 280–3.

Ryan, R.E. and Ryan, R.E. (1981) Migraine prophylaxis: a new approach. *Laryngoscope*, **91**, 1501–6.

Saito, K., Markowitz, S. and Moskowitz, M.A. (1988) Ergot alkaloids block neurogenic extravasation in dura mater: proposed action in vascular headaches. *Ann. Neurol.*, **24**, 732–7.

Sicuteri, F., Michelacci, S. and Anselmi, B. (1964) Characterisation of the vasoactive and anti-migraine properties of indomethacin, a new anti-inflammatory agent derived from indole. *Settim. Med. (Italy)*, **52**, 335.

Siemes, H. and Casaer, P. (1988) Alternating hemiplegia in childhood. Clinical report and single-photon emission computed tomography study. *Monatsschr-Kinderheilkd (German)*, **136**, 467–70.

Smith, M., Jerusalem, F., Rhyner, K. and Isler, H. (1984) Salicylate prophylaxis in migraine. *Schweiz. Arch. Neurol. Neurochir. Psychiatr.*, **135**, 273–5.

Steiner, T.J. and Clifford Rose, F. (1988) Problems encountered in the assessment of treatment of headache and migraine. In *Headache: Problems in Diagnosis and Management* (ed. A Hopkins), W.B. Saunders, London, pp. 307–48.

Steiner, T.J., Joseph, R. and Clifford Rose, F. (1985) Migraine is not a platelet disorder. *Headache*, **25**, 434–40.

Stensrud, P. and Sjaastad, O. (1974) Clinical trial of a new anti-bradykinin, anti-inflammatory drug ketoprofen in migraine. *Headache*, **14**, 96–100.

Tfelt-Hansen, P. and Olesen, J. (1980) Paracetamol (acetaminophen) versus acetylsalicylic acid in migraine. *Eur. Neurol.*, **19**, 163–5.

Tfelt-Hansen, P. and Olesen, J. (1984) Effervescent metoclopramide and aspirin (Migravess®) versus effervescent aspirin or placebo for migraine attacks: a double-blind study. *Cephalalgia*, **4**, 107–11.

Volans, G.N. (1974) Absorption of effervescent aspirin during migraine. *Brit. Med. J.*, **4**, 265–9.

Volans, G.N. (1975) The effect of metoclopramide on the absorption of effervescent aspirin in migraine. *Brit. J. Clin. Pharmac.*, **2**, 57–63.

Welch, K.M., Ellis, D.J. and Keenan, P.A. (1985) Successful migraine prophylaxis with naproxen sodium. *Neurology*, **35**, 1304–10.

Wind, J. and Punt, J. (1982) Low dose aspirin and migraine prophylaxis. *Laryngoscope*, **92**, 1198–9.

Wind, J. and Punt, J. (1989) Migraine prophylaxis with low-dose aspirin: a promising new approach. In *New Advances in Headache Research* (ed. F. Clifford Rose), Smith-Gordon, London, pp. 275–7.

15 *The use of aspirin in unstable angina with a supplement on atrial fibrillation*

J.A. CAIRNS

Unstable angina is a common condition intermediate between stable angina and acute myocardial infarction. Recent understanding about the pathophysiology of the acute complications of atherosclerotic coronary artery disease, and the benefits of aspirin in clinical trials have led to the widespread use of this agent in the management of these clinical syndromes.

15.1 DEFINITION

A spectrum of acute symptomatic manifestations of ischaemic heart disease lies between the well defined diagnosis of stable angina on the one hand and acute myocardial infarction on the other (Cairns, 1981). Although the predominant manifestation of all syndromes falling within this spectrum is that of ischaemic cardiac pain, a variety of terms (acute coronary insufficiency, intermediate coronary syndrome, crescendo angina, pre-infarction angina) has been employed, focusing on various aspects of the symptoms. The term unstable angina, in use since 1971 (Fowler, 1972) is the most simple, inclusive and descriptive that may be applied to this spectrum and is in general use.

Patients with the following syndromes are generally considered to have unstable angina:

1. angina of recent onset (previous 4 weeks);
2. angina with a progressively severe (crescendo) pattern (previous 4 weeks);
3. angina of prolonged duration (more than 15 min) at rest (includes patients with variant or Prinzmetal's angina);
4. angina occurring in the early period (4 weeks) after myocardial infarction.

Transient ST and T wave changes may occur, but the development

395

of fixed ECG abnormalities or significant myocardial enzyme elevation indicates that myocardial infarction has occurred.

15.2 CLINICAL COURSE AND PREVALENCE

Premonitory chest pain, as a sign of impending myocardial infarction, may have been recognized as early as 1799 by Parry (1799), although clear recognition of the syndromes of premonitory pain and of their clinical importance did not come until later (Feil, 1937; Sampson and Eliaser, 1937). Larger clinical studies published prior to 1970 (Nichol *et al.*, 1959; Beamish and Storrie, 1960; Wood, 1961; Vakil, 1964) of patients who received no long-acting nitrates, no anticoagulants, and no beta-blocking agents, observed that unstable angina was followed by acute myocardial infarction in from 21 to 80% of cases and by death in from 1 to 60%. With the recognition of the prognosis of these syndromes, the admission of patients to coronary care units, and the use of varying regimens of long-acting nitrates, beta-blockers, and anti-coagulation, the rate of acute myocardial infarction had fallen to 7–15% and of early sudden death to 1–2% by the 1970s (Fulton *et al.*, 1972; Kraus *et al.*, 1972). The patients at highest risk of acute myocardial infarction and sudden death were those with prolonged and recurrent rest pain in hospital, and with ST segment abnormalities accompanying the pain. Although the acute event rates had been sharply curtailed by the 1970s, patients continued to experience a high rate of vascular events over the year following hospitalization for unstable angina. Patients in the placebo groups in two large trials of anti-platelet drug therapy received varying combinations of long-acting nitrates, beta-blockers, anticoagulants, and calcium antagonists, and yet one year mortality was 9.6% in one trial (1974–81) (Lewis *et al.*, 1983) and 8.0% in the other (1979–84) (Cairns *et al.*, 1985).

The syndromes of unstable angina are common, accounting for approximately 25% of admissions to North American coronary care units (Cairns *et al.*, 1988).

15.3 PATHOPHYSIOLOGY

It has long been recognized that patients with unstable angina have extensive atherosclerotic coronary artery disease. Although a number of investigators have reported that coronary atherosclerosis is more extensive and severe in patients with unstable angina than in those with stable angina, the biases in such studies diminish their value, and the spectrum of fixed atherosclerotic lesions may be no different in patients with unstable angina (Maseri *et al.*, 1980; Rafflenbeul *et al.*, 1981). On the other hand, patients with unstable angina are more likely than those with stable angina to have had progression of coronary artery disease.

Moise and co-workers (1983) studied the progression of coronary artery disease in 38 patients who had undergone coronary angiography and after a mean of 44 months had developed unstable angina, followed by repeat coronary angiography. When these patients were compared to patients with stable angina, who had undergone a second angiogram after a mean of 35 months, progression of coronary artery disease was found to be much more marked in those with clinical unstable angina. It has been noted by other workers that patients with unstable angina may have less collateral formation (Rafflenbeul et al., 1979), and those who fail to respond to medical management may have more extensive and severe atherosclerosis (Hugenholtz et al., 1981; Bertrand 1985).

Increasingly, it appears that platelets play a role in the pathogenesis of coronary atherosclerosis and its complications. One of the normal functions of platelets is in haemostasis. Vessel injury results in collagen exposure, which stimulates platelet adhesion and aggregation. Eventually the platelets undergo a 'release reaction', with extrusion of active mediators of thrombosis from their cytoplasmic granules, including enzymatic liberation of arachidonic acid, and the sequential evolution of prostaglandins, culminating in the synthesis of thrombaxane A_2, an extremely potent vasoconstrictor and platelet aggregant. An irreversible stage of platelet aggregation is reached with fibrin and red blood cells incorporated in a haemostatic red thrombus.

The atherosclerotic plaque may have its origins in initial endothelial injury leading to platelet activation, release of a mitogenic factor that stimulates smooth muscle migration from media to subintima, and subsequent accumulation of lipids (Ross, 1986). Endothelial injury, particularly atherosclerotic plaque fracture, activates platelets, releasing thromboxane A_2 and may result in intraluminal thrombosis.

The observation of Moise et al., (1983) that progression of coronary atherosclerotic stenosis is a common feature of patients with unstable angina was confirmed by Ambrose et al., (1986). In addition, careful analysis of the morphology of these stenoses indicated that 71% of patients with unstable angina with progression of their coronary lesion to less than complete occlusion, had an eccentric stenosis, and very often the lesion was characterized by 'a narrow neck due to one or more overhanging edges or irregular, scalloped borders, or both', the so-called Ambrose Type II lesion (Fig. 15.1). It is very likely this is the angiographic appearance of a disrupted atherosclerotic plaque, a partially lysed thrombus, or both. Sherman et al., (1986) reported their observations from coronary angioscopy performed during coronary artery bypass surgery in 10 patients with unstable angina and

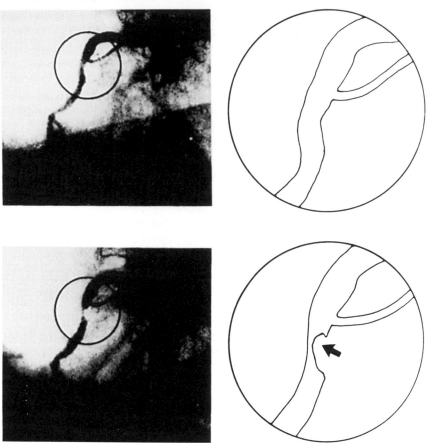

Figure 15.1 Selected angiographic frames from a patient with stable angina at the time of the upper study and unstable angina 4 months later, prompting the lower study. In the upper frame, there are only mild irregularities in the artery. In the lower frame, there is an eccentric stenosis with a convex intraluminal obstruction, overhanging edges, and irregular borders. It is likely this lesion represents plaque disruption, a partially occlusive thrombus, or both. (Reprinted from Ambrose *et al.*, 1986, with permission from the journal and author.)

10 patients with stable angina. Of the 17 arteries examined in the patients with stable angina, all had partially obstructive atheromas with a smooth surface free of haemorrhage, ulceration, or thrombus. Of the three patients with accelerated angina, all had a complex plaque characterized by ulceration and subendothelial haemorrhage, but no intraluminal thrombus. Of the seven patients with rest angina, all had either a partial or totally occlusive thrombus. The preceding

angiography was quite insensitive for the detection of complex plaque and intraluminal thrombosis. A number of reports of the angiographic anatomy of patients with unstable angina have shown considerable variation in the frequency of thrombosis (Suryapranata et al., 1988). However, the incidence is highest among those patients who undergo angiography within hours of the most recent episode of chest pain, suggesting that spontaneous lysis may have accounted for the relatively low incidence in earlier studies.

In the setting of acute myocardial infarction, abundant evidence from DeWood et al. (1980) indicates that occlusive coronary thrombosis is an early and important event in more than 80% of transmural infarcts. Falk (1985) has shown that patients experiencing sudden death preceded by serial episodes of unstable angina, may be shown at autopsy to have an occlusive thrombus composed of layers of platelet thrombi in different stages of organization, corresponding to the clinical episodes of ischaemia (Fig. 15.2). Platelet emboli distal to the site of the occlusive thrombosis have also been observed (Falk, 1985; Davies et al., 1986). Davies and Thomas (1984) have reported that coronary thrombosis and/or plaque injury have occurred in 95% of sudden death victims. Hence, a pathophysiologic sequence of atherosclerotic plaque fracture, platelet activation, and partial or complete coronary occlusion appears to underlie the development of the clinical syndromes of unstable angina and their complications of acute myocardial infarction and sudden death.

Recurrent episodes of pain at rest characterize the symptoms of many patients with unstable angina, and in some instances increased myocardial oxygen demand may underlie such pain patterns (Cannon et al., 1974). However, as a result of the work of Maseri and colleagues (1980), it is recognized that transient increases in coronary artery tone, usually in the region of an atherosclerotic plaque, are likely to account for many episodes of angina at rest. In a series of interrelated studies, these investigators showed that in patients with recurrent pain at rest, the initial change was myocardial and was followed by deviation of the ST segment and by chest pain, only if the ischaemic episode was sufficiently long and extensive. If alterations in blood pressure and heart rate occurred, they followed the changes in myocardial function. Other studies with thalium-201 showed that reversible defects of myocardial perfusion accounted for the changes in myocardial function and in the ECG (Maseri et al., 1976). Angiography done at the time of chest pain in patients with physiologic evidence of ischaemia showed severe coronary artery narrowing in the predicted location, yet when the test was repeated after administration of nitroglycerin and relief of ischaemic pain, substantial resolution of the narrowing was observed

Therapeutic applications

(Maseri *et al.*, 1977). A residual atherosclerotic lesion was usually detected in the area of the reversible stenosis. In some instances, the previously reversible spasm became prolonged, and acute myocardial infarction occurred (Maseri, *et al.*, 1978).

An extensive series of investigations make it very likely that platelet activation plays a role in the pathophysiology of recurrent ischaemic pain at rest. In a study of 19 patients with unstable angina at rest, Sobel and colleagues (1981) demonstrated that plasma levels of platelet-derived beta-thromboglobulin and platelet factor IV were significantly elevated in blood samples obtained during or within 4 h of an episode of angina. They were unable to observe such a clear association with plasma levels of thromboxane A_2. However, Fitzgerald and colleagues (1986) using measurements of 2,3 dinor-thromboxane B_2, a major urinary enzymatic metabolite of TXA_2, were able to show that, in hospital patients with unstable angina, 84% of episodes of chest pain were associated with phasic increases of this metabolite. Although platelet activation and thromboxane A_2 release are features of unstable

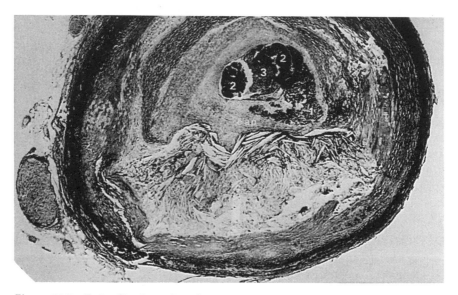

Figure 15.2 Episodic thrombus formation in a patient with unstable angina preceding fatal acute coronary thrombosis. This cross-section of an epicardial coronary artery depicts a large area of atheromatous 'gruel' in the lower half of the illustration. The thickened intima is then visible and occlusive thrombosis formed in three stages completely occludes the residual lumen. The oldest part of the thrombus (1) is incorporated into the fibrous cap covering the atheromatous 'gruel'. The acute thrombus associated with the fatal event is designated by (3). (Reprinted Falk, 1985, with permission from journal and author.)

400

angina, the administration of sufficient aspirin to almost completely suppress the TXA_2 synthesis does not decrease the episodes of recurrent ischaemia at rest, indicating that additional factors must play a role in the recurrence of ischaemia (Robertson et al., 1981; Chierchia et al., 1982). Folts et al., (1976) demonstrated in an experimental model of partial coronary occlusion and endothelial injury in the dog, a cyclic pattern of coronary blood flow decreases over a few minutes, to be followed by sudden restoration of flow, and repetition of the sequence. Microscopic examination of frozen sections revealed platelet plugging and subsequent dislodgement to underlie the cyclic blood flow variations (Fig. 15.3). Eventual sustained occlusion often occurs in this model. Administration of aspirin completely abolishes the cyclic flow variation. Ashton and colleagues (1989) have extended these observations to demonstrate abolition of the cyclic flow variations by the administration of a thromboxane A_2–prostaglandin H_2 receptor antagonist, or by a serotonin S_2 receptor antagonist. The effects of epinephrine to produce cyclic flow variations were overcome by the combined administration of the TXA_2 and the serotonin receptor antagonist. The sequence of platelet accumulation and release, if it occurs in humans, could account for episodic ischaemia at rest, and eventual complete occlusion could lead to coronary thrombosis and subsequently myocardial infarction or sudden death. Even in the absence of occlusive thrombosis, platelet embolization, analogous to that which precipitates transient cerebral ischaemic attacks in patients with carotid or vertebral atherosclerosis, may cause ischaemic complications. Experimental evidence in pigs showed that intracoronary infusion of adenosine diphosphate (ADP) or epinephrine results in platelet plugging and arrhythmic death (Jorgensen et al., 1967). Pretreatment with aspirin sharply reduced sudden death (Haft et al., 1972). Possibly analogous platelet emboli in the myocardial microcirculation have been noted in studies of human sudden death victims (Haerem 1974).

15.4 CLINICAL TRIALS OF ASPIRIN IN UNSTABLE ANGINA

Interest in the possible benefits of anti-thrombotic therapy in unstable angina extends back to the 1940s, when the first trials of anticoagulant therapy for these syndromes were initiated. Although there was a conclusion of efficacy in each of these early major trials (Nichol et al., 1959; Beamish and Storrie, 1960; Wood 1961; Vakil, 1964) none of them meets the criteria which are essential for such studies (Gifford and Feinstein, 1969). Uncertainties about the validity of these trials, and general improvements in medical management and outcomes in unstable angina, resulted in much less use of anti-coagulant treatment

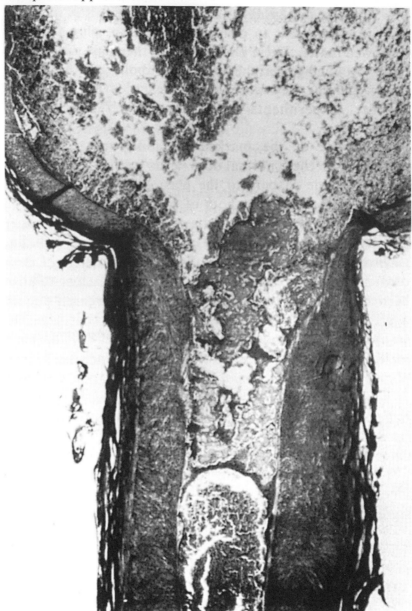

Figure 15.3 Canine coronary vessel showing site of partial constriction. At the low point of a cyclical flow reduction, the vessel was occluded proximal and distal to the partial constriction, excised, fixed and stained for platelets. This vessel shows platelet aggregates in the narrowed lumen. Vessels from dogs pretreated with ASA showed no cyclic flow and no platelet aggregates in the narrowed lumen. (Reprinted from Folts *et al.*, 1976, with permission from journal and author.)

for patients with unstable angina. However, with increasing experimental evidence for the role of thrombosis in the acute complications of coronary artery disease, the potential role for anticoagulation has been re-examined in several recent studies and appears to be efficacious (Telford and Wilson, 1981; Théroux et al., 1988; Neri Serneri et al., 1988; Cohen et al., 1990; The RISC Group, 1990).

Increasing evidence for the role of platelets in the pathogenesis of the complications of coronary artery disease, demonstration of the inhibitory effects of aspirin on platelet function, and the encouraging results from clinical trials in the secondary prevention of acute myocardial infarction and cerebrovascular disease stimulated the conduct of three major clinical trials of aspirin for the management of unstable angina (Table 15.1).

The Veterans' Administration Cooperative Study (Lewis et al., 1983) of aspirin was conducted in 12 Veterans' Administration medical centres between 1974 and 1981. A total of 1266 men entered the study and after 12 weeks of treatment, there was a marked benefit of aspirin in the reduction of death and myocardial infarction.

The target population consisted of patients hospitalized with a clinical diagnosis of unstable angina beginning within 1 month before and still present within the week before hospital admission. Patients had to have a good clinical history or ECG evidence of coronary artery disease, and an unstable angina pattern of either crescendo pain or prolonged pain at rest. Acute myocardial infarction was ruled out by ECG and enzymatic criteria. Of those patients with clinical unstable angina, 27.6% met the study criteria, and 18.3% entered the trial. Subsequently, 72 were found to have developed acute myocardial infarction and were excluded from the primary analysis, leaving 1266 patients.

Patients were randomly allocated to 324 mg of aspirin in an effervescent buffered powder (Alka-Seltzer) dissolved in water, or placebo. Coronary angiography was not performed routinely. Patients entered the study within 51 h of hospitalization. The principal outcome was death or acute myocardial infarction (AMI) which was reduced from 10.1% to 5.0% (51% reduction, $P = 0.0002$). The other major outcomes and the observed reductions were fatal or non-fatal AMI (55% reduction, $P = 0.001$), non-fatal AMI (51% reduction, $P = 0.005$) and all cause mortality (51% reduction, $P = 0.051$). An intention-to-treat analysis including all randomized patients indicated reductions in death or AMI (41% reduction, $P = 0.004$), and all cause mortality (34% reduction, $P = 0.17$). Eighty-six percent of patients were followed up to 1 year, with a reduction in mortality of 43% in the aspirin group, from 9.6% to 5.5% ($P = 0.008$).

The Canadian Multicentre Trial (Cairns et al., 1985) of aspirin or

Table 15.1 Randomized trials of aspirin in unstable angina

Author	Patients	mg/day⁻¹	Entry window	Follow-up	All-cause mortality			Cardiac death or nonfatal MI		
					ASA (%)	Placebo (%)	P	ASA (%)	Placebo (%)	P
Lewis et al., 1983	1266	324	51 h	3 months	1.6	3.3	0.054	5.0	10.1	0.005
Cairns et al., 1985	555	1300 + sulfinpyrazone	8 days	24 months	3.0	11.7	0.004	8.6	17.0	0.005
Théroux et al., 1988	479	650 + heparin	24 h	6 days	0	1.7		3.3	12	0.01

sulfinpyrazone, or both, in unstable angina was conducted in seven centres between 1979 and 1984. A total of 555 patients (73% men) entered the study, and after a mean follow-up of 18 months, there was a marked benefit from aspirin in the reduction of death and myocardial infarction. Sulfinpyrazone conferred no benefit.

The target population consisted of patients admitted to a coronary care unit with a clinical (non-angiographic) diagnosis of unstable angina. These patients underwent a detailed interview to determine whether there was good clinical or ECG evidence of myocardial ischaemia, and whether there was an unstable pain pattern, either crescendo pain or prolonged pain at rest. The study criteria were satisfied by 85% of the 817 patients interviewed after the exclusion process, among whom 159 refused study entry, leaving 555 who entered the trial. Patients were randomly allocated to one of four treatment regimens: aspirin (325 mg four times a day) or matching placebo, *plus* sulfinpyrazone (200 mg four times a day) or matching placebo, for a total of eight tablets daily to be taken with meals or milk. Coronary angiography was not a prerequisite for study entry.

The primary analysis was one of efficacy, with outcome to be assessed only among patients who met certain criteria established at the inception of the study, and applied without knowledge of treatment allocated or of clinical outcome. Patients in this analysis had to have been taking at least some study medication within the preceding month. The primary outcome event of cardiac death or non-fatal myocardial infarction occurred in 36 patients not given aspirin and in 17 taking aspirin, and by 2 years, the life table rate of these events was 17% versus 8.6%, a risk reduction of 50.8% ($P = 0.008$) (Fig. 15.4). The outcome event of cardiac death alone was reduced from 11.7% to 3%, a risk reduction of 71% ($P = 0.004$) (Fig. 15.5). All deaths were cardiac in this analysis.

In the intention-to-treat analysis, counting all randomized patients and all outcomes, the outcome of cardiac death or non-fatal myocardial infarction was observed in 70 patients, including 17 patients who were excluded from the primary analysis of efficacy. Again, sulfinpyrazone had no significant effect and no interaction with aspirin. The risk reduction with aspirin was 30% ($P = 0.072$). For the outcomes of cardiac death and death from any cause, the corresponding risk reductions with aspirin were 56.3% ($P = 0.009$) and 43.4% ($P = 0.035$), respectively.

A recently reported trial of aspirin, heparin or both in unstable angina, was conducted in two Canadian centres from 1986 to 1988 (Théroux *et al.*, 1988). A total of 479 patients (71% male) entered the study, and after a mean follow-up of 6 days, there was a marked benefit

Therapeutic applications

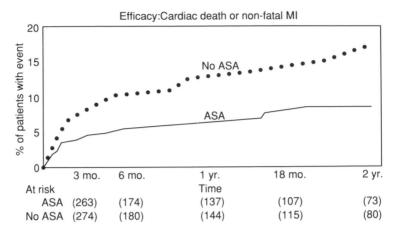

Efficacy:Cardiac death or non-fatal MI

At risk	3 mo.	6 mo.	1 yr.	18 mo.	2 yr.
ASA	(263)	(174)	(137)	(107)	(73)
No ASA	(274)	(180)	(144)	(115)	(80)

Figure 15.4 Occurrence of cardiac death or non-fatal myocardial infarction (MI) in the aspirin (ASA) and no aspirin groups of the Canadian multicenter trial of unstable angina. The graph is a life table depiction of the cumulative risk and time of first occurrence of an outcome event, according to aspirin allocation. The numbers of patients at risk are noted below the graph. (Reprinted from Cairns *et al.*, 1985, with permission from the journal and author.)

of heparin for a number of outcome events, with somewhat less benefit for the combination, or aspirin alone.

The target population consisted of patients hospitalized with a clinical diagnosis of unstable angina. The diagnosis was based upon a clinical history of accelerating chest pain or chest pain at rest, plus ECG or clinical evidence of underlying ischaemic heart disease. Acute myocardial infarction was ruled out by enzymatic and ECG criteria, and the patients entered the trial within 24 h of their most recent episode of pain. Of the patients admitted with unstable angina, 61.6% (479 patients) were randomized to one of four treatment regimens which were ASA 650 mg orally immediately, followed by 325 mg twice daily, or matching placebo, *plus* heparin 5000 units i.v., followed by an infusion of 1000 units h^{-1}, or matching placebo. Infusion rates were varied as necessary by the hospital pharmacist to maintain the coagulation time at 1.5–2 times control values, with similar adjustments of placebo infusions also undertaken. Coronary angiography was undertaken a mean of 4 days after randomization in 91% of patients in accordance with current clinical practice at the participating institutes. The study was ended when a final management decision was made, usually within 48 h after coronary angiography.

The three major end-points were: (1) refractory angina, defined as the presence of recurrent anginal chest pain with ischaemic ST-T changes occurring despite full medical therapy or the need for urgent intervention; (2) myocardial infarction; and (3) death.

Refractory angina occurred in 23% of placebo patients, and was reduced to 8% ($P = 0.002$) by heparin, 11% ($P = 0.011$) by aspirin plus heparin, and 17% ($P = 0.217$) by aspirin alone. Myocardial infarction was reduced from 11.9% on placebo to 0.8% ($P<0.0001$) by heparin, 1.6% ($P = 0.001$) by heparin plus aspirin, and 3.3% ($P = 0.012$) by aspirin alone. Mortality was 1.7% on placebo, while no deaths occurred on any of the study treatments. Although trends favoured heparin and the heparin plus aspirin combination over aspirin alone, there were no statistically significant differences between the treatment groups for any of the major end-points.

The principal side effect of concern was bleeding, most often at cardiac catheterization puncture sites. Bleeding occurred in 6.3% of all patients and was twice as common amongst patients receiving heparin. Serious bleeding occurred in 2.1% of patients.

The longer term trials of Lewis et al. (1983) and Cairns et al. (1985), did not demonstrate a reduction in the frequency of recurrent ischaemia in hospital (Lewis et al., 1984), and the striking benefits of aspirin appeared only over the next 3–24 months, presumably from the prevention of coronary thrombosis. On the other hand, in the short-term study of Théroux et al. (1988), where treatment lasted only 6 days, aspirin reduced the combined rate of fatal and non-fatal myocardial infarction by 72% as compared to placebo. Heparin appeared to be at least

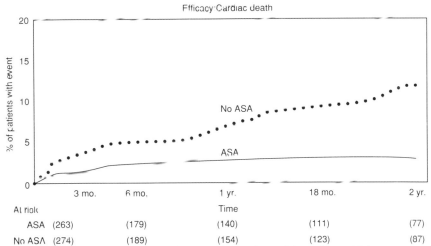

Figure 15.5 Occurrence of cardiac death in the ASA and no ASA groups of the Canadian multicenter trial of unstable angina. (Reprinted from Cairns et al., 1985, with permission from the journal and author.)

as efficacious, and in addition led to a significant reduction in the incidence of refractory angina.

Although gastrointestinal complaints occurred with remarkably similar frequency in the two longer term trials of aspirin in unstable angina (Lewis 38%, Cairns 39%), a significantly greater frequency of such side effects amongst aspirin-treated patients versus controls was observed only in the Cairns *et al.* (1985) trial ($P = 0.014$). In this trial, medication withdrawals were not more common among aspirin groups than non-aspirin groups. Nevertheless, overall withdrawal rate was 28% versus only 1.4% in the Lewis *et al.* (1983) study. This higher withdrawal rate may have arisen in part because the regimen required the ingestion of eight pills per day for 2 years, rather than only one pill a day for 12 weeks as in the Lewis trial, and the higher dose of aspirin itself may have contributed. In the UK-TIA Aspirin Trial (1988), the only randomized trial in vascular disease to compare two different doses of aspirin (300 mg versus 1200 mg day^{-1}), the smaller dose gave rise to fewer GI side effects ($2P < 0.001$) and less GI bleeding ($2P < 0.05$), yet was equally efficacious. It is clear therefore that a dose of aspirin of 325 mg daily is appropriate for patients with unstable angina. The hope of eliminating GI side effects almost completely, possibly limiting inactivation of PGI_2 synthesis, and the wish to use aspirin plus anticoagulation has led to trials employing lower dose aspirin regimens in conjunction with heparin and warfarin (Cohen *et al.*, 1990; The RISC Group, 1990).

In the RISC study (The RISC Group, 1990), 794 men hospitalized with unstable angina or non-Q wave infarction were randomized within 72 h to aspirin 75 mg day^{-1} or matching placebo, plus i.v. heparin 30 000 U day^{-1} or matching placebo in a factorial design. Aspirin significantly reduced the incidence of mycoardial infarction or death, and the addition of heparin appeared to further reduce the risk, particularly during the first days in hospital. Cohen *et al.* (1990) have also evaluated aspirin 325 mg alone, or at a dose of 80 mg in combination with heparin or warfarin in patients with unstable angina or non-Q wave infarction.

15.5 CURRENT MANAGEMENT AND RECOMMENDATIONS

The treatment of unstable angina has the following objectives: (1) minimize the acute risk of myocardial infarction and sudden death; (2) control ischaemia and chest pain by reducing myocardial oxygen demand and improving supply; (3) optimize subsequent patient function; (4) minimize long-term risk of myocardial infarction and sudden death.

Current approaches to therapy (Fig. 15.6) are directed toward achieving these objectives by CCU monitoring, bed rest, employment of nitrates, beta-blockers and calcium antagonists, and the judicious use of coronary angiography, PTCA and bypass surgery. Aspirin has become an integral part of this overall approach since the studies of Lewis *et al.* (1983) and Cairns *et al.* (1985) demonstrated a reduction in the incidence of myocardial infarction and death over the subsequent 3 months to 2 years. However, the study of Théroux *et al.* (1988) points to very early benefits of heparin and of aspirin in the reduction of refractory ischaemia and in-hospital myocardial infarction and death and appears to be confirmed by the RISC Study (The RISC Group, 1990). Evidence for superiority of heparin, or heparin plus aspirin over aspirin alone, is not clear as yet. However, it is clear that patients hospitalized with unstable angina who have no contraindications should be immediately started on either heparin or aspirin, with the expectation that the incidence of acute ischaemic events will be decreased. If heparin is used alone, aspirin should be initiated while the patient is still in hospital in conjunction with the heparin for a few days, then the heparin should be discontinued and the aspirin maintained out of hospital and probably indefinitely. The enteric coated form of aspirin results in fewer side effects.

The 15–20% of patients who fail medical therapy in hospital generally undergo coronary angiography, and angioplasty or aortocoronary bypass surgery are undertaken if feasible. The optimal long-term management of patients in whom ischaemic pain responds well to medical treatment in hospital is somewhat uncertain. Although a patient's prognosis may be predicted most accurately by the combination of the clinical course in hospital, non-invasive stress testing, and coronary angiography, resource constraints frequently dictate that coronary angiography will be done only for those patients who appear to have marked ischaemic abnormalities with initial non-invasive evaluation.

Whatever the patient's acute or chronic course, and whatever the physician's philosophy of investigation and therapy, aspirin treatment is an essential component of drug therapy. In the absence of contraindications, it should be started early in hospital in every patient and continued indefinitely.

15.6 ATRIAL FIBRILLATION SUPPLEMENT

There has been a long-standing consensus (Dunn *et al.*, 1989) that the risk of embolization in patients with atrial fibrillation and rheumatic heart disease, in particular, mitral stenosis, is sufficiently high to justify

409

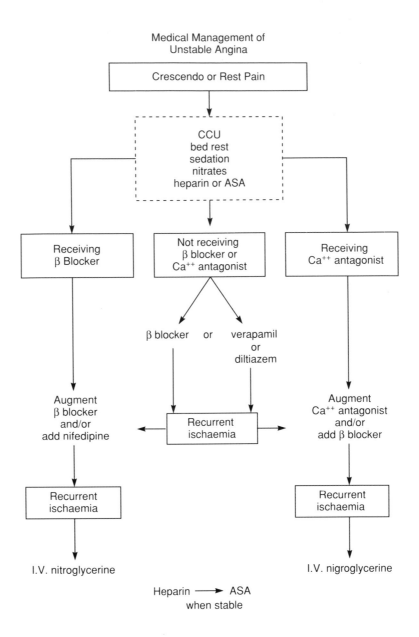

Figure 15.6 Medical management of unstable angina, a schematic approach.

anticoagulant prophylaxis. However, there has been no consensus in regard to non-rheumatic atrial fibrillation. The recognition that non-rheumatic atrial fibrillation is common and associated with a high risk of systemic embolization and stroke, as well as the suggestion of reduced embolism from both non-randomized trials of oral anticoagulation in atrial fibrillation and randomized trials of anticoagulant and antiplatelet drugs in vascular diseases, has heightened awareness of the potential efficacy of antithrombotic therapy. This recognition, together with evidence of the greater safety of lower dose warfarin, prompted the initiation of several randomized trials of anticoagulant and antiplatelet therapy in non-rheumatic atrial fibrillation. There are five recently published randomized clinical trials of warfarin among patients with non-rheumatic atrial fibrillation (Petersen et al., 1989; Petersen and Boysen, 1990; Stroke Prevention, 1990, 1991; Boston Area, 1990; Connolly et al., 1991; Ezekowitz et al., 1991.) In four of these (Petersen et al., 1989; Stroke Prevention, 1991; Boston Area, 1990; Ezekowitz et al., 1991), there were large and statistically significant reductions of the risk of stroke and systemic embolism, and in the fifth there was a trend favouring warfarin (Connolly et al., 1991). Two of the trials also evaluated aspirin, one of them observing no benefit (Petersen et al., 1989), while the second demonstrated a 42% reduction in the risk of stroke or systemic embolism with aspirin. (Stroke Prevention, 1990.)

The Danish AFASAK study (Petersen et al., 1989; Petersen and Boysen, 1990) enrolled patients who had chronic atrial fibrillation, while exclusion criteria included rheumatic heart disease, risk factors for bleeding, and a requirement for anticoagulation. There were 1007 patients (mean age 74 years) randomly allocated to warfarin (INR 2.8–4.2), aspirin (75 mg day^{-1}) or placebo. Aspirin therapy was double-blind, but warfarin therapy was open. Patients were followed for up to two years with the principal outcome being a composite of TIA, stroke (ischaemic or haemorrhagic), and systemic embolism among patients not permanently withdrawn from therapy. The observed reduction for warfarin compared to placebo was 64%, an absolute reduction of 3.5% yr^{-1} ($P<0.05$). There was no observed benefit with aspirin.

The Stroke Prevention and Atrial Fibrillation (SPAF) trial (Stroke Prevention, 1990, 1991) enrolled patients with paroxysmal (34%) and chronic atrial fibrillation, excluding those with possible haemorrhagic complications. The study examined two groups of patients defined on the basis of their eligibility for warfarin therapy. The 627 patients in Group 1 were judged by their physician to be eligible for warfarin therapy and were randomized equally to open-label warfarin (INR

2.0–4.5) or double blind to aspirin (enteric coated, 325 mg day^{-1}) or matching placebo. In Group 2, 703 patients were considered ineligible for warfarin therapy and were randomly allocated in double blind fashion to aspirin (enteric coated, 325 mg day^{-1}) or matching placebo. The patients were followed for a mean of 1.3 years, with the principal outcome being the composite of ischaemic stroke or systemic embolism. Among the Group 1 patients, compared with placebo, the rate of primary outcomes among the warfarin-treated patients was reduced by 67% ($P=0.01$), an absolute risk reduction of 5.1% yr^{-1}. Among the Groups 1 and 2 patients, by comparison with placebo, the rate of primary outcomes among the aspirin-treated patients was reduced by 42% ($P=0.02$) an absolute risk reduction of 2.7% per year.

Hence it appears that efficacy is demonstrated for aspirin in one major trial, but not in the other. The composite outcomes of the two trials differ and furthermore, the AFASAK trial was analysed using an efficacy approach, whereas the SPAF trial was analysed by intention-to-treat. It is possible to compare the outcomes of ischaemic stroke and systemic embolism by intention-to-treat (Petersen and Boysen, 1990; Cairns and Connolly, 1991). This outcome was significantly reduced in SPAF, but there was only a 13.6% (ns) reduction in AFASAK. The 95% confidence intervals of the estimates for risk reduction with aspirin in the two studies overlap, indicating that the results are, at least statistically, consistent with one another.

The results with aspirin observed in the AFASAK trial could be related to the lesser dosage of aspirin (75 mg vs 325 mg day^{-1}), and might also have resulted from the higher mean age of the patients (74 vs 67 years). The latter possibility is supported by a subgroup analysis from the preliminary report of the SPAF study, indicating that the benefit of aspirin was confined to patients under the age of 75 years (Stroke Prevention, 1990). The higher proportion of congestive heart failure patients in AFASAK compared to SPAF (50% vs 15%) may also have been a factor.

Aspirin is much simpler and cheaper to administer than warfarin, and has a lower risk of bleeding associated with its use. In the AFASAK study the risk of haemorrhage was much lower with aspirin than with warfarin. However, with the current low dose warfarin regimens, the risk of major bleeding is much less than it was formerly. In the SPAF trial, the risk of major bleeding was no different between warfarin and aspirin.

The prevalence of atrial fibrillation is 3–5% among patients over the age of 65 years, and the annual incidence of stroke is about 5%. The majority of these strokes have severe consequences. Low dose warfarin regimens (INR 2–3) markedly reduce the risk of stroke, while producing only a small risk of major bleeding (of 1000 atrial fibrillation patients treated with warfarin, the expectation is prevention of 15–50 occurrences per year of ischaemic stroke or systemic embolism, and a somewhat less reduction of disabling stroke or vascular death, at a cost of about five major bleeds per year).

Although aspirin can clearly benefit some patients, the benefits appear to be more modest than with warfarin, and there is uncertainty as to which patients are likely to benefit from aspirin. However, patients with paroxysmal atrial fibrillation are at lower risk of embolization than those with chronic atrial fibrillation (Kannel et al., 1983). Young patients with no evidence of cardiac abnormalities apart from atrial fibrillation (lone atrial fibrillation) are at very low risk of stroke and systemic emboli, in the range of 0.5% yr^{-1} (Kopecky et al., 1987). Aspirin may be the prudent choice in the young patient with lone atrial fibrillation. Among patients with paroxysmal atrial fibrillation, the choices are less clear; the young patient with minimal or no associated heart disease should probably receive aspirin, whereas the older patient should receive warfarin.

The SPAF study is continuing as SPAF–2. Patients originally randomized in Group 1 to warfarin or aspirin are being continued on the originally assigned therapy and will be followed to compare outcomes. There are two European trials (European Atrial Fibrillation Trial: EAFT, and Primary Prevention of Arterial Thromboembolism in Non-valvular Atrial Fibrillation: PATAF) which are comparing aspirin and warfarin in the management of patients with non–valvular atrial fibrillation. The results of all these trials should more clearly delineate the therapeutic role of aspirin in non-rheumatic atrial fibrillation.

REFERENCES

Ambrose, J.A., Winters, S.L., Arora, R.R. et al. (1986) Angiographic evolution of coronary artery morphology in unstable angina. J. Am. Coll. Cardiol., 7, 472–8.

Ashton, J.H., Golino, P., McNatt, J.M. et al. (1989) Serotonin S$_2$ and thromboxane A$_2$–prostaglandin H$_2$ receptor blockade provide protection against epinephrine-induced cyclic flow variations in severely narrowed canine coronary arteries. J. Am. Coll. Cardiol., 13, 755–63.

Beamish, R.E. and Storrie, V.M. (1960) Impending myocardial infarction. Recognition and management. Circulation, 21, 1107–15.

Bertrand, M.E. (1985) Diagnostic approach to unstable angina with coronary angiography. In Unstable Angina, Current Concepts and Management (eds P.G. Hugenholtz and B.S. Goldman), Schattauer, Stuttgart, pp. 119–25.

Boston Area Anticoagulation Trial in Atrial Fibrillation Investigators (1990) The effect of low dose warfarin on the risk of stroke in patients with non-rheumatic atrial fibrillation. N. Engl. J. Med.; 323, 1505–11.

413

Therapeutic applications

Cairns, J.A. (1981) Unstable angina – an overview. In *Unstable Angina* (eds A.G. Adelman and B.S. Goldman), PSG Publishing, Littleton, pp. 3–37.

Cairns, J. A. and Connolly, S. J. (1991) Non-rheumatic atrial fibrillation. Risk of stroke and role of antithrombotic therapy. *Circulation*, **84**, 469–81.

Cairns, J.A., Gent, M., Singer, J. *et al.* (1985) Aspirin, sulfinpyrazone, or both, in unstable angina. Results of a Canadian multicentre trial. *N. Engl. J. Med.*, **313**, 1369–75.

Cairns, J.A., Singer, J., Gent, M. *et al.* (1988) Coronary care unit utilization in Hamilton, Ontario, a city of 375,000 people. *Can. J. Cardiol.*, **4**, 25–32.

Cannon, D.S., Harrison, D.C. and Schroeder, J.S. (1974) Hemodynamic observations in patients with unstable angina pectoris. *Am. J. Cardiol.*, **33**, 17–22.

Chierchia, S., de Caterina, R., Crea, F. *et al.* (1982) Failure of thromboxane A$_2$ blockade to prevent attacks of vasospastic angina. *Circulation*, **66**, 702–5.

Cohen, M., Adams, P.C., Hawkins, L. *et al.* (1990) Usefulness of antithrombotic therapy in resting angina pectoris or non-Q-wave myocardial infarction in preventing death and myocardial infarction (a pilot study from the Antithrombotic Therapy in Acute Coronary Syndromes Study Group), *Am. J. Cardiol.*, **66**, 1287–92.

Connolly, S. J., Laupacis, A., Gent, M. *et al.* for the CAFA Study Coinvestigators (1991) Canadian Atrial Fibrillation Anticoagulation (CAFA) Study. *J. Am. Coll. Cardiol.*, **18**, 349–55.

Davies, M.J. and Thomas, A. (1984) Thrombosis and acute coronary artery lesions in sudden cardiac ischemic death. *N. Engl. J. Med.*, **310**, 1137–40.

Davies, M.J., Thomas, A.C., Knapman, P.A. and Hangartner, J.R. (1986) Intramyocardial platelet aggregation in patients with unstable angina suffering sudden ischemic cardiac death. *Circulation*, **73**, 418–27.

DeWood, M.A., Spores, J., Notske, R. *et al.* (1980) Prevalence of total coronary occlusion during the early hours of transmural myocardial infarction. *N. Engl. J. Med.*, **303**, 897–902.

Dunn, M.I., Alexander, J. K., de Silva, R. and Hildner F. (1989) Antithrombotic therapy in atrial fibrillation. *Chest*, **95**, 118S–27S.

Ezekowitz, M. D., Bridgers, S. L., James, K. E., and SPINAF Investigators (1991). Interim analysis of VA Cooperative Study, Stroke Prevention in Non-Rheumatic Atrial Fibrillation (abstr) *Circulation*, 84 (Suppl II): II–450.

Falk, E. (1985) Unstable angina with fatal outcome: dynamic coronary thrombosis leading to infarction and/or sudden death: autopsy evidence of recurrent mural thrombosis with peripheral embolization culminating in total vascular occlusion. *Circulation*, **71**, 699–708.

Feil, H. (1937) Preliminary pain in coronary thrombosis. *Am. J. Med. Sci.*, **193**, 42–8.

Fitzgerald, D.J., Roy, L., Catella, F. and FitzGerald, G.A. (1986) Platelet activation in unstable coronary disease. *N. Engl. J. Med.*, **315**, 983–9.

Folts, J.D., Crowell, E.B. Jr and Rowe, G.G. (1976) Platelet aggregation in partially obstructed vessels and its elimination with aspirin. *Circulation*, **54**, 365–70.

Fowler, N.O. (1972) Clinical diagnosis. *Circulation*, **46**, 1079–97.

Fulton, M., Lutz, W., Donald, K.W. *et al.* (1972) Natural history of unstable angina. *Lancet*, **1**, 860–5.

Gifford, R.H. and Feinstein, A.R. (1969) A critique of methodology in studies

414

of anticoagulant therapy for acute myocardial infarction. *N. Engl. J. Med.,* **280**, 351–7.

Haerem, J.W. (1974) Mural platelet microthrombi and major acute lesions of main epicardial arteries in sudden coronary death. *Atherosclerosis,* **19**, 529–41.

Haft, J.I., Gershengorn, K., Kranz, P.D. and Oestreicher, R. (1972) Protection against epinephrine-induced myocardial necrosis by drugs that inhibit platelet aggregation. *Am. J. Cardiol.,* **30**, 838–43.

Hugenholtz, P.G., Michels, H.R., Serruys, P.W. *et al.* (1981) Nifedipine in the treatment of unstable angina, coronary spasm and myocardial ischemia. *Am. J. Cardiol.,* **47**, 163–73.

Jorgensen, L., Rowsell, H.C., Hovig, T. *et al.* (1967) Adenosine diphosphate-induced platelet aggregation and myocardial infarction in swine. *Lab. Invest.,* **17**, 616–44.

Kannel, W. B., Abbott, R. D., Savage, D. D., and McNamara, P. M. (1983) Coronary heart disease and atrial fibrillation: The Framingham Study. *Am. Heart. J.,* **106**, 389–96.

Kopecky, S. L., Gersh, B. J., McGoon, M. D., *et al.* (1987): The natural history of lone atrial fibrillation. A population-based study over three decades. *N. Engl. J. Med.,* **317**, 669–74.

Krauss, K.R., Hutter, A.M. Jr and Desantis, R.W. (1972) Acute coronary insufficiency course and follow-up. *Circulation,* **45** (suppl. 1), I–66–71.

Lewis, H.D., Davis, J.W., Archibald, D.G. *et al.* (1983) Protective effects of aspirin against acute myocardial infarction and death in men with unstable angina: results of a Veterans' Administration Cooperative Study. *N. Engl. J. Med.,* **309**, 396–403.

Lewis, H.D. Jr, Davis, J.W. and Archibald, D.G. (1984) Aspirin and the risk of myocardial infarction. *N. Engl. J. Med.,* **310**, 122–3.

Maseri, A., Parodi, O., Severi, S. *et al,* (1976) Transient transmural reduction of myocardial blood flow demonstrated by thallium-201 scintigraphy as a cause of variant angina. *Circulation,* **54**, 280–8.

Maseri, A., L'Abbate, A., Pesola, A. *et al.* (1977) Coronary vasospasm in angina pectoris. *Lancet,* **1**, 713–17.

Maseri, A., L'Abbate, A., Baroldi, G. *et al.* (1978) Coronary vasospasm as a possible cause of myocardial infarction. A conclusion derived from the study of 'preinfarction' angina. *N. Engl. J. Med.,* **299**, 1271–7.

Maseri, A., Chierchia, S. and L'Abbate, A. (1980) Pathogenetic mechanisms underlying the clinical events associated with atherosclerotic heart disease. *Circulation,* **62**, V3-V13.

Moise, A., Théroux, P., Taeymans, Y. *et al.* (1983) Unstable angina and progression of coronary atherosclerosis. *N. Engl. J. Med.,* **309**, 685–9.

Neri Serneri, G.G., Abbate, R., Prisco, D. *et al.* (1988) Decrease in frequency of anginal episodes by control of thrombin generation with low-dose heparin; a controlled cross-over randomized study. *Am. Heart J.,* **115**, 60–6.

Nichol, E.S., Phillips, W.C. and Casten, G.G. (1959) Virtue of prompt anticoagulant therapy in impending myocardial infarction: experiences with 318 patients during a 10 year period. *Ann. Intern. Med.,* **50**, 1158–73.

Parry, C.H. (1799) *An Inquiry into the Symptoms and Causes of Syncope Anginosa, Commonly called Angina Pectoris,* Cadell and Davis, London, p. 28.

Therapeutic applications

Petersen, P. and Boysen, G. (1990). Letter to editor. *N. Engl. J. Med.*, **323**, 482–83.

Petersen, P., Boysen, G., Godtfredsen, J. *et al.* (1989), Placebo–controlled, randomized trial of warfarin and aspirin for prevention of thromboembolic complications in chronic atrial fibrillation. The Copenhagen AFASAK Study. *Lancet*, **i**, 175–9.

Rafflenbeul, W., Smith, L.R., Rogers, W.J. *et al.* (1979) Quantitative coronary arteriography. Coronary anatomy of patients with unstable angina pectoris re-examined 1 year after optimal therapy. *Am. J. Cardiol.*, **43**, 699–707.

Rafflenbeul, W., Russell, R. O. and Lichtlen, P.R. (1981) Angiographic anatomy of coronary arteries in unstable angina. In *Unstable Angina Pectoris* (eds W. Rafflenbeul, P.R. Lichtlen and R. Balcon), Thieme, Stuttgart, pp. 51–7.

Robertson, R.M., Robertson, D., Roberts, L.F. *et al.* (1981) Thromboxane A_2 in vasotonic angina pectoris: evidence from direct measurements and inhibitory trials. *N. Engl. J. Med.*, **304**, 988–1003.

Ross, R. (1986) The pathogenesis of atherosclerosis – an update. *N. Engl. J. Med.*, **314**, 488–500.

Sampson, J.J. and Eliaser, M. (1937) The diagnosis of impending acute coronary artery occlusion. *Am. Heart J.*, **13**, 676–86.

Sherman, C.T., Litvak, F., Grundfest, W. *et al.* (1986) Coronary angioscopy in patients with unstable angina pectoris. *N. Engl. J. Med.*, **315**, 913–19.

Sobel, M., Salzman, E.W., Davies, G.C. *et al.* (1981) Circulating platelet products in unstable angina pectoris. *Circulation*, **63**, 300–6.

Stroke Prevention in Atrial Fibrillation Study Group Investigators (1990) Preliminary report of the Stroke Prevention in Atrial Fibrillation Study. *N. Engl. J. Med.*, **322**, 863–68.

Stroke Prevention in Atrial Fibrillation Investigators (1991) The Stroke Prevention in Atrial Fibrillation Study: patient characteristics and final results. *Circulation*, **84**, 527–39.

Suryapranata, H., de Feyter, P.J. and Serruys, P.W. (1988) Coronary angioplasty in patients with unstable angina pectoris: is there is a role for thrombolysis. *J. Am. Coll. Cardiol.*, **12**, 69A–77A.

Telford, A.M. and Wilson, C. (1981) Trial of heparin versus atenolol in prevention of myocardial infarction in intermediate coronary syndrome. *Lancet*, **i**, 1225–8.

The RISC Group (1990) Risk of myocardial infarction and death during treatment with low-dose aspirin and intravenous heparin in men with unstable coronary artery disease. *Lancet*, **336**, 827–30.

Théroux, P., Ouimet, H., McCans, J. *et al.* (1988) Aspirin, heparin, or both to treat acute unstable angina. *N. Engl. J. Med.*, **319**, 1105–11.

UK-TIA Study Group (1988) United Kingdom transient ischaemic attack (UK-TIA) aspirin trial: interim results. *Brit. Med. J.*, **296**, 316–20.

Vakil, R.J. (1964) Preinfarction syndrome – management and follow-up. *Am. J. Cardiol.*, **14**, 55–63.

Wood, P. (1961) Acute and subacute coronary insufficiency. *Brit. Med. J.*, **1**, 1779–82.

416

16 The use of aspirin in grafts, coronary angioplasty and prosthetic heart valves

H. SINZINGER, P. FITSCHA and I. VIRGOLINI

16.1 INTRODUCTION

Thrombosis is a major cause of graft failure. The involvement of platelets both for the early and late consequences is well accepted. In view of the potential role of platelets in mediating thrombo-occlusive events, their possible prevention through the use of antiplatelet substances is of considerable interest. The oldest, most intensively studied member of this family is acetylsalicylic acid (aspirin).

Neo-intimal fibrous hyperplasia at the anastomoses of prosthetic vascular grafts (Hagen *et al.*, 1982) is thought to be a reparative process initiated by platelet-induced cellular proliferation in response to injury. The preparation of saphenous veins for bypass surgery is associated with a diminution of endothelial cells causing subsequent biochemical disturbances such as fibrinolysis and a decreased (anti-aggregatory) prostaglandin formation. These events further result in an exposure of underlying thrombogenic structures that lead to an accumulation of platelets *in vivo*. Experimental data have clearly indicated that a decreased patency of vascular prostheses is at least partly due to fibrous hyperplasia of the grafts (Weyman *et al.*, 1975). Inhibition of this mechanism may be achieved by decreasing platelet activity and adherence to the surface, as well as vascular wall cell proliferative activity, which has been related to mitogen release from platelets (Ross *et al.*, 1974).

16.1.1 Mechanism of Action

Aspirin is a relatively old drug, however, the knowledge about its antithrombotic properties is quite recent. In 1971 it was shown that aspirin and related compounds inhibit the synthesis of prostaglandins (Vane, 1971). Its inhibitory effect on platelet function has been recognized for many years. Aspirin blocks cyclo-oxygenase by irreversibly acetylating the active site of the enzyme. In contrast to endothelial

417

cells platelets do not have the capacity for *de novo* protein synthesis and therefore the acetylation of platelet cyclo-oxygenase lasts for the whole life-span of the platelet. The fractional dose of aspirin necessary to achieve a certain acetylation level equals the fractional daily platelet turnover of 10–15% (Patrono *et al.*, 1985). In addition, the platelet cyclo-oxygenase has been claimed to be more sensitive to the action of aspirin than the cyclo-oxygenase of endothelial or smooth muscle cells (Baenziger *et al.*, 1977). Consequently, attempts have recently been made to titrate aspirin to a dose resulting in thromboxane A_2 inhibition without significantly affecting prostaglandin I_2 production. This shifts the PGI_2/TXA_2 balance in favour of PGI_2 thus provoking disaggregation of platelets (Patrignani *et al.*, 1982) (Chapters 2 and 5).

There is some evidence, however, that alternative mechanisms may contribute to the antithrombotic action of aspirin. Platelet function is complex, involving several pathways of aggregation, the synthesis and action of thromboxane being only part of it. Furthermore, aspirin may have antithrombotic properties distinct from those of its inhibitory effects on platelets, such as fibrinolysis (Moroz, 1977) and increased bleeding time (O'Grady and Moncada, 1978). Last, but not least, knowledge about probably the most important beneficial influence of aspirin on thrombogenicity is still at a very early stage today.

Artificial prosthetic surfaces tend to activate circulating platelets and coagulation for a long period of time after implantation. Aspirin becomes more important as a graft reaches its critical limits which have previously been shown to be dependent on material characteristics and flow. Woven and more porous grafts (Goldman *et al.*, 1982) exclusively accumulate platelets which can be imaged by a gamma camera (Ritchie *et al.*, 1981) even for hours after reaching a steady state (Stratton *et al.*, 1982). Therefore, this methodology was used to elucidate pseudo-intimal production (Clagett *et al.*, 1982).

While there is controversy about the various antiplatelet properties of aspirin – not being completely understood even today – the monitoring of the *in vivo* platelet–vessel wall interaction and evaluation of platelet deposition on grafts (Fuster *et al.*, 1979; Christensen *et al.*, 1981a; Ritchie *et al.*, 1981) with radiolabelled platelets (using as a marker ^{51}Cr in the early days and nowadays ^{111}In) has been successfully used (Allen *et al.*, 1986; Megerman *et al.*, 1983) and provides a useful tool for a better understanding of the *in vivo* conditions.

16.1.2 Influence of Aspirin on Thrombogenicity

Experimental work has convincingly shown the stage of a non-thrombogenic vascular (prosthetic) surface which reflects (morphologically)

418

either a smooth muscle cell lining or the subendothelium covered with an intimal layer. Using radiolabelled platelets (^{111}In-oxine) it was clearly demonstrated that the extent of early platelet accumulation is related to graft occlusion (Christensen *et al.*, 1981b). In experimental animals (Hanson *et al.*, 1980) as well as in patients with implanted grafts a severely shortened platelet survival (Yui *et al.*, 1982) due to accelerated *in vivo* platelet consumption was demonstrated. The restoration of normal platelet survival correlates well with the development of a relatively non-thrombogenic surface.

ANIMAL EXPERIMENTS

In a series of extensive experimental studies, Dewanjee (1985) investigated the course of platelet deposition by evaluating the number of deposited platelets per surface area. He found a significantly ($P<0.01$) higher ^{111}In-oxine platelet deposition in prosthetic grafts compared to normal veins, its rate being always higher at the distal anastomosis compared to the proximal one, the well-known important site for thrombogenesis. Aspirin in this model induced a significant decrease in trapped platelets, the effect of the drug being most pronounced in the middle section of the graft, followed by the distal anastomosis showing a more marked effect than the proximal anastomosis.

In a canine femoral artery bypass model using ^{51}Cr-labelled platelets it was shown that platelet deposition on dacron grafts was significantly higher than on Gore-Tex grafts, while aspirin combined with dipyridamole caused a significantly diminished platelet deposition (Oblath *et al.*, 1978). In canine coronary venous bypass grafts aspirin combined with dipyridamole reduced platelet deposition (Fuster *et al.*, 1979; Josa *et al.*, 1981) while in a mongrel dog model the luminal surface of the prosthetic (PTFE) graft was rendered less thrombogenic by aspirin alone.

HUMAN STUDIES

In 42 patients undergoing femoro-popliteal bypass operation, the thrombogenicity index was calculated after autologous platelet labelling with ^{111}In-oxine. Thrombogenicity of dacron grafts was higher as compared to PTFE grafts, while autologous vein grafts accumulated only few, if any, labelled platelets. Aspirin (300 mg day^{-1}) combined with dipyridamole (75 mg day^{-1}) reduced thrombogenicity in prosthetic but not in autologous venous femoro-popliteal grafts (Goldman *et al.*, 1983). Aspirin (325 mg three times daily) plus dipyridamole (75 mg three times daily) significantly reduced platelet deposition on aorto-femoral dacron grafts, whereas no effect was observed when using PTFE grafts in the femoro-popliteal position (Pumphrey *et al.*, 1983). The authors (Sinzinger *et al.*, 1989) surprisingly found daily doses of 20, 50 or 1000 mg of aspirin to cause a significant improvement both in platelet survival (prolongation) and platelet uptake (reduction) in atherosclerotic human femoral arteries, while doses below or between were ineffective. It is noteworthy that the effect of aspirin persisted even after the end of therapy. The dose dependency on graft thrombogenicity in humans, however, has not been sufficiently examined so far.

16.1.3 Effect of Aspirin on Bypass Grafting in Experimental Dog Models (Table 16.1)

Bush *et al.* (1984) studied the effect of 3-week high or low dose aspirin therapy on thromboxane A_2 and prostacyclin release by the luminal surface of a prosthetic graft (PTFE) and the distal artery in 17 dogs. Both high and low dose aspirin therapy significantly reduced the release of thromboxane by the luminal surface of the PTFE graft and the distal artery indicating that the graft was rendered less thrombogenic compared to controls.

The effect of perioperative aspirin therapy (325 mg daily for 1–14 days) on the luminal structure and function of endarterectomized arteries was investigated in 28 dogs by Curl *et al.* (1985). Aspirin inhibited local and systemic generation of thromboxane and improved early patency by 95% versus 75% in controls. The same group also investigated the perioperative effect of aspirin (160 mg; given intravenously followed by 325 mg daily given orally) after PTFE grafting in 20 mongrel dogs. At the end of a 2-week study period all grafts in the aspirin group remained patent compared to two grafts out of 10 in the control group (Curl *et al.*, 1986).

Deen and Sundt reported in 1982 that aspirin (325 mg) in combination with dipyridamole (50 mg) significantly increased the early patency rate compared to heparin in dogs undergoing carotid endarterectomy.

Lane *et al.* (1986) showed in a placebo-controlled crossover study versus indobufen conducted in 24 greyhounds that aspirin in combination with dipyridamole had a comparably significant effect in reducing the thrombogenicity index after prosthetic grafting.

Zammit *et al.* (1984) investigated the effect of 3 mg kg^{-1} of aspirin on dacron grafts implanted in 20 mongrel dogs. A protective effect of aspirin on the early patency of small-calibre prostheses (patency rate 90% versus 56% in controls) was demonstrated.

Table 16.1 Aspirin (ASA) in experimental dog studies

Authors	n	Study design/dose	Results
Bush et al., 1984	17	(a) high-dose ASA (12 mg kg^{-1} day^{-1}) (b) low-dose ASA (minimum to inibit TXB$_2$-formation) duration: 3 wks, starting p.o.	Luminal surface of the prosthetic graft rendered less thrombogeric by both high and low ASA doses (sign. decrease PTFE grafts in TXB$_2$ and PGI$_2$ production versus controls)
Curl et al., 1985	28	ASA (325 mg day^{-1}) duration: 1 to 14 days p.o.	Early patency improved (90% versus 75% controls). sign. lower TXB$_2$ production in serum
Curl et al., 1986	20	ASA (160 mg i.v. initial and then 325 mg p.o.)	Serum TXB$_2$ and platelet aggregation sig. decreased PTFE graft patency improved (8/10 versus 2/10)
Deen and Sundt, 1982	20	ASA (325 mg)+DIP (50 mg) starting 2 weeks b.o. Cross-over study versus heparin	Patency sig. over the heparin-group
Lane et al., 1986	12	Indobufen versus ASA and DIP versus PL	Thrombogenicity index sig. lower
Zammit et al., 1984	28	Dacron carotid grafts ASA 3 mg kg^{-1}	Patency 90% versus controls 56% decreased platelet aggregation and diminished TXB$_2$ and PGI$_2$ formation

Table 16.2 Aspirin (ASA) and combination with dipyridamole (DIP) in the prevention of occlusion of aortocoronary vein grafts

Authors	Study design	Dose	Start	n	Effect
Pantely et al., 1979	Randomized versus no treatment	ASA (975 mg)+DIP (225 mg) versus warfarin	3rd day p.o.	65	Neg.
Mayer et al., 1981	Randomized versus no treatment	ASA (1300 mg)+DIP (100 mg)	1st day p.o.	175	Pos.
Chesebro et al., 1982/1984	DB versus PL	DIP (400 mg) ASA (975 mg)+DIP (225 mg)	2 days b.o. 1st day p.o.	407	Pos.
McEnany et al., 1982	Randomized versus PL	ASA (1200 mg) versus warfarin	3rd or 4th day p.o.	161	Neg.
Sharma et al., 1983	Randomized versus no treatment	ASA (975 mg) versus ASA (975 mg)+DIP (225 mg)	3rd or 4th day p.o.	223	Neg.
Lorenz et al., 1984	DB versus PL	ASA (100 mg)	1st day p.o.	83	Neg.
Brooks et al., 1985	DB versus PL	ASA (990 mg)+DIP (225 mg) warfarin first 3 mths	2nd to 3rd day p.o.	266	Neg.
Brown et al., 1985	DB versus PL	ASA (975 mg) versus ASA (975 mg)+DIP (225 mg)	2nd to 3rd day p.o.	107	Pos.
Rajah et al., 1985	DB versus PL	ASA (990 mg)+DIP (225 mg) warfarin first 3 mths	Evening b.o.	125	Pos.
Goldman et al., 1988/1989	DB versus PL	ASA (325 mg), ASA (975 mg) ASA (975 mg)+DIP (225 mg) sulfinpyrazone (801 mg)	ASA (325 mg) 12 h b.o. 2 days b.o.	772	Pos.
Sanz et al., 1989	DB versus PL	ASA (150 mg), ASA (150 mg)+DIP (225 mg)	DIP (400 mg) 2 days b.o. 1st day p.o.	947	Pos.

DB: double-blind; PL: placebo; b.o.: before operation; p.o.: post operation.

16.2 EFFECT OF ASPIRIN ON AORTOCORONARY BYPASS GRAFTS
(Tables 16.2 and 16.3)

16.2.1 Introduction

Early and late occlusions of aortocoronary artery venous bypass grafts compromise the surgical results. Occlusion rates are 10–15% per distal anastomosis at 1 month postoperatively and 16–26% at 12 months. At the end of 10 years, the cumulative occlusion rate is up to 50% (Brown *et al.*, 1977; Pantely *et al.*, 1979; Higginbotham *et al.*, 1980; Gohlke *et al.*, 1981; Bourassa *et al.*, 1982; Chesebro *et al.*, 1982, 1984; Verstraete *et al.*, 1986). There are two main phases of vein graft disease: an early postoperative phase of platelet thrombus formation and a late phase of smooth muscle cell proliferation (Unni *et al.*, 1974; Bulkley and Hutchins, 1977; Lie *et al.*, 1977; Fuster and Chesebro, 1985). Vascular injury starts with endothelial injury when the vein is removed from the leg. Surgical handling, delays before insertion and arterial shear rates may increase the endothelial damage preparing the source of thrombosis. The pathogenesis of the late phase of vein graft disease is multifactorial. As a result of chronic endothelial injury and release of mitogenic factors from platelets, smooth muscle cells start to proliferate, leading to intimal hyperplasia (Unni *et al.*, 1974; Lie *et al.*, 1977).

Occlusive or non-occlusive thrombus formation may occur at any point during this process (Unni *et al.*, 1974; Bulkley and Hutchins, 1977; Lie *et al.*, 1977; Solymoss *et al.*, 1988). Finally, months to years after graft implantation, intimal fibrous plaques indistinguishable from atherosclerotic plaques develop (Bulkley and Hutchins, 1977; Lie *et al.*, 1977). Because platelet–arterial wall interaction initiates the occlusion of vein grafts (Fuster and Chesebro, 1981) the choice of antiplatelet therapy is logical.

16.2.2 Results of Clinical Trials

The combination of aspirin and dipyridamole has been convincingly shown by the Mayo Clinic Study (Chesebro *et al.*, 1982, 1984) to prevent both early and late postoperative occlusion of aortocoronary bypass grafts. The randomized double-blind trial in 407 patients compared placebo with dipyridamole (100 mg, four times daily) for 2 days preoperatively, followed by aspirin (325 mg) and dipyridamole (75 mg) three times daily, started 7 h postoperatively and continued for 1 year. Angiography of vein grafts was performed early (median 8 days; range

423

Table 16.3 Positive trials of aspirin (ASA) and combination with dipyridamole (DIP) in the prevention of occlusion of aortocoronary vein grafts

Authors	Follow-up	Dose	Occluded grafts (%)		Pat. with >1 occluded graft (%)	
			CO	ASA	CO	ASA
Lorenz et al., 1984	4 mths	100 mg	32	10	62	27
Sanz et al., 1989	Early	150 mg	18	15	33	27
Goldman et al., 1988/1989	9 days	325 mg	15	8	30	17
		975 mg	15	7	30	19
	1 year	325 mg	23	13	44	35
		975 mg	23	17		
Brown et al., 1985	1 year	975 mg	21	12	41	26
Rajah et al., 1985	6 mths	990 mg	25	8	44	17
Chesebro et al., 1982/1984*	weeks	975 mg	10	3	21	8
	6 mths	975 mg	15	4	30	10
	1 year	975 mg	25	11	47	22
Mayer et al., 1981*	3 – 6 mths	1300 mg	23	8	30	3

CO: controls.
*Studies plus dipyridamole.

7 days to 6 months) after surgery in 360 patients (88%) and late (median 1 year; range 11–18 months) in 343 patients (84%). Within 1 month after surgery in the treatment group, 10 of 351 distal anastomoses (3%) were occluded compared to 38 of 362 (10%) in the placebo group. Correspondingly, 10 of 130 patients (8%) in the treated group had at least one occluded distal anastomosis as compared to 27 out of 130 (21%) in the placebo group. This difference between the groups was highly significant. Within 6 months after surgery in the treated patients 19 of 488 distal anastomoses (4%) were occluded as compared to 79 of 520 (15%) in the placebo group. In the treatment group, 17 of 176 patients (10%) had at least one occluded distal anastomosis, as compared with 56 of 184 (30%) in the placebo group, the difference being again highly significant. At the median of 1 year (range 11–18 months) 478 vein graft distal anastomoses (11%) were occluded in the treated group and 486 were occluded in the placebo group (25%). In the treatment group 37 of 171 patients (22%) had at least one occluded distal anastomosis

compared to 81 of 172 (47%) patients in the placebo group. The difference between the groups was significant. This large reduction in rates of occlusion in treated patients was present in various subgroups, including patients at high or low risk of occlusion as determined by flow in the vein graft, the diameter of the distal coronary artery lumen measured during arteriotomy or the presence or absence of endarterectomy. There was no increased incidence of bleeding complications in the treatment group.

The objective of the randomized double-blind Veterans Administration Cooperative Study (Goldman et al., 1988, 1989, 1990) was to compare graft patency when placebo and four antiplatelet treatments were begun before and continued after aortocoronary bypass surgery. The treatment regimens evaluated included: (1) aspirin (325 mg daily); (2) aspirin (325 mg, three times daily); (3) aspirin (325 mg) plus dipyridamole (75 mg) given together as a combination three times daily; (4) sulfinpyrazone (267 mg three times daily). Therapy, except for aspirin, was started 48 h before surgery. When aspirin was a treatment, one 325 mg dose was given 12 h before surgery. The study population consisted of 772 male patients who were randomized. Early aortocoronary bypass graft patency rate was assessed angiographically in 555 patients (72%) between 6 and 60 days (median 9) after surgery. The vein graft patency rate (1781 grafts) for distal anastomoses was significantly higher in the aspirin treatment groups (92–93.5%) compared to placebo (85%). The occlusion rate per patient (one or more occluded grafts) was 16.8% in the patients of the aspirin once daily group compared to 30.3% in the placebo group. This result approached statistical significance ($P = 0.067$). The occlusion rates of the other groups compared with placebo, however, were not significant: aspirin given three times daily – 19% ($P = 0.137$); aspirin plus dipyridamole – 21.1% ($P = 0.222$) and sulfinpyrazone – 22.1% ($P = 0.280$). It is important to note that aspirin given three times a day did not yield better results, and that dipyridamole conferred no additional benefit over aspirin alone. However, blood loss in all three aspirin groups exceeded significantly that of the placebo group. Transfusion requirements and re-operation rate were significantly higher in the aspirin treated patients, too. At 1 year (median 367 days, range 62–527 days) 555 of the initial 772 patients underwent recatheterization. The graft occlusion rates, defined for distal anastomoses, were 13.2% for the aspirin once daily group, 16.8% for the aspirin three times daily group, and 17.5% for the aspirin plus dipyridamole group. The graft occlusion rate in the sulfinpyrazone group was 18.2% and in the placebo group 22.6%. The difference in the occlusion rate was only significant ($P<0.05$) for patients receiving aspirin daily. Correspondingly, 34.8% of all aspirin treated patients had one or more occluded grafts as compared with 43.9% in the placebo group ($P = 0.101$). The beneficial effect of aspirin was most pronounced in grafts placed in vessels smaller than 2.0 mm in diameter. However, no improvement in new graft occlusions was observed in the patients with patent grafts at the early postoperative angiography. Again, the addition of dipyridamole conferred no benefit over the treatment with aspirin alone. In this study, a single daily dose of 325 mg aspirin was established to be efficacious in improving early occlusion of saphenous vein grafts. However, if a vein graft was patent early after bypass surgery, aspirin might not improve the reocclusion rate at 1 year.

In a further study by the same group (Goldman *et al.*, 1991), no difference in early graft patency was observed between pre-operative aspirin and 325 mg aspirin given 6 h after operation. This regimen also avoided bleeding complications.

The comparative efficacy of aspirin versus the combined therapy was also investigated by Brown *et al.* (1985). One hundred and forty-seven consecutive coronary bypass patients were enrolled in a randomized, double-blind, risk-stratified, placebo-controlled prospective trial evaluating the effect of graft patency after aspirin (325 mg) plus dipyridamole (75 mg) three times daily or aspirin (325 mg) alone. For the first 78 patients, drug treatment was scheduled to start on the third postoperative day. On average, therapy was initiated 67 h after the patient left the operating room. After 1 year 127 patients completed the protocol, including cardiac recatheterization. Fifty-nine per cent of 44 patients taking placebo had all grafts patent, compared with 67% of 45 patients taking aspirin plus dipyridamole and 74% of 38 taking aspirin only. The proportion of the 399 total grafts which occluded was 21% in the placebo group, 14% in the patients treated with aspirin plus dipyridamole, and 12% for the group receiving aspirin alone. The reduction in the risk of occlusion in the treated groups compared to the placebo group was significant. However, no significant difference between the treated groups could be detected. The benefit was principally due to reduction of occlusion in the most common and presumably most important groups of grafts, those in which flow exceeded 40 ml min^{-1}, or those supplying arteries having luminal diameters greater than 1.5 mm.

Lorenz *et al.* (1984) reported a small study in which 100 mg of aspirin daily started within 24 h of operation significantly reduced the number of occluded grafts. The study was designed as a prospective, randomized, double-blind, placebo controlled trial. Of 83 patients eligible, 60 (72%) were randomized and 46 (77%) had repeat angiography at 4 months. Following aspirin therapy, 4 of 40 grafts (10%) were occluded, as compared with 17 of 53 (32%) in the placebo group. Correspondingly, at least one anastomosis was occluded in 6 of 22 patients (27%) on aspirin compared to 15 of 24 patients (62%) on placebo. The difference between the groups was statistically significant. Although these results are particularly interesting in view of the low dose of aspirin, this study requires independent confirmation, because of the relatively small number of patients with inequality in baseline characteristics, and because of the exceptionally high frequency of graft occlusion in the untreated control group and even in the treated group.

An open, prospective randomized trial was performed by Mayer et al. (1981). One hundred and seventy-four patients entered the study, and 113 were analysed. On the first postoperative day patients were randomized to receive either aspirin (650 mg) and dipyridamole (50 mg) twice daily or neither drug. Repeated angiography was performed 3–6 months after aortocoronary bypass operation. In the control group 22 (18%) of 120 grafts (internal mammary artery and saphenous vein) were occluded compared to 6 (6%) of 93 grafts in the treatment group. In the control group, 21 (23%) of 93 saphenous vein grafts were occluded compared to 6 (8%) of 75 in the treatment group. The difference between the groups was significant. The results were similar when patients rather than grafts were analysed. In the treatment group 6 (13%) of 47 patients had one graft occluded compared to 20 (30%) of 66 in the control group, who had one or more grafts occluded.

In the GESIC Study (Sanz, 1989) the efficacy of low dose aspirin alone or in combination was investigated. Nine hundred and twenty-seven consecutive patients were enrolled in this multicentre, randomized, double blind, placebo-controlled trial. All patients received dipyridamole (100 mg, four times daily) 48 h preoperatively and were allocated 7 h postoperatively to receive aspirin (50 mg, three times daily) alone, aspirin (50 mg, three times daily) plus dipyridamole (75 mg three times daily) and placebo. Early occlusion rate of distal anastomosis was 18% in the placebo group compared to 14.9% in the aspirin group and 12.9% in the patients treated with aspirin plus dipyridamole. The difference between treatment and placebo was significant. However, only aspirin plus dipyridamole reduced significantly the number of patients with at least one occluded graft (24.3%) compared to placebo (33%). The reduction following aspirin alone (27.1%) was not significant.

Rajah et al. (1985) reported an improvement of early patency of saphenous vein aortocoronary bypass grafts in patients given warfarin for the first 3 months postoperatively. In this double blind study, a total of 125 patients were randomized to receive either aspirin (330 mg) plus dipyridamole (75 mg) three times daily or placebo for 6 months, the first dose starting the evening prior to operation. Repeated angiography was performed at 6 months in 103 patients. In the treatment group 8.4% grafts were occluded, as compared to 22.4% in the placebo group, the difference between the groups being significant.

There are four studies reporting that aspirin plus dipyridamole confer no benefit on patency of aortocoronary saphenous vein bypass grafts (Pantely *et al.*, 1979; McEnany *et al.*, 1982; Sharma *et al.*, 1983; Brooks *et al.*, 1985). However, in one study (McEnany *et al.*, 1982), only 50% of the patients underwent repeat angiography, which was performed in one third of patients more than 2 years after surgery. In the study published by Sharma *et al.* (1983) there was no placebo control group. Pantely *et al.* (1979) investigated only a small number of patients. Brooks and his colleagues (1985) administered warfarin as additional treatment for the first 3 months after operation. It is noteworthy that in all the four negative studies antiplatelet therapy was started late (2–3 days postoperatively).

16.2.3 Conclusions

The difference between aspirin alone (McEnany *et al.*, 1982; Sharma *et al.*, 1983; Lorenz *et al.*, 1984; Brown *et al.*, 1985; Goldman *et al.*, 1988, 1989; Sanz, 1989) and in combination with dipyridamole (Pantely *et al.*, 1979; Chesebro *et al.*, 1982, 1984; Sharma *et al.*, 1983; Brooks *et al.*, 1985; Rajah *et al.*, 1985; Goldman *et al.*, 1988; Sanz, 1989) on postoperative occlusion of saphenous vein bypass grafts was investigated in 13 prospective randomized trials (Table 16.2). Of these, nine were designed double blind, placebo controlled and four compared treated with untreated patients. In two studies warfarin was given to all patients in the first 3 months postoperatively (Pantely *et al.*, 1979; McEnany *et al.*, 1982).

It has been convincingly shown that aspirin alone or in combination with dipyridamole is effective in preventing early thrombotic occlusion of saphenous vein bypass grafts if therapy is started preoperatively or on the first postoperative day (Mayer *et al.*, 1981; Chesebro *et al.*, 1982, 1984; Lorenz *et al.*, 1984; Rajah *et al.*, 1985; Goldman *et al.*, 1988, 1989; Sanz, 1989). One study (Brown *et al.*, 1985) reported that the beneficial effect of aspirin occurs in grafts with good flow, whereas four other studies (Bulkley and Hutchins, 1977; Chesebro *et al.*, 1982, 1984; Goldman *et al.*, 1989) found the major benefit in vein grafts placed in smaller vessels. Once treatment is started 2 days or later after surgery, antiplatelet therapy fails to confirm beneficial effects on occlusion rate (Pantely *et al.*, 1979; McEnany *et al.*, 1982; Sharma *et al.*, 1983; Brooks *et al.*, 1985). These results are not unexpected since early vein graft occlusion is mainly of thrombotic origin and platelet deposition begins intraoperatively (Josa et al., 1981). Preoperative application of aspirin was associated with an increased risk of bleeding (Goldman et al., 1988, 1989; Rajah et al., 1985), whereas starting platelet inhibitor therapy on the first postoperative day was both safe and well tolerated (Goldman et al.., 1991). However, no firm clinical data are available on the bleeding risk of low doses of aspirin (e.g. 100 mg day^{-1} or below) started the evening preceding aortocoronary bypass surgery. Because preoperative aspirin is associated with increased intraoperative blood loss, the preoperative use of dipyridamole was recommended (Rajah et al., 1985; Sanz, 1989) although its clinical benefit still needs firm proof. It is also doubtful whether the addition of dipyridamole adds benefit to the efficacy of aspirin in aortocoronary bypass surgery. The optimal dose of aspirin is still unanswered. A daily dose between 100 mg and 1300 mg of aspirin was given in a single or multiple dose as treatment in the trials discussed above. There is no firm evidence that higher aspirin doses yield better clinical results nor that multiple dosing is superior to aspirin given once daily (Table 16.3). Therefore further studies with low dose of aspirin (0.5–1 mg kg^{-1} day^{-1}) alone or in combination with dipyridamole, starting before or on the day of coronary artery bypass surgery should be performed. It is not yet clear how long patients undergoing aortocoronary bypass surgery should be treated. The Mayo Clinic Study (Chesebro et al., 1982, 1984) reported a decreased incidence of new graft occlusion rates between 1 week and 1 year following surgery whereas in the Veterans Adminstration Study (Goldman et al., 1988, 1989) the rate of progression of graft occlusion was unaffected by aspirin. It may be that a different modification of risk factors provoked a different progression of coronary atherosclerosis (Blankenhorn et al., 1987). The influence of aspirin on graft occlusion beyond the first year of operation still needs evaluation. However, it is rational not to stop aspirin 1 week after surgery, because this may cause a rebound effect leading to an increased occlusion rate (Goldman et al., 1989). Furthermore, thrombus formation which is not an uncommon event in chronically injured grafts (Solymoss et al., 1988), and aspirin may suppress lipid incorporation into the venous wall, another mechanism that seems to be involved in the progression of venous graft disease (Bonchek et al., 1982; Campeau et al., 1984).

A meta-analysis of 13 randomized trials, examining the efficacy of anti-platelet or anti-coagulant therapy in preventing coronary graft occlusion, concluded that all active treatment was beneficial (Henderson et al., 1989).

16.3 EFFECT OF ASPIRIN ON THE PATENCY OF LOWER EXTREMITY BYPASS GRAFTS (Table 16.4)

16.3.1 Introduction

In patients with prosthetic vascular grafts of the lower limbs a substantial number of grafts fail during the first year after operation. Re-occlusion is dependent on the segment of vascular reconstruction and the material used for the graft. Long term patency rate of aortofemoral bypass grafts is 85% at 5 years and 65% at 10 years (Malone *et al.*, 1975; Nevelsteen *et al.*, 1980). Following femoropopliteal bypass operation, 20–40% of grafts fail during the first year after operation (Whittemore *et al.*, 1981), whereas 45% of bypasses to the tibial arteries are occluded within 5 years after surgery (Maini and Mannick, 1978; Reichle *et al.*, 1979). Primary patency rates for saphenous vein bypasses are significantly better than those with synthetic material (Veith, 1986).

In contrast to aortocoronary bypass surgery, relatively few data are available to clarify the effect of aspirin alone or in combination with dipyridamole on graft patency following peripheral vascular reconstruction surgery.

16.3.2 Results of Clinical Trials

The largest randomized, prospective study was reported recently by Clyne *et al.* (1987). One hundred and forty patients with 148 distal grafts were randomized as controls, or to receive 200 mg dipyridamole twice daily for 48 h prior to surgery, 200 mg dipyridamole with premedication, 10 mg dipyridamole intravenously three times daily on the first postoperative day, and then 200 mg dipyridamole plus 300 mg aspirin twice daily for 6 weeks. Following active treatment overall graft occlusion was 16%, and in grafts below the knee 17% compared to 35% and 32%, respectively, in the control group. The occlusion for all saphenous vein grafts was 17% in the treated patients versus 28% in the control group, and for saphenous vein grafts below the knee 17% versus 27%, respectively. However, these beneficial effects did not reach statistical significance. There was a significant reduction in occlusions among treated patients who had prosthetic reconstructions. Of all prosthetics 15% were occluded in the treated and 47% in the control group, of all below knee prosthetics 17% versus 42%, respectively. The higher patency rate was obtained in expanded PTFE prostheses and umbilical vein grafts, but not in dacron grafts.

Table 16.4 Aspirin (ASA) and combination with dipyridamole (DIP) in the prevention of occlusion of peripheral bypasses

Authors	Study design	Dose	Start	n	Effect
Green et al., 1982	DB versus PL	ASA (975 mg) ASA (975 mg)+DIP (225 mg)	1st day b.o.	49	Pos.
Kohler et al., 1984	DB versus PL	ASA (975 mg)+DIP (225 mg)	1st day p.o.	88	n.s.
Goldman and McCollum, 1984	DB versus PL	ASA (900 mg)+DIP (225 mg)	2nd day b.o.	53	Pos.
Archer et al., 1985	Random. versus no treatment	ASA (300 mg)+DIP (400 mg)	2nd day b.o	94	Pos.
Clyne et al., 1987	Random. versus no treatment	ASA (900 mg)+DIP (600 mg)	2nd day b.o.	140	Pos.

DB: double-blind; PL: placebo; b.o.: before operation; p.o.: post operation.

Therapeutic applications

The beneficial effects of the combined aspirin dipyridamole treatment were confirmed in a smaller placebo-controlled, double-blind study reported by Goldman and McCollum (1984). Fifty-three patients undergoing femoropopliteal bypass operation using either dacron or expanded PTFE prostheses were randomized to receive either 300 mg aspirin plus 75 mg dipyridamole three times daily or placebo. Treatment was started 48 h prior to surgery. During the follow-up period of 12 months 33% of grafts were occluded in the active treatment group as compared to 64% in the placebo group ($P<0.05$).

Similar results were obtained by Archer et al. (1985). Ninety-four patients undergoing femorodistal bypass grafting (52 autologous vein, 42 prosthetic material) were allocated randomly to treatment or control groups. Patients were given 200 mg dipyridamole twice daily and 300 mg aspirin daily for 6 weeks, commencing 48 h preoperatively. On the first postoperative day 10 mg dipyridamole was given intravenously three times daily. Antiplatelet therapy failed to provoke beneficial effects in venous grafts. However, in the follow-up period of 1 year 14% of prosthetic grafts were occluded in the treated and 55% in the control group ($P<0.002$).

To investigate the efficacy of dipyridamole plus aspirin, Green et al. (1982), randomized in a double-blind study 49 patients to receive either placebo, aspirin 325 mg three times daily, or aspirin 325 mg and dipyridamole 75 mg three times daily 24 h prior to PTFE graft surgery of the lower limbs. Patients were followed for 1 year, and the cumulative patency rate of the entire series was 59%. There were no occlusions in the patients with above knee grafts treated with aspirin alone or aspirin plus dipyridamole, as compared to 50% occlusions in the placebo group. The difference between active and placebo treatment was significant ($P<0.05$). Of the below knee grafts 35% were occluded following aspirin treatment, as compared to 79% in the aspirin plus dipyridamole group and 81% in the placebo group. However, the difference failed to reach statistical significance.

The beneficial effects of aspirin alone or in combination reported by the four studies discussed (Green et al., 1982; Goldman and McCollum, 1984; Archer et al., 1985; Clyne et al., 1987) are in contrast to the results of a large randomized double-blind study reported by Kohler et al. (1984). One hundred patients undergoing infra-inguinal bypass surgery with either autologous saphenous vein or expanded PTFE grafts were randomized. However, only 88 entered the study, and were treated on the first postoperative day either with aspirin (325 mg) plus dipyridamole (75 mg) or placebo three times daily. During the follow-up period of 24 months 38% of all grafts were occluded. These findings were not statistically different for the treatment (43%) versus control

432

(33%) group. On subgroup analysis there was a non-significant trend suggesting that patients with infrapopliteal bypasses had lower rates of occlusion.

16.3.3 Conclusions

There are five randomized, prospective studies on aspirin alone or in combination with dipyridamole in patients undergoing reconstructive surgery of the lower limb. Two are open (Archer *et al.*, 1985; Clyne *et al.*, 1987) and three are double-blind placebo-controlled (Green *et al.*, 1982; Goldman and McCollum, 1984; Kohler *et al.*, 1984). The available data provide no firm evidence that aspirin alone or in combination provokes a beneficial effect by reducing the rate of occlusion of autologous saphenous vein grafts. However, when a synthetic graft was implanted, a significant improvement in patency was observed (Green *et al.*, 1982; Goldman and McCollum, 1984; Kohler *et al.*, 1984; Archer *et al.*, 1985) as long as antithrombotic therapy was started preoperatively. When drug therapy was initiated postoperatively and only one third of the patients received prosthetic bypasses, negative results were obtained (Kohler *et al.*, 1984). It is still unproven whether the addition of dipyridamole adds further benefit to aspirin. Furthermore, the optimal dose of aspirin has yet to be determined.

16.4 EFFECTS OF ASPIRIN ON AV SHUNTS

16.4.1 Introduction

Thrombi frequently occur in arterio-venous (AV) shunts such as those used in patients on long term haemodialysis. The management of this life threatening thrombosis is hardly contested (Kohler, 1977; Friedman, 1980). However, the currently used Cimino shunt is much less subject to thrombotic occlusion than the Scribner shunt used before. The risk of clotting in these patients is related to poor arterial blood flow, female sex and the number of unsuccessful previous fistula operations (Andrassy *et al.*, 1974). Vascular access grafts used for chronic haemodialysis even of the Cimino-type exhibit an increased deposition of platelets (Ritchie *et al.*, 1981) as evidenced by radiolabelling of autologous platelets.

16.4.2 Results of Clinical Trials

In a double-blind placebo-controlled trial conducted in 92 uraemic patients, Andrassy *et al.* (1974) provided the first evidence that aspirin given in a dose of 1 g daily starting the day prior to operation and continued for 28 days significantly prevents postoperative clotting of AV Cimino fistulae.

In 1976, Harter *et al.* (1979) conducted one of the first double-blind placebo-controlled studies using low dose aspirin (160 mg daily) in 44 patients on chronic dialysis. The study was conducted until there were 24 patients with thrombosis and both groups had been under observation for a mean of 5 months. Thrombosis occurred in 18 out of 25 patients on placebo (72%) and in 6 out of 19 patients (32%) treated with aspirin. The difference was significant giving a P-value of less than 0.01. This study provided convincing evidence that low-dose aspirin is effective in reducing thrombosis in external shunts for maintenance of haemodialysis, a procedure no longer used.

The same group reported that aspirin reduces thrombosis in human extracorporeal shunts (Harter *et al.*, 1979). Aspirin at 1 g every second day given to patients with Brescia-Cimino AV fistula resulted in less occlusions than in patients on placebo (4 versus 23% during the first month after surgery).

In a prospective controlled study Livio *et al.* (1986), tested the effect of 100 mg aspirin on haemostatic function in 29 patients on chronic haemodialysis who had a normal or only slightly prolonged bleeding time. Following aspirin, in 12 out of 29 uraemic patients bleeding for longer than 15 min was observed. Therefore, a careful risk-benefit estimation is necessary before giving aspirin to uraemic patients on haemodialysis to prevent thrombosis of the shunt.

Schulz *et al.* (1981) treated 10 patients on haemodialysis with increased risk of recurring shunt venous thrombosis for a period of 2 years with a combination of aspirin plus dipyridamole. The average preservation of shunts was prolonged from 3 up to 12 months per surgical intervention. If prosthetic material was used, the shunt remained open five times as long as usual.

Wizeman *et al.* (1983) concluded from a study in 19 haemodialysis patients and two patients with chronic ambulatory peritoneal dialysis that aspirin is not preferable to sulfinpyrazone for the prevention of shunt thrombosis because of the propensity for gastrointestinal bleeding.

16.4.3 Conclusions

These days, haemodialysis shunt occlusion is no longer a central problem. Therefore, actual randomized, double-blind, placebo-controlled trials examining the efficacy of aspirin in this particular indication are lacking. Furthermore, the risk of bleeding in this group of patients has to be carefully considered. Nevertheless, aspirin is not infrequently used in a small subgroup of patients suffering recurrent shunt problems due to different reasons. Again, the dose administered varies considerably and thus does not allow any valid general conclusion.

It would be highly desirable to identify patients at risk of platelet mediated events in order to administer a drug specifically inhibiting their reactivity. Some clinicians believe that any aspirin dose blocking thromboxane formation is antithrombotic, some others believe in selective blockade of platelet thromboxane synthesis without affecting vascular prostacyclin generation, while others think that high-dose aspirin possesses additional cyclo-oxygenase-independent antithrombotic properties. Although even clinical results using lower aspirin doses indicate comparable clinical benefit, the clinical proof of the hypothesis put forward most recently that lower doses reduce the side effects of the drug without diminishing its antithrombotic activity remains to be established. Furthermore, the individual bleeding risk still has to be evaluated.

16.5 EFFECTS OF ASPIRIN AFTER CORONARY ANGIOPLASTY

16.5.1 Introduction

Coronary angioplasty has become a successful and widely used treatment for patients with coronary artery disease within the last decade. Although continuing improvements have occurred in angioplasty technique, the problem of restenosis after the procedure has proved enduring and formidable. A restenosis rate of 30–40% within the first 6 to 12 months has been reported (Fleck et al., 1982; Jutzy et al., 1982; Dangoisse et al., 1982; Levine et al., 1985; Holmes et al., 1984). A multifactorial pathophysiological progress accounts for acute reocclusion: thrombosis, intimal dissection with fibrocellular proliferation, platelet activation, thrombin generation and the release of mitogens (John et al., 1991; Califf et al., 1991). Given the importance of platelet deposition and mural thrombosis in the pathogenesis of restenosis, it appears logical to use aspirin for its prevention.

16.5.2 Results of Clinical Trials

There are two randomized placebo-controlled double-blind studies published. Finci and coworkers (1988) randomized 40 patients before coronary angioplasty for therapy with either aspirin (100 mg day^{-1}) or placebo (beginning before angioplasty). Control angiography at 6 months revealed a restenosis rate of 33% following aspirin and 14% in the placebo group (ns). In a recent study (Taylor *et al.*, 1991), 216 patients were randomized to treatment with aspirin (100 mg daily) or placebo. After 6 months, restenosis occurred in 35% aspirin and 45% placebo treated patients (ns). Concordantly, restenosis occurred in 42 of 168 (25%) aspirin and 51 of 135 (38%) placebo-treated lesions ($P<0.025$). Thornton *et al.* (1984) randomized 248 patients, in whom coronary angioplasty was successfully performed, to either 325 mg aspirin daily or coumarin treatment sufficient to maintain a prothrombin time 2 to 2.5 times the control value. Follow-up coronary angiography was performed after 3 to 6 months. Of the 122 patients randomized to coumarin 36% had recurrent stenoses as opposed to 27% of patients on aspirin (ns). However, patients with at least a 6 months history of angina showed a significantly ($P<0.05$) different response: 44% of coumarin patients had recurrent stenoses as compared to 21% of aspirin patients.

When aspirin was combined with dipyridamole the following results were observed in comparison to placebo. A randomized, double-blind, placebo-controlled study conducted in 376 patients was reported by Schwartz *et al.* in 1988. The active treatment consisted of an oral aspirin–dipyridamole combination (330 mg–75 mg three times daily), beginning 24 h before percutaneous coronary angioplasty. Out of 249 patients who underwent follow-up angiography 4 to 7 months after angioplasty, 37.7% of patients receiving active drug had restenosis at least in one segment, as compared with 38.6% of patients taking placebo (ns). Among the 376 randomized patients, 6.9% developed a myocardial infarction during or soon after the angioplastic procedure, as compared to 1.6% in the active group ($P=0.0113$). Similar findings were observed by Chesebro *et al.* (1989). To study the effect of aspirin (975 mg day^{-1}) in combination with dipyridamole (225 mg day^{-1}) on acute complications and restenosis, 207 patients were randomized double-blind to active treatment or placebo starting one day prior to angioplasty. Acute complications (occlusion, myocardial infarction, repeat percutaneous angioplasty or urgent surgical revascularization) occurred in 20% of placebo and 11% of active treatment ($P=0.07$). Repeated angiography was performed in 171 patients 5 months later, and no difference in prevention of restenosis found. When aspirin in combination with dipyridamole was compared with ticlopidine and placebo (White *et al.*, 1987) in a randomized, double-blind study in 333 patients, a significant ($P<0.005$) reduction in the incidence of immediate complications of coronary angioplasty (abrupt occlusion, thrombosis, major dissection) was observed (placebo 14%, ticlopidine 2%, combination 4%). However, reocclusion was not an endpoint in this study. To study the effect of the addition of dipyridamole to aspirin as pretreatment for patients undergoing percutaneous coronary angioplasty, 232 patients were randomized to receive either aspirin (975 mg daily) or aspirin (975 mg daily) plus dipyridamole (225 mg daily) before elective coronary angioplasty (Lembo et al., 1990). The addition of dipyridamole did not significantly reduce acute complications compared to aspirin alone: myocardial infarction occurred in 1.7% of the aspirin group and in 4.3% following combination therapy. Emergency coronary bypass grafting was required in 2.6% after mono and in 6.1% after combination therapy. A non-randomized study (Barnathan et al., 1987) suggested a significant reduction of acute coronary thrombosis during coronary angioplasty when aspirin was administered before hospital admission. A further reduction in thrombus formation was observed when dipyridamole was added to aspirin.

Three studies were reported addressing the question of high and low aspirin dose. Mufson et al. (1988) could find no significant difference in acute complications and restenosis in patients randomized to 80 mg aspirin daily ($n=253$) or 1500 mg daily ($n=242$). Schanzenbächer et al. (1988) reported a clinically significant restenosis rate of 18% in 40 patients on 100 mg and 21% in 39 patients on 1000 mg daily aspirin after 6 months follow-up. In a preliminary report (Dyckmans et al., 1988) a better effect of 1500 mg aspirin daily (restenosis 21%) in comparison to 320 mg daily (restenosis 31%) was suggested, when reangiography was performed 6 months after coronary angioplasty in 86 patients (ns).

16.5.3 Discussion

Percutaneous transluminal coronary angioplasty is an established technique providing immediate relief of symptoms in patients with angina pectoris and restoring blood flow in acute myocardial infarction. Although continuing improvements have occurred in the angioplastic technique, the possibility of restenosis after the procedure has proved to be a problem. Given the importance of platelet deposition and mural thrombosis in the pathogenesis of postangioplasty restenosis, it was suggested that aspirin might be useful for prevention. However, no beneficial effect on restenosis was shown with the use of aspirin in 5 placebo-controlled randomized trials, with or without the use of dipyridamole (Taylor et al., 1991; Finci et al., 1988; Chesebro et al., 1989; Schwartz et al., 1988; White et al., 1987). However, when the data from 4 studies (Thornton et al., 1984; White et al., 1987; Schwartz et al., 1988; Finci et al., 1988) were analysed by means of meta-analysis, an insignificant 11% reduction of restenosis by the use of aspirin was reported (Oluman et al., 1990). There is no firm evidence that high aspirin doses are superior to low doses in the prevention of postangioplasty restenosis. It is noteworthy, that the combination of aspirin and dipyridamole significantly reduced the acute complications of angioplasty in 3 randomized placebo-controlled studies (White et al., 1987; Chesebro et al., 1989; Schwartz et al., 1988). There is no study for aspirin monotherapy published with acute complications as an endpoint. Therefore this effect cannot be excluded, as there is no difference between aspirin and the combination with dipyridamole in the incidence of acute complications during and after coronary angioplasty (Lembo et al., 1990). Therefore studies with hard clinical events are clearly needed for aspirin. Although mural thrombosis with a subsequent fibroproliferative response is important in the pathophysiology of restenosis, adhesion and aggregation of platelets to the vascular wall with release of mitogens and chemo-attractants for smooth muscle cells may be sufficient to initiate intimal hyperplasia. This process cannot be inhibited completely by aspirin. Probably the combination of aspirin with antithrombin agents will provoke a better reduction of restenosis. Until the results of future clinical trials are available, the best empirical antithrombotic therapy for the prevention of acute occlusion may be aspirin, started before angioplasty. All patients should receive a bolus of heparin (100 U kg h^{-1}), which should be continued for several hours; the length of heparin therapy will depend on whether a thrombus or a large vessel wall dissection is detected at the end of the procedure (Stein et al., 1989).

16.6 THE USE OF ASPIRIN IN PROSTHETIC HEART VALVES

16.6.1 Introduction

Thromboembolic disease is a major problem in patients with mechanical heart valves (Fuster et al., 1982; Edmunds, 1987). Conventional anticoagulant therapy significantly reduces the incidence of valvular thrombosis and embolism (Chaux et al., 1984; Fuster et al., 1981; Myers et al., 1989). Bioprostheses are less thrombogenic than mechanical devices. However, thromboembolism still occurs (Edmunds, 1987).

16.6.2 Clinical Studies

There are three randomized studies in which aspirin was added to anticoagulant therapy for prevention of thromboembolic complications in patients with substitute heart valves. Anticoagulation therapy with acenocoumarin or with anticoagulants plus 500 mg aspirin daily was

438

given to 65 and 57 patients, respectively, with cardiac valve replacements (Altman *et al.*, 1976). The frequency of embolic accidents was significantly ($P<0.005$) lower in the group taking aspirin: 5.2% vs 20.3%. There was no difference in the haemorrhagic risk between the two groups. Dale *et al.* (1977) randomized 169 patients with cardiac valve replacements to 1000 mg aspirin daily or placebo in combination with anticoagulants. Within the follow-up period of two years, embolic episodes per year occurred in 12% of the patients on placebo as compared to 2% in the group on aspirin ($P<0.01$). Bleeding complications were the same in the two groups. However, an increased incidence of bleeding complications in the aspirin group was reported by Chesebro and coworkers (1983), when 534 patients receiving one or more mechanical prosthetic heart valves were randomized to therapy with warfarin plus dipyridamole (400 mg day^{-1}) or warfarin plus aspirin (500 mg day^{-1}) and followed up with a concurrent, non-randomized control group taking warfarin alone. Excessive bleeding was noted in the warfarin plus aspirin group (14%) compared with warfarin plus dipyridamole (4%), or warfarin alone (5%). A trend was evident towards a reduction in thromboembolism in the warfarin plus dipyridamole group (1%) as compared with warfarin plus aspirin (4%) or warfarin alone (4%).

16.6.3 Discussion

Patients with mechanical prosthetic valves are at considerable risk of developing thromboembolism (Fuster *et al.*, 1982; Edmunds, 1987; Chaux *et al.*, 1984; Myers *et al.*, 1989), which can be reduced significantly by anticoagulant treatment. Aspirin in combination with anticoagulant therapy was found to be beneficial in two trials (Altman *et al.*, 1976; Dale *et al.*, 1977) but not in a third one (Chesebro *et al.*, 1983), in which an increased incidence of gastrointestinal bleeding was found. Therefore no general recommendation can be made at present.

REFERENCES

Allen, B.T., Mathias, C.J., Sicard, G.A. *et al.* (1986) Platelet deposition on vascular grafts. The accuracy of *in vitro* quantification and the significance of *in vivo* platelet reactivity. *Ann. Surg.*, **203**, 318–28.

Altman, R., Boullon, F., Rouvier, J. *et al.* (1976) Aspirin and prophylaxis of thromboembolic complications in patients with substitute heart valves. *J. Thorac. Cardiovasc. Surg.*, **72**, 127–9.

Andrassy, M., Malluche, H., Bornefeld, H. *et al.* (1974) Prevention of p.o. clotting of a.v. Cimino fistulae with acetylsalicyclic acid: results of a prospective double blind study. *Klin. Wschr.*, **52**, 348–9.

Archer, T.J., Atuhaire, L.K. and Clyne, C.A.C. (1985) Does dipyridamole and aspirin therapy prevent early failure of femorodistal bypass grafts? *Brit. J. Surg.*, **5**, 402–3.

Baenziger, N.L., Dillender, M.J. and Majerus, P.W. (1977) Cultured human skin fibroblasts and arterial cells produce a labile platelet inhibitory prostaglandin. *Biochem. Biophys. Res. Commun.*, **78**, 294–301.

Barnathan, E.S., Schwartz, J., Taylor, L. *et al.* (1987) Aspirin and dipyridamole in the prevention of acute coronary thrombosis complicating coronary angioplasty. *Circulation* **76**, 125–34.

Blankenhorn, D.H. Nessim, S.A., Johnson, R.L. *et al.* (1987) Beneficial effects of combined colestipol-niacin therapy on coronary atherosclerosis and coronary venous bypass grafts. *J. Am. Med. Assoc.*, **257**, 3233–40.

Bonchek, L.I., Boerboom, L.E., Olinger, G.N. *et al.* (1982) Prevention of lipid accumulation in experimental vein bypass grafts by antiplatelet therapy. *Circulation*, **66**, 338–41.

Bourassa, M.G., Campeau, L., Lesperance, J. and Grondin, C.M. (1982) Changes in grafts and coronary arteries after saphenous vein aortocoronary bypass surgery: results at repeat angiography. *Circulation*, **65** (suppl.), 90–7.

Brooks, N., Wright, J., Sturridge, M. *et al.* (1985) Randomized placebo controlled trial of aspirin and dipyridamole in the prevention of coronary vein graft occlusion. *Brit. Heart. J.*, **53**, 201–7.

Brown, B.G., Bolson, E., Frimer, M. and Dodge, H.T. (1977) Quantitative coronary angiography. Estimation of dimensions, hemodynamic resistance, and atheroma mass of coronary artery lesions using the arteriogram and digital computation. *Circulation*, **55**, 329–37.

Brown, B.G., Cukingnam, R.A, De Rouen, T. *et al.* (1985) Improved graft patency in patients treated with platelet-inhibiting therapy after coronary bypass surgery. *Circulation*, **72**, 138–46.

Bulkley, B.H. and Hutchins, G.M. (1977) Accelerated 'atherosclerosis': a morphologic study of 97 saphenous vein coronary artery bypass grafts. *Circulation*, **55**, 163–9.

Bush, H.L., Jakubowski, J.A., Deykin, D. *et al.* (1984), Efficacy of low dose aspirin therapy in prosthetic graft surgery. *Circulation*, **70**, 164 (abstract).

Califf, M., Fortin, D.F., Frid, D.J. *et al.* (1991). Restenosis after coronary angioplasty: An overview. *J. Am. Coll. Cardiol.*, **17**, 2B–13B.

Campeau, L., Enjalbert, M., Lesperance, J. *et al.* (1984) The relation of risk factors to the development of atherosclerosis in saphenous vein bypass grafts and the progression of disease in the native circulation. A study 10 years after aortocoronary bypass surgery. *N. Engl. J. Med.*, **311**, 1329–32.

Chaux, A., Czer, L.S.C., Matloff, J.M. *et al.* (1984) The St. Jude bileaflet valve prosthesis: A 5–year experience. *J. Thorac. Cardiovasc. Surg.*, **88**, 706–17.

Chesebro, J.H., Clements, I.P., Fuster. V. *et al.* (1982) A platelet inhibitor drug trial on coronary artery bypass operations. Benefit of perioperative dipyridamole and aspirin therapy on early postoperative vein graft patency. *N. Engl. J. Med.*, **307**, 73–8.

Chesebro J., Fuster V., Elveback, L.R. *et al.* (1983) Trial of combined warfarin plus dipyridamole or aspirin therapy in prosthetic heart valve replacement: danger of aspirin compared with dipyridamole. *Am. J. Cardiol.*, **51**, 1537–41.

Chesebro, J.H., Fuster, V., Elveback, L.R. *et al.* (1984) Effect of dipyridamole and aspirin on late vein-graft patency after coronary bypass operation. *N. Engl. J. Med.*, **310**, 209–14.

Chesebro, J.H., Webster, M.W.I., Reeder, G. S. *et al.* (1989). Coronary angioplasty: antiplatelet therapy reduces acute complications but not restenosis. *Circulation*, **80** (suppl. II), II–64.

Christenson, J.T., Mergerman, J. and Hanel, K.C. (1981a) Prediction of early graft occlusion using Indium-111 labelled platelets. *J. Cardiovasc. Surg.*, **22**, 464 (abstract).

Christenson, J.T. Mergerman, J., Hanel, K.C. *et al.* (1981b) The effect of blood flow rates on platelet deposition in PTFE arterial bypass grafts. *Trans. Am. Soc. Artif. Intern. Organs*, **27**, 188–91.

Clagett, G.P., Robinowitz, M., Maddox, Y. *et al.*, (1982) The antithrombotic nature of vascular prosthetic pseudointima. *Surgery*, **91**, 87–94.

Clyne, A.C., Archer, T.J., Atuhaire, L.K. *et al.* (1987) Random control trial of a short course of aspirin and dipyridamole (persantin) for femorodistal grafts. *Brit. J. Surg.*, **74**, 246–8.

Curl, G.R., Jakubowski, J.A., Deykin, D. and Bush, H.L. (1985) Eicosanoid production and morphology after carotid endarterectomy: influence of aspirin therapy. *Stroke*, **16**, 140(abstract).

Curl, G.R., Jakubowski, J.A., Deykin, D. and Bush, H.L. (1986) Beneficial effect of aspirin in maintaining the patency of small caliber prosthetic grafts after thrombolysis with urokinase or tissue type plasminogen-activator. *Circulation*, **74** (Suppl. I), I 21–4.

Dale, J., Myhre, E., Storstein, O. *et al.* (1977) Prevention of arterial thromboembolism with acetylsalicylic acid. *Am. Heart. J.*, **94**, 101–111.

Dangoisse, V., Guiteras, V. and David, P.R. (1982) Recurrence of stenosis after successful percutaneous transluminal coronary angioplasty (PTCA). *Circulation*, **66** (suppl. II), II–331.

Deen, H.G. and Sundt, T.M. (1982) The effect of combined aspirin and dipyridamole therapy on thrombus formation in an arterial thrombogenic lesion in the dog. *Stroke*, **13**, 179–84.

Dewanjee, M.R. (1985) Indium 111 platelets in bypass grafts: experimental and clinical applications. In *Radiolabelled Cellular Blood Elements* (ed. M.L. Thakur), Plenum Press, New York, pp. 229–63.

Dyckmans, J., Thonnes, W., and Otzbeck, C. (1988) High vs low dosage of acetylsalicylic acid for prevention of restenosis after successful PTCA: preliminary results of a randomized trial. *Eur. Heart. J.*, **9** (suppl. 1), 58.

Edmunds, L.H., (1987) Thrombotic and bleeding complications of prosthetic heart valves. *Ann. Thorac. Surg.*, **44**, 430–45.

Finci L., Meier, B., Steffenio, C., and Rutishauser, W. (1988) Aspirin versus placebo after coronary angioplasty for prevention of restenosis *Eur. Heart. J.*, **9** (suppl. 1), 156.

Fleck, E., Dancian, S., Dirschinger, J. *et al.* (1982) Quantitative changes in stenotic coronary artery lesions during follow-up after PTCA. *Circulation*, **66** (suppl II), 11–331.

Friedman, E.A. (1980) Prevention of thrombosis by low-dose aspirin in patients on hemodialysis. *N. Engl. J. Med.*, **302**, 179.

Fuster, V. and Chesebro, J.H. (1981) Current concepts of thrombogenesis: role of platelets. *Mayo Clin. Proc.*, **56**, 102 12.

Therapeutic applications

Fuster, V. and Chesebro, J.H. (1985) Coronary artery bypass grafting. A model for the understanding of the progression of atherosclerotic disease and the role of pharmacological intervention. *Adv. Prostagl. Thrombox. Leukotr. Res.*, **13**, 285–99.

Fuster, V. and Chesebro, J.H. (1986) Role of platelets and platelet inhibitors in aortocoronary artery vein graft disease. *Circulation*, **73**, 227–32.

Fuster, V., Dewanjee, M.K., Kaye, M.P. *et al.*, (1979) Noninvasive radioisotopic technique for detection of platelet deposition in coronary artery bypass grafts in dogs and its reduction with platelet inhibitors. *Circulation*, **60**, 1508–12.

Fuster, V., Pumphrey, C.W., McGoon, M.D. *et al.* (1982) Systemic thrombo-embolism in mitral and aortic Starr-Edwards prostheses. A 10–19 year follow-up. *Circulation*, **66** (suppl I) I–157–161.

Gohlke, H., Gohlke-Barwolf, G., Sturzenhofecker, P. *et al.* (1981) Improved graft patency with oral anticoagulant therapy after aortocoronary bypass surgery: a prospective randomized study. *Circulation*, **64** (suppl. II), II 22–7.

Goldman, M. and McCollum, C. (1984) A randomized study to examine the effect of aspirin plus dipyridamole on the patency of prosthetic femoro-popliteal grafts. *Vasc. Surg.*, **18**, 217–22.

Goldman M.D., McCollum, C.N., Hawker, R.J. *et al.* (1982) Dacron arterial grafts: the influence of porosity, velour and maturity on thrombogenicity. *Surgery*, **92**, 947–51.

Goldman, M.D., Simpson, D., Hawker, R.J. *et al.* (1983) Aspirin and dipyrida-mole reduce platelet deposition on prosthetic femoro-popliteal grafts in man. *Ann. Surg.*, **198**, 713–16.

Goldman, S., Copleland. J., Moritz, T. *et al.* (1988) Improvement in early saphe-nous vein graft patency after coronary bypass surgery with antiplatelet therapy: results of a Veterans Administration Cooperative Study. *Circulation*, **77**, 1324–32.

Goldman, S., Copeland, J., Moritz, T. *et al.* (1989) Saphenous vein graft patency 1 year after coronary bypass surgery and effects of antiplatelet therapy. Results of a Veterans Administration Cooperative Study. *Circulation*, **80**, 1190–7.

Goldman, S., Copeland, J., Moritz, T. *et al.* (1990) Internal mammary artery and saphenous vein graft patency: effects of aspirin. *Circulation*, **82** (suppl. IV), IV-237–IV–242.

Goldman, S., Copeland, J., Moritz, T. *et al.* (1991) Starting aspirin therapy after operation: effects on early graft patency. *Circulation*, **84**, 520–6.

Green, R.M., Roederscheimer, L.R. and De Weese, J.A. (1982) Effects of aspirin and dipyridamole on expanded polytetrafluoroethylene graft patency. *Surgery*, **92**, 1016–26.

Hagen, P.O., Wang, Z.G., Mikat, E.M. and Hacket, D.B. (1982) Antiplatelet therapy reduces aortic intimal hyperplasia distal to small diameter vascular prosthesis (PTFE) in nonhuman primates. *Ann. Surg.*, **195**, 328–39.

Hanson, S.R., Harker, L.A., Ratner, B.D. and Hoffman, A.S. (1980) *In vivo* evaluation of artificial surfaces with a non-human primate model of arterial thrombosis. *J. Lab. Clin. Med.*, **95**, 289–304.

Harter, H.R., Burch, J.W., Majerus, P.W. *et al.* (1979) Prevention of thrombosis in patients on hemodialysis by low-dose aspirin. *N. Engl. J. Med.*, **301**, 577–9.

442

Henderson, W.G., Goldman, S., Copeland, J.G. *et al.* (1989) Antiplatelet or anticoagulant therapy after coronary artery bypass surgery: a meta-analysis of clinical trials. *Ann. Intern. Med.*, **111**, 743–50.

Higginbotham, M., Hunt, D., Stuckey, J. and Sloman, G. (1980) Prospective angiographic assessment of factors affecting early patency of saphenous vein-coronary artery bypass grafts. *Aust. NZ J. Med.*, **10**, 295–9.

Holmes, D.R., Vliestra, R.E., and Smith, H.C. (1984) Restenosis after percutaneous transluminal coronary angioplasty (PTCA): a report from the PTCA registry of the NHLBI. *Am. J. Cardiol.*, **53**, 77C–81C.

Huang, T.W. *et al.* (1981) In-111 platelet imaging for detection of platelet deposition in abdominal aneurysms and prosthetic arterial grafts. *Am. J. Cardiol.*, **47**, 882–6.

John, H., Fuster, V., Isreal, D. *et al.* (1991) The role of platelets, thrombin and hyperplasia in restenosis after coronary angioplasty. *J. Am. Coll. Cardiol.*, **17**, 77B–88B.

Josa, M., Lie, J. T., Bianco, R.L. and Kaye, M.P. (1981) Reduction of thrombosis in canine coronary bypass vein grafts with dipyridamole and aspirin. *Am. J. Cardiol.*, **47**, 1248–54.

Jutzy, K. R., Berte, L. E., Alderman, E. L. *et al.* (1982) Coronary restenosis rates in a consecutive patient series one year post successful angioplasty. *Circulation*, **66** (suppl II) II–331.

Kohler, H. (1977) Prophylaxis and therapy of shunt thrombosis in terminal renal insufficiency. *Klin. Wschr.*, **55**, 49–56.

Kohler, T.R., Kaufmann, J.L., Kacoyanis, G. *et al.* (1984) Effect of aspirin and dipyridamole on the patency of lower extremity bypass grafts. *Surgery*, **96**, 462–6.

Lane, I.F., Irwin, J.T., Jennings, S.A. *et al.* (1986) Effect of cyclooxygenase inhibitor indobufen on platelet accumulation in prosthetic vascular grafts. *Brit. J. Surg.*, **73**, 563–5.

Lembo, N.J., Black, A.J.R., Roubin, G. S. *et al.* (1990) Effect of pretreatment with aspirin versus aspirin plus dipyridamole on frequency and type of acute complications of percutaneous transluminal coronary angioplasty. *Am. J. Cardiol.*, **65**, 422–6.

Levine, S., Ewels, C.J., Rosing, D.R., and Kent, K.M. (1985) Coronary angioplasty: clinical and angiographic follow-up. *Am. J. Cardiol.*, **55**, 673–9.

Lie, J.T., Lawrie, G.M., Morris, G.C. (1977) Aortocoronary bypass saphenous vein graft atherosclerosis. *Am. J. Cardiol.*, **40**, 906–14.

Livio, M., Benigni, A., Vigano, G. *et al.* (1986) Moderate doses of aspirin and risk of bleeding in renal failure. *Lancet*, **i**, 414–16.

Lorenz, R.L., Weber, M., Kotzur, J. *et al.* (1984) Improved aortocoronary bypass patency by low dose aspirin (100 mg daily): effects on platelet aggregation and thromboxane formation. *Lancet*, **i**, 1261–64.

Maini, B.G. and Mannick, J.A. (1978) Effect of arterial reconstruction on limb salvage: a ten-year appraisal. *Arch. Surg.*, **113**, 1297–304.

Malone, J.M., Moore, W.S. and Goldstone, J. (1975) The natural history of bilateral aortofemoral bypass grafts for ischaemia of the lower extremities. *Arch. Surg.*, **110**, 1300–6.

Mayer, J.E. Jr., Lindsay, W.G., Castaneda, W. and Nicoloff, D.M. (1981) Influence of aspirin and dipyridamole on patency of coronary artery bypass grafts. *Ann. Thorac. Surg.*, **31**, 204–10.

Megerman, J., Christenson, J. T., Hanel, K.C. *et al.* (1983) Imaging vascular grafts *in vivo* with Indium-111-labelled platelets. Influence of timing on image interpretation. *Ann. Surg.* **198**, 178–84.

McEnany, M.T., Salzman, E.W., Mundth, E.D. *et al.* (1982) The effect of antithrombotic therapy on patency rates of saphenous vein coronary bypass grafts. *J. Thorac. Cardiovasc. Surg.*, **83**, 81–9.

Moroz, L.A. (1977) Increased fibrinolytic activity after aspirin ingestion. *N. Engl. J. Med.*, **296**, 525–9.

Mufson, L., Black, A., Roubin, G. *et al.* (1988) A randomized trial of aspirin in PTCA: effect of high vs low dose aspirin on major complications and restenosis. *J. Am. Coll. Cardiol.*, **11**, 236A (Abstract).

Myers, M.L., Lawrie, G.M., Crawford, E.S. *et al.* (1989) The St Jude valve prosthesis: Analysis of the clinical results in 815 implants and the need for systemic anticoagulation. *J. Amer. Coll. Cardiol.*, **13**, 57–62.

Nevelsteen, A., Suy, R., Daenen, W. *et al.* (1980) Aorto-femoral grafting. Factors influencing late results. *Surgery*, **88**, 642–53.

Oblath R.W., Buckley, F.O., Green, R.M. *et al.* (1978) Prevention of platelet aggregation and adherence to prosthetic vascular grafts by aspirin and dipyridamole. *Surgery*, **84**, 37–44.

O'Grady, J. and Moncada, S. (1978) Aspirin: a paradoxical effect on bleeding time (letter). *Lancet*, **ii**, 780.

Ohman, E.M., Califf, R.M., Lee, K.L. *et al.* (1990), Restenosis after angioplasty: overview of clinical trials using aspirin and omega–3 fatty acids. *J. Am. Coll. Cardiol.*, **15** (suppl A): 88A (abstract).

Pantely, G.A., Goodnight, S.H., Rahimtoola, S.H. *et al.* (1979) Failure of antiplatelet and anticoagulant therapy to improve patency of grafts after coronary-artery bypass: a controlled, randomized study. *N. Engl. J. Med.*, **301**, 962–6.

Patrignani, P., Filabozzi, P. and Patrono, C. (1982) Selective cumulative inhibition of platelet thromboxane production by low-dose aspirin in healthy subjects. *J. Clin. Invest.*, **69**, 1366–72.

Patrono, C., Ciabattoni, G., Patrignani, P. *et al.* (1985) Clinical pharmacology of platelet cyclooxygenase inhibition. *Circulation*, **72**, 1177–84.

Pumphrey, C.W., Chesebro, J.H., Dewanjee, M.K. *et al.* (1983) *In vivo* quantification of platelet deposition on human peripheral arterial bypass grafts using indium-111-labelled platelets. *Am. J. Cardiol.*, **51**, 796–801.

Rajah, S.M., Salter, M.C., Donaldson, D.R. *et al.* (1985) Acetylsalicylic acid and dipyridamole improve the early patency of aorto-coronary bypass grafts – a double blind, placebo-controlled randomized trial. *J. Thorac. Cardiovasc. Surg.*, **90**, 373–7.

Reichle, F.A., Rankin, K.P., Tyson, R.R. *et al.* (1979) Long-term results of 474 arterial reconstructions for severely ischaemic limbs: a fourteen year follow-up. *Surgery*, **85**, 93–100.

Ritchie, J.L., Stratton, J.R., Thiele, B. *et al.* (1981) Indium–111 platelet imaging for detection of platelet deposition in abdominal aneurysms and prosthetic arterial grafts. *Am. J. Cardiol.*, **47**, 882–9.

Ross, R., Glomset, J., Kariya, B. and Harker, L. (1974) A platelet–dependent serum factor that stimulates the proliferation of arterial smooth muscle cells *in vitro*. *Proc. Natl Acad. Sci. USA*, **71**, 1207–10.

Sanz, G. (1989) Does low dose aspirin prevent aortocoronary vein bypass graft occlusion? *Circulation*, **80** (suppl. II), 628.

Schanzenbächer, P., Grimme, M., Maish, B. and Kochsiek, K. (1988) Effect of high dose and low dose aspirin on restenosis after primary successful angioplasty. *Circulation*, **78** (suppl II) II–98.

Schulz, V., Zehle, A., Kindler, S. and Sieberth, H.G. (1981) Dipyridamole-acetylsalicylic acid for prophylaxis of shunt thrombosis with chronic dialysis patients. *Nieren- und Hochdruckkrankheiten*, **10**, 49–52.

Schwartz, L., Bourassa, M. G., Lesperance, J. *et al.* (1988) Aspirin and dipyridamole in the prevention of restenosis after percutaneous trans-luminal coronary angioplasty. *N. Engl. J. Med.*, **318**, 1714–19.

Sharma, G.V., Khuri, S.F., Josa, M. *et al.* (1983) The effect of antiplatelet therapy on saphenous vein coronary artery bypass graft patency. *Circulation*, **68** (suppl. II), II 218–21.

Sinzinger, H., O'Grady, J., Fitscha, P. and Kaliman, J. (1989) Diminished platelet residence time on active human atherosclerotic lesion *in vivo* – evidence for an optimal dose of aspirin? *Prostagl. Leucotr. Ess. Fatty Acids*, **34**, 89–93.

Solymoss, B.C., Nadeau, P., Millette, D. and Campeau, L. (1988) Late thrombosis of saphenous vein coronary bypass grafts related to risk factors. *Circulation*, **78** (suppl. I), I 140–3.

Stein, B., Fuster V., Isreal, D.H. *et al.* (1989) Platelet inhibitor agents in cardiovascular disease: an update. *J. Am. Coll. Cardiol.*, **14**, 813–36.

Stratton, J.R., Thiele, B.L. and Ritchie, J.L. (1982) Platelet deposition on dacron aortic bifurcation grafts in man: quantitation with indium-111 platelet imaging. *Circulation*, **66**, 1287–93.

Taylor, R. R., Gibbons, F. A., Cope, G. D. *et al.* (1991) Effects of low-dose aspirin on restenosis after coronary angioplasty. *Am. J. Cardiol.*, **68**, 874–8.

Thornton, M. A., Gruenzig, A. R., Hollman, J. *et al.* (1984) Coumadin and aspirin in prevention of recurrence after transluminal coronary angioplasty: a randomized study. *Circulation*, **69**, 721–7.

Unni, K.K., Kottke, B.A., Titus, J.L. *et al.* (1974) Pathologic changes in aortocoronary saphenous vein grafts. *Am. J. Cardiol.*, **34**, 526–32.

Vane, J.R. (1971) Inhibition of prostaglandin synthesis as a mechanism of action for aspirin like drugs. *Nature (New Biol.)*, **231**, 232–9.

Veith, F.J. (1986) Six-year prospective multicenter randomized comparison of autologous saphenous vein and expanded polytetra-fluoro-ethylene grafts in infrainguinal arterial reconstructions. *J. Vasc. Surg.*, **3**, 104–13.

Verstraete, M., Brown, B G., Chesebro, J.H. *et al.* (1986) Evaluation of antiplatelet agents in the prevention of aorto-coronary bypass occlusion. *Eur. Heart J.*, **7**, 4–13.

Weyman, A.K., Plume, S.K., De Weese, J.A. (1975) Bovine heterografts and autogenous veins as canine arterial bypass grafts. *Arch. Surg.*, **110**, 746–50.

White, C. W., Knudson, M., Schmidt, D. *et al.* (1987) Neither ticlopidine nor aspirin-dipyridamole prevents restenosis post PTCA: results from

Therapeutic applications

a randomized placebo-controlled multicenter trial. *Circulation*, **76** (Suppl IV), IV–213 (Abstract).

Whittemore, A.D., Clowes, A.W., Couch, N.P. and Mannick, J.A. (1981) Secondary femoropopliteal reconstruction. *Ann. Surg.*, **193**, 35–42.

Wizeman, V., Buddensiek, P. and deBoor, J. (1983) Gastrointestinal blood loss in patients on maintenance dialysis. *Kidney Int.*, **24** (suppl.), 218–20.

Yui, J., Uchida, T., Matsuda, S. *et al.* (1982) Detection of platelet consumption in aortic graft with In-111-labeled platelets. *Eur. J. Nucl. Med.*, **7**, 77–9.

Zammit, M., Kaplan, S., Sauvage, L.R. *et al.* (1984) Aspirin therapy in small-caliber arterial prostheses: long-term experimental observations. *J. Vasc. Surg.*, **1**, 839–51.

17 *Pre-eclampsia and intra-uterine growth retardation*

M. DE SWIET

For many years it has been realized that women are at specific risk of developing epileptic seizures during pregnancy, a condition known as eclampsia; when this occurs the prognoses for the mother and foetus are poor. Eclampsia is often preceded by a condition called pre-eclampsia or pre-eclamptic toxaemia that was formerly characterized by albuminuria, hypertension and oedema. More recently it has been realized that pre-eclampsia is a multi-system disease which can, for example, variably affect the kidneys, liver, uterine circulation, formed elements of the blood, and the brain; and that hypertension is a rather variable manifestation of the condition. Other abnormalities such as consumption coagulopathy or liver or renal failure may also indirectly harm the mother. To use or demand hypertension as the sole marker of the condition invites confusion particularly because blood pressure is so variable and because hypertension may be present before pregnancy and be unconnected with the appearance of pre-eclampsia. Even more recently it has been realized that pre-eclampsia starts early in pregnancy, before there are any clinical manifestations. At about 14 weeks gestation in normal pregnancy, trophoblast from the materno-foetal unit invades the maternal spiral arteries in the placental bed. These arteries supply blood to the chorio-decidual space where the foetal placental villi are perfused. Invasion of the spiral arteries by trophoblast converts them from narrow thick-walled vessels to wide, dilated conduits and must be associated with a marked increase in maternal placental blood flow which occurs at this time and subsequently in pregnancy. At the same time, or earlier in normal pregnancy, there is a generalized systemic vasodilatation manifested as an increase in circulating blood volume and a decreased sensitivity of resistance of blood vessels to certain vaso-constrictor agents such as angiotensin. Neither of these physiological changes occur in patients destined to develop pre-eclampsia. They also do not occur in patients who suffer with recurrent foetal intra-uterine growth retardation whether this is associated with pre-eclampsia or not.

Therapeutic applications

This suggests that pre-eclampsia and intra-uterine growth retardation have a similar basic pathology and that they differ only in the degree to which mother and foetus are affected. Prophylactic treatment for pre-eclampsia might well be effective in reducing the risk of intra-uterine growth retardation.

17.1 THE SIGNIFICANCE OF PRE-ECLAMPSIA AND INTRA-UTERINE GROWTH RETARDATION

Pre-eclampsia affects about 10% of women in their first pregnancies. Of those who get pre-eclampsia in the first pregnancy, about 10% will get it in subsequent pregnancies. The maternal and foetal consequences of pre-eclampsia vary between patients and between pregnancies from trivial to catastrophic. In the developed world pre-eclampsia has become the leading cause of maternal mortality as other obstetric problems such as haemorrhage and sepsis have been overcome. Pre-eclampsia kills about 10 women per year in the UK. In under-developed countries pre-eclampsia kills proportionately far more women and is only relatively less important than haemorrhage, sepsis and obstetric trauma since these kill even more women. In the UK pre-eclampsia is the commonest cause of iatrogenic pre-term delivery. Patients may be delivered as early as 26 weeks' gestation for severe pre-eclampsia in which case the foetus, if it survives, will have a stormy first few months of life in a special care baby unit. It will require ventilation and every other resource-consuming aid that the special care baby unit has to offer. Perhaps half of all ante-natal care in the second half of pregnancy is directed towards early detection, monitoring and 'treatment' of pre-eclampsia. It is difficult to be so precise concerning intra-uterine growth retardation without pre-eclampsia since this is a less common condition; but again if the foetus does not die *in utero* it may be delivered as soon as it is viable when it will require intensive special care baby unit treatment; and much effort is put into detecting growth-retarded foetuses in the ante-natal clinic.

17.2 THE CURRENT MANAGEMENT OF PRE-ECLAMPSIA AND INTRA-UTERINE GROWTH RETARDATION

At present the only treatment for the maternal syndrome of pre-eclampsia is delivery. Anti-hypertensive and anti-convulsant treatment must reduce the maternal risks of eclampsia and intra-cerebral haemorrhage but they do not alter the other manifestations of the disease which continue through delivery. It is possible that anti-hypertensive and anti-convulsive treatment will allow the obstetrician to delay delivery until the foetus is more mature, but the effect is not marked and there is no other way by which anti-hypertensive and anti-convulsant therapy can improve the foetal prognosis. Indeed, it is quite possible that by lowering perfusion pressure, the anti-hypertensive therapy may reduce maternal placental blood flow still further. The place of hospital admission is to allow closer monitoring of the foetus rather than directly to improve foetal well-being by bed rest. No drug therapy has helped patients with intra-uterine growth retardation without pre-eclampsia. Hyperalimentation or giving increased inspired oxygen concentrations to the mother has not had consistent effects. Once again, timely delivery when the risk to the foetus seems greater inside the uterus than inside the special care baby unit is all that can be offered at present.

So a form of therapy that could either stop pre-eclamptic toxaemia and/or intra-uterine growth retardation occurring or that could treat the early stages of these conditions would have much to offer. Such a therapy is low-dose aspirin.

17.3   RATIONALE OF LOW-DOSE ASPIRIN THERAPY

It was probably the coagulopathy of pre-eclampsia that first attracted Goodlin *et al.* (1978) to use the drug. Since pre-eclampsia is associated with increased platelet activation (Greer *et al.*, 1988) and hence increased platelet consumption, aspirin, a drug that was known to inhibit platelet activation, might modulate disease activity. More recently it has been realized that in pre-eclampsia and intra-uterine growth retardation the placenta (Walsh, 1985) and platelets (Wallenburg and Rotmans, 1982) produce more thromboxane than is seen in normal pregnancy. The values for thromboxane B_2 in maternal plasma are variable with reports of increased (Koullapis *et al.*, 1982) and normal (Yamaguchi and Mori, 1985) levels in pre-eclampsia. However, the levels of metabolites of thromboxane B_2 in the urine of women with pregnancy-induced hypertension were significantly higher than in a normotensive pregnant group (Fitzgerald *et al.*, 1990). Prostacyclin production by maternal vascular endothelium (Bussolino *et al.*, 1980) and the level of prosta-cyclin metabolites in the urine are decreased (Goodman *et al.*, 1982). Complementary data have been collected from investigating the foetal condition where there is a reduction in amniotic fluid prostacyclin metabolites and from the ability of cord blood vessels to synthesize prostacyclin (Ylikorkala and Makila, 1985). Since these eicosanoids are not circulating hormones but appear to act locally at a tissue level, information about the activity of prostacyclin and thromboxane is only being inferred from the 'spill-over' of the substances into the circulation.

Therapeutic applications

However, it is interesting to observe that Greenland Eskimos eat a lot of fish, have a diet with a high content of polyunsaturated fatty acids of the n-3 family, especially eicosapentaenoic acid, which shifts the balance of prostaglandin production away from platelet production, and have one quarter the incidence of pre-eclampsia compared to an urban Danish population (Dyerberg and Bang, 1985). As has been described in earlier chapters, it is attractive to postulate that low-dose aspirin could act by irreversibly inactivating platelet cyclo-oxygenase in the portal circulation. Inhibition of cyclo-oxygenase reduces the level of cyclic endoperoxide synthesis from arachidonic acid. Platelets are not nucleated and once their cyclo-oxygenase has been inactivated they do not have the ability to regenerate it. The platelet cyclo-oxygenase responsible for the synthesis of thromboxane remains inactive for the remainder of the life of the platelet. By contrast, the endothelial cells of blood vessels are nucleated. So, endothelial prostacyclin synthesis, depressed by relatively high salicylate levels at the time of aspirin ingestion, could recover when the salicylate level drops. But perhaps more importantly at low doses of aspirin most of the salicylate will only be active in the portal circulation since it is largely metabolized at first-pass through the liver. Systemic vasodilatation and anti-platelet effects of prostacyclin should be maintained. It is uncertain to what extent this effect of low-dose aspirin sparing prostacyclin is important in pregnancy or in other therapeutic conditions. However, an additional benefit of first-pass metabolism to pregnancy is that at low doses little aspirin should enter the uterine circulation from where it would otherwise pass to the foetus. Aspirin might have harmful anti-platelet effects predisposing to bleeding in the foetus. Thus these could be obviated by first-pass metabolism at low doses.

The effects of low-dose aspirin in high risk pregnancy have been demonstrated by Schiff *et al.* (1989). These authors treated high risk patients with either aspirin 100 mg daily ($n=34$) or placebo ($n=31$). Maternal thromboxane B_2 was markedly reduced in the treated group compared to the placebo-treated group. There was no significant change in the level of 6-keto-prostaglandin $F_{1\alpha}$, a metabolite of prostacyclin (Table 17.1). Similar results were found by Wallenberg and Rotmans (1987), Spitz *et al.* (1988) and Benigni *et al.* (1989). Benigni *et al.* (Table 17.2) gave aspirin 60 mg day^{-1} to women with a history of previous hypertension in pregnancy or to patients presenting with hypertension early in pregnancy. Again thromboxane synthesis was inhibited and prostacyclin production was spared; but despite the low dose (60 mg) of aspirin and the possibility of first-pass metabolism before aspirin could reach the umbilical circulation (above), foetal blood showed impaired thromboxane B_2 synthesis which did not recover until at least day 5

450

Table 17.1 Mean serum thromboxane B_2 and 6-keto-prostaglandin $F_{1\alpha}$ concentrations in 64 high-risk pregnant patients before and after 21 days treatment with aspirin or placebo (Schiff *et al.*, 1989)

	Aspirin n = 34	Placebo n = 31
Thromboxane B_2 nmol l^{-1}		
Pre-treatment	0.105	0.097
During treatment	0.056	0.125
% change	−47	+29
6-keto-prostaglandin $F_{1\alpha}$		
Pre-treatment	1.09	1.15
During treatment	0.89	0.98
% change	−18	−15
Pregnancy induced hypertension	4(11.8%)	11(35.5%)
Proteinuric pre-eclampsia	1(2.9%)	7(22.6%)
Gestational age at delivery (days)	272	261

(Table 17.2). However, the significance of depressed foetal and maternal thromboxane production is uncertain since even a 10% capacity to form thromboxane may fully sustain thromboxane-dependent platelet aggregation (Di Minno *et al.*, 1983; Reilly and FitzGerald, 1987). On the other hand Forrestier *et al.* (1985) were able to study the effect of single doses of aspirin 50–600 mg given to the mother 3 hours before cord sampling for pre-natal diagnosis of toxoplasmosis. At all doses of aspirin there was complete absence of arachidonic acid platelet aggregation in foetal blood. In maternal blood aspirin 50 mg induced 70% inhibition, aspirin 100 mg 85% inhibition and higher doses 100%. This suggests that even low doses of aspirin may affect foetal platelets but this may not necessarily equate with increased bleeding risk.

Not only does aspirin reduce maternal thromboxane levels, it also decreases sensitivity to angiotensin (above) when given in a single low dose (80 mg acetylsalicylic acid) to normotensive pregnant patients (Sanchez-Ramos *et al.*, 1987). The concept is that even a single low dose of aspirin alters the balance between thromboxane and vasodilator agents in favour of vasodilatation so that more exogenous angiotensin is necessary to cause a given rise in blood pressure. By contrast, high doses of aspirin (two doses of 600 mg given 6 h apart) increase the sensitivity to angiotensin, presumably by blocking the production of prostacyclin and/or other vasodilator substances (Everett *et al.*, 1978).

17.4 EFFICACY OF LOW-DOSE ASPIRIN IN PRE-ECLAMPSIA

Against the above background what is the effect of low-dose aspirin in pre-eclampsia? In 1978, Goodlin *et al.* (1978) reported the beneficial effect of aspirin 1800 mg day^{-1} in the third pregnancy of a woman who had lost two previous pregnancies from pre-eclampsia in association with thrombocytopenia. The effect of aspirin was monitored by noting the reversal of thrombocytopenia and the pregnancy was successful. This is probably the first report of aspirin success in pregnancy but it was by no means low dose aspirin that was used. This report stimulated Crandon and Isherwood (1979) to analyse retrospectively the incidence of pre-eclampsia in primagravid patients participating in a drug consumption study. Only 4% of 48 patients taking aspirin developed pre-eclampsia compared to 12% of 98 patients who did not take any aspirin ($P = 0.027$).

Goodlin (1983) and Jespersen (1980) who used aspirin 1500 mg in a patient presenting early in pregnancy with pre-eclampsia both report that thrombocytopenia and other manifestations of pre-eclampsia (Jespersen, 1980) might improve but that the foetal condition remains poor. Even though Goodlin used aspirin 85 mg day^{-1}, the foetuses often died when aspirin was given to patients who already had thrombocytopenia.

Current opinion is that aspirin is more effective in the prevention

Table 17.2 Maternal urinary thromboxane B_2 and 6-keto-prostaglandin $F_{1\alpha}$ and neonatal serum thromboxane B_2 after giving aspirin 60 mg or placebo from 12 weeks gestation to women at high risk in pregnancy. Values are means $\pm$ SD (from Benigni *et al.*, 1989)

	Aspirin *n = 17*	*Placebo* *n = 16*
Maternal urinary excretion (ng l^{-1})		
Thromboxane B_2		
12 weeks	8.6±5.4	9.1±3.9
Term	4.6±2.0*	13.9±7.1*
6-keto-prostaglandin $F_{1\alpha}$		
12 weeks	11.0±6.1	12.2±5.8
Term	13.7±7.6	13.6±7.2
Neonate serum		
Thromboxane B_2		
Cord blood	157±82*	423±215*
1 day	175±106†	352±195†
5 days	254±130	386±310

* Significant difference between aspirin and placebo group ($P < 0.01$).
† Significant difference between aspirin and placebo group ($P < 0.05$).

Table 17.3 Outcome of pregnancy following aspirin 150 mg daily and dipyridamole 300 mg daily compared to no treatment in high risk pregnant patients (from Beaufils et al., 1985)

	Treatment $n = 48$	No treatment $n = 45$	n
Normal	29	12	< 0.005
Isolated hypertension	19	22	n.s.
Proteinuric pre-eclampsia	0	6	< 0.01
Foetal and neonatal loss	0	5	< 0.01
Growth retardation < 3rd centile	0	7	< 0.005
Duration of pregnancy (weeks)	38.6	36.5	< 0.001

of pre-eclampsia, than in its treatment once the patient has already developed thrombocytopenia.

Two papers laid the foundation for low-dose aspirin use in the prevention of pre-eclampsia; one from Paris by Beaufils et al. (1985) and the other from Rotterdam by Wallenberg et al. (1986). Beaufils et al. selected 102 patients judged at particularly high risk because of their previous bad obstetric and/or medical history or because they had hypertension early in pregnancy (non-toxaemic hypertension, a known risk factor for the subsequent development of pre-eclampsia). Starting in the first trimester, the treated group received aspirin 150 mg day^{-1} and dipyridamole 300 mg day^{-1}. The control group did not receive placebo. The study was not blind.

Although the study design has been criticized, the results were outstandingly good in the treatment group and equally bad in the no-treatment group (Table 17.3). There were no cases of proteinuric pre-eclampsia or foetal loss in the treated group as opposed to six and five respectively in the no-treatment group

Wallenburg's study was designed very differently (Wallenburg et al., 1986). He took patients known to be at risk of developing pre-eclampsia because of their blood pressure sensitivity to angiotensin. Patients who will develop pre-eclampsia are sensitive to angiotension infusion (above). The infusion of angiotensin in pregnancy as a predictor of the subsequent development of pre-eclampsia had been formally studied by Gant et al. (1973). Wallenburg found 46 patients sensitive to angiotensin at 28 weeks gestation out of 207 women infused. These 46 patients were randomized to receive aspirin 60 mg daily or placebo. The study was double blind. Once again the results were good (Table 17.4). There was no severe pre-eclampsia in the treated group, and significantly fewer patients were delivered by caesarean section. Since treatment was not started until 28 weeks, and the abnormalities of pre-eclampsia begin to occur at 14 weeks, this must be considered a therapeutic trial even though the patients were normotensive at the time they started taking aspirin. But the angiotensin infusion test is not a practical way to select patients for aspirin treatment; it is too invasive and too time-consuming for normal clinical practice. Therefore this study, like that of Beaufils *et al.* (1985), must be considered a pilot study.

As an alternative to the angiotension infusion test Schiff *et al.* (1989) used the 'roll-over test' to predict patients at risk from pre-eclampsia. This test looks at the rise in blood pressure which occurs when patients roll over from the lateral to the supine position (Gant *et al.*, 1974). A rise in diastolic blood pressure of at least 15 mm Hg maintained after 15 min in the supine position is considered predictive of pre-eclampsia. The test is generally discredited (Phelan *et al.*, 1977) because of concern that in the original observations insufficient attention was paid to the haemodynamic consequences of measuring blood pressure in the arm above the heart in the lateral position and beside the heart in the supine position. Be that as it may, the incidence of pre-eclampsia was still high, 35% in the placebo treated roll-over positive group. On the basis of a positive roll-over test at 28 weeks gestation Schiff *et al.* (1989) randomized 65 women; 34 received aspirin 100 mg daily and 31 placebo. As we have already seen (Table 17.1) aspirin treatment had a favourable influence on eicosanoid metabolism. But also there were marked reductions in the incidence of hypertension and pre-eclampsia in the aspirin treated group compared to controls (Table 17.1). The mothers were delivered significantly later (11 days) in pregnancy in the aspirin group compared to controls (Table 17.1). The study of Benigni *et al.* (1989) previously referred to (Table 17.2) also showed some advantage

Table 17.4 Effect of aspirin (60 mg daily) or placebo given from 28 weeks gestation in women at risk of pre-eclampsia because of positive angiotensin infusion test (Wallenburg *et al.*, 1986)

	Aspirin n = 21	Control n = 23	n
Hypertension	2	4	
Pre-eclampsia	0	7	< 0.01
Eclampsia	0	1	
Delivery before 37 weeks	0	4	
Caesarian section	1	7	< 0.01
Birth weight < 2.3 centile	0	3	

for high-risk women randomized to receive aspirin 60 mg day^{-1} or placebo because of previous bad obstetric history of hypertension at the onset of pregnancy. Mothers were delivered significantly later (4 weeks on average) of significantly larger babies (658 g increase).

In a later study (McParland *et al.*, *1990*), women at risk of pregnancy-induced hypertension were selected in early pregnancy on the basis of doppler interoplacental flow-velocity waveforms, and treated with 75 mg aspirin daily. There was a significant reduction in the frequency of proteinuric hypertension and hypertension occurring before 37 weeks gestation in the aspirin-treated compared to the placebo group.

17.5   EFFECT OF LOW-DOSE ASPIRIN IN GROWTH RETARDATION

Growth retardation is a feature of pre-eclampsia; so measures that reduce the risk of pre-eclampsia might well reduce the risk of growth retardation. This was reported in some of the studies considered already, e.g. Beaufils *et al.* (1985), Wallenburg *et al.* (1987), Benigni *et al.* (1989), Schiff *et al.* (1989); but does aspirin affect birth weight in pregnancies selected primarily because of a risk of intra-uterine growth retardation rather than because of a risk of pre-eclampsia? It has been shown that abnormalities of the umbilical artery flow velocity wave form detected non-invasively by Doppler ultrasound predict growth retardation, almost certainly, because the umbilical artery resistance is high in this condition (Fleischer *et al.*, 1985; Trudinger *et al.*, 1985, 1987). Therefore, the ratio of systolic to diastolic flow velocity is high in affected foetuses and the resistance may be so high as to stop blood flow in diastole, 'absent end-diastolic flow'. In extreme cases blood flow may even reverse in diastole. In this context, systole and diastole of course refer to the foetal cardiac cycle.

Trudinger *et al.* (1988) took 46 women with abnormal umbilical wave forms and randomized them to receive aspirin 150 mg day^{-1} or placebo. None were hypertensive at the time of randomization. In those patients with moderately abnormal wave forms there were significant improvements in birth weight, head circumference and placental weight in favour of aspirin therapy. In the most severely affected foetuses, aspirin did not significantly improve foetal outcome. It was assumed that these pregnancies were so severely affected that they were 'past redemption'; but unfortunately the differentiation between very severely and less severely affected foetuses was only made after the results were being analysed, and this puts some doubt on the study's credibility.

By the time Wallenburg and Rotmans (1987) studied women who were at risk for recurrent growth retardation because they had had two previously severely growth retarded pregnancies, they were unable to obtain a control group. These 24 women had such bad obstetric histories that they insisted on being in the therapeutic group, whatever the risk. They were treated with daily aspirin 1–1.6 mg kg^{-1} and dipyridamole 225 mg from 16 to 34 weeks gestation. The controls were historical: all those who had had recurrent growth retardation in the previous 5 years at the same hospital. There was a striking difference in outcome, 13% growth retardation in the treated group compared to 61% in the controls; no cases of severe growth retardation in the treated group compared to 27% in controls.

Perhaps not surprisingly, low-dose aspirin does not affect birth weight in otherwise uncomplicated twin pregnancy (Trudinger et al., 1989). It is assumed that the relatively low birth weight in twin pregnancy relates to the overall inability of the uterus to sustain such a large foeto-placental mass, rather than to any pathological process.

In an uncontrolled study Elder et al. (1988) reviewed their experience with the use of low-dose aspirin in pregnancy. Thirty-eight women had been treated with aspirin 75 mg daily because of recurrent pre-eclampsia, growth retardation or lupus, another condition showing similar placental histology to pre-eclampsia where the foetus is affected adversely (Lubbe, 1988). The women had between them lost 76 pregnancies in the past and only had eight successful pregnancies. With aspirin therapy there were 35 live births and five pregnancy losses.

A recent multicentre trial (Uzan et al., 1991) of 323 women in 25 centres compared 150 mg day^{-1} aspirin plus 225 mg day^{-1} dipyridamole or 150 mg day^{-1} aspirin with placebo. Mean birthweight was 225 g higher in the treated than in the placebo group and the frequency of fetal growth retardation in the placebo group was twice that in the treated group. No significant differences were found between the aspirin only and the aspirin plus dipyridamole groups.

The results of these studies emphasize the necessity for large trials not only to establish the precise possible benefits of aspirin therapy but also its risks.

17.6 POSSIBLE ADVERSE EFFECTS OF SALICYLATE IN PREGNANCY

Salicylates cross the placenta (Perkin et al., 1980) and equilibrate between the mother and foetus 60–90 min after ingestion (Heymann, 1985). So, in addition to any adverse effects of salicylates that are observed in the non-pregnant state (and any specific maternal side effects), the possibility of some specific effects(s) on the foetus should be considered.

17.6.1 Teratogenesis

Although early studies suggested an increased risk of congenital defects (McNeil, 1973), in particular talipes (Richards, 1969), this was not confirmed in a larger epidemiological study involving over 14 000 patients exposed to aspirin (Slone *et al.*, 1976). A more recent study of 300 children with congenital heart disease suggested that there may be an increased risk of certain types of congenital heart disease – in particular aortic stenosis, coarctation and hypoplastic left heart syndrome (Zierler and Rothman, 1985). This was not confirmed in a much larger case control study of 1381 infants with congenital heart disease (Werler *et al.*, 1989). In practice, aspirin therapy is usually initiated after 12 weeks of pregnancy when organogenesis is complete. So, even if aspirin were teratogenic, this is unlikely to be a problem.

17.6.2 Foetal Lung Impairment

Experimental work on animals would suggest that prostaglandin synthetase inhibitors might, at least in theory, impair surfactant formation, increase foetal respiratory movements and decrease the pulmonary vascular dilatation that occurs at birth (Heymann, 1985). There is, however, no evidence that any such clinically significant effects occur in patients taking aspirin.

17.6.3 Inhibition of Labour

Prostaglandins are involved in the initiation and maintenance of labour, and prostaglandin synthetase inhibitors, particularly indomethacin, have been used to arrest premature labour (Nierbyl *et al.*, 1980). Women taking aspirin appear to have a longer mean duration of pregnancy than those that do not (Collins and Turner, 1975), but this difference may have been due to an increased rate of induction (perhaps for pre-eclampsia) in the group not taking aspirin.

17.6.4 Blood Clotting Defects

Part of the rationale for the use of aspirin is to decrease platelet thromboxane production, and thereby to discourage thrombogenesis. Although it is hoped that the benefits of this will outweigh the disadvantages, some maternal and foetal bleeding tendency must be anticipated.

Collins and Turner (1975) noted an increased incidence of ante- and post-partum haemorrhage and transfusion at delivery in women who had taken aspirin therapy every day during pregnancy. Likewise, Stuart *et al.* (1982) noted bleeding problems in neonates and their mothers

457

where aspirin had been taken in the 5 days preceding delivery. Finally, Forrestier *et al.* (1985) noted inhibition of foetal platelet aggregation after the mothers had taken 50 mg of aspirin. But in the studies where bleeding recurred (Collins and Turner, 1975; Stuart *et al.*, 1982), the mothers had been taking analgesic doses of aspirin, at least 500 mg day^{-1}, and sometimes much more. Most investigators are now using 75 mg or less of aspirin per day for prophylaxis of pre-eclampsia and intra-uterine growth retardation. Thus risk of bleeding should be much less.

17.6.5 Foetal Circulation

Patency of the ductus arteriosus is maintained in part by prostaglandins, in particular prostaglandin E_2 and prostacyclin (Heymann, 1985). The effect of prostaglandin synthetase inhibitors on the ductal circulation is, therefore, clearly an important potential complication of aspirin therapy, and there are clinical reports suggesting an association with certain forms of congenital heart disease (Zierler and Rothman, 1985), congestive heart failure presenting *in utero*, and severe persistent pulmonary hypertension syndrome (Levin *et al.*, 1978). But, even though most of these reports are in relation to indomethacin treatment (Heymann, 1985), clinical trials of indomethacin in premature labour have not shown any association between prostaglandin synthetase inhibition and persistent pulmonary hypertension syndrome (Nierbyl *et al.*, 1980). Furthermore, the Collaborative Perinatal Project did not show any excess perinatal mortality in the children of over 26 000 mothers taking aspirin in pregnancy compared to those of nearly 15 000 who were not exposed to aspirin (Shapiro *et al.*, 1976).

17.6.6 Reye's Syndrome

MATERNAL CONSIDERATIONS

Reye's Syndrome has not been described in women of child-bearing age; however, the very rare condition of acute fatty liver of pregnancy (AFLP) has a rather similar presentation and histological appearance in the liver. Nevertheless, no association between aspirin use and AFLP has been reported, and there are sufficient differences in the clinical features and histology (Weber *et al.*, 1979) to conclude that AFLP and Reye's syndrome are probably different.

FOETAL CONSIDERATIONS

Typically, Reye's Syndrome occurs at a median age of 14 months in children who have been taking about 10 mg kg^{-1} of aspirin daily for a febrile illness (Lancet, 1986). Neonates do not appear to be at risk of developing the condition, nor has any association with maternal use of aspirin been described in large case-controlled studies (Collins and Turner, 1975; Stuart *et al.*, 1982). In practice, the foetus is exposed to very low levels of aspirin (perhaps, less than 1 mg kg^{-1} daily) without any antecedent febrile illness. It seems very unlikely, therefore, that there is any increased risk of Reye's Syndrome.

In conclusion, adverse effects from low-dose aspirin therapy though possible, are likely to be uncommon. Indeed, none of the trials of low-dose aspirin therapy published so far (Beaufils *et al.*, 1985; Wallenburg *et al.*, 1986; Wallenburg and Rotmans, 1987; Trudinger *et al.*, 1988; Benigni *et al.*, 1989; Schiff *et al.*, 1989; Sibai *et al.*, 1989) has shown any increased risks of side effects; nor have the two recent studies of aspirin versus aspirin and dipyridamole versus placebo, and aspirin versus aspirin and dipyridamole (Uzan *et al.*, 1991).

17.7 CONCLUSION

There have been eight published randomized, placebo-controlled trials of low-dose aspirin in pregnancy given for prophylaxis or treatment of pre-eclampsia and/or growth retardation. About 324 patients have been in the experimental groups and 240 patients have taken placebo. Meta-analysis by Breart (Personal communication), showed only one case of proteinuric pre-eclampsia in the treated group, and 23 in controls. Birth weight was increased by 396 g in the treated group. The incidence of growth retardation below the 10th centile was reduced from 27% to 10% (the expected incidence in a healthy population). The caesarian section rate was reduced from 50% to 29%. Two further meta-analyses (Collins, 1991; Imperiale and Petrulis, 1991) presented promising evidence of the protective action of aspirin in pre-eclampsia and growth retardation.

To be confident of these very worthwhile improvements we need the results of larger studies. These should also tell us about the possibility of important rare but adverse side effects occurring at the less than 1% level that the current published studies are too small to detect. Such large studies are in progress organized by the National Institutes of Health in the USA and the Medical Research Council in the UK (CLASP study). Their publication in the next few years should establish the place of low-dose aspirin in pregnancy.

REFERENCES

Beaufils, M., Uzan, S., Donsimoni, R. and Colau, J.C. (1985) Prevention of pre-eclampsia by early anti-platelet therapy. *Lancet*, i, 840–2.

Therapeutic applications

Benigni, A., Gregorini, G., Frusca, T. *et al.* (1989) Effect of low-dose aspirin on fetal and maternal generation of thromboxane by platelets in women at risk for pregnancy induced hypertension. *N. Engl. J. Med.*, **321**, 357–62.

Bussolino, F., Benedetto, C., Massobrio, M. and Camussi, G. (1980) Maternal vascular prostacyclin activity in pre-eclampsia. *Lancet*, **ii**, 702.

Collins, R. (1991) Antiplatelet agents for IUGR and pre-eclampsia. In *Oxford Database of Perinatal Trials* (ed. I. Chalmers), Version 1.2, Disk Issue 5, Record 4000.

Collins, E. and Turner, G. (1975) Maternal effects of regular salicylate ingestion in pregnancy. *Lancet*, **ii**, 335–8.

Crandon, A.J. and Isherwood, D.M. (1979) Effect of aspirin on incidence of pre-eclampsia. *Lancet*, **i**, 1356.

Di Minno, G., Silver, M.J. and Murphy, S. (1983) Monitoring the entry of new platelets into the circulation after ingestion of aspirin. *Blood*, **61**, 1081–5.

Dyerberg, J. and Bang, H.O. (1985) Pre-eclampsia and prostaglandins. *Lancet*, **i**, 1267–8.

Elder, M.G., de Swiet, M., Robertson, A. *et al.* (1988) Low-dose aspirin in pregnancy. *Lancet*, **i**, 410.

Everett, R.B., Worley, R.J., Macdonald, P.C. and Gant, N.F. (1978) Effects of prostaglandin synthetase inhibitors on pressor response to angiotension II in human pregnancy. *J. Clin. Endocrinol. Metab.*, **46**, 1007–10.

Fitzgerald, D.J., Rocki, W., Murray, R. *et al.* (1990) Thromboxane A_2 synthesis in pregnancy-induced hypertension. *Lancet*, **335**, 751–4.

Fleischer, A., Schulman, H., Farmakides, G. *et al.* (1985) Umbilical velocity wave ratios in intrauterine growth retardation. *Am. J. Obstet. Gynecol.*, **151**, 502–6.

Forrestier, F., Daffos, F. and Rainaut, M. (1985) Pre-eclampsia and prostaglandins. *Lancet*, **1**, 1268.

Gant, N.F., Daley, G.L., Chand, S. *et al.* (1973) A study of angiotensin II pressor response throughout primigravid pregnancy. *J. Clin. Invest.*, **52**, 2682–9.

Gant, N.F., Chand, S., Worley, R.J. *et al.* (1974) A clinical test for predicting the development of active hypertension in pregnancy. *Am. J. Obstet. Gynecol.*, **120**, 1–7.

Goodlin, R.C. (1983) Connection of pregnancy-related thrombocytopenia with aspirin without improvement in fetal outcome. *Am. J. Obstet. Gynecol.*, **146**, 862–4.

Goodlin, R.C., Haesslein, H.O. and Fleming, J. (1978) Aspirin for the treatment of recurrent toxaemia. *Lancet*, **ii**, 51.

Goodman, R.P., Killam, A.P., Brash, A.R. and Branch, R.A. (1982) Prostacyclin production during pregnancy: comparison of production during normal pregnancy and pregnancy complicated by hypertension. *Am. J. Obstet. Gynecol.*, **142**, 817–22.

Greer, I.A., Calder, A.A., Walker, J.J. and Lunan, C.B. (1988) Increased platelet reactivity in pregnancy-induced hypertension and uncomplicated diabetic pregnancy: an indication for antiplatelet therapy? *Brit. J. Obstet. Gynaecol.*, **95**, 1204–8.

Heymann, M.A. (1985) Non-steroidal anti-inflammatory agents. In *Drug Therapy during Pregnancy* (eds T.K.A.B Eskes and M. Finster), Butterworths, London, pp. 85–99.

Imperiale, T.F. and Petrulis, A.S. (1991) A meta-analysis of low-dose aspirin for the prevention of pregnancy-induced hypertensive disease. *J. Am. Med. Assoc.*, **266**, 260–5.

Jespersen, J. (1980) Disseminated intravascular coagulation in toxaemia of pregnancy. Connection of the decreased platelet counts and raised levels of serum uric acid and fibrin(ogen) degradation products by aspirin. *Thromb. Res.*, **17**, 743–6.

Koullapis, E.N., Nicholaides, K.H., Collins, W.P. *et al.* (1982) Plasma prostanoids in pregnancy-induced hypertension. *Brit. J. Obstet. Gynaecol.*, **89**, 617–21.

Lancet Notes and News (1986) Reye's syndrome and the giving of aspirin to children. *Lancet*, **i**, 1396.

Levin, D.L., Fixler, D.E., Moriss, F.C. and Tyson, J. (1978) Morphologic analysis of the pulmonary vasculature in infants exposed *in utero* to prostaglandin synthetase inhibitors. *J. Pediat.* **92**, 478–83.

Lubbe, W.F. (1988) Low-dose aspirin in prevention of toxaemia of pregnancy. Does it have a place? *Drugs*, **34**, 515–18.

McNeil, J.R. (1973) The possible teratogenic effect of salicylates on the developing fetus: brief summaries of eight suggestive cases. *Clin. Pediat.*, **12**, 347–50.

McParland, P., Pearce, J.M. and Chamberlain, G.V.P. (1990) Doppler ultrasound and aspirin in recognition and prevention of pregnancy-induced hypertension. *Lancet*, **335**, 1552–5.

Nierbyl, J.R., Blake, D.A., White, R.D. *et al.* (1980) The inhibition of premature labor with indomethacin. *Am. J. Obstet. Gynecol.*, **136**, 1014–19.

Perkin, R.M., Levin, D.L. and Clark, R. (1980) Serum salicylate levels and right-to-left ductal shunts in newborn infants with persistent pulmonary hypertension. *J. Pediat.*, **96**, 721–6.

Phelan, J.P., Everidge, G.J., Wilder, T.L. and Newman, C. (1977) Is the supine pressor test an adequate means of predicting acute hypertension in pregnancy? *Am. J. Obstet. Gynecol.*, **128**, 173–6.

Reilly, I.A. and FitzGerald, G.A. (1987) Inhibition of thromboxane formation *in vivo* and *ex vivo*: implication for therapy with platelet inhibitory drugs. *Blood*, **69**, 180–6.

Richards, I.D. (1969) Congenital malformations and environmental influence in pregnancy. *Brit. J. Prevent. Social Med.*, **23**, 218–25.

Sanchez-Ramos, L., O'Sullivan, M.J. and Garrido-Calderon, J. (1987) Effect of low-dose aspirin in angiotensin II pressor response in human pregnancy. *Am. J. Obstet. Gynecol.*, **156**, 193–4.

Schiff, E., Peleg, E., Goldenberg, M. *et al.* (1989) The use of aspirin to prevent pregnancy-induced hypertension and lower the ratio of thromboxane A_2 to prostacyclin in relatively high risk pregnancies. *N. Engl. J. Med.*, **321**, 351–6.

Shapiro, S., Siskind, V., Monson, R.R. *et al.* (1976) Perinatal mortality and birth-weight in relation to aspirin taken during pregnancy. *Lancet*, **i**, 1375–6.

Sibai, B.M., Mirro, R., Chesney, C.M. and Leffler, C. (1989) Low-dose aspirin in pregnancy. *Obstet. Gynecol.*, **74**, 551–7.

Slone, D., Siskind, V., Heinonen, O.P. *et al.* (1976) Aspirin and congenital malformations. *Lancet*, **i** 1373–5.

Therapeutic applications

Spitz, B., Magness, R.R., Cox, S.M. *et al.* (1988) Low dose aspirin. 1. Effect on angiotensin II pressor responses and blood prostacyclin concentrations in pregnant women sensitive to angiotensin II. *Am. J. Obstet. Gynecol.*, **159**, 1035–43.

Stuart, M.J., Gross, S.J., Ellad, M. and Graeber, J.E. (1982) Effects of acetylsalicylic-acid ingestion on maternal and neonatal hemostasis. *N. Engl. J. Med.*, **307**, 909–12.

Trudinger, B.J. Giles, W.B., Cook, C.M. *et al.* (1985) Fetal umbilical artery flow velocity wave forms and placental resistance: clinical significance. *Brit. J. Obstet. Gynaecol.*, **92**, 23–30.

Trudinger, B.J., Cook, C.M., Giles, W.B. *et al.* (1987) Umbilical artery flow velocity wave forms – a randomized controlled trial. *Lancet*, **i**, 188–90.

Trudinger, B.J., Cook, C.M., Thompson, R.S. *et al.* (1988) Low-dose aspirin therapy improves fetal weight in umbilical placental insufficiency. *Am. J. Obstet. Gynecol.*, **159**, 681–5.

Trudinger, B.J., Cook, C.M., Giles, W.B. *et al.* (1989) Low dose aspirin and twin pregnancy. *Lancet*, **ii**, 1214.

Uzan, S., Beaufils, M., Breart, G. *et al.* (1991) Prevention of fetal growth retardation with low-dose aspirin: findings of the EPREDA trial. *Lancet* **337**, 1427–31.,

Wallenburg, H.C.S. and Rotmans, N. (1982) Enhanced reactivity of the platelet thromboxane pathway in normotensive and hypertensive pregnancies with insufficient fetal growth. *Am. J. Obstet. Gynecol.*, **144**, 523–8.

Wallenburg, H.C.S. and Rotmans, N. (1987) Prevention of recurrent idiopathic fetal growth retardation by low-dose aspirin and dipyridamole. *Am. J. Obstet. Gynecol.*, **157**, 1230–5.

Wallenburg, H.C.S., Dekker, G.A., Makovitz, J.W. and Rotmans, P. (1986) Low dose aspirin prevents pregnancy-induced hypertension and pre-eclampsia in angiotensin-sensitive primigravidae. *Lancet*, **i**, 1–3.

Walsh, S.W. (1985) Pre-eclampsia: An imbalance in placental prostacyclin and thromboxane production. *Am. J. Obstet. Gynecol.*, **152**, 335–40.

Weber, F.L.Jr, Snodgrass, P.J., Powell, D.E. *et al.* (1979) Abnormalities of hepatic mitochondrial urea-cycle enzyme activities and hepatic ultrastructure in acute fatty liver in pregnancy. *J. Lab. Clin. Med.*, **94**, 27–41.

Werler, M.M., Mitchell, A.A. and Shapiro, S. (1989) The relation of aspirin use during the first trimester of pregnancy to congenital cardiac defects. *N. Engl. J. Med.*, **321**, 1639–42.

Yamaguchi, M. and Mori, N. (1985) 6-keto-prostaglandin $F_{1\alpha}$, thromboxane B_2, and 13, 14-dihydro-15-keto-prostaglandin F concentrations of normotensive and pre-eclamptic patients during pregnancy, delivery and the post partum period. *Am. J. Obstet. Gynecol.*, **151**, 121–7.

Ylikorkala, O. and Makila, U.M. (1985) Prostacyclin and thromboxane in gynecology and obstetrics. *Am. J. Obstet. Gynecol.*, **152**, 318–29.

Zierler, S. and Rothman, K.J. (1985) Congenital heart disease in relation to maternal use of bendectin and other drugs in early pregnancy. *N. Engl. J. Med.*, **313**, 347–52.

PART FIVE
Unwanted effects

18 Unwanted effects of aspirin and related agents on the gastrointestinal tract

B.J.R. WHITTLE

18.1 INTRODUCTION

One of the most frequent iatrogenic diseases encountered in clinical practice is gastrointestinal irritation and distress induced by anti-inflammatory agents, notably those of the non-steroid class. This reflects the extensive use of such non-steroid anti-inflammatory agents, obtained by both prescription and over-the-counter sales. Indeed, it has been suggested from consideration of prescription analysis, that sufficient of these drugs are prescribed in the USA to allow for daily use by over 1.2% of its total population, with an annual incidence of serious gastrointestinal reactions of 2–4% in patients receiving such drugs (Fries *et al.*, 1989). These side effects can present as a wide spectrum of upper gastrointestinal symptoms encompassing dyspepsia, mild epigastric pain, gastritis, nausea, vomiting or frank haemorrhage, while blood loss detected in the stools may increase up to 20 times the normal limits as a result of gastric mucosal damage.

Gastrointestinal symptoms and haemorrhage are also the major side effects reported in most clinical trials using aspirin not only as an anti-inflammatory agent, but as a potential anti-thrombotic agent. Thus, in a study on transient ischaemic attack in the UK, oral ingestion of aspirin (300 and 1200 mg daily over 4 years) gave an incidence of indigestion, nausea, vomiting and heartburn of 29% and 39% respectively compared with the incidence in the placebo group of 24%, while the incidence of actual gastrointestinal bleeding increased from 1.6% to 2.6% and 4.7% with the lower and higher doses of aspirin respectively (UK-TIA group, 1988). In a more recent study on the beneficial effects of low-dose aspirin (75 mg daily) on the risk of myocardial infarction, an increase in gastrointestinal symptoms compared with placebo (from 2% to 7%) was observed after a 3-month treatment period, but no haemorrhage was reported with this low-dose regimen (RISC group, 1990).

Early studies had also suggested that the frequent and heavy intake

465

of aspirin may be a factor underlying major gastrointestinal bleeding and peptic ulceration (Duggan, 1972; Levy, 1974; Piper *et al.*, 1981). Although some investigators challenged the contribution of such agents to peptic ulcer disease (Rees and Turnberg, 1980), more recent studies firmly support this contention (Walt *et al.*, 1986; Faulkner *et al.*, 1988). Several dozen newer non-steroid anti-inflammatory drugs of different chemical classes have been introduced into therapeutic practice, whose potencies are many times that of aspirin itself. However, the majority of these newer aspirin substitutes in clinical use still retain gastric mucosal toxicity, although this is usually less than that seen with aspirin.

A number of clinical studies have supported the relationship between the ingestion of non-steriod anti-inflammatory agents and the incidence of haemorrhage and ulceration in the stomach (Duggan *et al.*, 1986; Somerville *et al.*, 1986) and a correlation between life-threatening complications such as ulcer perforation is also evident (Collier and Pain, 1985). In one study, 80% of all deaths associated with peptic ulcer occurred in patients using non-steroid anti-inflammatory drugs (Armstrong and Blower, 1987). Furthermore, it is apparent that elderly patients, particularly women, are at risk from developing these severe gastrointestinal effects (Clinch *et al.*, 1987; Griffin *et al.*, 1988; Fries *et al.*, 1989). Overall, the gastropathies associated with the ingestion of non-steriod anti-inflammatory drugs have been estimated to account for some 2600 deaths and 20 000 hospital admissions in the USA, even when considering only those patients who were taking these drugs specifically for the treatment of rheumatoid arthritis (Fries *et al.*, 1989). Furthermore, it was also concluded that an enteropathy consisting of changes in intestinal permeability with local inflammation occurs in over 60% of patients on long-term therapy with these agents (Bjarnason *et al.*, 1987a, b).

Several studies have attempted to rank the incidence and severity of the gastrointestinal side effects of the newer non-steroid anti-inflammatory drugs, although there is as yet no clear clinical evidence for a significant therapeutic–safety ratio benefit with any of these agents (Pemberton and Strand, 1979; Caruso and Bianchi-Porro, 1980; Rainsford, 1982; Biour *et al.*, 1987; Langman, 1989). Thus, the search for an anti-inflammatory drug completely devoid of such toxic actions appears not to have ended. The rational development of safer compounds will clearly depend upon a fuller understanding of the processes initiating and promoting such gastric injury by the current non-steroid anti-inflammatory agents. Over the past 50 years, many concepts have been elaborated concerning these mechanisms and although many have not withstood rigorous experimental study, it

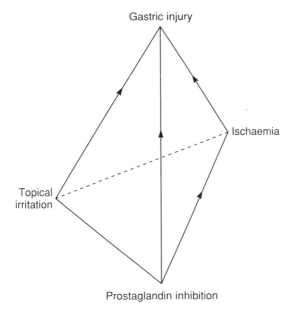

Gastric injury

Ischaemia

Topical
irritation

Prostaglandin inhibition

Figure 18.1 Interactive mechanisms in the pathogenesis of gastric mucosal damage induced by aspirin and other non-steroid anti-inflammatory drugs.

is clear that such mechanisms are complex and no single process can explain all of the events leading to mucosal damage.

General consideration of the more promoted and investigated theories on the mechanisms of damage by the aspirin-like drugs indicates that they can be categorized into several distinct classes relating to topical irritancy following local intragastric administration, leading to biochemical, metabolic and structural changes within the mucosa, and the sequence of events resulting from inhibition of gastric prostaglandin synthesis. In this chapter, the involvement and interaction between these factors (Fig. 18.1) in the overall gastric toxicity of aspirin and its substitutes will be analysed.

18.2 CLINICAL MEASUREMENTS OF GASTRIC MUCOSAL INJURY

Ever since the introduction of salicylates into medicine at the beginning of this century, side effects on the stomach and intestine have been documented, though much of the early evidence was somewhat anecdotal. Several methods for determining gastrointestinal damage and bleeding have been used, including the faecal output of radiotagged erythrocytes, measurement of back-diffusion or acid-loss, and ion flux across the mucosa with accompanying changes in transepithelial

467

potential difference (Domschke and Domschke, 1984). In a recent study to determine the output of haemoglobin into gastric luminal washings following aspirin ingestion (300 mg daily) over 12 days by healthy volunteers, a six-fold increase in mucosal bleeding was observed after 5 days of treatment, which was similar to that after 12 days (Kitchingman et al., 1989). Furthermore, low-dose aspirin (75 mg daily by mouth) increased the gastric bleeding into the luminal washings two-fold when measured 5 and 12 days after the start of treatment (Prichard et al., 1989).

It is now clear that direct visual inspection by endoscopy is of major importance in determining the toxic effects of non-steroid anti-inflammatory drugs on the gastric and duodenal mucosa. However, experiences from experimental studies have taught that simple macroscopic observation may not reveal mucosal defects that would be apparent on histological examination of biopsy samples (Lacy and Ito, 1982). Thus, some caution must be applied to the interpretation of all such macroscopic data especially regarding claims for absence of toxic effects on the stomach with novel agents.

Over 40 years ago, a gastroscopic study of the effect of aspirin on the human stomach showed the deleterious properties of this compound in the gastric mucosa (Douthwaite and Lintott, 1935). Over the past decade, the direct gastric effects of many of the clinically used anti-inflammatory agents such as aspirin, naproxen, indomethacin and phenylbutazone have been investigated by endoscopic techniques (Lanza et al., 1979; Silvoso et al., 1979; Caruso and Bianchi-Porro, 1980; Lanza, 1984, 1989). All of these compounds caused visible gastric mucosal damage and erosion formation to various degrees, depending on the dosage regimen. One interesting and important finding which has emerged from these studies is that the patient is a poor judge of gastrointestinal irritancy by these drugs, since in many cases, the development of gastric damage was clearly observed in the absence of any correlation with upper abdominal symptoms. This has emphasized that judicious care must be exercised in the prescribing of high doses of anti-inflammatory analgesics for prolonged periods of time (Barrier and Hirschowitz, 1989).

18.3 TOPICAL IRRITATION AND GASTRIC MUCOSAL DAMAGE

An important concept concerning the effects of topically applied salicy-lates on the gastric mucosa was developed by Davenport and colleagues in the mid-1960s, and this has remained a key issue since that time (Davenport, 1964, 1965, 1966; Davenport et al., 1964). It was proposed that the normal resistance of the gastric mucosa to the back-diffusion of gastric acid from the lumen into the mucosal tissue can be disrupted by the topical administration of aspirin and similar compounds. Although of major importance, such a topical action cannot be the sole mechanism, since many such compounds, including aspirin and indomethacin, can cause gastric damage when administered parenterally in experimental animals including the rat, cat and monkey (Brodie and Hooke, 1971; Main and Whittle, 1975; Bugat et al., 1976; Kauffman and Grossman, 1978; Whittle et al., 1985a; Shea-Donohue et al., 1990) and humans (Grossman et al., 1961). Indeed, in one 2-year survey on the incidence of severe gastrointestinal bleeding, the most toxic non-steroid anti-inflammatory agents were non-oral preparations, administered via the rectal or intramuscular route (Biour et al., 1987). However, the local action is of primary concern in therapeutic use, since the vast majority of the aspirin substitutes are administered orally.

18.3.1 Histological Detection of Damage

There have been many histological and ultrastructural studies on the actions of aspirin and related compounds. In an early study using transmission electron microscopy, aspirin-induced erosions in the rat appeared as mucosal excavations with cellular debris and erythrocyte fragments in the lumen and substratum when measured 2–8 h after administration (Yeomans, 1976). Other studies in the rat have shown that within 5 min of intragastric administration of aspirin, focal structural changes to the basement membrane of capillary and post-capillary endothelial cells are induced. These result in destruction of the microvessels, with the subsequent ischaemic areas developing into the erosion site (Robins, 1980). The predominant cellular changes, which occurred some 15 min after administration of aspirin and after the primary vascular damage, were localized in the mitochondria of the parietal cells, which became swollen with disrupted cristea.

Studies in the pig with indomethacin likewise have demonstrated red blood cell extravasation from damaged capillaries, with parietal cell damage following 15 min after intragastric administration (Rainsford and Willis, 1982; Rainsford et al., 1982) and similar actions of both agents have been observed in the rat (Rainsford et al., 1984). A common feature of these ultrastructural investigations is the detection of microvascular changes and capillary damage at an early stage in the formation of the erosions (Rainsford, 1983).

Luminal challenge of the gastric mucosa of mice with acidified aspirin was also found to induce macroscopically detectable cell injury, with lysis and exfoliation of epithelial cells (Hingson and Ito, 1971). Furthermore, studies in the dog stomach using freeze-fracture techniques have

469

demonstrated adverse actions of aspirin on the cellular tight junctions, with the appearance of focal discontinuity and disorganization (Meyer et al., 1986).

18.3.2 Gastric Barrier Changes

The ability of topically administered aspirin and related salicylates to promote acid back-diffusion into the canine gastric mucosa was clearly demonstrated in early experiments (Davenport, 1964) and has been amply confirmed by many workers using different species and models, both *in vivo* and *in vitro*. The increase in acid loss is accompanied by an increase in luminal sodium ion concentrations (Davenport et al., 1964). The efflux of potassium ions into the gastric lumen can also be detected following application of local acidified irritants such as salicylic acid (Morris et al., 1984). In the rabbit isolated antral mucosa, where salicylate also increases acid back-diffusion, the increase in cation flow was initially associated with a decreased anion permeability, but subsequently a non-specific increase in permeability to ions was noted (Fuhro and Fromm, 1978). Changes in cation transport by aspirin in isolated gastric mucosal cells have also been reported (Koelz et al., 1978).

The transmucosal flux of non-ionic moieties can also be enhanced by topical irritants. Thus, in the cat stomach, aspirin increased the absorption of inulin, while in the frog isolated gastric mucosa aspirin increased the permeability to dextran (Flemstrom and Marsden, 1974). Furthermore, in his early studies on the mucosal barrier, Davenport (1966) detected an increase of albumin in the luminal contents following salicylate-induced damage in the dog stomach. The latter changes may in part be a result of the intramucosal release of permeability-inducing mediators such as histamine. The release of other pro-inflammatory mediators such as 5-hydroxytryptamine, bradykinin, PAF-acether and the leukotrienes under these conditions has not yet been explored. However, it is likely that their release will result from damage to the cellular components of the mucosa, including resident or invading inflammatory cells. Such cellular injury, as well as the change in intramucosal pH, may also release or activate tissue destructive lysosomal enzymes (Himal et al., 1975) or proteases, which will augment the cell damage and necrosis.

The transmural electropotential difference (PD) across the gastric mucosa has been used as an index of the integrity of the gastric mucosa in animals and man (Geall et al., 1970; Chvasta and Cooke, 1972; Anderson and Grossman, 1965). The ionic basis for the gastric PD is not clearly defined but involves the flux of H^+, Na^+ and Cl^- ions. A reduction in gastric PD has been observed after the topical application of irritants such as aspirin, bile salts, and ethanol in animals and in man (Murray *et al.*, 1974; Cochrane *et al.*, 1975; Morris *et al.*, 1984). These effects occur concurrently with the other characteristics of gastric 'barrier' damage such as the back-diffusion of acid from the gastric lumen into the mucosa, and correlate with histologically demonstrable damage to the human mucosa after aspirin ingestion (Bowen *et al.*, 1977; Smith *et al.*, 1971). It is likely that changes in PD reflect damage to the superficial epithelial cells, while restoration of PD accompanies the process of rapid restitution of the damaged epithelium following local injury (Wallace and Whittle, 1986).

The 'barrier changes' to the mucosa following aspirin or salicylate extend not only to other non-steroid anti-inflammatory drugs such as indomethacin, but also to other local irritants such as bile acids and salts or ethanol (Chvasta and Cooke, 1972; Morris *et al.*, 1984). The action of these agents, not generally regarded as cyclo-oxygenase inhibitors, suggests that this 'barrier-breaking' activity is not related to the inhibition of prostaglandin biosynthesis (Whittle, 1977). Furthermore, intravenous administration of aspirin to cats, dogs or humans failed to elicit barrier damage as determined by luminal acid-loss or potential difference measurements indicating that such changes are the result of local contact with the mucosal tissue and not a reflection of cyclo-oxygenase inhibition (Bugat *et al.*, 1976; Ivey *et al.*, 1980; Kauffman *et al.*, 1980).

Since early studies indicated that such barrier-breaking activities of aspirin and salicylate occurred under acid conditions in the stomach, absorption of the un-ionized form of these carboxylic acids has been suggested to be involved with the damage, although the presence of hydrogen ions in the gastric lumen appears important. It was proposed from early studies that salicylate anions could be trapped in the mucosal cells during absorption (Martin, 1963). Indeed, autoradiographic studies with ^{14}C-salicylate suggested that initial accumulation of salicylate may occur in the parietal cells, although extremely rapid passage of the radiolabelled compound through the mucosa was noted, indicating that absorption and clearance of the drug from gastric tissue occurred within 15 min of exposure (Brune *et al.*, 1977). Aspirin may be de-acetylated in the mucosal cells to yield high intracellular concentrations of salicylate, which may be more toxic then aspirin itself to those cells (Szabo *et al.*, 1989).

Other topical irritants such as ethanol are unlikely to act in this manner. Thus, in the dog, a low intragastric concentration of ethanol which lowered PD induced morphological changes in the surface epithelial cells, but not in the deeper parietal cells, initially without disruption of the apical cells or cellular tight junction (Eastwood and Erdmann,

1978). It has been proposed, however, that bile acids may disrupt gastric integrity by entering apical mucosal cells, whereas bile salts can exert a detergent action by promoting the dissolution of mucosal lipids (Duane *et al.*, 1982). Whether the changes in mucosal integrity resulting from accumulation within parietal or other cells could lead to or account for all the characteristics of barrier damage with aspirin, and whether other anti-inflammatory agents are likewise accumulated, remains to be fully established.

18.4   GASTRIC METABOLIC CHANGES

In the guinea-pig isolated gastric mucosa, aspirin and taurocholate produced a slow reduction in total mucosal ATP levels, and a fall in PD, both occurring over a 2 h period (Ohe *et al.*, 1980a). Earlier studies had shown a small reduction in mucosal ATP content following a 1 h exposure of the isolated amphibian mucosa to salicylic acid, while a 30 min exposure to aspirin has been shown to reduce both mucosal ATP and phosphocreatine content in a similar preparation, perhaps by uncoupling or inhibiting mitochondrial oxidative phosphorylation (Kasbekar, 1973; Spenney and Bhown, 1977). Furthermore, uncoupling of oxidative phosphorylation by aspirin and salicylate in gastric mucosal mitochondria has been reported (Glarborg-Jorgensen *et al.*, 1976).

It has also been proposed that the reduction in mucosal ATP levels following application of aspirin to a dog isolated chambered mucosa could underly the observed changes in ion transport and changes in mucosal permeability, which reflect alterations in cellular integrity (Kuo and Shanbour, 1976). However, in the absence of detailed studies on the temporal relationship between such metabolic changes and the effects on ion flux, it is difficult to interpret whether such changes in energy metabolism are simply a consequence of the rapid sequence of events following primary damage to the tissue. Furthermore, evaluation of the effects of the newer anti-inflammatory agents on these metabolic processes in the stomach *in vivo* and in isolated mucosal cells could provide further information on the relevance of such events to gastric injury.

18.5   ROLE OF LUMINAL FACTORS

18.5.1   Intraluminal pH and Chemical Modifications

A low luminal pH provides a non-dissociated form of the acidic anti-inflammatory compounds which, being lipid soluble, will be more readily absorbed into and through the mucosa. Furthermore, back-diffusion of luminal acid appears intimately connected with the pathogenesis of gastric damage by topical irritants. Buffering of a solution of aspirin to pH 7 with sodium bicarbonate abolished the fall in PD in human subjects, suggesting that formulations of aspirin or similar compounds may show less superficial irritancy if buffered (Bowen *et al.*, 1977). Aspirin and sodium salicylate also reduced the PD across the human buccal mucosa when applied in acid solution, but not when buffered to neutral pH (Whittle *et al.*, 1981b). However, the buffering of aspirin will also dramatically alter rates of gastric absorption and may additionally alter the rate of its gastric emptying, factors which will have a clinical bearing on the pharmacokinetics of these agents. Furthermore, the buffering capacity of such formulations must take into account the low pH of the gastric lumen, and the chronic ingestion of high levels of buffering solutions, especially those with sodium salts, may not be desirable.

Although acute administration of a relatively low dose of buffered aspirin mixture has been reported to cause negligible damage to the gastric mucosa, as assessed by histological examination, other studies have indicated that higher doses (3.9 g day^{-1}) of a buffered aspirin preparation offer little or no protection to the gastric and duodenal mucosa (Bowen *et al.*, 1977; Lanza *et al.*, 1980). Enteric coated tablets did appear, however, to cause less gastro-duodenal irritation (Hoftiezer *et al.*, 1980; Lanza *et al.*, 1980).

Other approaches to reducing the direct topical gastric damage by the salicylates concern modification to the free carboxyl substituents on the salicylate, which have been implicated as a factor in these toxic actions (Fuhro and Fromm, 1978). Esterification of this moiety, as in methyl aspirin, has apparently provided compounds with less acute ulcerogenic actions following intragastric administration, while anti-inflammatory activity is retained, presumably following liberation of the free acid by the action of plasma esterases (Rainsford and Whitehouse, 1980). While such modifications may reduce direct local irritancy, these compounds, once activated in the systemic circulation, could retain their biochemical actions, including actions on gastric cyclo-oxygenase, which may lead to more chronic development of gastrointestinal disturbances.

18.5.2 Pepsinogen Activation

During acid secretion, the gastric contents can contain high concentrations of the proteolytic enzyme, pepsin. Early studies suggested that rat gastric mucosal pepsinogens were activated by unbuffered suspensions of aspirin *in vitro*, as found with other acids, including HCl (Mangla *et*

473

al., 1974). In other investigations, changes in the ratio of acid-labile to total pepsinogen levels following application of aspirin and taurocholate were taken as an indication of pepsin activation within the mucosa during the development of gastric erosions (Ohe *et al.*, 1980b). In another study, aspirin and hyperosmotic topical irritants likewise caused a small increase in pepsinogen output into the rat gastric lumen (Puurunen *et al.*, 1980). Aspirin can also augment the proteolytic actions of pepsin on gastric gel mucus (Sarosiek *et al.*, 1986).

It is not yet clear whether pepsin contributes to the pathogenesis of mucosal injury following ingestion of aspirin and like compounds. Local changes in the pH of the mucosal micro-environment following the induction of acid back-diffusion could conceivably initiate pepsinogen activation within the mucosa and thus proteolytic digestion may contribute to the subsequent development of the gastric erosion. However, further work is necessary before such autodigestion can be fully implicated in the gastric damage associated with other non-steroid anti-inflammatory agents.

18.5.3 Luminal Surface Layers

The mucus layer offers little buffering capacity and appears readily permeable to acid. However, it can act as a lubricant and barrier to physical damage such as that induced by local tissue contact with fragments of anti-inflammatory tablets. This layer can also impede the back-diffusion of hydrogen ions by creating an unstirred layer of water and electrolytes, notably bicarbonate, at the apical membrane (Allen and Garner, 1980; Flemstrom, 1981, 1986; Ross *et al.*, 1981; Starlinger and Schiessel, 1988). Inhibition of mucus biosynthesis, as well as alkaline secretion, could therefore contribute to the process of ulceration by attenuating the elaboration of this local more-alkaline environment, making the underlying tissue more susceptible to damage.

Early studies with aspirin demonstrated the reduction of mucus biosynthesis by superficial epithelial cells and mucus neck cells (Menguy and Masters, 1965). Inhibition of the biosynthesis of sulphated gastric mucus glycoproteins by aspirin and salicylate *in vitro* and following oral administration of aspirin, salicylate and indomethacin in the rat has also been reported (Rainsford, 1978). Aspirin can also alter the physiochemical and biochemical characteristics of mucus, with a substantial decrease in its viscosity (Sarosiek *et al.*, 1986).

Aspirin and indomethacin can also inhibit bicarbonate secretion from isolated gastric amphibian or rabbit mucosa (Garner, 1977; Garner *et al.*, 1979; Rees *et al.*, 1982), and from guinea-pig mucosa and rat duodenum *in vivo* (Garner, 1978; Isenberg *et al.*, 1985; Flemstrom,

1986). In addition, aspirin and indomethacin can suppress gastric and duodenal bicarbonate secretion in man (Rees et al., 1984; Sellings et al., 1987). Thus, aspirin and other non-steroid anti-inflammatory agents may interfere with this provision of a mucus-alkaline layer under physiological conditions.

Following superficial damage to the gastric mucosa, a mucoid cap consisting of mucus, fibrin and cell debris with a relatively high pH is formed over the injured area (Morris and Harding, 1984). This cap appears to provide a micro-environment conducive to the rapid repair of the epithelial continuity by the process of restitution under these conditions of mucosal injury (Wallace and Whittle, 1986). However, the pH gradient across this mucoid cap, produced by bicarbonate secretion and plasma flux, is dissipated following the acute parenteral administration of indomethacin and naproxen in the rat. Such effects could thus compromise this process of rapid repair, and hence would tend to augment any concurrent damage (Wallace and McKnight, 1990). In man, however, oral administration of indomethacin, in sufficient doses to induce acute mucosal damage after 24 h, increased the mucosal-luminal pH gradient (Shorrock et al., 1990). This could reflect a species difference, or the subsequent more chronic protective response of the mucosa to injury over the 24-h period following the initial challenge with the anti-inflammatory agent.

It has also been proposed that the mucosa is protected from attack by luminal acid by the water-repellent properties of the luminal surface. This hydrophobicity of the mucosal surface, previously attributed to a layer of surface-active phospholipids (Lichtenberger et al., 1985), has now been shown to be largely dependent on surface mucus gel (Goddard et al., 1990). This hydrophobicity was substantially reduced by topical application of aspirin, which may reflect the inhibition of mucus and bicarbonate secretion (Goddard et al., 1990). Such changes could thus augment acid back-diffusion and contribute to the local irritant actions of aspirin and other non-steroid anti-inflammatory drugs.

18.5.4 Bile Reflux

The reflux of bile into the gastric lumen has been considered as a possible factor in the aetiology of peptic ulceration and in the pathogenesis of gastric erosions induced by non-steroid anti-inflammatory agents (Djahanguiri et al., 1973; Semple and Russell, 1975; Whittle, 1977). Although this topical irritant could disrupt mucosal integrity by allowing acid back-diffusion, this in itself may cause only limited damage in a functionally intact tissue. However, bile salt-induced injury to the gastric mucosa is significantly enhanced by the administration of

Unwanted effects

aspirin, indomethacin and other such agents in both rat (Cochrane *et al.*, 1975; Semple and Russell, 1975; Whittle, 1977, 1983) and dog (Lewi and Carter, 1981; Whittle and Moncada, 1983). Thus, it is likely that the injurious effects of anti-inflammatory agents on the gastric mucosa will be augmented in patients that exhibit bile reflux.

18.6 INHIBITION OF GASTRIC PROSTANOID SYNTHESIS

18.6.1 Gastric Cyclo-oxygenase

The ability of gastrointestinal tissue to generate substantial levels of prostanoids, notably prostacyclin and prostaglandin E_2 (PGE_2) (Whittle and Vane, 1987), coupled with their many potent biological actions, has led to the concept that these endogenous lipids, derived from arachidonic acid, play a significant role in the local modulation of gastrointestinal function and integrity (Robert, 1976, 1981; Chaudhury and Jacobson, 1978; Miller, 1983; Hawkey and Rampton, 1985; Whittle and Vane, 1987). The discovery by Vane and his colleagues in 1971 that aspirin and its substitutes potently inhibited the formation of prostaglandins (Vane, 1971; Flower, 1974) gave new insight into the understanding of the mechanisms by which such anti-inflammatory agents exert both their therapeutic actions and associated side effects.

18.6.2 Gastric Cyclo-oxygenase Inhibition

Early studies in the rat had shown that indomethacin in ulcerogenic doses could reduce the level of prostaglandins in gastric mucosal homogenates bioassayed as PGE_2 (Main and Whittle, 1975) and the levels of both PGE_2 and $PGF_{2\alpha}$ in the stomach estimated by radioimmunoassay (RIA) (Fitzpatrick *et al.*, 1976). In an initial study on the temporal relationship between the healing of gastric erosions induced by indomethacin and the inhibition of gastric mucosal prostacyclin formation, the rate of disappearance of the erosions over the ensuing 48 h closely paralleled the recovery of the ability of the mucosa to generate prostacyclin (Whittle, 1981). In a study on the early time-course of mucosal injury in the rat, oral administration of aspirin or indomethacin induced near-maximal inhibition of mucosal cyclo-oxygenase within 5 min, with ultrastructural signs of mucosal damage being seen 10–60 min after administration (Rainsford *et al.*, 1984).

Following either oral or parenteral administration, indomethacin, aspirin, naproxen and flurbiprofen in anti-inflammatory doses caused a dose-related inhibition of gastric mucosal prostaglandin production, determined *ex vivo*, in the rat (Whittle *et al.*, 1980) as shown in Fig. 18.2. Others have confirmed, using similar techniques, that intragastric or intravenous administration of aspirin inhibits both PGE_2 and prostacyclin production by the rat gastric mucosa *ex vivo* (Konturek *et al.*, 1981b; Kobayashi *et al.*, 1985).

In the dog, irrigation of the denervated fundic gastric pouch with aspirin caused a concentration-related inhibition of cyclo-oxygenase activity in gastric mucosal biopsies (Ligumsky *et al.*, 1982). In the cat, bolus intravenous injection of aspirin significantly inhibited *ex-vivo* gastric mucosal 6-oxo-$PGF_{1\alpha}$ and PGE_2 synthesis when determined after 4 h (Whittle *et al.*, 1985a). Studies in the pig involving 10-day intragastric treatment with several anti-inflammatory drugs, including aspirin and indomethacin, caused a significant fall in the freeze-clamped mucosal 'levels' of both PGE_2 and 6-keto-$PGF_{1\alpha}$ determined by RIA (Rainsford and Willis, 1982). In the hamster, subcutaneous administration of indomethacin or oral administration of aspirin reduced mucosal PGE_2 and 6-keto-$PGF_{1\alpha}$ formation in doses producing antral ulcers (Kolbasa *et al.*, 1988).

Non-steroid anti-inflammatory agents such as indomethacin also inhibit gastric cyclo-oxygenase *in vitro* in a variety of mucosal preparations from rat, rabbit and human stomach (Peskar, 1977; Peskar *et al.*, 1980; Boughton-Smith and Whittle, 1983; Jeremy *et al.*, 1985; Melarange and Rashbrook, 1986).

18.6.3 Consequences of Cyclo-oxygenase Inhibition

The major products of arachidonate metabolism by cyclo-oxygenase in the gastric mucosa, prostacyclin and PGE_2, exert potent actions on several aspects of gastric function. Thus, these prostanoids are potent vasodilators in the mucosal microcirculation, they can stimulate mucus-alkaline secretion and inhibit gastric acid secretion and can affect transmucosal ion flux (Robert, 1981; Whittle and Vane, 1987). They exert potent anti-ulcer effects in a wide range of experimental ulcer models and can protect the mucosa from haemorrhagic damage induced by local irritants such as aspirin, acid and ethanol (Robert *et al.*, 1979; Whittle and Vane, 1987). These so-called 'cytoprotective' actions may reflect an action on the mucus–bicarbonate and phospholipid layer and importantly, effects on mucosal blood flow and microvascular integrity. Thus, by interference with such processes, cyclo-oxygenase inhibitors can potentially alter a number of critical factors that regulate mucosal integrity.

An adequate blood flow in the mucosal microcirculation is essential for the mucosa to maintain its cellular and functional status. Parenteral

Unwanted effects

administration of indomethacin has been demonstrated to reduce gastric mucosal blood flow using indirect clearance techniques in the rat and dog (Main and Whittle, 1975; Whittle, 1977, 1980; Kauffman *et al.*, 1980). In studies using flow probes or the determination of gastric vascular resistance, intravenous indomethacin has been shown to reduce gastric blood flow in the dog (Gerkens *et al.*, 1977; Whittle and Moncada, 1983). Furthermore, direct microscopic visualization of rat submucosal microvessels (Guth and Moler, 1982) and studies on microsphere distribution in the rat and rabbit (Skarstein, 1979; Hierton, 1981) likewise have shown a reduction in gastric blood flow following indomethacin administration, suggesting inhibition of endogenous vasodilator prostanoids. Aspirin also decreases blood flow in the canine gastric mucosa (Gerkens *et al.*, 1977), while in a study utilizing hydrogen gas clearance, aspirin was shown to selectively decrease mucosal blood flow at the sites of damage (Ashley *et al.*, 1985). Such changes in the microcirculation may thus lead to areas of focal ischaemia which could

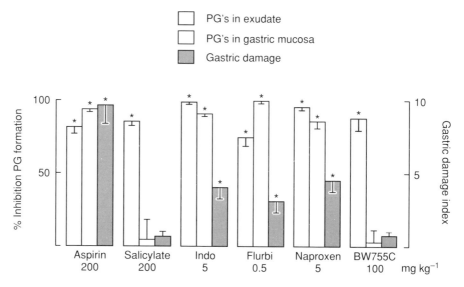

Figure 18.2 Gastric mucosal damage and the inhibition of cyclo-oxygenase products in the rat gastric mucosa and inflammatory exudate induced by non-steroid anti-inflammatory drugs. The compounds (Indo=indomethacin, Flurbi=flurbiprofen) were administered orally three times over 24 h, and prostacyclin formation in gastric mucosal strips *ex vivo* and PGE_2 levels in carrageenin-induced inflammatory exudate in an implanted sponge was determined by bioassay. Gastric mucosal damage was assessed macroscopically in terms of a damage score. Results are shown as mean ± s.e.mean of 5–12 experiments where significant difference from control is shown as * $P<0.01$. (Data are adapted from Whittle *et al.*, 1980.)

478

eventually ulcerate. Furthermore, such blood flow changes would also make the mucosa more susceptible to damage, particularly by local irritants, especially if concurrent alterations in mucus and bicarbonate secretion occur as a consequence of cyclo-oxygenase inhibition.

18.6.4 Tissue Selective Inhibition of Cyclo-oxygenase

Prostaglandin E_2 and prostacyclin, which are the predominant cyclo-oxygenase products found in acute inflammatory exudates, have potent pro-inflammatory actions, and are likely to be involved in the mediation of the acute inflammation process. These prostanoids can, however, exert protective actions on the gastrointestinal tract and may have physiological roles in the gastric mucosa. Thus, to develop a less toxic anti-inflammatory agent, it would be desirable to inhibit cyclo-oxygenase only at the site of inflammation and not in the gastrointestinal tract.

In one study, a range of the newer non-steroid anti-inflammatory agents reduced cyclo-oxygenase products in both the inflammatory exudate induced by carrageenin and the gastric mucosa when administered in anti-inflammatory doses (Fig. 18.2). Thus, these compounds showed no tissue selectivity in their actions towards gastric cyclo-oxygenase (Whittle et al., 1980). In contrast, sodium salicylate and BW755C (a dual lipoxygenase–cyclo-oxygenase inhibitor), in doses causing a significant reduction in prostanoids in the inflammatory exudate, failed to inhibit mucosal cyclo-oxygenase activity (Fig. 18.2). This tissue selectivity of BW755C, also demonstrated in vitro in homogenates of rat gastric mucosa (Boughton-Smith and Whittle, 1983) has also been observed by others (Peskar et al., 1982). Likewise, the lack of inhibition of gastric mucosal cyclo-oxygenase by sodium salicylate has also been confirmed in studies on the cat (Whittle et al., 1985a) and dog (Ligumsky et al., 1982).

Studies with tiaprofenic acid in the rat suggested that the apparent reduced potential for mucosal irritation with this agent compared with indomethacin resulted from a relative lack of potency on mucosal prostacyclin synthesis, although PGE_2 synthesis was potently inhibited (Kobayashi et al., 1985). Furthermore, no such selectivity on gastric cyclo-oxygenase from rat, rabbit or human mucosal biopsies could be seen with this agent in vitro (Jeremy et al., 1985).

It is not yet known whether the failure of certain anti-inflammatory agents to inhibit gastric mucosal cyclo-oxygenase in vivo in doses that suppress prostanoid production in other tissues is a reflection of differences in the pharmacokinetic profile of these agents, although following oral administration, high local concentrations in the mucosa would be expected to be achieved. Furthermore, the failure of agents such as BW755C to inhibit cyclo-oxygenase activity in mucosal homogenates, but to be active in other isolated tissue prepartions including gastric muscle homogenates (Boughton-Smith and Whittle, 1983), implies some fundamental differences in the enzyme's susceptibility to such inhibitors. Full characterization of the isolated enzymes from gastric mucosa and other tissues should resolve this question and may aid in the identification and development of novel tissue-selective cyclo-oxygenase inhibitors.

18.7 CORRELATION OF CYCLO-OXYGENASE INHIBITION WITH GASTRIC DAMAGE

18.7.1 Laboratory Studies

Attempts at correlating the potency of non-steroid anti-inflammatory agents in inducing gastric mucosal damage with their potency as inhibitors of cyclo-oxygenase from tissues other than the mucosa (Rainsford, 1988) are clearly inappropriate in the light of tissue-selective actions. Furthermore, comparison of the rank potency of such agents as inhibitors of mucosal cyclo-oxygenase *in vitro* with their ulcerogenic potential *in vivo* disregards the possibility of major differences in pharmacokinetic distribution and metabolism. Thus, *in-vitro* studies to determine gastric damage and concurrent cyclo-oxygenase inhibition provide an initial approach to understanding the interrelationship between these events, although as discussed below, there may be pitfalls in interpretation of the data.

The findings from early *in-vivo* studies on the formation of gastric erosions in the rat following oral administration of aspirin and its substitutes in anti-inflammatory doses are shown in Fig. 18.2. Indomethacin, flurbiprofen and naproxen induced a comparable degree of gastric erosion formation, which paralleled their efficacy in inhibiting mucosal prostacyclin production in the doses used, supporting an association between these events. Aspirin, however, was more active in inducing gastric damage in doses causing a similar mucosal cyclo-oxygenase inhibition to the other compounds (Whittle *et al.*, 1980).

Sodium salicylate, which failed to inhibit mucosal prostacyclin production in anti-inflammatory doses, caused little gastric damage in the rat following oral administration (Fig. 18.2). This finding is similar to early observations in man that sodium salicylate produced far less gastrointestinal irritation than aspirin, as determined by faecal blood loss (Leonards and Levy, 1973). Although salicylate is known to induce

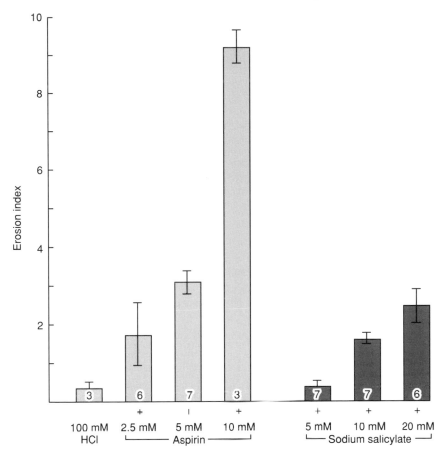

Figure 18.3 Gastric mucosal injury in the pentobarbitone-anaesthetized rat following a 3 h continuous luminal perfusion with aspirin (2.5–10mM) or sodium salicylate (5–20 mM), both acidified with 100 mM HCl. The mucosal damage expressed as an erosion index that takes into account the incidence and severity of the macroscopic haemorrhagic damage, is expressed as mean±s.e.m of (*n*) studies.

acid back-diffusion following mucosal application, topical irritation alone seems insufficient to induce extensive gastric bleeding. Thus, Ligumsky and co-workers (1982) have confirmed that sodium salicylate, unlike aspirin, failed to inhibit prostanoid production, yet both compounds reduced PD and enhanced hydrogen ion back-diffusion and sodium and potassium ion flux following intragastric instillation in the canine fundic pouch. Likewise in the anaesthetized rat, a 3-h luminal perfusion with acidified aspirin induced significantly greater incidence of gastric damage than did higher concentrations of acidified sodium salicylate, as shown in Fig. 18.3, suggesting that local 'barrier' actions do not solely account for the differences in mucosal injury seen with these salicylates. Furthermore, such luminal perfusion should have reduced initial differences in uptake and distribution between these salicylates.

In a study in the cat, single bolus intravenous injection of aspirin, which inhibited the antral formation of prostanoids *ex vivo*, produced gastric antral ulcers during stimulated acid secretion (Hansen *et al.*, 1980), as shown in Fig. 18.4 (See colour plate). This model is therefore of significant interest since in man, gastric lesions induced by non-steroid anti-inflammatory agents are often located in the antrum. Intravenous injection of sodium salicylate under these conditions in the cat did not, however, significantly inhibit antral mucosal prostanoid generation and failed to induce these extensive antral lesions (Whittle *et al.*, 1985a).

Studies in the pig have confirmed an overall association between the inhibition of gastric cyclo-oxygenase and the potential to induce gastric lesions with seven out of eight anti-inflammatory agents tested (Rainsford and Willis, 1982). Of these seven compounds, azapropazone, fenclofenac and flufenamic acid failed to significantly inhibit mucosal prostanoid formation and did not induce gastric damage, whereas indomethacin, aspirin, diclofenac and the pro-drug sulindac, all inhibited mucosal prostanoid production and induced gastric erosions, with aspirin producing the most extensive gastric damage. Meseclazone, however, inhibited gastric prostanoids but did not induce mucosal damage (Rainsford *et al.*, 1982). In a similar study in the rat, indomethacin and aspirin reduced mucosal prostanoid levels and induced injury, azapropazone neither inhibited prostanoid formation nor induced damage, while benoxaprofen induced a variable inhibition of prostanoids but did not cause substantial mucosal damage (Rainsford *et al.*, 1984).

In other studies in the rat, the experimental compound BW755C, in doses some tenfold of its anti-inflammatory dose, failed to inhibit mucosal cyclo-oxygenase activity following both intragastric and parenteral administration and did not induce the formation of mucosal lesions (Whittle *et al.*, 1980). The antipyretic analgesic drug paracetamol, which is not considered a gastric irritant, inhibited prostanoid formation in rat gastric mucosal homogenates *in vitro* only at high concentrations (Boughton-Smith and Whittle, 1983), and had little action on prostanoid formation following administration in the rat gastric mucosa *ex vivo* (Van Kolfscholten *et al.*, 1981).

18.7.2 Human Studies

In studies on the effects of a single oral dose of aspirin (2.5 g) in healthy subjects and duodenal ulcer patients, substantial inhibition of prostanoid formation by mucosal biopsies was observed (Konturek et al., 1981a). This dose of aspirin was sufficient to induce extensive endoscopically detectable haemorrhage and erosions, while oral ingestion of paracetamol in that study induced minimal mucosal injury and inconsistent inhibition of gastric prostanoid formation. In a 5-day study in healthy subjects, aspirin (2.6 g each day) inhibited gastroduodenal prostanoid formation and induced endoscopic and histologically detectable damage (Cohen and MacDonald, 1982). No correlation between the degree of cyclo-oxygenase inhibition and damage was observed, but whether tolerance to the injurious effects of repeated challenge with aspirin had developed, allowing rapid restitution to repair the mucosal damage over this time period, is not known.

Other studies have also attempted to correlate inhibition of gastric cyclo-oxygenase with mucosal damage, but interpretation of these findings are apparently confounded by technical problems. Thus, in a study of the effects of a 4-day oral course of indomethacin (50 mg, t.i.d.), significant inhibition of mucosal levels of PGE_2, $PGF_{2\alpha}$ or 6-oxo-$PGF_{1\alpha}$ could not be detected, but this regimen also did not damage the mucosa (Redfern et al., 1987a). Following ingestion of a single oral dose of indomethacin (100 mg) however, significant inhibition of PGF_2 and $PGF_{2\alpha}$ levels in antral and fundic mucosa was observed, although the failure of 6-keto-$PGF_{1\alpha}$ to be likewise reduced requires some consideration. There was considerable variability between prostanoid levels in the subjects, which could thus preclude a valid correlation of cyclo-oxygenase inhibition with the endoscopic damage observed with this single dose of indomethacin (Redfern et al., 1987a). In a further study on the effects of orally ingested indomethacin (25 mg, t.i.d.) or carprofen over 8 days, no significant inhibition of gastric mucosal PGE_2 or 6-oxo-$PGF_{1\alpha}$ formation by either of these agents was observed, although urinary output of these prostanoids was reduced by indomethacin (Levine et al., 1988). Indomethacin did however, induce damage to the duodenal mucosa, but the failure to correlate the severity of such endoscopic duodenal injury with the overall non-significant actions on gastric prostanoid formation may not therefore be too unexpected (Levine et al., 1988).

Although dose-response clinical studies with a number of non-steroid anti-inflammatory agents are clearly warranted, it is unlikely that a direct correlation between mucosal damage and cyclo-oxygenase inhibition in the gastrointestinal tract will be observed. A simple two-way analysis between these parameters ignores the contribution of other local injurious factors of aspirin and its substitutes, especially since many of these actions synergistically interact (Whittle *et al.*, 1980; Whittle and Vane, 1984).

18.8 INTERACTIONS BETWEEN MECHANISMS OF DAMAGE

It will be apparent that local irritant actions on the gastric mucosa or inhibition of mucosal cyclo-oxygenase following parenteral administration both have the potential to induce superficial injury or extensive haemorrhagic damage in the stomach. However, experimental studies have indicated that, following inhibition of prostanoid biosynthesis, the mucosa is considerably more susceptible to damage by local irritants. Thus, both mechanisms can synergistically interact to provoke more extensive mucosal injury than by either process alone.

18.8.1 Potentiation of Bile Salt Damage

Since blood flow is a critical determinant of the ability of the mucosa to withstand challenge, direct gastric vasoconstriction will greatly augment the damage and ulceration with endogenous local irritants such as bile. Thus, intra-arterial infusion of vasopressin significantly enhanced gastric necrosis following acid-taurocholate instillation in the canine chambered fundic segment *in situ* (Ritchie, 1975). Local generation of the vasoconstrictor thromboxane A_2 or intra-arterial infusion of a stable epoxy-methano-thromboxane mimetic, likewise induced substantial necrosis following acid-taurocholate exposure of the canine mucosa (Whittle *et al.*, 1981a; Whittle and Moncada, 1983). In the rat, intravenous infusion of noradrenaline was also found to augment the mucosal erosions following gastric perfusion of acidified taurocholate (Whittle, 1983). Thus, under conditions of low microvascular flow in the stomach, induced either by direct gastric vasoconstriction or by systemic hypotension (Hamza and Den Besten, 1972; Mersereau and Hinchey, 1978; Svanes *et al.*, 1979; Morris *et al.*, 1990), extensive mucosal damage can be readily induced by agents promoting luminal acid flux.

In the dog and rat, parenteral administration of indomethacin in doses which inhibit mucosal prostanoid formation, substantially potentiated the gastric damage induced by topical acidified taurocholate

(Whittle, 1977; Lewi and Carter, 1981; Whittle and Moncada, 1983). In these doses, indomethacin significantly reduced gastric mucosal blood flow in the rat and elevated gastric vascular resistance in the dog, which may reflect the inhibition of vasodilator prostanoids such as prostacyclin. These effects were not accompanied by a further significant increase in acid back-diffusion (Whittle, 1977, 1983; Whittle and Moncada, 1983). Thus the potentiation of bile salt damage by parenteral indomethacin is likely to reflect the fall in mucosal blood flow leading to an inability of the mucosal tissue to dispose effectively of the excess intramucosal acid. This would allow a fall in intramural pH with subsequent necrosis, as also found in shocked states (Kivilaakso *et al.*, 1978).

Parenteral administration of aspirin, flurbiprofen and naproxen, in doses which significantly inhibited prostacyclin formation *ex vivo*, was also found to potentiate bile-salt induced damage (Whittle, 1983). The degree of gastric damage was significantly greater than that caused by bile-salt perfusion alone or by these agents during gastric perfusion of acid saline. In that study, doses of these agents inducing inhibition of cyclo-oxygenase greater than 75% potentiated taurocholate-induced damage, while in another study in the rat, doses of aspirin inhibiting prostanoid formation by 80% potentiated acidified bile salt mucosal injury (Ligumsky *et al.*, 1983). Mucosal damage produced by low concentrations of acidified ethanol in the lumen can also be substantially augmented by parenteral administration of indomethacin or aspirin (Whittle, 1984). Local tissue anoxia induced by cyclo-oxygenase inhibition, with its resulting alterations in mucosal cell metabolism, may underlie the increased susceptibility of the gastric tissue to necrosis.

In contrast, sodium salicylate or BW755C, which failed to inhibit mucosal prostacyclin synthesis also failed to potentiate gastric damage induced by acidified taurocholate (Whittle, 1983). In a study in which the actions of intravenously administered high doses of aspirin and salicylate were compared, both agents were observed to induce mucosal damage, but only in the presence of luminal acid (Rowe *et al.*, 1987). It was suggested that the failure to observe damage with salicylate in most other studies was the result of inhibition of acid secretion. However, such antisecretory actions could not account for the lack of potency of acidified salicylate when perfused through the gastric lumen (Fig. 18.3) or the failure of intravenous salicylate to potentiate damage induced by luminal perfusion with acidified bile salts (Whittle, 1983). Furthermore, it is difficult to reconcile the rapid hydrolysis of aspirin to salicylate following both oral or parenteral administration with such proposed differential effects on acid secretion between these two agents as a factor to explain their different propensities to induce mucosal damage. The mechanisms underlying the toxic action of parenteral salicylate in that study therefore requires clarification, but may reflect its inhibitory actions on other metabolic functions (Rowe *et al.*, 1987).

18.8.2 Potentiation of Salicylate-induced Damage

The protective responses of the gastric mucosa to topical irritation such as the local hyperaemia seen after challenge with taurocholate or acidfied salicylate (Whittle, 1977; Bruggerman *et al.*, 1979), could be offset by the concurrent inhibition of vasodilator prostanoid bio-synthesis. To investigate the interaction between the local irritancy of salicylate and the concurrent inhibition of cyclo-oxygenase by non-steroid anti-inflammatory agents, experiments were performed to evaluate the potentiation of gastric damage induced by oral administration of sodium salicylate by parenteral pretreatment with indomethacin or naproxen. The doses of these agents, injected subcutaneously, were sufficient to induce near-maximal inhibition of gastric mucosal cyclo-oxygenase, determined *ex vivo*, and themselves induced a low degree of macroscopically assessed mucosal injury when assessed after 3 h (Figs 18.5 and 18.6). These findings confirm that local mucosal contact by these agents is not necessarily required for the induction of erosion formation. However, the low degree of erosion formation observed 3 h after oral administration of sodium salicylate, which presumably reflects local irritation, was substantially potentiated in animals pretreated parenterally with the cyclo-oxygenase inhibitors (Figs 18.5 and 18.6). This pretreatment schedule to inhibit prostanoid formation prior to oral challenge was necessary since sodium salicylate can prevent these other non-steroid anti-inflammatory agents from inhibiting cyclo-oxygenase when administered concurrently (Ligumsky *et al.*, 1985).

The synergistic interaction of local and systemic actions of salicylates were further demonstrated by the use of parenteral aspirin. Thus, relatively low doses of aspirin, administered subcutaneously, which did not themselves induce macroscopic mucosal injury over the 3-h study period, dose-dependently potentiated the damage induced by oral sodium salicylate (Fig. 18.7). Thus, prior cyclo-oxygenase inhibition in the gastric mucosa confers the full ulcerogenic potential of aspirin on sodium salicylate following its oral administration.

18.8.3 Synergistic Interactions

The potency of anti-inflammatory agents for inducing gastric lesions could therefore depend on both their activity as barrier-breakers and as cyclo-oxygenase inhibitors, with both actions independently having the potential to lead to gastric damage, but interacting synergistically to provoke more extensive ulceration. Other factors such as the luminal pH and the molecular form of the compound would also be expected to influence the severity of the local mucosal injury. Relative to its anti-inflammatory dose, aspirin appears the more active of the more commonly used non-steroid anti-inflammatory agents in inducing gastric damage in both animals and man when administered orally (Pemberton and Strand, 1979; Whittle *et al.*, 1980; Rainsford and Willis, 1982). Since all of these compounds can inhibit cyclo-oxygenase to a comparable degree this could reflect the greater local irritancy of aspirin compared to the newer aspirin substitutes.

Mucosal lesions induced by aspirin have been shown to be potentiated by experimental stress, such as that induced by restraint or cold (Senay and Levin, 1967; Rainsford, 1975; Meeroff *et al.*, 1975). In a more recent study, it was concluded that the synergism between cold stress and aspirin resulted from the combined effects of increased acid secetion and reduced gastric mucosal blood flow in the mucosa, made vulnerable to damage following cyclo-oxygenase inhibition (Robert *et al.*, 1989). It has also been suggested that changes in gastric motility contribute to the mechanisms by which indomethacin induces mucosal erosions (Okada *et al.*, 1989).

Because of potentiating interactions between different mechanisms, it will therefore be apparent that any attempt to correlate the potential of such anti-inflammatory agents to induce gastric mucosal injury with either one of these parameters, or indeed any other single determinant, is unlikely to yield meaningful data. This may well explain the early apparent discrepancies in the overall relationship between inhibition of prostanoid biosynthesis with mucosal damage with some such agents, which may have led to the inappropriate underestimation by some investigators of the importance of cyclo-oxygenase inhibition as a fundamental mechanism contributing to the pathogenesis of gastric injury and ulceration (Rainsford, 1988; Szabo *et al.*, 1989).

18.9 THROMBOSIS AND HAEMOSTASIS IN THE STOMACH

Since aspirin and other cyclo-oxygenase inhibitors will inhibit platelet thromboxane formation, the possibility that inhibition of platelet aggregation by such agents could contribute to mucosal bleeding has

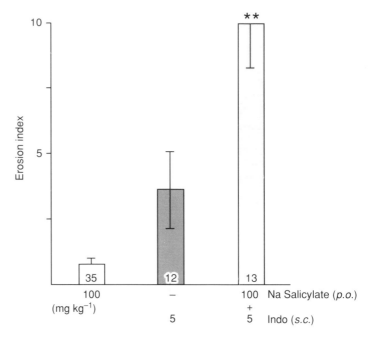

Figure 18.5 Potentiation of the low degree of gastric mucosal damage induced by oral administration of sodium salicylate (100 mg kg⁻¹) by prior (1 h) parenteral administration of indomethacin (5 mg kg⁻¹ s.c.) in the unanaesthetized rat. The mucosal injury, assessed 3 h after challenge with sodium salicylate, is shown in terms of an erosion index, that takes into account both the incidence and severity of the macroscopic haemorrhagic lesions, and is shown as the mean±s.e.mean of (*n*) experiments. The significance of the increase in damage from that induced by subcutaneous administration of indomethacin alone, is given by $**P<0.01$.

been considered. However, in studies utilizing *in vivo* microscopy, topically-applied acidified aspirin in a concentration that reduced blood flow in the superficial gastric microvessels of the rat, induced the appearance of white thrombi, probably platelet aggregates, and focal damage was subsequently observed (Kitahora and Guth, 1987). Using histological techniques others have likewise observed the appearance of subepithelial platelet thrombi in the mucosal microvasculature following aspirin challenge (Morris *et al.*, 1990).

In a study on bleeding time from a standard incision made in the gastric mucosa of rat, rabbit and dog, neither topical aspirin nor intravenous indomethacin augmented the rates of bleeding (Whittle *et al.*, 1986), as shown in Fig. 18.8. Other anti-platelet agents such as prostacyclin or thromboxane synthase inhibitors likewise had no effect on bleeding time, while heparin substantially prolonged bleeding. It

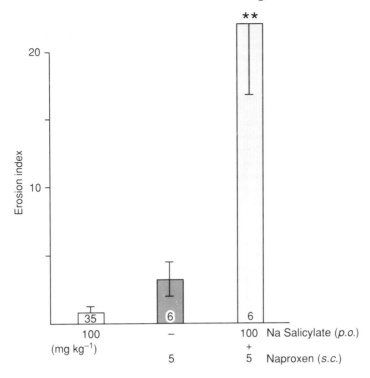

Figure 18.6 Potentiation of the low degree of gastric mucosal damage induced by oral administration of sodium salicylate (100 mg kg⁻¹) by prior (1 h) parenteral administration of naproxen (5 mg kg⁻¹ s.c.) in the unanaesthetized rat. The mucosal injury, assessed 3 h after challenge with sodium salicylate, is shown in terms of an erosion index, that takes into account both the incidence and severity of the macroscopic haemorrhagic lesions, and is shown as the mean ± s.e.mean of (n) experiments. The significance of the increase in damage from that induced by subcutaneous administration of naproxen alone, is given by **$P < 0.01$.

was concluded, in contrast to the skin and larger blood vessels, that the haemostatic mechanisms in the gastric mucosa were independent of platelet aggregation but involved the coagulation system (Whittle *et al.*, 1986).

These findings thus explain the clinical observations that acute or chronic administration of aspirin, in doses sufficient to prolong skin bleeding time, had no effect on bleeding from gastric biopsy sites in human volunteers (O'Laughlin *et al.*, 1981). Although inhibition of platelet aggregation by aspirin thus does not appear to enhance bleeding from such mucosal wounds, bleeding induced by low aspirin dosage (75 mg daily for 12 days) was not augmented by concurrent

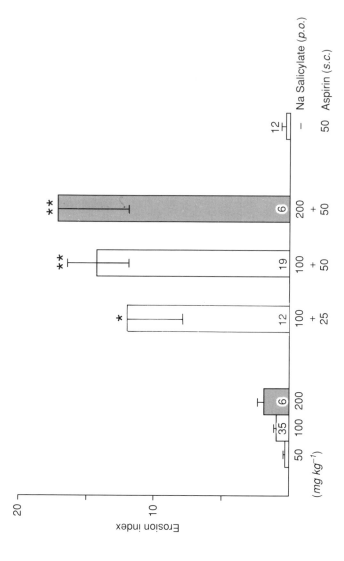

Figure 18.7 Potentiation of the low degree of gastric mucosal damage induced by oral adminstration of sodium salicylate (100–200 mg kg⁻¹) by prior parenteral administration of aspirin (25–50 mg kg⁻¹ s.c.), in doses not significantly inducing mucosal injury by this route. The mucosal injury, assessed 3 h after challenge in the unanaesthetized rat, is expressed in terms of an erosion index, which takes into account both the incidence and severity of the haemorrhagic lesions, and is shown as the mean ± s.e.mean of (n) experiments. Significant increases in mucosal damage compared to salicylate alone are shown as *$P<0.05$, **$P<0.01$.

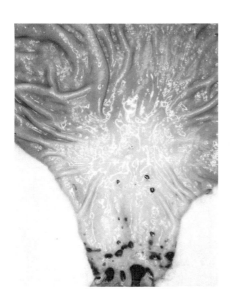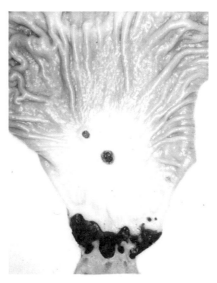

Figure 18.4 Induction of gastric ulceration in the antral region of the cat, 4 h following bolus intravenous injection of aspirin (40 mg kg^{-1}) in a dose causing 92±3% inhibition ($n=5$) of mucosal prostacyclin formation *ex vivo*. Near maximal rate of gastric acid secretion was induced by continuous intravenous infusion of histamine (160 µg kg^{-1} h^{-1}). Two examples of the macroscopic appearance of the stomachs are shown, that exhibit deep penetrating ulcers in the antral mucosa and extensive haemorrhagic injury at the gastro-duodenal junction. Overall, the macroscopically assessed area of antral damage was increased from the control (histamine alone) value of 1±0.8 mm^2 ($n=4$) to 91±34 mm^2 ($n=5$; $P<0.05$). (Data derived from the studies reported in Whittle *et al*, 1985a.)

administration of warfarin (Prichard *et al.*, 1989). The mechanisms of haemostasis that arrest bleeding from the gastric erosion sites induced by non-steroid anti-inflammatory drugs may thus require further elucidation.

18.10 EFFECTS ON MUCOSAL REPAIR AND ULCER HEALING

Following superficial mucosal injury, the process of restitution provides for the rapid repair of the surface cell continuity (Morris and Wallace, 1981; Morris and Harding, 1984; Svanes *et al.*, 1984; Silen and Ito, 1985). This re-epithelialization by rapid migration of cells along the intact basal lamina, which is accompanied by restoration of the transmucosal PD, is not affected by cyclo-oxygenase inhibition (Svanes *et al.*, 1984).

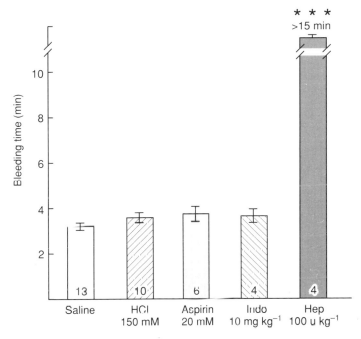

Figure 18.8 Effect of local application of acidified aspirin (20 mM) or acid (100 mM HCl), or the parenteral administration of indomethacin (10 mg kg⁻¹ i.v.) or heparin (100 units kg⁻¹ i.v.), on gastric mucosal haemostasis. Mucosal bleeding was induced in the chambered stomach of the pentobarbitone-anaesthetized rat by a 2 mm scalpel incision at a rugal fold. Bleeding time was estimated as the period for haemoglobin output to cease, as determined spectrophotometrically. Results, expressed as bleeding time (min) are the mean±s.e.mean of (*n*) studies, where significant prolongation of mucosal bleeding by heparin is shown as ***$P<0.001$. (Data are adapted from Whittle *et al.*, 1986.)

Unwanted effects

This process of restitution thus could account for the scarcity of epithelial damage that can be observed 30 min after exposure to aspirin in early studies (Hingson and Ito, 1971).

Repair of the more severe mucosal injury including deep haemorrhagic lesions and ulcers requires a protracted healing process involving cell division. In studies in the rat, non-steroid anti-inflammatory agents produced an initial decrease in cell proliferation in the gastric mucosa followed by an increase, as a consequence of exaggerated repair in response to the initial cell shedding (Eastwood and Quimby, 1982; Kuwayama and Eastwood, 1985; Baumgartner et al., 1986). In recent studies in man, the rate of mitosis in the gastric glands at the edge of ulcer sites was significantly lower in those patients that were taking non-steroid anti-inflammatory drugs (Levi et al., 1990).

Studies on experimental ulcers have also suggested that non-steroid anti-inflammatory agents can delay mucosal healing. Thus indomethacin could delay the healing of rat gastric ulcers induced by serosal injection of acetic acid or application of a cryoprobe (Szelenyi et al., 1980; Inauen et al., 1988; Levi et al., 1990). The size of the cryo-ulcer was greater in those animals receiving indomethacin (Inauen et al., 1988), while a reduction in proliferative zone and the number of mitotic cells at the ulcer edge could also be noted (Levi et al., 1990). Such effects may well contribute to the adverse effects of chronic ingestion of aspirin and its substitutes on the gastrointestinal tract and to the elevated relapse rates of patients with peptic ulcer receiving such drugs.

18.11 LIPOXYGENASE PRODUCTS, FREE RADICALS AND LIPID PEROXIDATION

Inhibition of cyclo-oxygenase by non-steroid anti-inflammatory drugs could theoretically lead to the metabolic diversion of the substrate, arachidonic acid, towards the formation of lipoxygenase products. Such a process would require the presence of lipoxygenase enzymes in the appropriate cells and tissues. One pro-inflammatory metabolite of the 5-lipoxygenase pathway, leukotriene C_4 (LTC_4) has been demonstrated to exert potent vasoconstrictor actions on the gastric submucosal microcirculation (Whittle et al., 1985b). Furthermore local infusion of LTC_4 can aggravate mucosal injury induced by local irritation, and histological examination has demonstrated extensive disruption of the microcirculation (Pihan et al., 1988). Although such findings implicate this leukotriene as a potential mediator of inflammatory damage of the mucosa (Whittle et al., 1985b), there is no experimental evidence to support the increased formation of 5-lipoxygenase products following cyclo-oxygenase inhibition (Peskar et al., 1988; Wallace et

492

al., 1990). Furthermore, although in early studies the non-selective lipoxygenase inhibitor BW755C reduced indomethacin-induced gastric damage (Wallace and Whittle, 1985), as did other inhibitors of 5-lipoxygenase (Rainsford, 1988), more recent studies with selective 5-lipoxygenase inhibitors failed to show such protection (Boughton-Smith and Whittle, 1988; Boughton-Smith, 1989). The possible involvement of other products of the 12- or 15-lipoxygenase enzymes, such as the hydroperoxy intermediates, in the mechanism of gastric mucosal injury has yet to be explored. Whether the elevation of such mediators in the intestinal mucosa following cyclo-oxygenase inhibition could contribute to the known damage and inflammation in the human small intestine (Bjarnason *et al.*, 1987 a,b) requires consideration.

The role of the local release of free radicals in the tissue damage induced by aspirin or indomethacin has also been considered. Thus, mucosal injury induced by such agents has been demonstrated to be reduced by a number of inorganic free-radical scavengers (Van Kolfsholten *et al.*, 1984; Rainsford, 1984; Pihan *et al.*, 1987), as well as by systemic infusion of superoxide dismutase and catalase (Pihan *et al.*, 1987). The potential cellular source of this putative release of free radicals during tissue damage has not yet been determined. However, neutrophils release free radicals on activation, and have been implicated in the mechanisms underlying oxidant damage following ischaemia–reperfusion in the gastric mucosa (Smith *et al.*, 1987). Indeed, depletion of circulating neutrophils has recently been shown also to reduce mucosal damage injury induced by indomethacin or naproxen (Wallace *et al.*, 1990).

Lipid peroxidation of cell membrane constituents is considered one primary event in the process of cellular disruption by free radicals. However, elevated mucosal formation of lipid peroxides following acute aspirin challenge in the rat could not be detected (Pihan *et al.*, 1987). The involvement of free radical formation as a primary event in the mucosal injury seen with these agents is therefore not clear and the mechanisms by which anti-oxidants may protect the mucosa from injury needs careful evaluation.

18.12 EFFECTS ON THE INTESTINE

18.12.1 Animal Studies

Although the actions of aspirin and related compounds on the gastric or duodenal mucosa have been more extensively studied and reported, such agents are also well known to cause or promote damage in the small and large intestine. In rats, indomethacin induces the chronic development of lesions in the jejunum and ileum after 1–3 days of acute or chronic administration, leading to extensive inflammation and eventual intestinal perforation and death (Kent *et al.*, 1969; Brodie *et al.*, 1970a; Robert, 1975; Fang *et al.*, 1977; Whittle, 1981). Bacterial invasion from the lumen appears to be involved in the eventual process of tissue damage (Robert, 1975; Fang *et al.*, 1977) which may be aided by a reduction in prostanoid biosynthesis. Aspirin, in doses sufficient to cause a comparable degree of cyclo-oxygenase inhibition, however, does not cause a similar enteropathy, although some macroscopic damage to the rat intestine following aspirin has been recorded in an early study (Brodie *et al.*, 1970b). Thus, other factors including enterohepatic recirculation of indomethacin and similar agents may interact to bring about this enteropathy.

18.12.2 Human Studies

Acute administration of aspirin suspension rapidly produces erythrocyte extrusion and focal erosion of the jejunal villi as determined by electron microscopy (Ivey *et al.*, 1979). Chronic ingestion of non-steroid anti-inflammatory agents has also been associated with damage to the small intestinal mucosa. Thus, oral ingestion of aspirin, ibuprofen or indomethacin by healthy volunteers increased the permeability of the small intestine to radiolabelled markers (Bjarnason *et al.*, 1986). This effect was also observed after rectal administration of these agents, indicating that this was a systemic action and not just a reflection of any local irritation. Moreover, in studies on patients receiving non-steroid anti-inflammatory drugs for the treatment of rheumatoid arthritis or osteoarthritis, over 60% exhibited blood and protein loss with demonstrable inflammation of the small intestine (Bjarnason *et al.*, 1987 a,b). The degree of mucosal inflammation was milder than that observed in patients with Crohn's ileitis, although the radiologically detected abnormalities in the ileum suggest that ulceration and structures could ultimately develop on chronic administration of these agents (Bjarnason *et al.*, 1987a).

There have been some reports that non-steroid anti-inflammatory agents can induce damage to the colon (Rampton, 1987). However, the deleterious effects of these agents on the bowel have usually been associated with relapse in patients with inflammatory bowel disease, particularly those with ulcerative colitis (Rampton and Sladen, 1981; Kauffman and Taubin, 1987; Rampton *et al.*, 1983; Rampton, 1987). Such an induction of relapse could reflect the removal of protective prostaglandins in the colon or the diversion of substrate arachidonic acid towards the pro-inflammatory lipoxygenase products such as LTB_4 and LTC_4.

18.13 CONCLUSIONS

Over the past half decade, convincing evidence has accumulated from epidemiological studies and direct clinical trials to confirm that chronic use of aspirin and the other non-steroid anti-inflammatory agents gives rise to serious toxic actions in the gastro-intestinal tract including haemorrhage and ulcers in a large proportion of the patient population, particularly the elderly. These recent advances in clinical knowledge and recognition of the substantial problems associated with such compounds has not been matched by a significant change in our understanding of the basic mechanisms underlying these damaging actions.

The major insight into the mechanisms by which these agents can induce local irritancy in the stomach and duodenum has come from the original proposals of Davenport and his collegues in the mid-1960s and the early studies on ion flux, salicylate uptake and local metabolic actions. These concepts have not been greatly modified or advanced since that time. The more recent identification of the importance of the mucus, bicarbonate and phospholipid lining of the mucosa as luminal protective factors has, however, allowed further speculation as to the nature of the deleterious actions of aspirin and the other agents on the resistance of the mucosa to acid, pepsin and chemical attack.

The mechanisms by which these anti-inflammatory agents can provoke and enhance gastrointestinal damage following parenteral administration is likely to involve cyclo-oxygenase inhibition, although there have been experimental pointers to implicate other, as yet undefined processes, in such injury. The role of prostaglandin depletion in gastrointestinal damage has attracted much support, as well as some criticism. Failure to correlate cyclo-oxygenase inhibition directly with mucosal injury has been taken by some as evidence that the effects on prostaglandin biosynthesis have no involvement in the gastrointestinal damage. However such interpretation is probably inappropriate since it is unlikely that the effects of these agents on any one parameter could underlie such a complex pathology, as has been previously pointed out (Whittle et al., 1980; Whittle and Vane, 1984). Given the wide spectrum of potentially protective pharmacological actions that prostanoids can exert on the gastrointestinal tract, it would seem somewhat unlikely that inhibition of their endogenous formation would be without any effect on mucosal function or tissue integrity. Moreover, most experimental

495

studies suggest that cyclo-oxygenase inhibition can make the mucosa considerably more susceptible to challenge by a wide variety of topical irritants including salicylates, and to the damaging actions of systemic pro-ulcerogenic agents.

Strong support for the involvement of endogenous prostanoids in the modulation of mucosal integrity comes from studies using specific antibodies directed towards the protective prostaglandins PGE_2 or prostacyclin. Thus, in the dog, active immunization with a PGE_2-conjugate induced endoscopic evidence of gastric and duodenal erosions, and in one case a deep penetrating ulcer was observed (Redfern et al., 1987b). Likewise, active immunization with prostaglandin conjugates in the rabbit induced both acute and chronic gastric ulcers, and the damage was considered to resemble the acute gastric lesions in humans induced by non-steroid anti-inflammatory drugs (Redfern and Feldman, 1989). Such immunization against endogenous prostanoids also led to the chronic development of lesions in the rabbit small intestine. Furthermore, passive sensitization of rabbits by administration of PGE_2-hyperimmune rabbit plasma also led to the development of gastric ulcers. These observations indicate that the induction of mucosal damage was likely to be the consequence of binding of the specific antibodies with their endogenous ligand to prevent the physiological actions of these prostanoids (Redfern and Feldman, 1989).

The comparable findings with prostaglandin neutralizing antibodies and cyclo-oxygenase inhibitors thus support the contention that inhibition of the activity of endogenous prostanoids in the gastric mucosa can lead to damage and ulceration. However, it is very clear that cyclo-oxygenase inhibition may not always induce gastrointestinal damage, and that mucosal injury does not have to involve inhibition of prostanoid biosynthesis.

Recent studies have suggested that prostaglandins act in concert with other endogenous protective mediators in the gastric mucosa. Thus, prevention of the release of sensory local neuropeptides from primary afferent neurones located in the submucosa in association with microvessels, augments the damage induced by indomethacin (Holzer and Sametz, 1986; Whittle et al., 1990). Furthermore, recent studies have shown that inhibition of the biosynthesis of the endothelium-derived vasodilator, nitric oxide, also augments mucosal damage induced by indomethacin, which is further potentiated by depletion of sensory neuropeptides (Whittle et al., 1990). Thus, endogenous prostaglandins interact with these other mediators in the regulation of mucosal integrity, while concurrent suppression of these vasoactive mediators potentiates the mucosal damage following cyclo-oxygenase inhibition. Under disease conditions where interference with the biosynthesis or actions of sensory neuropeptides or nitric oxide could occur, non-steroid anti-inflammatory drugs would therefore be anticipated to be far more injurious to the gastrointestinal mucosa.

The unifying hypothesis of the synergistic interactions between local irritation and cyclo-oxygenase inhibition attempts to provide a coherent explanation for the primary events in mucosal injury, leading to the multitude of subsequent events that characterize the damage induced by these anti-inflammatory agents. There will no doubt be specific experimental conditions that will argue against the universal applicability of the concept, and it is likely that it represents an over-simplification of the actual mechanisms involved. It would be therefore unwise to propose that all forms of mucosal damage induced by non-steroid anti-inflammatory agents result either from topical irritation with its attendant acid back-diffusion, intramucosal acidification and metabolic changes, or from the sequelae of events following inhibition of cyclo-oxygenase, or a combination of both. Indeed, the permissive or obligatory role of the neutrophil in such injury (Wallace et al., 1990) perhaps interacting with the vascular endothelium and its locally-released mediators such as nitric oxide, will need to be clarified However, such a concept does provide a working model on which to base the rational development of better-tolerated anti-inflammatory drugs. These newer compounds should lack topical irritancy, which may be achieved by the development of a basic compound rather than one of the more usual acidic nature, or by esterification and other molecular modifications, or by appropriate formulation procedures. The compounds may inhibit the metabolism of arachidonate either by the cyclo-oxygenase and lipoxygenase enzymes at the site of inflammation and in inflammatory cells, but should not prevent prostanoid biosynthesis by gastrointestinal tissue, or indeed reduce the activity of the other protective mediators in the mucosa, either directly or indirectly.

As discussed earlier, experimental compounds conforming to such specifications do indeed show a reduced potential for inducing gastric damage. Thus, detailed structure–activity studies with anti-inflammatory compounds, in which both these major injurious processes have been reduced or eliminated, will be useful in revealing any further tissue damaging and pro-ulcerogenic components not yet characterized. This should allow the design of molecules that do not exhibit the usual gastrointestinal side effects associated with agents for the treatment of the inflammatory process. The need for superior and safer anti-inflammatory drugs is emphasized by the failure of gastric anti-secretory agents such as the histamine H_2-receptor antagonists or locally acting anti-ulcer agents such as sucralfate to be effective in the

Unwanted effects

clinical control of such gastric mucosal damage. In a recent study however, involving 420 osteo-arthritic patients receiving either ibuprofen, piroxicam or naproxen daily for 3 months, the high incidence (22%) of gastric ulcer was significantly reduced by co-administration of the prostaglandin analogue, misoprostol (Graham *et al.*, 1988). It could be argued though, that prevention of drug-induced toxicity is better than its subsequent cure, both in terms of benefit to the patient and eventual cost. Thus, a greater understanding of the relative importance of the analgesic and the anti-inflammatory properties to the perceived therapeutic value of this class of drug, coupled with further fundamental knowledge of the interactions between the mediators and mechanisms of inflammation, should allow for the identification of more effective and safer drugs for both acute and chronic use in the clinic.

REFERENCES

Allen, A. and Garner, A. (1980) Mucus and bicarbonate secretion in the stomach and their possible role in mucosal protection. *Gut*, **21**, 249–62.

Anderson, S. and Grossman, M.I. (1965) Profile of pH, pressure and potential difference at gastroduodenal junction in man. *Gastroenterology*, **49**, 364–71.

Armstrong, C.P. and Blower, A.L. (1987) Non-steroidal anti-inflammatory drugs and life-threatening complications of peptic ulceration. *Gut*, **28**, 527–32.

Ashley, S.W., Sonnenschein, L.A. and Cheung, L.Y. (1985) Focal gastric mucosal blood flow at the site of aspirin-induced ulceration. *Am. J. Surg.*, **149**, 53–9.

Barrier, C.H. and Hirschowitz, B.I. (1989) Controversies in the detection and management of nonsteroidal antiinflammatory drug-induced side effects of the upper gastrointestinal tract. *Arthritis Rheum*, **32**, 926–32.

Baumgartner, A., Koelz, H.R. and Halter, F. (1986) Indomethacin and turnover of gastric mucosal cells in the rat. *Am. J. Physiol.*, **250**, G830–5.

Biour, M., Balnquart, A., Moore, N. *et al.* (1987) Incidence of NSAID-related, severe gastrointestinal bleeding. *Lancet*, **ii**, 340–1.

Bjarnason, I., Williams, P., Smethurst, P. *et al.* (1986) Effect of non-steroidal anti-inflammatory drugs and prostaglandins on the permeability of the human small intestine. *Gut*, **27**, 1292–7.

Bjarnason, I., Prouse, P., Smith, T. *et al.* (1987a) Blood and protein loss via small-intestinal inflammation induced by non-steroidal anti-inflammatory drugs. *Lancet*, **ii**, 711–14.

Bjarnason, I., Zanelli, G., Smith, T. *et al.* (1987b) Nonsteroidal anti-inflammatory drug-induced intestinal inflammation in humans. *Gastroenterology*, **93**, 480–9.

Bowen, B.K., Krause, W.J. and Ivey, K.J. (1977) Effect of sodium bicarbonate on aspirin-induced damage and potential difference changes in human gastric mucosa. *Brit. Med. J.*, **2**, 1052–5.

Boughton-Smith, N.K. (1989) Involvement of leukotrienes in acute gastric damage. *Meth. Find. Exp. Clin. Pharmacol.*, **11** (suppl.), 53–9.

Boughton-Smith, N.K. and Whittle, B. J. R. (1983) Stimulation and inhibition of prostacyclin formation in the gastric mucosa and ileum *in vitro* by anti-inflammatory agents. *Brit. J. Pharmacol.*, **78**, 173–80.

Boughton-Smith, N.K. and Whittle, B.J.R. (1988) The role of leukotrienes in the pathogenesis of gastric ulceration. *Pharmacol. Res. Comm.*, **20**, 919–34.

Brodie, D.A. and Hooke, K.F. (1971) Effects of route of administration on the production of gastric hemorrhage in the rat by aspirin and sodium salicylate. *Am. J. Dig. Dis.*, **16**, 985–9.

Brodie, D.A., Cook, P.G. and Bauer, B.J. (1970a) Indomethacin-induced intestinal lesions in the rat. *Toxicol. Appl. Pharmac.*, **17**, 615–24.

Brodie, D.A., Tate, C.L. and Hooke, K.F. (1970b) Aspirin: intestinal damage in rats. *Science*, **170**, 183–5.

Bruggeman, T.M., Wood, J.G. and Davenport, H.W. (1979) Local control of blood flow in the dog's stomach: Vasodilatation caused by acid back-diffusion following topical application of salicylic acid. *Gastroenterology*, **77**, 736–44.

Brune, K., Schwietzer, A. and Eckert, H. (1977) Parietal cells of the stomach trap salicylates during absorption, *Biochem. Pharmacol.*, **26**, 1735–40.

Bugat, R., Thompson, M.R., Aures, D. and Grossman, M.I. (1976) Gastric mucosal lesions produced by intravenous infusion of aspirin in cats. *Gastroenterology*, **71**, 754–9.

Caruso, I. and Bianchi-Porro, G. (1980) Gastroscopic evaluation of anti-inflammatory agents. *Brit. Med. J.*, **280**, 75–8.

Chaudhury, T.K. and Jacobson, E.D. (1978) Prostaglandin cytoprotection of gastric mucosa. *Gastroenterology*, **74**, 58–63.

Chvasta, T.E. and Cooke, A.R. (1972) The effect of several ulcerogenic drugs on the canine gastric mucosal barrier. *J. Lab. Clin. Med.*, **79**, 302–15.

Clinch, D., Banerjee, A.K., Levy, D.W. *et al.* (1987) Non-steroidal anti-inflammatory drugs and peptic ulceration. *J. R. Coll. Physicians Lond.*, **21**, 183–7.

Cochrane, K.M., Mackenzie, J.F. and Russell, R.I. (1975) Role of taurocholic acid in production of gastric mucosal damage after ingestion of aspirin. *Brit. Med. J.*, **1**, 183–5.

Cohen, M.M and MacDonald, W.C. (1982) Mechanism of aspirin injury to the human gastroduodenal mucosa. *Prost. Leuk Med.*, **9**, 241–55.

Collier, D.S. and Pain, J.A. (1985) Nonsteroidal anti-inflammatory drugs and peptic ulcer perforation. *Gut*, **26**, 359–63.

Davenport, H.W. (1964) Gastric mucosal injury by fatty and acetylsalicylic acids. *Gastroenterology*, **16**, 245–53.

Davenport, H.W. (1965) Damage to the gastric mucosa: Effects of salicylates and stimulation. *Gastroenterology*, **49**, 184–96.

Davenport, H.W. (1966) Fluid production by the gastric mucosa during damage by acetic and salicylic acids. *Gastroenterology*, **50**, 487–99.

Davenport, H.W., Warner, H.A. and Code, C.F. (1964) Functional significance of gastric mucosal barrier to sodium. *Gastroenterology*, **457**, 142–51.

Djahanguiri, B., Abtahi, F.S. and Hemmati, M. (1973) Prevention of aspirin-induced gastric ulceration by bile-duct or pylorus ligation in the rat. *Gastroenterology*, **65**, 630–3.

Domschke, S. and Domschke, W. (1984) Gastroduodenal damage due to drugs, alcohol and smoking. *Clinics Gastroenterol.*, **13**, 405–36.

Douthwaite, A.H. and Lintott, G.M. (1935) Gastroscopic observation of the effect of aspirin and certain other substances on the stomach. *Lancet*, **ii**, 1222–5.

Duane, W.C., Wiegand, D.M. and Sievert, C.E. (1982) Bile acid and bile salt disrupt gastric mucosal barrier in the dog by different mechanisms. *Am. J. Physiol.*, **242**, G95–9.

Duggan, J.A. (1972) Aspirin ingestion and perforated peptic ulcer. *Gut*, **13**, 631–3.

Duggan, J.M., Dobson, A.J., Johnson, H. and Fahey, P. (1986) Peptic ulcer and non-steroidal anti-inflammatory agents. *Gut*, **27**, 929–33.

Eastwood, G.L. and Erdmann, K.R. (1978) Effect of ethanol on canine gastric epithelial ultrastructure and transmucosal potential difference. *Dig. Dis. Sci.*, **23**, 429–35.

Eastwood, G.L. and Quimby, G.F. (1982) Effect of chronic aspirin ingestion on epithelial proliferation in rat fundus, antrum and duodenum. *Gastroenterology*, **82**, 852–6.

Fang, W.F., Broughton, A. and Jacobson, E.D. (1977) Indomethacin-induced intestinal inflammation. *Am. J. Dig. Dis.*, **22**, 749–60.

Faulkner, G., Prichard, P., Sommerville, K. and Langman, M.J.S. (1988) Aspirin and bleeding peptic ulcers in the elderly. *Brit. Med. J.*, **297**, 1311–13.

Fitzpatrick, F.A. and Wynalda, M.A. (1976) *In vivo* suppression of prostaglandin biosynthesis by non-steroidal anti-inflammatory agents. *Prostaglandins*, **12**, 1037–51.

Flemstrom, G. (1981) Gastric secretion of bicarbonate. In *Physiology of the Gastrointestinal Tract* (ed. L.R. Johnson), Raven Press, New York, pp. 603–16.

Flemstrom, G. (1986). Gastroduodenal mucosal secretion of bicarbonate and mucus: Physiological control and stimulation by prostaglandins. *Am. J. Med.*, **81**, 18–22.

Flemstrom, G. and Marsden, N.V.B. (1974) Increased inulin absorption from the cat stomach exposed to acetyl-salicyclic acid. *Acta Physiol. Scand.*, **92**, 517–25.

Flower, R.J. (1974) Drugs which inhibit prostaglandin biosynthesis. *Pharmacol. Rev.*, **26**, 33–67.

Fries, J.F., Miller, S.R., Spitz, P.W. *et al.* (1989) Toward an epidemiology of gastropathy associated with nonsteroidal antiinflammatory drug use. *Gastroenterology*, **96**, 647–55.

Fuhro, R. and Fromm, D. (1978) Effects on compounds chemically related to salicylate on isolated antral mucosa of rabbits. *Gastroenterology*, **75**, 661–7.

Garner, A. (1977) Effects of acetylsalicylate on alkalization, acid secretion and electrogenic properties in isolated gastric mucosa. *Acta Physiol. Scand.*, **99**, 281–91.

Garner, A. (1978) Mechanisms of action of aspirin on the gastric mucosa of the guinea-pig. *Acta. Physiol. Scand (suppl.).*, *Gastro. Ion. Transp.*, 101–10.

Garner, A., Flemstrom, G. and Heyling, J.R. (1979) Effects of antiinflammatory agents and prostaglandins on acid and bicarbonate secretions in the amphibian-isolated gastric mucosa. *Gastroenterology*, **77**, 451–7.

Geall, M.G., Phillips, S.F. and Summerskill, D.M. (1970) Profile of gastric potential difference in man – effects of aspirin, alcohol, bile and endogenous acid. *Gastroenterology*, **38**, 437–43.

Gerkens, J.F., Shand, D.G., Flexner, C. *et al.* (1977) Effect of indomethacin and aspirin on gastric blood flow and acid secretion. *J. Pharmacol. Exp. Ther.*, **203**, 646–52.

Glarborg-Jorgensen, T., Weis-Fogh, U.S., Neilsen, H.H. and Olsen, H.P. (1976) Salicylate- and aspirin-induced uncoupling of oxidative phosphorylation in mitochondria isolated from the mucosal membrane of the stomach. *Scand. J. Clin. Lab. Invest.*, **36**, 649–53.

Goddard, P.J., Kao, Y.J. and Lightenberger, L.M. (1990) Luminal surface hydrophobicity of canine gastric mucosa is dependent on a surface mucous gel. *Gastroenterology* **98**, 361–70.

Graham, D., Agrawal, N. and Roth, S. (1988) Prevention of NSAID-induced gastric ulcer with the synthetic prostaglandin, misoprostol: a multicentre, double-blind, placebo-controlled trial. *Lancet*, **ii**, 1277–80.

Griffin, M.R., Ray, W.A. and Schaffner, W. (1988) Nonsteroidal anti-inflammatory drug use and death from peptic ulcer in elderly persons. *Ann. Intern. Med.*, **109**, 359–63.

Grossman, M.I., Matsumota, K.K. and Lichter, R.J. (1961) Fecal blood loss by oral and intravenous administration of various salicylates. *Gastroenterology*, **40**, 383–8.

Guth, P.H. and Moler, T.L. (1982) The role of endogenous prostanoids in the response of the rat gastric microcirculation to vasoactive agents. *Microvasc. Res.*, **25**, 336–42.

Hamza, K.N. and Den Besten, K. (1972) Bile salts producing stress ulcers during experimental shock. *Surgery*, **71**, 161–7.

Hansen, D., Aures, D. and Grossman, M.I. (1980) Comparison of intravenous and intragastric aspirin in production of antral gastric ulcers in the cat. *Proc. Soc. Exp. Biol. Med.*, **164**, 589–92.

Hawkey, C.J. and Rampton, D.S. (1985) Prostaglandins and the gastro-intestinal mucosa: are they important in its function, disease or treatment? *Gastroenterology*, **89**, 1162–8.

Hierton, C. (1981) Effects of indomethacin, naproxen and paracetamol on regional blood flow in rabbits: a microsphere study. *Acta Pharmacol. Toxicol.*, **49**, 327–33.

Himal, H.S., Greenberg, L., Boutros M.I.R. and Waldon-Edward, D. (1975) Effect of aspirin on ionic movement and acid hydrolase activity of explants of canine antral and duodenal mucosae. *Gastroenterology*, **69**, 439–47.

Hingson, D.J. and Ito, S. (1971) Effect of aspirin and related compounds on the fine structure of mouse gastric mucosa. *Gastroenterology*, **61**, 156–77.

Hoftiezer, J.W., Silvoso, G.K., Burks, M. and Ivey, K.J. (1980) Comparison of the effects of regular and enteric-coated aspirin in gastro-duodenal mucosa of man. *Lancet*, **ii**, 609–12.

Holzer, P. and Sametz, W. (1986) Gastric mucosal protection against ulcerogenic factors in the rat mediated by capsicin-sensitive afferent neurones. *Gastroenterology*, **91**, 975–81.

Inauen, W., Wyss, P.A., Kayser, S. *et al.* (1988) Influence of prostaglandins, omprazole, and indomethacin on healing of experimental gastric ulcers in the rat. *Gastroenterology*, **95**, 636–41.

Isenberg, J.I., Smedfors, B. and Johansson, C. (1985) Effect of graded doses of intraluminal H^+, prostaglandin E_2, and inhibition of endogenous prostaglandin synthesis on proximal duodenal bicarbonate secretion in unanesthetized rat. *Gastroenterology*, **88**, 303–7.

Ivey, K.J., Baskin, W.N., Krause, W.J. and Terry, B. (1979) Effect of aspirin and acid on human jejunal mucosa. An ultrastructural study. *Gastroenterology*, **76**, 50–6.

Ivey, K.J., Poane, D.B. and Krause, W.J. (1980) Acute effect of systemic aspirin on gastric mucosa in man. *Dig. Dis. Sci.*, **25**, 97–9.

Jeremy, J.Y., Mikhailidis, D.P. and Dandona, P. (1985) The effect of tiaprofenic acid and indomethacin on in vitro prostaglandin synthesis by rat, rabbit and human stomach tissue. *Agents Actions* **17**, 205–8.

Kasbekar, D.K. (1973) Effects of salicylate and related compounds in gastric HCl secretion. *Am. J. Physiol.*, **225**, 521–7.

Kauffman, G.L. Jr and Grossman, M.I. (1978) Prostaglandin and cimetidine inhibit the formation of ulcers produced by parenteral salicylates. *Gastroenterology*, **75**, 1099–102.

Kauffman, G.L., Aures, D. and Grossman, M.I. (1980) Intravenous indomethacin and aspirin reduce basal gastric mucosal blood flow in dogs. *Am. J. Physiol.*, **238**, G131–4.

Kauffman, H.J. and Taubin, H.L. (1987) Nonsteroidal anti-inflammatory drugs activate quiescent inflammatory bowel disease. *Ann. Intern. Med.*, **107**, 513–16.

Kent, T.H., Cardelli, R.M. and Stamler, F.W. (1969) Small intestinal ulcers and intestinal flora in rats given indomethacin. *Am. J. Pathol.*, **54**, 237–49.

Kitahora, T. and Guth, P.H. (1987) Effect of aspirin plus hydrochloric acid on the gastric mucosal microcirculation. *Gastroenterology*, **93**, 810–17.

Kitchingman, G.K., Prichard, P.J., Daneshmend, T.K. *et al.* (1989) Enhanced gastric mucosal bleeding with doses of aspirin used for prophylaxis and its reduction by ranitidine. *Brit. J. Clin. Pharmac.*, **28**, 581–5.

Kivilaakso, E., Fromm, D. and Silen, W. (1978) Relationship between ulceration and intramural pH of gastric mucosa during hemorrhagic shock. *Surgery*, **94**, 70–8.

Kobayashi, K., Arakawa, T., Satoh, H. *et al.* (1985) Effect of indomethacin, tiaprofenic acid and diclofenac on rat gastric mucosal damage and content of prostacyclin and prostaglandin E_2. *Prostaglandins*, **30**, 609–18.

Koelz, H.R., Fischet, J.A., Sachs, G. and Blum, A.L. (1978) Specific effect of acetylsalicylic acid on cation transport of isolated gastric mucosal cells. *Am. J. Physiol.*, **235**, E16–21.

Kolbasa, K.P., Lancaster, C., Olafsson, A.S. *et al.* (1988) Indomethacin-induced gastric antral ulcers in hamsters. *Gastroenterology*, **95**, 932–44.

Konturek, S.J., Obtulowicz, W., Sito, E. *et al.* (1981a) Distribution of prostaglandins in gastric and duodenal mucosa of healthy subjects and duodenal ulcer patients: effects of aspirin and paracetamol. *Gut*, **22**, 283–9.

Konturek, S.J., Piastlucki, I., Brzozowski, T. *et al.* (1981b) Role of prostaglandins in the formation of aspirin-induced gastric ulcers. *Gastroenterology*, **80**, 4–9.

Kuo, Y.-J. and Shanbour, L.L. (1976) Mechanism of action of aspirin on canine gastric mucosa. *Am. J. Physiol.*, **230**, 762–7.

Kuwayama, H. and Eastwood, G.L. (1985) Effects of water immersion, restraint, stress and chronic indomethacin ingestion on gastric antral and fundic epithelial proliferation. *Gastroenterology*, **88**, 362–5.

Lacy, E.R. and Ito, S. (1982) Microscopic analysis of ethanol damage to rat gastric mucosa after treatment with a prostaglandin. *Gastroenterology*, **83**, 619–25.

Langman, M.J.S. (1989) Epidemiologic evidence on the association between peptic ulceration and anti-inflammatory drug use. *Gastroenterology*, **96**, 640–6.

Lanza, F.L. (1984) Endoscopic studies of gastric and duodenal injury after the use of ibuprofen, aspirin, and other nonsteroidal anti-inflammatory agents. *Am. J. Med.*, **77**, 19–24.

Lanza, F.L. (1989) A review of gastric ulcer and gastroduodenal injury in normal volunteers receiving aspirin and other non-steroidal anti-inflammatory drugs. *Scand. J. Gastroenterol.*, **24** (suppl. 63), 24–31.

Lanza, F.L., Royer, G.L., Nelson, R.S. *et al.* (1979) The effects of ibuprofen, indomethacin, aspirin, naproxen and placebo on the gastric mucosa of normal volunteers – a gastroscopic and photographic study. *Dig. Dis. Sci.*, **24**, 823–8.

Lanza, F.L., Royer, G.R. and Nelson, A.S. (1980) Endoscopic evaluation of the effects of aspirin, buffered aspirin, and enteric coated aspirin on gastric and duodenal mucosa. *N. Engl. J. Med.*, **303**, 136–8.

Leonards, J.R. and Levy, G. (1973) Gastrointestinal blood loss from aspirin and sodium salicylate tablets in man. *Clin. Pharmacol. Ther.*, **14**, 62–6.

Levi, S., Goodlad, R.A., Lee, C.Y. *et al.* (1990) Inhibitory effect of non-steroidal anti-inflammatory drugs on mucosal cell proliferation associated with gastric ulcer healing. *Lancet*, **336**, 840–3.

Levine, R.A., Petokas, S., Nandi, J. and Enthoven, D. (1988) Effects of nonsteroidal, anti-inflammatory drugs on gastrointestinal injury and prostanoid generation in healthy volunteers. *Dig. Dis. Sci.*, **33**, 660–6.

Levy, M. (1974) Aspirin use in patients with major upper gastrointestinal bleeding and peptic ulcer disease. *N. Engl. J. Med.*, **290**, 1158–62.

Lewi, H.J. and Carter, D.C. (1981) Intravenous prostaglandin synthetase inhibitors potentiate the effect of topical taurocholate on transmucosal ion flux. In *Gastrointestinal Mucosal Blood Flow* (ed. L.P. Fielding), Churchill Livingstone, London, pp. 192–201.

Lichtenberger, L.M., Richards, J.E. and Hills, B.A. (1985) Effect of 16, 16-dimethyl prostaglandin E$_2$ on the surface hydrophobicity of aspirin-treated canine gastric mucosa. *Gastroenterology*, **88**, 308–14.

Ligumsky, M., Grossman, M.I. and Kauffman, G.L. (1982) Endogenous gastric mucosal prostaglandins: their role in mucosal integrity. *Am. J. Physiol*, **242**, G337–41.

Ligumsky, M., Golanska, E.M. Hansen, D.G. and Kauffman, G.L. (1983) Aspirin can inhibit gastric mucosal cyclo-oxygenase without causing lesions in the rat. *Gastroenterology*, **84**, 756–61.

Ligumsky, M., Guth, P.J., Elashoff, J. *et al.* (1985) Salicylic acid blocks indomethacin-induced cyclo-oxygenase inhibition and lesion formation in rat gastric mucosa. *Proc. Soc. Exp. Biol. Med.*, **178**, 250–3.

Main, I.H.M. and Whittle, B.J.R. (1975) Investigation of the vasodilator and antisecretory role of prostaglandins in the rat gastric mucosa by use of non-steroidal anti-inflammatory drugs. *Brit. J. Pharmcol.*, **53**, 217–24.

Unwanted effects

Mangla, J.C., Kim, Y.M. and Turner, M.D. (1974) Are pepsinogens activated in gastric mucosa after aspirin-induced injury? *Experientia*, **30**, 727–9.

Martin, B. (1963) Accumulation of drug anions in gastric mucosal cells. *Nature (London)*, **198**, 896–7.

Meeroff, J.C., Paulsen, G. and Guth, P.H. (1975) Parenteral aspirin produces and enhances gastric mucosal lesions and bleeding in rats. *Am. J. Dig. Dis.*, **20**, 847–52.

Melarange, R. and Rashbrook, L.C. (1986) A rat gastric mucosal preparation for studying agents which affect the *in vitro* production of prostanoids. *Prostagland. Leuko. Med.*, **22**, 89–100.

Menguy, R. and Masters, Y.F. (1965) Effects of aspirin on gastric mucus secretion. *Surg. Gynec. and Obstet.*, **120**, 92–8.

Mersereau, W.A. and Hinchey, E.J. (1978) Interactions of gastric blood flow, barrier breaker, and hydrogen ion back diffusion during ulcer formation in the rat. *Surgery*, **83**, 248–51.

Meyer, R.A., McGinley, D. and Posalaky, Z. (1986) Effects of aspirin on tight junction structure of the canine gastric mucosa. *Gastroenterology*, **91**, 351–9.

Miller, T.A. (1983) Protective effects of prostaglandins against gastric mucosal damage: Current knowledge and proposed mechanisms. *Am. J. Physiol.*, **245**, G601–23.

Morris, G.P. and Wallace, J.L. (1981) The roles of ethanol and of acid in the production of gastric mucosal erosions in rats. *Virchows Arch. [Cell Pathol.]*, **38**, 23–38.

Morris, G.P. and Harding, P.L. (1984) Mechanisms of mucosal recovery from acute gastric damage: the roles of extracellular mucus and cell migration. In *Mechanisms of Mucosal Protection in the Upper Gastrointestinal Tract* (eds A. Allen, G. Flemstrom, A. Garner, W. Silen and L.A. Turnberg), Raven Press, New York, pp. 209–14.

Morris, G.P., Wallace, J.L., Harding, P.L. *et al.* (1984) Correlations between changes in indicators of gastric mucosal barrier integrity at time of exposure to 'barrier breakers' and extent of hemorrhagic erosions one hour later. *Dig. Dis. Sci.*, **29**, 6–11.

Morris, G.P., Williamson, T.E. and Hynna, T.T. (1990) Prostaglandins and mucosal defensive mechanisms. *Can. J. Gastroenterol.*, **4**, 95–107.

Murray, H.S., Strottman, M.P. and Cooke, A.R. (1974) Effect of several drugs on gastric potential difference in man. *Brit. Med. J.*, 19–21.

Ohe, K., Hayashi, K., Shirakawa, T., Yamada, K. *et al.* (1980a) Aspirin- and taurocholate-induced metabolic damage in mammalian gastric mucosa *in vitro*. *Am. J. Physiol.*, **239**, G457–62.

Ohe, K., Yokoya, H., Kitaura, T. (1980b) Increase in pepsin content in gastric mucosa during the course of aspirin and taurocholate-induced gastric ulceration in rats. *Dig. Dis. Sci.*, **25**, 849–56.

O'Laughlin, J.C., Hoftiezer, J.W., Mahoney, J.P. and Ivey, K.J. (1981) Does aspirin prolong bleeding from gastric biopsies in man? *Gastrointest. Endosc.*, **27**, 1–5.

Okada, M., Niida, H., Takeuchi, K. and Okabe, S. (1989) Role of prostaglandin deficiency in pathogenetic mechanism of gastric lesions induced by indomethacin in rats. *Dig. Dis. Sci.*, **34**, 694–702.

504

Pemberton, R.E. and Strand, L.J. (1979) A review of the upper-gastrointestinal effects of the new non-steroidal anti-inflammatory agents, *Dig. Dis. Sci.*, **24**, 53–64.

Peskar, B.M. (1977) On the synthesis of prostaglandins by human gastric mucosa and its modification by drugs. *Biochim. Biophys. Acta*, **487**, 307–14.

Peskar, B.M., Seyberth, H.W. and Peskar, B.A. (1980) Synthesis and metabolism of endogenous prostaglandins by human gastric mucosa. In *Adv. Prostaglandin Thromboxane Res.*, **8** 1511–14.

Peskar, B.M., Weiler, H. and Peskar, B.A. (1982) Effect of BW755C on prostaglandin synthesis in the rat stomach. *Biochem. Pharmacol.*, **331**, 1652–3.

Peskar, B.M., Hoppe, U., Lange, K. and Peskar, B.A. (1988) Effects of non-steroidal anti-inflammatory drugs on rat gastric mucosal leukotriene C_4 and prostanoid release: relation to ethanol-induced injury. *Brit. J. Pharmacol.*, **93**, 937–43.

Pihan, G., Regillo, C. and Szabo, S. (1987) Free radicals and lipid peroxidation in ethanol or aspirin-induced gastric mucosal injury. *Dig. Dis. Sci.*, **32**, 1395–401.

Pihan, G., Rogers, C. and Szabo, S. (1988) Vascular injury in acute gastric mucosal damage. Mediatory role of leukotrienes. *Dig. Dis Sci.*, **33**, 625–32.

Piper, D.W., McIntosh, J.H., Arioti, D.E. *et al.* (1981) Analgesic ingestion and chronic peptic ulcer. *Gastroenterology*, **80**, 427–32.

Prichard, P.J., Kitchingman, G.K., Walt, R.P. *et al.* (1989) Human gastric mucosal bleeding induced by low dose aspirin, but not warfarin. *Brit. Med. J.*, **298**, 493–6.

Puurunen, J., Huttmunen, P. and Hirvonen, J. (1980) Is ethanol-induced damage of the gastric mucosa a hyperosmotic effect? Comparative studies on the effects of ethanol, some other hyperosmotic solutions and acetylsalicylic acid on rat gastric mucosa. *Acta Pharmacol. Toxicol.*, **47**, 312–27.

Rainsford, K.D. (1975) A synergistic interaction between aspirin, or other nonsteroidal anti-inflammatory drugs, and stress which produces severe gastric mucosal damage in rats and pigs. *Agents Actions*, **5**, 553–8.

Rainsford, K.D. (1978) The effects of aspirin and other non-steroid anti-inflammatory/analgesic drugs on gastrointestinal mucus glycoprotein biosynthesis *in vivo*: relationship to ulcerogenic actions. *Biochem. Pharmacol.*, **27**, 877–85.

Rainsford, K.D. (1982) An analysis of the gastro-intestinal side-effects of non-steroidal anti-inflammatory drugs, with particular reference to comparative studies in man and laboratory species. *Rheumatol. Int.*, **2**, 1–10.

Rainsford, K.D. (1983) Microvascular injury during gastric mucosal damage by anti-inflammatory drugs in pigs and rats. *Agents Actions*, **13**, 457–60.

Rainsford, K.D. (1984) The mechanisms of gastro-intestinal ulceration by non-steroidal anti-inflammatory drugs. In *Side Effects of Anti-inflammatory/Analgesic Drugs* (eds K.D. Rainsford and G.P. Velo), Raven Press, New York, pp. 51–64.

Rainsford, K.D. (1988) Interplay between anti-inflammatory drugs and eicosanoids in gastrointestinal damage. In *Eicosanoids and the Gastrointestinal Tract* (ed. K. Hillier), MTP Press, Lancaster, pp.111–28.

Rainsford, K.D. and Whitehouse, M.W. (1980) Anti-inflammatory antipyretic salicylic acid esters, with low gastric ulcerogenic activity. *Agents Actions*, **10**, 451–6.

Rainsford, K.D. and Willis, C. (1982) Relationship of gastric mucosal damage induced in pigs by anti-inflammatory drugs to their effects on prostaglandin production. *Dig. Dis. Sci.*, **27**, 624–35.

Rainsford, K.D., Willis, C.M., Walker, S.A. and Robins, P.G. (1982) Electron microscopic observations comparing the gastric mucosal damage induced in rats and pigs by benoxaprofen and aspirin, reflecting their differing actions as prostaglandin-synthesis-inhibitors. *Brit. J. Exp. Pathol.*, **63**, 25–34.

Rainsford, K.D., Fox, S.A. and Osborne, D.J. (1984) Comparative effects of some non-steroidal anti-inflammatory drugs on the ultrastructural integrity and prostaglandin levels in the rat gastric mucosa: Relationship to drug uptake. *Scand. J. Gastroenterol.*, **19** (suppl. 101), 55–68.

Rampton, D. (1987) Non-steroidal anti-inflammatory drugs and lower gastrointestinal tract. *Scand. J. Gastroenterol.*, **22**, 1–4.

Rampton, D.S. and Sladen, G.E. (1981) Prostaglandin synthesis inhibitors in ulcerative colitis. Flurbiprofen compared with conventional treatment. *Prostaglandins.*, **21**, 417–25.

Rampton, D.S.. McNeil, N.I. and Sarner, M. (1983) Analgesic ingestion and other factors preceding relapse in ulcerative colitis. *Gut*, **24**, 187–9.

Redfern, J.S. and Feldman, M. (1989) Role of endogenous prostaglandins in preventing gastrointestinal ulceration: Induction of ulcers by antibodies to prostaglandins. *Gastroenterology*, **96**, 596–605.

Redfern, J.S., Lee, E. and Feldman, M. (1987a) Effect of indomethacin on gastric mucosal prostaglandins in humans. Correlation with mucosal damage. *Gastroenterology*, **92**, 969–77.

Redfern, J.S., Blair, A.J., Clubb, F.J. *et al.* (1987b) Gastroduodenal ulceration following active immunization with prostaglandin E_2 in dogs. Role of gastric acid secretion. *Prostaglandins*, **34**, 623–32.

Rees, W.D.W. and Turnberg, L.A. (1980) Reappraisal of the effects of aspirin on the stomach. *Lancet*, **ii**, 410–13.

Rees, W.D.W., Garner, A., Turnberg, L.A. and Gibbons, L.C. (1982) Studies of acid and alkaline secretion by rabbit gastric fundus *in vitro*. Effect of low concentrations of sodium taurocholate. *Gastroenterology*, **83**, 435–40.

Rees, W.D.W., Gibbons, L.C., Warhurst, G. and Turnberg, L.A. (1984) Studies of bicarbonate secretion by the normal human stomach *in vivo* – effect of aspirin, sodium taurocholate and prostaglandin E_2. In *Mechanisms of Mucosal Protection in the Upper Gastrointestinal tract* (eds A. Allen, G. Flemstrom, A. Garner, W. Silen and L.A. Turnberg), Raven Press, New York, pp. 119–24.

RISC Group (1990) Risk of myocardial infarction and death during treatment with low dose aspirin and intravenous heparin in men with unstable coronary artery disease. *Lancet*, **336**, 827–30.

Ritchie, W.P. (1975) Acute gastric mucosal damage induced by bile salts, acid and ischemia. *Gastroenterology*, **68**, 699–707.

Robert, A. (1975) An intestinal disease produced experimentally by a prostaglandin deficiency. *Gastroenterology*, **69**, 1045–7.

Robert, A. (1976) Antisecretory, antiulcer, cytoprotective and diarrhoegenic properties of prostglandins. *Adv. Prostaglandin Thromboxane Res.*, **2**, 507–20.

Robert, A. (1981) Prostaglandins and the gastrointestinal tract. In *Physiology of the Gastrointestinal Tract* (ed. L.R. Johnson), Raven Press, New York, pp. 1407–34.

Robert, A., Nezamis, J.E., Lancaster, C. and Hanchar, A.J. (1979) Cytoprotection by prostaglandins in rats – prevention of gastric necrosis produced by alcohol, HCl, NaOH, hypertonic NaCl and thermal injury. *Gastroenterology*, **77**, 433–43.

Robert, A., Leung, F.W., Kaiser, D.G. and Guth, P.H. (1989) Potentiation of aspirin-induced gastric lesions by exposure to cold in rats. *Gastroenterology*, **97**, 1147–58.

Robins, P.G. (1980) Ultra-structural observations on the pathogenesis of aspirin-induced gastric erosions, *Brit. J. Exp. Pathol.*, **61**, 497–504.

Ross, I.R., Bahari, H.M.M. and Turnberg, L.A. (1981) The pH gradient across mucus adherent to rat fundic mucosa *in vivo* and the effect of potential damaging agents. *Gastroenterology*, 713–18.

Rowe, P.H., Starlinger, M.J., Kasdon, E. *et al.* (1987) Parenteral aspirin and sodium salicylate are equally injurious to the rat gastric mucosa. *Gastroenterology*, **93**, 863–71.

Sarosiek, J., Mitzuta, K., Slomiany, A. and Slomiany, B.L. (1986) Effect of acetylsalicylic acid on gastric mucin viscosity, permeability to hydrogen ion, and susceptibility to pepsin. *Biochem. Pharmacol.*, **35**, 4291–5.

Sellings, J.A., Hogan, D.L., Aly, A. *et al.* (1987) Indomethacin inhibits duodenal mucosal bicarbonate secretion and endogenous PGE_2 output in human subjects. *Ann. Intern. Med.*, **106**, 368–71.

Semple, P.F. and Russell, R.I. (1975) Role of bile acids in the pathogenesis of aspirin-induced gastric mucosal haemorrhage in rats. *Gastroenterology*, **68**, 67–70.

Senay, E.C. and Levin, R.J. (1967) Synergism between cold and restraint for rapid production of stress ulcers in rats. *Proc. Soc. Biol. Med.*, **124**, 1221–3.

Shea-Donohue, T., Steel, L., Montcalm-Mazzilli, E. and Dubois, A. (1990) Aspirin-induced changes in gastric function: Role of endogenous prostaglandins and mucosal damage. *Gastroenterology*, **98**, 284–92.

Shorrock, C.J., Prescott, R.J. and Rees, W.D.W. (1990) The effects of indomethacin on gastroduodenal morphology and mucosal pH gradient in the healthy human stomach. *Gastroenterology*, **99**, 334–9.

Silen, W. and Ito, S. (1985) Mechanisms for rapid re-epithelialization of the gastric mucosal surface. *Ann. Rev. Physiol.*, **47**, 217–29.

Silvoso, G.R., Ivey, K.J., Butt, J.H. *et al.* (1979) Incidence of gastric lesions in patients with rheumatic disease on chronic aspirin therapy. *Ann. Intern. Med.*, **91**, 517–20.

Skarstein, A. (1979) Effect of indomethacin on blood flow distribution in the stomach of cats with gastric ulcer. *Scand. J. Gastroenterol.*, **14**, 905–11.

Smith, B.M., Skillman, J.J., Edwards, B.G. and Silen, W. (1971) Permeability of the human gastric mucosa: alteration by acetylsalicylic acid and ethanol. *N. Engl. J. Med.*, **285**, 716.

Smith, S.M., Holm-Rutili, L., Perry, M.A., *et al.* (1987) Role of neutrophils in hemorrhagic shock-induced gastric mucosal injury in the rat. *Gastroenterology*, **93**, 466–71.

Somerville, K., Faulkner, G. and Langman, M. (1986) Non-steroidal anti-inflammatory drugs and bleeding peptic ulcer. *Lancet*, **i**, 462–4.

Spenney, J.G. and Bhown, M. (1977) Effect of acetylsalicylic acid on gastric mucosa. II. Mucosal ATP and phosphocreatine content and salicylic effects on mitochondrial metabolism. *Gastroenterology*, **73**, 995–9.

Starlinger, M. and Schiessel, R. (1988) Bicarbonate (HCO_3) delivery to the gastroduodenal mucosa by the blood: its importance for mucosal integrity. *Gut*, **29**, 647–54.

Svanes, K., Leiknes, K.A., Varhaug, J.E. and Soreide, O. (1979) Aspirin damage to ischemic gastric mucosa in shocked cats. *Scand. J. Gastroenterol.*, **14**, 633–9.

Svanes, K., Critchlow, J., Takeuchi, K., *et al.* (1984) Factors influencing reconstitution of frog gastric mucosa: role of prostaglandins. In *Mechanisms of Mucosal Protection in the Upper Gastrointestinal Tract*, (eds A. Allen, G. Flemstrom, A. Garner, W. Silen and L.A. Turnberg), Raven Press, New York, pp.33–8.

Szabo, S., Spill, W.F. and Rainsford, K.D. (1989) Non-steroidal anti-inflammatory drug-induced gastropathy. *Med. Tox. Adverse Drug Exper.*, **4**, 77–94.

Szelenyi, I., Engler, H., Herzog, P., *et al.* (1980) Influence of non-steroidal anti-inflammatory compounds on healing of chronic gastric ulcers in rats. *Agents Actions*, **12**, 180–2.

UK-TIA Study Group (1988) United Kingdom transient ischaemic attack (UK-TIA) aspirin trial: interim results. *Brit. Med. J..*, **296**, 316–20.

Vane, J.R. (1971) Inhibition of prostaglandin synthesis as a mechanism of action of aspirin-like drugs. *Nature (New Biol.)*, **231**, 232–5.

Van Kolfscholten, A.A., Dembinska-Kiec, A. and Basista, M. (1981) Interaction between aspirin and paracetamol on the production of prostaglandins in the rat gastric mucosa. *J. Pharm. Pharmacol.*, **33**, 462–3.

Van Kolfscholten, A.A., Hagelen, F. and Van Noordwijk, J. (1984) Butyl hydroxy toluene antagonizes the gastric toxicity but not the pharmacological activity of acetylsalicyclic acid in rats. *Naunyn-Schmiedeberg's Arch. Pharmacol.*, **327**, 283–5.

Wallace, J.L. and Whittle, B.J.R. (1985) Role of prostanoids in the protective actions of BW755C on the gastric mucosa. *Eur. J. Pharmacol.*, **115**, 45–52.

Wallace, J.L. and Whittle, B.J.R. (1986) Role of mucus in the repair of gastric epithelial damage in the rat. *Gastroenterology*, **91**, 603–11.

Wallace, J.L. and McKnight, G.W. (1990) The mucoid cap over superficial gastric damage in the rat. A high-pH microenvironment dissipated by nonsteroidal antiinflammatory drugs and endothelin. *Gastroenterology*, **99**, 295–304.

Wallace, J.L., Keenan, C.M. and Granger, D.N. (1990) Gastric ulceration induced by non-steroidal anti-inflammatory drugs is a neutrophil-dependent process. *Am. J. Physiol.*, **259**, G462–7.

Walt, R., Katschinski, B., Logan, R., Ashley, J. and Langman, M.J.S. (1986) Rising frequency of ulcer perforation in elderly people in the United Kingdom. *Lancet*, **i**, 489–92.

Whittle, B.J.R. (1977) Mechanisms underlying gastric mucosal damage induced by indomethacin and bile salt, and the actions of prostaglandins. *Brit. J. Pharmacol.*, **60**, 455–60.

Whittle, B.J.R. (1980) Actions of prostaglandins on gastric mucosal blood flow. In *Gastro-Intestinal Mucosal Blood Flow*, (ed. L.P. Fielding), Churchill Livingstone, Edinburgh, pp. 180–91.

Whittle, B.J.R. (1981) Temporal relationship between cyclo-oxygenase inhibition, as measured by prostacyclin biosynthesis, and the gastrointestinal damage induced by indomethacin in the rat. *Gastroenterology*, **80**, 94–8.

Whittle, B.J.R. (1983) The potentiation of taurocholate-induced rat gastric erosions following parenteral administration of cyclo-oxygenase inhibitors. *Brit. J. Pharmacol.*, **80**, 545–51.

Whittle, B.J.R. (1984) Cellular mediators in gastric damage: Actions of thromboxane A_2 and its inhibitors. In *Mechanisms of Mucosal Protection in the Upper Gastrointestinal Tract* (eds A. Allen, A. Garner, G. Flemstrom, W. Silen and L.A. Turnberg), Raven Press, New York, pp. 295–301.

Whittle, B.J.R. and Moncada, S. (1983) Ulceration induced by an endoperoxide analogue and by indomethacin in the canine stomach. *Adv Prostaglandin, Thromboxane Leukotriene Res.*, **12**, 373–8.

Whittle, B.J.R. and Vane, J.R. (1984) A biochemical basis for the gastrointestinal toxicity on non-steroid antirheumatoid drugs. *Arch. Toxicol. Suppl.*, **7**, 315–22.

Whittle, B.J.R. and Vane, J.R. (1987) Prostanoids as regulators of gastrointestinal function. In *Physiology of the Gastrointestinal Tract Vol.* **I**, 2nd Edn (ed. L.R. Johnston), Raven Press, New York, pp. 143–80.

Whittle, B.J.R., Higgs, G.A., Eakins, K.E. *et al.* (1980) Selective inhibition of prostaglandin production in inflammatory exudates and gastric mucosa. *Nature (Lond.)*, **284**, 271–3.

Whittle, B.J.R., Kauffman, G.L. and Moncada, S. (1981a) Vasoconstriction with thromboxane A_2 induces ulceration of the gastric mucosa. *Nature (Lond.)*, **292**, 472–4.

Whittle, B.J.R., Makki, K.A. and O'Grady, J. (1981b) Changes in potential difference across the human buccal mucosa with buffered or unbuffered aspirin and salicylate. *Gut*, **22**, 798.

Whittle, B.J.R., Hansen, D. and Salmon, J.A. (1985a) Gastric ulcer formation and cyclo-oxygenase inhibition in cat antrum follows parenteral administration of aspirin but not salicylate. *Eur. J. Pharmacol.*, **115**, 153–7.

Whittle, B.J.R., Oren-Wolman, N. and Guth, P.H. (1985b) Gastric vasoconstrictor actions of leukotriene C_4, $PGF_{2\alpha}$, and thromboxane mimetic U-46619 on rat submucosal microcirculation *in vivo. Am. J. Physiol.*, **248**, G580–6.

Whittle, B.J.R., Kauffman, G.L. and Moncada, S. (1986). Hemostatic mechanisms, independent of platelet aggregation arrest gastric mucosal bleeding. *Proc. Natl Acad Sci. USA*, **83**, 5683–7.

Whittle, B.J.R., Lopez-Belmonte, J. and Moncada, S. (1990) Regulation of gastric mucosal integrity by endogenous nitric oxide: interactions with prostanoids and sensory neuropeptides in the rat. *Brit. J. Pharmacol.*, **99**, 607–11.

Yeomans, N.E. (1976) Electron microscopic study of the repair of aspirin-induced gastric erosions. *Dig. Dis.*, **21**, 533–41.

19 *Renal effects of aspirin*

E.J. ZAMBRASKI and M.J. DUNN

19.1 INTRODUCTION

To understand the potential effects of acetylsalicylic acid (ASA) on the kidney it is necessary to have some awareness of renal prostaglandin (PG) biochemistry and the processes within the kidney that PGs influence. This chapter will first review these aspects. Experimental animal studies will then be discussed to illustrate the situations in which PGs are important in determining kidney function, i.e. settings in which ASA treatment would be predicted to significantly alter renal function. Following this, studies specifically examining the effects of ASA in man will be reviewed. Lastly, the issue of ASA versus non-acetylated salicylic acid (SA) will be discussed.

19.2 RENAL PROSTAGLANDIN SYNTHESIS

The kidney has a large capacity to produce various eicosanoids from the metabolism of arachidonic acid. Our understanding of renal prostanoid synthesis and the site-specific functions of PGs has been greatly advanced by studies using isolated tissue and tissue culture methodology, as well as studies employing whole organ/animal techniques. It has become apparent that within the kidney, and along the various structures of the nephron, there are large differences in PG synthetic capacity, as well as in the production of individual PGs. This regional heterogeneity of PG synthesis has supported the concept that within the kidney PGs are truly autacoids; they are produced and act locally. Functionally a compartmentalization of the renal PG system appears to exist, with the two major compartments representing the cortical versus medullary regions. PGs produced in cortical structures (i.e. glomeruli, arterioles) influence events which are cortical in nature. A similar situation exists for the medulla. There appears to be very little interaction or transport of PGs between these two compartments.

510

Reviews detailing renal PG biochemistry have been published (Dunn, 1983; Schlondorff and Ardaillou, 1986). In general, the major PGs synthesized by the kidneys are PGE_2, PGI_2, $PGF_{2\alpha}$ and thromboxane A_2 (TXA_2). Cyclo-oxygenase is found in the endoplasmic reticulum of collecting tubules, medullary interstitial and arterial endothelial cells. Although the highest PG biosynthetic capacity is in the medulla, it has become apparent that the cortical synthesis of PG is significant and extremely important in determining various aspects of renal function.

19.2.1 Cortical Synthesis

Various studies using isolated nephron segments (Sraer et al., 1982; Farman et al., 1987), isolated glomeruli (Hassid et al., 1979; Sraer et al., 1979) and various cultured cell preparations (Petrulis et al., 1981; Kreisberg et al., 1982; Currie et al., 1983) have evaluated cortical PG synthesis. Within the cortex the major PGs produced are PGE_2 and PGI_2. Arterioles and human glomeruli synthesize predominantly PGI_2. Glomerular epithelial and mesangial cells both have the capacity to produce PGI_2 and PGE_2. In normal kidneys reports vary as to the amount of TXA_2 synthesis, however, the relative TXA_2 synthetic rates are low compared to PGE_2 and PGI_2. Cortical collecting tubules synthesize predominantly PGE_2. Within the renal cortex certain structures, such as the proximal tubule and the thick ascending loop of Henle appear to possess relatively low PG synthetic capacity.

The results of many studies demonstrating the cortical synthesis of PGs, particularly in the glomeruli and arterioles, have assisted in delineating a role for PGs in mediating several cortical events. These include the control of renal blood flow (RBF)/vascular resistance, glomerular filtration rate (GFR), and the release of renin.

19.2.2 Medullary Synthesis

Within the medulla the two major cell types responsible for the large PG synthetic capacity are the collecting tubules and medullary interstitial cells. The predominant PG produced in the medulla is PGE_2 (Zusman and Keiser, 1977). The medullary capacity to produce PGE_2 may be as high as 20–25-fold of that measured in the cortex. Site-specific roles for medullary PGE_2 include: determination of the medullary tonicity by influencing both medullary blood flow and sodium/chloride reabsorption, and the attenuation of the hydro-osmotic effects of arginine vasopressin (AVP). An important point concerning the control of intrarenal PG synthesis is that several factors, including angiotensin II (Ang II), AVP, catecholamines, and renal sympathetic nerve activity, all have the capacity to stimulate renal prostanoid production (Dunn, 1983).

19.2.3 Assessment of Renal PG Production *in vivo*

Although *in-vitro* techniques have determined that various structures within the kidney can synthesize PGs, a method to quantify renal PG synthesis *in vivo* is required. This is especially true when trying to assess the effects of ASA or other cyclo-oxygenase inhibitors, on kidney function *in vivo*.

The measurement of PG excretion has been generally accepted as an appropriate indirect assessment of intrarenal PG synthesis. Advantages, as well as the limitations of this measure, and factors which may significantly influence its validity, have been pointed out (Patrono and Dunn, 1987). There are several factors, however, that one must consider when using measurements of PG excretion to estimate intrarenal synthesis.

The amount of PG excreted represents only a small fraction of the total renal PG generated. Renal secretion of PGs into renal venous effluent is another major component, although when cyclo-oxygenase inhibitors are administered decrements in renal secretion and excretion parallel each other (Zambraski and Dunn, 1979). PGE_2 and PGI_2 entering the kidney from the arterial circulation may be excreted in the urine. Quantitatively, the excretion of extrarenal PGI_2 (as 6-keto-$PGF_{1\alpha}$) exceeds that of PGE_2, as 80% or more of PGE_2 is metabolized by the kidney, whereas only 25% of 6-keto-$PGF_{1\alpha}$, appears to be metabolized (Bugge *et al.*, 1987). Certain PGs (PGE_2 or PGI_2) generated within the kidney may selectively enter the vascular versus tubular compartments (Boyd *et al.*, 1986). The degree to which renal PGs enter the vascular compartment would clearly influence the sensitivity of the measurement of PG excretion to reflect intrarenal synthesis. Extensive tubular handling of intrarenal PGs may also influence the amount excreted. Lastly, the relative contributions of PGs of cortical versus medullary origin to the total amount excreted is not known. The fact that chemical medullectomy of the kidney may reduce PGE_2 excretion by 75% suggests that the PGE_2 excreted may largely represent PGE_2 of medullary origin (Bing *et al.*, 1983).

Nonetheless, all of these limitations notwithstanding, the assessment of intrarenal PG synthesis by the measurement of PG excretion has been an important tool in elucidating the role of PGs in kidney function. As will be discussed, changes in PG excretion, due to the administration of ASA or other cyclo-oxygenase inhibitors, for the most part correlate with and predict changes in renal function anticipated due to a decrease in intrarenal PG synthesis.

19.3 PROSTAGLANDIN REGULATION OF RENAL FUNCTION

19.3.1 Haemodynamic, Tubular and Glomerular Actions

PGs have the capacity to influence essentially all elements of renal function. They have the potential to control renal haemodynamics, glomerular filtration, tubular electrolyte transport, water reabsorption, and the release of renal hormones. The difficulty, however, in actually pinpointing a regulatory role of PGs over various aspects of renal function is because their effects, and importance, are dependent upon the conditions that exist. As will be pointed out, in normal animals and healthy man the control of renal function by PGs is minor. However, with perturbations in fluid/electrolyte balance, and/or the activation of other hormone systems, PG control of specific aspects of renal function becomes significant. This is largely due to the fact that renal PGs are modulatory in nature. They interact with, and can alter the resultant effects of, both neural and endocrine control systems operative within the kidney (Dunn and Zambraski, 1980). Also, in various disease states PGs play a more consistent and dominant role in determining kidney function; a role which for the most part is protective and beneficial in nature.

PGE$_2$ and PGI$_2$ are renal vasodilators. In contrast, TXA$_2$ is a vaso-constrictor. Intrarenal infusion of PGE$_2$, or arachidonic acid, increases RBF. PGs are also natriuretic, inhibiting tubular sodium reabsorption, and in the thick ascending limb they limit chloride transport. PGs are important modulators of neural, Ang II, and AVP vasoconstriction (Dunn, 1983). This effect is extremely important, both in minimizing reductions in RBF and GFR and attenuating glomerular mesangial cell contraction induced by these compounds (Scharschmidt and Dunn, 1983). In the absence of elevated vasoconstrictors, PGs probably do not normally influence mesangial cell contractility, or determine the glomerular ultrafiltration coefficient (Baylis and Brenner, 1978). PGs also attenuate the hydro-osmotic effects of AVP (Orloff and Zusman, 1978).

19.3.2 Endocrine Release

Intrarenal PGs (PGI$_2$, PGE$_2$) are important in the release of renin. Several, but not all, pathways for renin release are PG-dependent (Henrich, 1981). PGs are also coupled to the actions of the renal

Unwanted effects

kallikrein–kinin system (McGiff, 1980). PGs do not appear to influence the natriuretic effects of atrial natriuretic peptide (Salazar *et al.*, 1988).

19.4 RENAL EFFECTS OF ASPIRIN – ANIMAL STUDIES

19.4.1 Effect on Prostaglandin Synthesis

ASA significantly decreases renal PG production. It has been shown that ASA acetylates both cortical and medullary PG synthetase (Caterson, 1978). In animal studies ASA treatment significantly decreases PGE_2 excretion (Oliw *et al.*, 1978; Quilley *et al.*, 1987; Gafni *et al.*, 1978). ASA also attenuates the renal vasodilatation which is normally seen with intrarenal administration of arachidonic acid, which is a functional test indicative of a decrease in renal PG synthesis (Anderson *et al.*, 1983).

As discussed in earlier chapters, ASA is a significantly weaker inhibitor of cyclo-oxygenase, as compared to other anti-inflammatory drugs such as indomethacin. In various animal, as well as human studies, reductions in PG excretion with ASA compared to indomethacin are often similar, with decrements ranging from 60 to 80%. A far greater number of studies have evaluated the renal effects of PG inhibition with compounds like indomethacin or meclofenamate, as compared to ASA. Because ASA and other anti-inflammatory drugs both may decrease renal PG synthesis, where data are not available on the effects of ASA, results of studies using indomethacin or other similar compounds can be extrapolated to predict the potential effects of high doses of ASA. This is especially true in some of the animal models of various disease states.

19.4.2 Effects in Normal Animals

In normal animals the acute administration of ASA has little or no effect on the kidney. The ASA induced reduction of renal PG is of little physiological consequence. In some studies increased renal vascular resistance, decreased sodium excretion, and increased urine osmolarity have been reported. However, these effects are usually minimal and transient. In contrast, if normal animals are stressed (i.e. anaesthesia, surgical trauma) ASA treatment may decrease the RBF, and sodium and water excretion. These different results, depending on experimental conditions, suggest that these disturbances either increase renal PG synthesis or modify some other neural or endocrine stimuli which PGs normally modulate or attenuate. Both circumstances would amplify the renal effects of ASA treatment.

514

19.4.3 Animals with Volume Disturbances

The support for renal PGs as modulators of other factors in healthy animals was initially derived from important studies in normal animals with experimentally induced volume/electrolyte disturbances. Blasingham and Nasjletti (1980), Blasingham et al. (1980) and DeForrest et al. (1980) clearly demonstrated that sodium depletion increases the adverse effects of renal PG inhibition. In anaesthetized, as well as conscious dogs, renal PG inhibition with meclofenamate decreases RBF and GFR selectively in sodium-depleted animals. Decrements in renal haemodynamics were inversely correlated with plasma renin levels. Izumi et al. (1985) also reported decreases in GFR and free water clearance only in sodium-depleted rats with indomethacin treatment. More recently, Podjarny et al. (1988) reported similar responses in sodium-depleted rats with ASA treatment.

Although sodium depletion, via an activation of the renin–angiotensin system, sensitizes the kidneys to the adverse effects of ASA, it is not clear as to whether sodium depletion actually increases renal PG synthesis. Many of the studies utilizing sodium depletion have observed no increase in renal PGE_2 excretion (Blasingham and Nasjletti, 1980; Blasingham et al., 1980; Izumi et al., 1985) or glomerular/papillary PG synthesis (Chaumet-Riffaud et al., 1981), whereas, other studies employing sodium depletion have reported increases in PGE_2 synthesis (Kramer et al., 1985; Schlondorff et al., 1987; Podjarny et al., 1988; Oliver et al., 1980). This emphasizes the point that since PGs play a modulatory role, in situations where renal vasoconstrictor stimuli are elevated (i.e. sympathetic nerve activity, Ang II, AVP), deleterious effects of ASA may occur in the absence of measurably increased renal PG synthesis or excretion.

The results of studies with ASA seen with sodium depletion are similar to those in studies inducing low cardiac output states (Oliver et al., 1981, Echthenkamp et al., 1981; Riegger et al., 1989). Inhibition of renal cyclo-oxygenase, which would eliminate PG antagonism to both sympathetic and renin–angiotensin constrictor activity, causes significant renal vasoconstriction in animals with low cardiac output.

19.4.4 Animal Models of Various Disease States

Although in healthy animals the importance of renal PG, and thus the response to ASA, may depend upon the experimental conditions or the degree to which other renal vasoconstrictor systems are activated, an important and dominant role of PGs controlling renal function has

Table 19.1 Conditions or disease states in animal models where renal function is PG-dependent

Hepatic cirrhosis
Heart failure
Glomerular disease
Diabetes
Papillary necrosis
Reduction in renal mass
Renal ischaemia/decreased perfusion pressure
Ureteral obstruction
Hydronephrosis
Aminoglycoside nephrotoxicity

been shown for various abnormal and disease states. Table 19.1 lists some of the conditions in which renal function is PG-dependent, states in which ASA treatment will significantly alter kidney function.

In bile-duct-ligated cirrhotic animals renal PGE_2 synthesis is increased. In this model of hepatic cirrhosis cyclo-oxygenase inhibition has a deleterious effect on renal function, reducing RBF, GFR and sodium excretion (Zambraski and Dunn, 1984; Zambraski *et al.*, 1984).

Increases in prostanoid synthesis accompany experimentally induced glomerular disease, such as nephrotoxic serum nephritis (Lianos *et al.*, 1983; Kaizu *et al.*, 1985). Vasodilatory PGE_2 assists in maintaining GFR and a role for increased TXA_2-mediated vasoconstriction has been postulated (Scharschmidt and Dunn, 1983).

Diabetes is associated with changes in glomerular function and morphology. In streptozotocin-induced diabetic rats the initial increase in GFR is mediated by PGs (Kirschenbaum and Chaudhari, 1986). In addition, the longer term control of GFR is also PG dependent (Jensen *et al.*, 1986). Glomerular PGE_2 synthesis is increased in this model (Barnett *et al.*, 1987). ASA prevents the early hyperfiltration and reduces the thickening of the glomerular basement membrane (Moel *et al.*, 1987).

ASA treatment has been used to induce papillary necrosis in normal and hyperbilirubinaemic Gunn rats (Molland, 1978). This effect may be due to the removal by ASA of vasodilatory PG maintenance of papillary blood flow (Ganguli *et al.*, 1989).

The experimental reduction of renal mass in the rodent has been used extensively as a model of chronic renal disease. The hyperfiltration seen in this model is accompanied by significant increases in prostanoid synthesis. PG inhibition decreases the GFR of the remaining nephrons by 40–60% (Stahl *et al.*, 1986; Kirschenbaum and Serros, 1981).

With acute reductions in renal perfusion pressure there are increases in renal PG synthesis. PGs attenuate the vasoconstriction of simultaneously released Ang II (Goto *et al.*, 1987). In response to an ischaemic challenge PGs also assist in protecting against acute tubular necrosis (Kaufman *et al.*, 1987).

With unilateral ureteral obstruction vasodilatory PGs mediate the whole kidney hyperaemic response (Cadnapaphornchai *et al.*, 1978). During partial obstruction PGs also regulate single nephron function, with PG inhibition significantly decreasing filtration rate and plasma flow (Ichikawa and Brenner, 1979).

Gentamicin-induced nephrotoxicity causes an increase in renal PG synthesis. ASA treatment exacerbates the decline in GFR observed with aminoglycoside-induced acute renal failure (Higa *et al.*, 1985).

These studies in various animal disease models have demonstrated an important protective role of renal PGs. In these conditions the effects of large doses of ASA, or other compounds that inhibit renal PG cyclo-oxygenase, are clearly deleterious to the kidney.

19.5 RENAL EFFECTS OF ASPIRIN – HUMAN STUDIES

19.5.1 Tubular Damage

Hanzlik *et al.* (1917) were the first to report alterations of renal function and abnormalities of urinalysis after SA administration. In normal volunteers, as well as subjects with rheumatoid arthritis, they administered a 10% SA solution orally until 'toxicity' was reached (generally 8–14 g of SA administered) and noticed the appearance of leukocytes and casts in the urine as well as the development of albuminuria. In 28 patients, urinary albumin increased from 0.02 g over the 10-h period of observation to 0.13 g. Scott and coworkers (1963) administered ASA or SA in doses of 2.7–3.3 g day $^{-1}$ and found an acute but transient increase of cells in the urine. The shedding of cells peaked on the fourth day after initiation of ASA or SA and returned to normal over 1 week despite continued administration of the drug. This 'desensitization' was also apparent with intermittent dosing of ASA as subsequent doses showed little toxicity to the kidney after the initial dose. Prescott (1965) compared ASA, phenacetin, paracetamol and caffeine for their effects on renal tubular epithelium. Studying ten normal volunteers who received 3.6 g of ASA in four divided doses, Prescott confirmed earlier observations of increased renal tubular epithelial cells in the urine (ten-fold increment) as well as increased numbers of red blood cells (three-fold increment) without any significant leukocyturia.

Unwanted effects

ASA induced greater increments of renal tubular epithelial shedding than paracetemol, caffeine, phenacetin or mixtures of aspirin, phenacetin and caffeine. Burry *et al.* (1976) studied 18 volunteers (10 normals and 8 patients with rheumatoid arthritis) who, over a 10-day period, received $4 \, g \, day^{-1}$ of aloxiprin and confirmed the transient increase of epithelial cells in the urine at 3 days of therapy but with cessation of tubular shedding after 10 days of treatment. The renal tubular enzyme, N-acetyl-β-glucosaminidase (NAG), was increased at 3 and 10 days, indicative of continuing tubular injury. Other studies (Lockwood and Bosmann, 1979) confirmed these results and concluded that ASA increased the excretion of NAG in a dose-dependent fashion, indicative of ASA-induced renal tubular injury.

These studies, in the aggregate, indicate a toxic effect of ASA and SA on renal tubular epithelium although the portion of the tubule which is injured is unknown. These changes are transient and probably have no long-lasting significance (below under Chronic Studies). It also is unlikely that these changes are related to inhibition of renal PG synthesis since subsequent studies have shown that ASA is more potent than SA in inhibiting PG synthesis, whereas the shedding of renal tubular epithelium can be induced by either class of compounds.

19.5.2 Effects on Glomerular Filtration Rate and Renal Blood Flow

NORMAL SUBJECTS

Most investigators have found negligible or only transient effects of ASA and SA on GFR and RBF. In his pioneering studies in 1917, Hanzlik noted transient increases of blood urea nitrogen and decreases of phenolsulfophthalein excretion, albeit after very large doses of SA orally (8–14 g over 10 h). Robert and colleagues (1972) administered ASA intravenously with a bolus dose of 0.9 g and a sustaining infusion of $1 \, mg \, kg^{-1} \, min^{-1}$ for 40 min achieving blood SA levels of $10 \, mg \, dl^{-1}$. In this study, ASA transiently decreased GFR (creatinine clearance and inulin clearance) and RBF (PAH clearance) by 30–33%. Berg (1977) did not find any decrease of creatinine clearance in normal volunteers administered ASA, $70 \, mg \, kg^{-1}$ of body weight, over a 24-h period. The studies of Muther and Bennett (1980) confirm those of Berg as they observed no effects on GFR of ASA 650 mg every 4 h in nine normal volunteers. In a subsequent study, they showed that if normal volunteers were sodium-depleted, ASA reduced GFR and RBF by 10–15%. Reimann *et al.* (1985) evaluated the effects of intravenous ASA, 2 g over 3 h and intravenous SA, 1.8 g over 3 h in normal volunteers and found no changes in GFR (inulin clearance and creatinine clearance) or in RBF (clearance of PAH). It is noteworthy that ASA reduced urinary PGE_2 excretion by 60% whereas SA had no effect on urinary PGE_2. Lastly, Arroyo and his colleagues (1983), while studying patients with hepatic disease, also evaluated the effects of intravenous ASA in normal controls. Lysine ASA 450 mg (equivalent to 250 mg of ASA) administered intravenously did not reduce GFR despite significant reductions in urinary PGE_2 excretion. In summary, the majority of studies do not show any acute renal haemodynamic effects of ASA or SA in normal subjects.

SUBJECTS WITH RENAL/CARDIOVASCULAR DISEASE

Patients with cardiovascular, hepatic and renal disease, unlike normal subjects, do suffer decrements of renal function after the administration of ASA. Berg (1977) administered 750 mg of ASA i.v. to patients with chronic renal insufficiency and a mean GFR of 23 ml min^{-1}. Under these circumstances, GFR and RBF fell 35–50% over 90 min; these changes were totally reversible over 6–10 h. Kimberly et al (1978) studied women with systemic lupus erythematosus and only mild renal involvement. Treatment with 4.8 g of ASA per day (mean SA level 30 mg dl^{-1}) induced transient increments of blood urea nitrogen and serum creatinine accompanied by decrements of creatinine and inulin clearance (19% and 14%, respectively) as well as PAH clearance (29%). These changes were transient and reversible during a 3-day recovery period. Urinary excretion of PGE_2 decreased 45% over the course of ASA therapy. Studies by Arroyo et al. (1983) show that the effects of ASA on renal function in patients with liver disease are quite dramatic. Lysine ASA did not reduce renal function in patients with hepatic disease without ascites, but 11 of 19 ascitic patients showed a reduction of GFR from 95 ml min^{-1} to 47 ml min^{-1} after ASA. These patients with a reduction of GFR showed substantially greater decrements of urinary PGE_2 after ASA than did the patients with cirrhosis and ascites who showed no decrease of GFR. As will be discussed, in this setting the effects of SA may be uniquely different from those of ASA. Mirouze and coworkers (1983) found no change in GFR after 900 mg of ASA in cirrhotic patients, but comparing the effects of ASA to the effects of indomethacin and other non-steroidal anti-inflammatory drugs, it was clear that the deleterious renal effects of indomethacin are far greater than those of ASA in this clinical setting. Patients with cardiovascular disease, particularly with congestive heart failure, also show large decreases of GFR (41%) after intravenous administration of 1 g of ASA (Bock et al., 1986). However, patients recovering from a myocardial infarct who have stable cardiovascular function showed no changes of renal function during ASA therapy (30 mg three times daily over 7 days) (Lijnen et al., 1984).

Functional or haemodynamic acute renal failure after ASA/SA therapy in patients with cardiovascular, hepatic and renal disease is very rare. One case of acute renal failure after salsalate therapy in a 73-year-old woman with chronic renal failure and arteriosclerotic cardiovascular disease has been reported (Abraham and Stillman, 1987). Comprehensive reviews on the topic of non-steroidal anti-inflammatory drug-induced renal failure do not mention ASA as a cause of functional or haemodynamic reversible renal insufficiency (Dunn and Zambraski, 1980; Blackshear et al., 1983; Corwin and Bonventre, 1984; Pirson and van Ypersele de Strihou, 1986). Clearly, indomethacin, ibuprofen, naproxen and the other 'modern' inhibitors of PG synthesis are both more potent and, hence, involve more renal risk (Whelton et al., 1990; Sandler et al., 1991; Wagner, 1991). However, if ASA is administered intravenously in large doses, it is clear from the aforementioned studies that certain susceptible patients could suffer transient acute renal failure.

19.5.3   Effects on Electrolyte and Water Excretion

The effects of SA on water and electrolyte balance were studied by Hanzlik et al. (1917) who noted the development of oedema and weight gain in normal volunteers receiving large doses of SA. ASA 70 mg kg^{-1} of body weight for 1 day reduced urinary sodium excretion in the studies by Berg (1977) whereas Reimann et al. (1985) found no changes of either sodium or water excretion after either ASA or SA infusions over 3 h. Arroyo and colleagues (1983, 1986) have extensively evaluated the effects of intravenous lysine ASA on electrolyte excretion in normal volunteers as well as cirrhotic patients. Urine volume and sodium excretion did not change in normal subjects whereas similar doses of ASA reduced urine volume, free water clearance and sodium excretion in cirrhotic patients, particulary those with ascites. ASA may also interfere with the natriuretic effects of spironolactone both in normal volunteers (Tweeddale and Ogilvie, 1973) and in patients with cirrhosis and ascites (Mirouze et al., 1983). Berg (1977) has made similar observations in six patients with chronic renal failure who showed 60–70% reductions of urine volume and urinary sodium excretion after intravenous ASA. The natriuretic efficacy of furosemide is also attenuated by ASA therapy (Kimberly et al., 1978), however, these acute changes were transient and, after 7 days of ASA therapy in patients with SLE, free water clearance and sodium excretion had returned to normal. Patients in an intensive care setting, particularly those with cardiovascular disease, are also susceptible to ASA therapy as manifested by 50–80% reductions in water and sodium excretion (Bock *et al.*, 1986).

In summary, the effects of ASA on electrolyte and water excretion generally parallel those of the changes of RBF and GFR. The reductions of electrolyte excretion undoubtedly reflect both a reduction of filtered sodium and water combined with enhanced tubular reabsorption, secondary to the inhibition of PGE_2 synthesis.

19.5.4 Chronic Effects of Aspirin

Does chronic ASA therapy pose any increased risk of renal disease in rheumatoid arthritis patients? Autopsy series have noted microscopic evidence of renal papillary necrosis in 20–50% of patients with rheumatoid arthritis (Lawson and Maclean, 1966; Nanra and Kincaid-Smith, 1975). The New Zealand Rheumatism Study (1974) evaluated 763 rheumatoid arthritis patients and 145 osteo-arthritis patients who had received chronic ASA therapy. No evidence of chronic renal injury was found by examination of urine, serum urea, serum creatinine, and urine protein. Other reports have reached the same conclusion, namely that chronic ASA therapy in arthritic patients does not cause chronic renal disease (Macklon *et al.*, 1974; Akyol *et al.*, 1982). Emkey and Mills (1982) analysed 46 rheumatoid patients after 13–38 years of ASA therapy and segregated the cases into low (0–10 mg dl^{-1}) and high (11–30 mg dl^{-1}) plasma SA groups. There was little evidence of chronic renal disease and no differences of blood urea nitrogen (BUN), serum creatinine or urinalyses between the two groups. It should be noted that both groups had similar mean total doses of ASA (32 and 36 kg). Burry *et al.* (1976) reached similar conclusions, based upon measurements of GFR, protein excretion and urinalyses in 20 rheumatoid patients divided equally into high (14 kg) and low (0.125 kg) ASA groups. Bonney *et al.* (1986) evaluated 1468 patients with rheumatoid arthritis or osteo-arthritis who took daily therapeutic doses of either ASA, ibuprofen or oxaprozin. ASA dosages ranged from 2.6 to 3.9 g daily. There were no significant elevations of either BUN or creatinine in any of the ASA-treated patients and the incidence of potentially serious changes in renal function were 1% or less with the other non-steroidal anti-inflammatory drugs.

In summary, there are no persuasive data indicative of a 'chronic aspirin nephropathy' in patients who have been treated with kg of ASA over 10–20 years.

Chronic use of ASA combined with phenacetin undoubtedly plays a role in the genesis of analgesic nephropathy. Analgesic nephropathy defines a clinical and pathological picture of chronic interstitial nephritis, papillary necrosis, tubular atrophy with interstitial fibrosis, and eventual chronic renal failure (Murray and Goldberg, 1975; Kincaid-Smith, 1978; Gonwa *et al.*, 1981). This syndrome has not been definitively associated with ASA as a single drug whereas phenacetin or acetaminophen, combined with ASA, can cause analgesic nephropathy (Plotz and Kimberley, 1981). The tentative explanation for the deleterious interaction of ASA with phenacetin includes the PG inhibitory effects of ASA coupled with the direct tubular toxicity of phenacetin which is concentrated in the renal medulla. As discussed earlier, chronic ASA therapy may reduce renal medullary blood flow and potentiate phenacetin or acetaminophen-induced tubular damage.

19.6 NON-ACETYLATED SALICYLATES

In the literature, the terms aspirin (ASA) and SA are often used interchangeably, with comments referring to SA when aspirin was utilized, and vice versa. In the last few years it has become clear that non-acetylated SAs have many different properties from ASA. In terms of the kidney, in PG-dependent states the responses to ASA versus SA are significantly different, and some of the unique properties of SA warrant further study.

SA is clearly a 'renal PG- sparing' anti-inflammatory drug. Most of the studies in man have shown no significant decrease in renal PG excretion with SA (Reimann *et al.*, 1985; Rosenkranz *et al.*, 1986). Because of our interest in identifying an effective anti-inflammatory agent which does not adversely affect the kidney in PG-dependent states, a series of studies were undertaken to evaluate the effects of sodium salicylate on renal function in normal, sodium-depleted, and cirrhotic animals (Zambraski *et al.*, 1988a, b). In sodium-depleted dogs SA did not cause a significant fall in GFR, RBF or sodium excretion, responses that are always observed when indomethacin is administered. More importantly, as shown in Fig. 19.1, in groups of normal and common bile duct-ligated cirrhotic swine SA (40 mg kg^{-1} i.v.) did not cause any changes in RBF or GFR. In addition, in both groups SA caused a significant diuresis and natriuresis. In the six cirrhotic animals, four of whom had ascites, these effects of SA were seen despite the fact that PGE$_2$ excretion was significantly decreased. A natriuretic effect of SA has been reported in other animal studies (Ramsay and Elliott, 1967; Quintanilla and Kessler, 1973; Bartha and Hably, 1978), however, this effect has not been seen in man. Of note in Fig. 19.1 is the fact that renal PG inhibition with meclofenamate, administered after SA, did not cause a reduction of RBF or GFR in the cirrhotic animals. This may

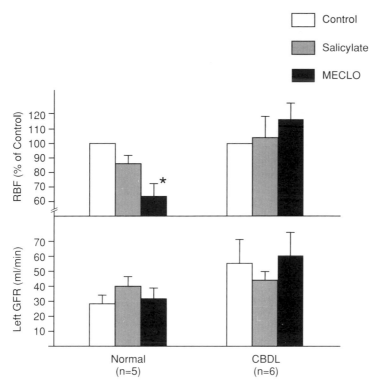

Figure 19.1 Effects of non-acetylated salicylate (40 mg kg^{-1} i.v.) and subsequent meclofenamate (MECLO) (2 mg kg^{-1} i.v.) on renal blood flow (RBF) and glomerular filtration rate (GFR) in normal and cirrhotic (CBDL) swine (*$P<0.05$ versus Control) (from Zambraski *et al.*, 1988b).

be due to an SA-mediated interference of meclofenamate's inhibition of cyclo-oxygenase.

These studies suggest that SA may offer a therapeutic advantage in treating patients who are in a renal PG-dependent state. This possibility has been supported by the very recent work of Antillon *et al.* (1989) who compared the effects of the non-acetylated SA, diflunisal, versus indomethacin in nine patients with alcoholic cirrhosis and ascites. A single dose of indomethacin caused a significant fall in GFR and PGE_2 excretion, and blunted the natriuretic response to furosemide. In contrast, with diflunisal there were no changes in GFR or PGE_2 excretion, and the natriuretic response to furosemide was unaltered. In these patients the extremely low basal sodium excretion (3 ± 1 mEq h^{-1}) was not changed by diflunisal.

For safety reasons, the study of Antillon *et al.* (1989) tested only

523

a single dose of diflunisal. Obviously, the effects of longer term non-acetylated SA treatment must be evaluated. In that regard, a very recent experiment in the authors' laboratory did evaluate the effects of 4 days of the non-acetylated salsalate (Disalcid), administered orally (1.5 g day^{-1}) in cirrhotic swine. Renal function tests performed at the end of the treatment period revealed no decrements in RBF or GFR. Urine flow rates and sodium excretion rates were at least twice that seen in another group of untreated cirrhotic swine.

Salicylate, especially when taken chronically and in large doses, clearly has the capacity to be nephrotoxic. These studies, however, showing the lack of an adverse renal effect of non-acetylated SA in cirrhotic subjects are extremely important. They clearly demonstrate that there is a requirement to differentiate between the renal effects of ASA versus non-acetylated SA.

19.7 SUMMARY

Under normal conditions, in healthy animals or man, intact renal PG synthesis is not necessary for the maintenance of renal function. Hence, the acute inhibition of renal PG synthesis by aspirin, or other compounds, does not adversely affect the kidney. In various diseases a state of PG dependence develops, due to either an increase in renal PG synthesis and/or increased PG attenuation of sympathetic or renin–angiotensin vasoconstrictor activity. In these situations there may be detrimental effects with aspirin, however, changes are clearly less severe than those seen with more effective PG synthesis inhibitors (i.e. non-steroidal anti-inflammatory drugs). Lastly, in PG-dependent disease states non-acetylated salicylates may have even less adverse renal effects than aspirin.

ACKNOWLEDGEMENT

The authors thank and acknowledge the secretarial assistance of Jan Houtman in the preparation of this chapter.

REFERENCES

Abraham, P.A. and Stillman, M.T. (1987) Salsalate exacerbation of chronic renal insufficiency. Relation to inhibition of prostaglandin synthesis. *Arch. Int. Med.*, **147**, 1674–6.

Akyol, S.M., Thompson, M. and Kerr, D.N.S. (1982) Renal function after prolonged consumption of aspirin. *Brit. Med. J.*, **284**, 631–2.

Anderson, W.P., Bartley, P.J., Casley, D.J. and Selig, S.E. (1983) Comparison of aspirin and indomethacin pretreatments on responses to reduced renal artery pressure in conscious dogs. *J. Physiol.* **336**, 101–12.

Antillon, M., Cominelli, F., Reynolds, T.B. and Zipser, R.D. (1989) Comparative acute effects of diflunisal and indomethacin on renal function in patients with cirrhosis and ascites. *Am. J. Gastroenterol.*, **84**, 153–5.

Arroyo, V., Planas, R., Gaya, J. *et al.* (1983) Sympathetic nervous activity, renin–angiotensin system and renal excretion of prostaglandin E_2 in cirrhosis. Relationship to functional renal failure and sodium and water excretion. *Eur. J. Clin. Invest.*, **13**, 271–8.

Arroyo, V., Gines, P., Rimola, A. and Gaya, J. (1986) Renal function abnormalities, prostaglandins, and effects of nonsteroidal anti-inflammatory drugs in cirrhosis with ascites. An overview with emphasis on pathogenesis. *Am. J. Med.*, **81 (2B)**, 104–22.

Barnett, R., Scharschmidt, L., Ko, Y.H. *et al.* (1987) Comparison of glomerular and mesangial prostaglandin synthesis and glomerular contraction in two rat models of diabetes mellitus. *Diabetes*, **36**, 1468–75.

Bartha, J. and Hably, C. (1978) Comparative study of the effects of indomethacin and sodium salicylate on the renal circulation. *Acta Physiol. Acad. Sci. Hung.*, **52**, 355–66.

Baylis, C. and Brenner, B.M. (1978) Modulation by prostaglandin synthesis inhibitors of the action of exogenous angiotensin II on glomerular ultrafiltration in the rat. *Circ. Res.*, **43**, 889–98.

Berg, K.J. (1977) Acute effects of acetylsalicylic acid in patients with chronic renal insufficiency. *Eur. J. Clin. Pharm.*, **11**, 111–16.

Bing, R.F., Russel, G.I., Thurston, H. *et al.* (1983) Chemical renal medullectomy. Effect on urinary PGE_2 and plasma renin in response to variations in sodium intake and in relation to blood pressure. *Hypertension*, **5**, 951–7.

Blackshear, J.L., Davidman, M. and Stillman, M.T. (1983) Identification of risk for renal insufficiency from nonsteroidal anti-inflammatory drugs. *Arch. Intern. Med.*, **143**, 1130–4.

Blasingham, M.C. and Nasjletti, A. (1980) Differential renal effects of cyclooxygenase inhibition in sodium-replete and sodium-deprived dog. *Am. J. Physiol*, **239**, F360–5.

Blasingham, M.C., Shade, R.E., Share, L. *et al.* (1980) The effect of meclofenamate on renal blood flow in the unanesthetized dog: Relation to renal prostaglandins and sodium balance. *J. Pharmacol. Exp. Ther.*, **214**, 1–4.

Bock, H.A., Frolich, J.C., Ritz, R. and Brunner, F.P. (1986) Effects of intravenous aspirin on prostaglandin synthesis and kidney function in intensive care patients. *Nephrol. Dial. Transplant*, **1**, 164–9.

Bonney, S.L., Northington, R.S., Hedrich, D.A. and Walker, B.R. (1986) Renal safety of two analgesics used over the counter: ibuprofen and aspirin. *Clin. Pharm. Ther.*, **40(4)**, 373–7.

Boyd, R.M., Nasjletti, A., Heerdt, P.M. and Baer, P.G. (1986) PGI_2 synthesis and excretion in dog kidney: evidence for renal PG compartmentalization. *Am. J. Physiol.*, **250**, F58–F65.

Bugge, J.F., Vikse, A., Dahl, E. and Kiil, F. (1987) Renal degradation and distribution between urinary and venous output of prostaglandins E_2 and I_2. *Acta Physiol. Scand.*, **130**, 467–74.

Unwanted effects

Burry, H.C., Dieppe, P.A., Bresnahand, F.B. and Brown, C. (1976) Salicylates in renal function and rheumatoid arthritis. *Brit. Med. J.*, **1**, 613–15.

Cadnapaphornchai, P., Aisenbrey, G., McDonald, K.M. *et al.* (1978) Prostaglandin-mediated hyperemia and renin-mediated hypertension during acute ureteral obstruction. *Prostaglandins*, **16**, 965–71.

Caterson, R.J., Duggin, G.G., Horvath, J. *et al.* (1978) Aspirin, protein transacetylation and inhibition of prostaglandin synthetase in the kidney. *Brit. J. Pharmac.*, **64**, 353–8.

Chaumet-Riffaud, P., Oudinet, J.P., Sraer, J. *et al.* (1981) Altered PGE_2 and $PGF_{2\alpha}$ production by glomeruli and papilla of sodium-depleted and sodium loaded rats. *Am. J. Physiol.*, **241**, F517–24.

Corwin, H.L. and Bonventre, J.V. (1984) Renal insufficiency associated with nonsteroidal anti-inflammatory agents. *Am. J. Kidney Dis.*, **4**(2), 147–52.

Currie, M.G, Cole, B.R., DeSchryver-Kecskemeti, K. *et al.* (1983) Cell culture of renal epithelium derived from rabbit microdissected cortical collecting tubules. *Am. J. Physiol.*, **244**, 724–8.

DeForrest, J.M., Davis, J.O., Freeman, R.H. *et al.* (1980) Effects of indomethacin and meclofenamate on renin release and renal hemodynamic function during chronic sodium depletion in conscious dogs. *Circ. Res.*, **47**, 99–107.

Dunn, M.J. (1983) Renal prostaglandins. In *Renal Endocrinology*, William and Wilkins, Baltimore, Maryland, pp. 1–74.

Dunn, M.J. and Zambraski, E.J. (1980) Renal effects of drugs that inhibit prostaglandin synthesis. *Kidney Int.*, **18**, 609–22.

Ecthenkamp, S.F., Davis, J.O., DeForrest, J.M. *et al.* (1981) Effects of indomethacin, renal denervation and propranolol on plasma renin activity in conscious dogs with chronic caval constriction. *Circ. Res.*, **49**, 492–500.

Emkey, R.D. and Mills, J.A. (1982) Aspirin and analgesic nephropathy. *J. Am. Med. Assoc.*, **247**, 55–7.

Farman, N., Pradelles, P. and Bonvalet, J.P. (1987) PGE_2, $PGF_{2\alpha}$, 6-keto-$PGF_{1\alpha}$, and TXB_2 synthesis along the rabbit nephron. *Am. J. Physiol.*, **252**, F53–9.

Gafni, Y. Schwartzman, M. and Raz, A. (1978) Prostaglandin biosynthesis in rabbit kidney medulla: inhibition *in vitro* vs. *in vivo* by aspirin, indomethacin and meclofenamic acid. *Prostaglandins*, **15**, 759–72.

Ganguli, M. Tobian, L., Ferris, T. *et al.* (1989) Acute prostaglandin reduction with indomethacin and chronic prostaglandin reduction with an essential fatty acid deficient diet both decrease plasma flow to the renal papilla in the rat. *Prostaglandins*, **38**, 3–19.

Gonwa, T.A., Hamilton, R.W. and Buckalew, V.M. Jr (1981) Chronic renal failure and end-stage renal disease in northwest North Carolina. Importance of analgesic-associated nephropathy. *Arch. Intern. Med.*, **4**, 462–5.

Goto, F., Jackson, E.K., Ohnishi, A. *et al.* (1987) Effect of cyclooxygenase and thromboxane synthase inhibition on the response to angiotensin II in the hypoperfused canine kidney. *J. Pharmacol. Exp. Ther.*, **243**, 799–803.

Hanzlik, P.J. and Karsner, H.T. (1917) The salicylates. VI. Renal functional and morphologic changes in animals following administration of salicylates. *Arch. Intern. Med.*, **19**, 1029–41.

Hanzlik, P.J., Scott, R.W. and Reycraft, J.L. (1917) The salicylates. VIII. Salicyl edema. *Arch. Intern. Med.*, **20**, 329–40.

Hassid, A., Konieczkowski, M. and Dunn, M.J. (1979) Prostaglandin synthesis in isolated rat kidney glomeruli. *Proc. Natl. Acad. Sci. USA*, **76**, 1155–9.

Henrich, W. (1981) Role of prostaglandins in renin secretion. *Kidney Int.*, **19**, 822–30.

Higa, E.M., Schor, N., Boim, M.A. *et al.* (1985) Role of the prostaglandin and kallikrein–kinin systems in aminoglycoside-induced acute renal failure. *Braz. J. Med. Biol. Res.*, **18**, 355–65.

Ichikawa, I. and Brenner, B.M. (1979) Local intrarenal vasoconstrictor–vasodilator interactions in mild partial ureteral obstruction. *Am. J. Physiol.*, **236**, F131–F40.

Izumi, Y., Franco-Saenz, R. and Mulrow, P.J. (1985) Effect of prostaglandin synthesis inhibitors on the renin–angiotensin system and renal function. *Hypertension*, **7**, 791–6.

Jensen, P.K., Steven, K., Blaehr, H. *et al.* (1986) Effects of indomethacin on glomerular hemodynamics in experimental diabetes. *Kidney Int.*, **29**, 490–5.

Kaizu, K., Marsh, D., Zipser, R. *et al.* (1985) Role of prostaglandins and angiotensin II in experimental glomerulonephritis. *Kidney Int.*, **28**, 629–35.

Kaufman, R.P. Anner, H., Kobzik, L. *et al.* (1987) Vasodilator prostaglandins (PG) prevent renal damage after ischemia. *Ann. Surg.*, **205**, 195–8.

Kimberly, R.P., Gill, J.R., Bowden, R.E. *et al.* (1978) Elevated urinary prostaglandins and the effects of aspirin on renal function in lupus erythematosus. *Ann. Intern. Med.*, **89**, 336–41.

Kincaid-Smith, P. (1978) Analgesic nephropathy. *Kidney Int.*, **13**, 1–4.

Kirschenbaum, M.A. and Chaudhari, A. (1986) Effect of experimental diabetes on glomerular filtration rate and glomerular prostanoid production in the rat. *Miner. Electrolyte Metab.*, **12**, 352–5.

Kirschenbaum, M.A. and Serros, E.R. (1981) Effect of prostaglandin inhibition on glomerular filtration rate in normal and uremic rabbits. *Prostaglandins*, **22**, 245–54.

Kramer, H.J. Stinnesbeck, B., Klautke, G. *et al.* (1985) Interaction of the renal prostaglandins with the renin–angiotensin and renal adrenergic nervous systems in healthy subjects during dietary changes in sodium intake. *Clin. Sci.*, **68**, 387–93.

Kreisberg, J.I. Karnovsky, M.J. and Levine, L (1982) Prostaglandin production by homogeneous cultures of rat glomerular epithelial and mesangial cells. *Kidney Int.*, **22**, 355–9.

Lawson, A.A. and Maclean, N. (1966) Renal disease and drug therapy in rheumatoid arthritis. *Ann. Rheum. Dis.*, **25**, 441–9.

Lianos, E.A., Andres, G.A. and Dunn, M.J. (1983) Glomerular prostaglandin and thromboxane synthesis in rat nephrotoxic serum nephritis. *J. Clin. Invest.*, **72**, 1439–48.

Lijnen, P., Boelaert, J., Van Eeghem, P. *et al.* (1984) Effect of aspirin on renal function and the prostaglandin–kallikrein systems early after myocardial infarction. *J. Cardiovasc. Pharm.*, **6**, 455–9.

Lockwood, T.D. and Bosmann, H.B. (1979) The use of urinary N-acetyl-B-glucosaminidase in human renal toxicology II. Elevations in humans and excretion after aspirin and sodium salicylate. *Toxicol. Appl. Pharmacol.*, **49**, 337–45.

Unwanted effects

Macklon, A.F., Craft, A.W., Thompson, M. and Kerr, D.N. (1974) Aspirin and analgesic nephropathy. *Brit. Med. J.*, **1**, 597–600.

McGiff, J.F. (1980) Interactions of prostaglandins with the kallikrein–kinin and renin–angiotensin systems. *Clin. Sci.*, **59**, 105s–16s.

Mirouze, D., Zipser, R.D. and Reynolds, T.B. (1983) Effect of inhibitors of prostaglandin synthesis on induced diuresis in cirrhosis. *Hepatology*, **3**, 50–5.

Moel, D.I., Safirstein, R.L., McEvoy, R.C. *et al.* (1987) Effect of aspirin on experimental diabetic nephropathy. *J. Lab. Clin. Med.*, **110**, 300–7.

Molland, E.A. (1978) Experimental renal papillary necrosis. *Kidney Int.*, **13**, 5–14.

Murray, T. and Goldberg, M. (1975) Analgesic abuse and renal disease. *Ann. Rev. Med.*, **26**, 537–50.

Muther, R. and Bennett, W. (1980) Effects of aspirin on glomerular filtration rate in normal humans. *Ann. Intern. Med.*, **92**, 386–7.

Nanra, R.S. and Kincaid-Smith, P. (1975) Renal papillary necrosis in rheumatoid arthritis. *Med. J. Aust.*, **1**, 194.

New Zealand Rheumatism Study (1974) Aspirin and the kidney. *Brit. Med. J.*, **1**, 593–6.

Oliver, J.A., Pinto, J., Sciacca, R.R., *et al.* (1980) Increased renal secretion of norepinephrine and prostaglandin E_2 during sodium depletion in the dog. *J. Clin. Invest.*, **66**, 748–56.

Oliver, J.A., Sciacca, R.R., Pinto, J. *et al.* (1981) Role of the prostaglandins in norepinephrine release during augmented renal sympathetic nerve activity in the dog. *Circ. Res.*, **48**, 835–43.

Oliw, E., Lunden, I. and Anggard, E. (1978) *In vivo* inhibition of prostaglandin synthesis in rabbit kidney by non-steroidal anti-inflammatory drugs. *Acta Pharmacol. Toxicol.*, **42**, 179–84.

Orloff, J. and Zusman, R. (1978) Role of prostaglandin E (PGE) in the modulation of action of vasopressin on water flow in the urinary bladder of the toad and mammalian kidney. *J. Membr. Biol.*, **40**, 297–304.

Patrono, C. and Dunn, M.J. (1987) The clinical significance of inhibition of renal prostaglandin synthesis. *Kidney Int.*, **32**, 1–12.

Petrulis, A.S., Aikawa, M. and Dunn, M.J. (1981) Prostaglandin and thromboxane synthesis by rat glomerular epithelial cells. *Kidney Int.*, **20**, 469–74.

Pirson, Y. and van Ypersele de Strihou, C. (1986) Nonsteroidal anti-inflammatory agents: Renal side effects of nonsteroidal anti-inflammatory drugs: clinical relevance. *Am. J. Kidney Dis.*, **VIII**(5), 338–44.

Plotz, P.H. and Kimberly, R.P. (1981) Acute effects of aspirin and acetaminophen on renal function. *Arch. Intern. Med.*, **141**, 343–8.

Podjarny, E., Rathaus, M., Pomeranz, A. *et al.* (1988) Prostanoids in renal failure induced by converting enzyme inhibition in sodium-depleted rats. *Am. J. Physiol.*, **254**, F358–63.

Prescott, L.F. (1965) Effects of ASA, phenacetin, paracetamol and caffeine on renal tubular epithelium. *Lancet*, **ii**, 91–5.

Quilley, C.P., McGiff, J.C. and Quilley, J. (1987) Failure of chronic aspirin treatment to inhibit urinary prostaglandin excretion in spontaneously hypertensive rats: comparison with indomethacin and flurbiprofen. *J. Pharmacol. Exp. Ther.*, **240**, 916–21.

Quintanilla, A. and Kessler, R.H. (1973) Direct effects of salicylate on renal function in the dog. *J. Clin. Invest.*, **52**, 3143–53.

Ramsay, A.G. and Elliott, H.C. (1967) Effect of acetylsalicylic acid on ionic reabsorption in the renal tubule. *Am. J. Physiol.*, **213**, 323–7.

Reimann, I.W., Golbs, E., Fischer, C. and Frolich, J.C. (1985) Influence of intravenous acetylsalicylic acid and sodium salicylate on human renal function and lithium clearance. *Eur. J. Clin. Pharmacol.*, **29**, 435–41.

Riegger, G.A., Eisner, D. and Kromer, E.P. (1989) Circulatory and renal control by prostaglandins and renin in low cardiac output dogs. *Am. J. Physiol.*, **256**, H1079–86.

Robert, M., Fellastre, J.P., Berger, H. and Malandain, H. (1972) Effects of intravenous infusion of acetylsalicylic acid on renal function. *Brit. Med. J.*, **2**, 466–7.

Rosenkranz, B., Fischer, C., Meese, C.O. *et al.* (1986) Effects of salicylic and acetylsalicylic acid alone and in combination on platelet aggregation and prostanoid synthesis in man. *Brit. J. Clin. Pharm.*, **21**, 309–17.

Salazar, F.J., Bolterman, R. and Fiksen-Olsen, M.J. *et al.* (1988) Role of prostaglandins in mediating the renal effects of atrial natriuretic factor. *Hypertension*, **12**, 274–8.

Sandler, D.P., Burr, R. and Weinberg, C.R. (1991) Nonsteroidal anti-inflammatory drugs and the risk for chronic renal disease. *Ann. Intern. Med.*, **115**, 165–71.

Scharschmidt, L.A. and Dunn, M.J. (1983) Prostaglandin synthesis by rat glomerular mesangial cells in culture. Effects of angiotensin II and arginine vasopressin. *J. Clin. Invest.*, **71**, 1756–64.

Schlondorff, D. and Ardaillou, R. (1986) Prostaglandins and other arachidonic metabolites in the kidney. *Kidney Int.*, **29**, 108–19.

Schlondorff, D., Aynedjian, H.S., Satriano, J.A. *et al.* (1987) *In vivo* demonstration of glomerular PGE$_2$ responses to physiological manipulations and experimental agents. *Am. J. Physiol.*, **252**, F717–23.

Scott, J.T., Denman, A.M. and Darling, J. (1963) Renal irritation caused by salicylates *Brit. Med. J.*, **1**, 344–8.

Sraer, J., Sraer, J.D., Chansel, D. *et al.* (1979) Prostaglandin synthesis by isolated rat renal glomeruli. *Molec. Cell Endocrinol.*, **16**, 29–37.

Sraer, J., Siess, W., Moulonguet-Doleris, L. *et al.* (1982) *In vitro* prostaglandin synthesis by various rat renal preparations. *Biochim. Biophys. Acta*, **15**, 45–52.

Stahl, R.A., Kudelka, S., Paravicini, M. *et al.* (1986) Prostaglandin and thromboxane formation in glomeruli from rats with reduced renal mass. *Nephron*, **42**, 252–7.

Tweeddale, M.G. and Ogilvie, R.I. (1973) Antagonism of spironolactone-induced natriuresis by aspirin in man. *New Engl. J. Med.*, **289**, 198–200.

Wagner, E.H. (1991) Nonsteroidal anti-inflammatory drugs and renal disease – still unsettled. *Ann. Intern. Med.*, **115**, 227–8.

Whelton, A., Stout, R.L., Spilman, P.S. and Klassen, D.K. (1990) Renal effects of ibuprofen, piroxicam and sulindac in patients with symptomatic renal failure. *Ann. Intern. Med.*, **112**, 568–76.

Zambraski, E.J. and Dunn, M.J. (1979) Renal prostaglandin E$_2$ secretion and excretion in conscious dogs. *Am. J. Physiol.*, **236**, F552–8.

Unwanted effects

Zambraski, E.J. and Dunn, M.J. (1984) Importance of renal prostaglandin in control of renal function after chronic ligation of the common bile duct in dogs. *J. Lab. Clin. Med.*, **103**, 549–59.

Zambraski, E.J., Chremos, A.N. and Dunn, M.J. (1984) Comparison of the effects of sulindac with other cyclooxygenase inhibitors on prostaglandin excretion and renal function in normal and chronic bile duct-ligated dogs and swine. *J. Pharmacol. Exp. Ther.*, **228**, 560–5.

Zambraski, E.J., Atkinson, D.C. and Diamond, J. (1988a) Effect of salicyclate vs. aspirin on renal prostaglandins and function in normal and sodium-depleted dogs. *J. Pharmacol. Exp. Ther.*, **247**, 96–103.

Zambraski, E.J., Guidotti, S., Atkinson, D.C. *et al.* (1988b) Salicylic acid causes a diuresis and natriuresis in normal and common bile duct-ligated cirrhotic miniature swine. *J. Pharmacol. Exp. Ther.*, **247**, 983–8.

Zusman, R.M. and Keiser, H.R. (1977) Prostaglandin biosynthesis by rabbit renomedullary interstitial cells in tissue culture. Stimulation by angiotensin II, bradykinin, and arginine vasopressin. *J. Clin. Invest.*, **60**, 215–23.

20 *Reye's Syndrome and aspirin*

A.P. MOWAT

20.1 INTRODUCTION

Reye's Syndrome is a rare, acute, sporadic liver disorder which presents as an encephalopathy. This clinico-pathological entity was first described by Reye and his colleagues in 1963. Since then an ever-increasing number of inherited metabolic disorders have been recognized as presenting with similar clinical features. The differential diagnosis also includes many acquired infectious or toxic conditions in which the liver and brain may be affected. In the cryptogenic variety the pathogenesis is unique. There is a severe self-limiting disturbance of hepatic mitochondrial structure with decreased mitochondrial enzymatic activity lasting up to 6 days. The function and structure of other subcellular organelles are unaffected. Similar structural changes may occur in muscle and neural tissue but are less well documented and mitochondrial enzymatic activity is relatively well preserved. There is no hepatocellular necrosis but marked microvesicular fat deposition occurs. An acute intense catabolic state aggravates the mitochondrial dysfunction and its sequelae.

Death or permanent brain damage is caused by cerebral oedema. The relationship between the liver lesion and the central nervous system manifestations is obscure. If cerebral oedema is controlled there is complete recovery. Unfortunately between 20 and 60% of recognized cases die. As many as 50% of survivors have permanent brain damage (Wood, 1988).

The cause of idiopathic Reye's Syndrome is unknown and how it develops is not clear but recent epidemiological and experimental studies have implicated aspirin ingestion as a possible contributory factor. In order to evaluate the evidence supporting this contention it is essential to be conversant with the main clinico-pathological features of this unusual syndrome and to consider the difficulties in reaching a precise diagnosis in a disorder with a marked range of severity.

531

20.2 CLINICAL FEATURES

20.2.1 Children and Adults

Reye's Syndrome has been recognized mainly in infants and children with only a few cases in adults. The clinical picture of Reye's Syndrome in the child and adult is similar (Ede and Williams, 1988). Typically it occurs in a child with a previously unremarkable medical history, during the recovery phase of what seems to be an unexceptional or ordinary viral infection. This may take the form of a respiratory or gastrointestinal tract infection or an exanthematous illness such as chicken pox (Glasgow, 1984).

The clinical features are dominated by pernicious vomiting and disturbed consciousness – the main signs of encephalopathy. Initially the neurological change is the onset of a quiet, withdrawn, unresponsive state or a confused, argumentative, combative one, with irrational behaviour, sometimes with visual hallucinations and agitated delirium. There are no focal neurological signs and no meningeal irritation. Ophthalmological features of increased intracranial pressure are rarely evident. Thirty percent of cases develop convulsions. In progressive cases deepening coma is associated with decerebrate posturing, opisthotonous, dilated, slowly responsive pupils, deep and rapid respiration and variations in pulse rate which precede a flaccid apnoeic state with fixed dilated pupils. The neurological status may stabilize or improve and recover completely, spontaneously or with therapy, at any stage short of brain death after an illness lasting from 6 hours to 5 days.

In contrast to the overt encephalopathy and vomiting the acute disturbance of liver function has little or no clinical features. It is suspected by the finding of disturbed coagulation (prolonged prothrombin time) and abnormal biochemical tests of liver function, particularly raised serum transaminases and ammonia, and hypoglycaemia. Hepatomegaly may be noted. Jaundice is very rare. If the patient does not die of cerebral oedema, laboratory evidence of liver involvement resolves within 4–6 days.

20.2.2 Infants

Infants with Reye's Syndrome have a somewhat different presentation. Initial features are respiratory, namely tachypnoea, respiratory distress, hyper-inflation and apnoea. There may be temperature instability. Seizures are more common but vomiting may be absent and is rarely pernicious. Hypoglycaemia and hepatomegaly are more commonly identified in infants than in older children. A history of preceding viral infection is less commonly obtained (Huttenlocher and Trauner, 1978). In this age group it is always essential to assume that an inborn error of metabolism is responsible for the features. Serum and urine collected at the time of presentation and stored at $-70\,°C$, may be invaluable in providing evidence for the diagnosis, particularly of organic acidurias and disorders of ketogenesis.

20.2.3 Hepatic Pathology

In the first 24 h after the onset of vomiting or neurological abnormalities hepatic abnormalities seen on light microscopy are limited to glycogen depletion and cytoplasmic swelling, most evident at the periphery of the hepatic lobule. In severe cases the glycogen depletion may be panlobular (Partin, 1988). If frozen sections are stained with Sudan Red, tiny lipid droplets are found throughout the hepatic parenchyma. These cannot be detected by stains performed on paraffin-fixed tissues. Over the course of 1–4 days the fat droplets coalesce and become evident as micro-vacuolization in the periphery of the hepatocytes. Hepatic necrosis is absent or minimal. In severe cases mild portal tract inflammation is evident.

Electron microscopy of liver tissues obtained early in the course of encephalopathy shows loss of glycogen, proliferation of the smooth endoplasmic reticulum and an increase in peroxisomes. The mitochondria are swollen, deformed and pleomorphic but at this stage still have an intact matrix. There may be proliferation of the smooth endoplasmic reticulum and an increase in peroxisomes. Ultrastructural alterations appear first in individual cells. Surrounding cells may be nearly normal. In comatose patients virtually all liver cells are affected. The mitochondrial matrix becomes less dense and disorganized. Some hepatocytes lose electron density except in residual bodies and peroxisomes. In fulminant cases such clear cells dominate the liver histology. The outer membranes of the mitochondria are often disrupted. After 4–5 days of the illness the mitochondrial injury resolves, glycogen is restored in those cells, small fat droplets coalesce to large globules. The ultrastructural diagnosis of Reye's syndrome is then impossible.

Histochemical techniques or biochemical assays show a severe reduction of all mitochondrial enzymes (e.g. cytochrome oxidase or succinate dehydrogenase) but cytoplasmic enzyme activity is normal. Within 4–7 days of onset enzymatic activity is restored.

20.2.4 Cerebral Lesions

In fatal cases the brain is swollen with flattened gyri and narrow sulci. There may be herniation of the brain stem through the foramen magnum and secondary compression. There is no significant inflammatory reaction in the brain or meninges. The cerebrospinal fluid is normal. Microscopic changes are secondary to cerebral oedema and hypoxia.

Ultrastructural studies of the few brain biopsies performed at the time of craniotomy, a manoeuvre used for alleviating severe cerebral oedema, have shown unusual diffuse neuronal mitochondrial swelling, somewhat similar to that seen in hepatocytes. Astrocytes are swollen, devoid of granules and vacuolated. Small blebs or vesicles may be found in the myelin sheath.

20.2.5 Skeletal Muscle

Glycogen deposition and fat deposition are apparent. The mitochondria show matrix expansion and a degree of pleomorphism (Partin, 1988).

20.2.6 Biochemical and Metabolic Features

Serum aspartate aminotransferase values are elevated to between 2 and 100 times normal. Hyperammonaemia with values at between 2 and 40 times the upper limit of normal is found in almost all cases except those with grade one encephalopathy. Its occurrence may be transient. Prothrombin time is prolonged, sometimes by a few seconds but in other instances coagulopathy may be severe. Hypoglycaemia occurs particularly in those of less than 2 years of age.

Massive tissue breakdown occurs in Reye's syndrome. Enormous losses of protein and nitrogen occur. Serum amino acids increase including substrates of the enzymes of the urea cycle. Amongst these is carbamyl phosphate. This diffuses from mitochondria into the cytoplasm where it is changed to orotic acid, a substance which, in some species at least, decreases lipoprotein synthesis and may thereby contribute to fatty acid retention within the liver.

Another important feature is increased lipolysis from adipose tissue stores. It is thought to be caused by a very high concentration of glucocorticoids, growth hormones and glucagon. Lipolysis causes high concentrations of fatty acids in serum and a raised serum glycerol level. The presentation of these to a liver incapable of fully metabolizing them may result in an accumulation of triglycerides in the parenchymal cells. There is frequently a defect in beta oxidation of fatty acids with accumulation of fatty acids and Co-A esters in plasma and liver. Omega oxidation may occur with the production of dicarboxylic acids. Long chain ones may aggravate the primary mitochondrial injury by acting as uncouplers of oxidative phosphorylation. Thus, mitochondrial energy production will be decreased together with the mitochondrial processes which are energy dependent.

The abnormal products of the amino acid or fatty acid metabolism may undergo reversible conjugation with glycine and carnitine. Relative carnitine deficiency may develop further impairing fatty acid transfer into mitochondria and thereby further decreasing energy production (Crocker, 1982; Kilpatrick-Smith et al., 1989).

The precise role and pathogenesis of the many metabolic aberrations reported in children with this syndrome is at present not unravelled. The confusion may be due to observers failing to relate the findings to the stage of the disease. In addition, there may be very different metabolic effects depending on the relative degree of hepatic impairment and the amount of tissue destruction and catabolism. Undoubtedly, an important factor in the pathogenesis of Reye's syndrome is the transient depression of mitochondrial function. It is important to remember that mitochondria contain enzymes that are essential in such pathways of intermediate metabolism as urea synthesis, gluconeogenesis, organic acid oxidation and oxidative phosphorylation. In addition, efficient mitochondrial function is required for drug detoxification. The mechanism underlying this is unclear. There is no evidence of a defect in biosynthesis. There is some experimental evidence which suggests that dicarboxylic acids could aggravate mitochondrial dysfunction and modify mitochondrial structure.

20.3 AETIOLOGICAL CONSIDERATIONS

20.3.1 Epidemiological Problems

All epidemiological studies of the syndrome are severely limited by four factors (Sullivan-Bolya and Corey, 1981; Anon, 1982; Kilpatrick-Smith et al., 1989).

1. Lack of a specific practical diagnostic laboratory test, positive at all stages of the illness and in all grades of severity.

As a result epidemiologists have had to use relatively non-specific measures for case definition, namely encephalopathy of unknown cause with no sign of infection or inflammation in the central nervous system in the presence of raised serum transaminases, blood ammonia or refined fatty infiltration in liver biopsy. There should be no other reasonable explanation for the condition.

Diagnostic criteria on which epidemiological data depend fall into three levels of specificity. Least specific is a typical clinical illness with abnormal biochemical tests of liver function. Second is such an illness with, in addition, the demonstration of microvesicular fat accumulation in hepatocytes. The most specific are these features with, in addition, the characteristic structural and enzymatic changes in liver mitochondria.

The vast majority of cases in epidemiological studies are in the least specific diagnostic category. Very few of the reported cases of Reye's syndrome have had the necessary highly technical diagnostic investigations to identify inborn errors of metabolism such as urea cycle defects and recently recognized disorders such as defects in fatty acid oxidation. Relatively few have had electron microscopy of liver mitochondria in the acute phase.

2. Epidemiologists must rely on voluntary reporting of cases.
3. Retrospective case control studies.

   The low incidence, between 0.2 and 4.0 cases per 100,000 aged 17 years and less, has resulted in all epidemiological studies being retrospective. Usually they take the form of case control studies. Biases are difficult to avoid in such studies, even with meticulous planning, and well-trained investigators.
4. Grade 1 cases with minimal evidence of encephalopathy.

   A further problem came to light during prospective studies (Heubi *et al.*, 1984) in an area with a very high public and professional awareness of Reye's Syndrome. Investigators at Cincinnati Children's Hospital, during periods when Reye's Syndrome occurred commonly in their community, studied 85 children with a preceding viral upper respiratory tract infection or chicken pox and vomiting, who had on investigation a three-fold aspartate aminotransferase but none of the neurological features of Reye's Syndrome, other than being quiet or withdrawn. On percutaneous liver biopsy, typical liver mitochondrial changes of Reye's Syndrome were observed. The severity of change in the liver mitochondria and the degree of decrease and histochemical evidence of enzymatic activity in the mitochondria was no less than that observed in children with deep coma. Of the 83 patients treated only with glucose and electrolyte infusion, only five progressed to a deeper grade of coma. These five had significant elevation of blood ammonia or prolongation of the prothrombin time at presentation. Had these children not presented to investigators who were studying this disorder prospectively, it is very unlikely that the diagnosis of Reye's Syndrome would have been considered and it certainly would not have been confirmed. Such cases do not appear in most epidemiological surveys.

20.3.2 Current Hypothesis

The epidemiological information on which current aetiological hypotheses are based must therefore be viewed with some reservation

(Anon., 1982; Kilpatrick-Smith *et al.*, 1989). It is a very rare sequela of common viral infections. The sex incidence is equal. The geographical distribution is worldwide. Case prevalence may be increased in rural and suburban areas. The frequency of recognition of cases in any one area increases from time to time, sometimes in relation to epidemics of viral infection, particularly influenza.

Experimental studies are limited by the absence of an animal model which accurately mimics the idiopathic disorder in man.

Both epidemiological and experimental studies in small laboratory rodents suggest that Reye's Syndrome is a stereotypic reversible reaction in mitochondria arising from an interaction of viral and toxic environmental factors in the developing child. Genetic factors have been implicated. Starvation may aggravate the pathological process.

20.3.3 Viral Factors in the Aetiology

Reye and his colleagues found no clear evidence of current infection in their cases. Since then at least 19 different viruses have been implicated in the prodromal illness (Sullivan-Boya and Corey, 1981; Crocker, 1982; Kilpatrick-Smith *et al.*, 1989). They include examples of the major groups of DNA and RNA viruses, with the sole exception of measles, and live viral vaccines. Influenza B, influenza A and varicella, having easily recognizable epidemiological or clinical features, are most commonly implicated, with estimated attack rates of 50, 3 and 0.3 per 100 000 cases respectively. Viruses are rarely recovered from affected tissues. Should we now be looking for other viruses or other infectious agents? Could Reye's Syndrome be produced by a virus such as the HIV virus? Could an incomplete virus cause it? An example of such a virus is the Delta virus, a small RNA virus which can only function if the hepatitis B virus supplies it with a coat. Delta virus causes severe hepatitis in those infected with hepatitis B. Do we need to consider something of the nature of a bacteriophage, since mitochondria have features of bacteria?

Could the connection with viral infection be related to exogenous factors influencing the immunological response? This is a complex process involving the co-ordinate action of a whole host of cells in the immune system. Many details of their interaction are poorly understood. The sera of patients with Reye's Syndrome have both complement and fibronectin depletion. Interferon production by the lymphocytes is decreased. Whether these immune changes are primary or secondary is unclear (Mowat, 1988). There have, to my knowledge, been no studies of the other intracellular messengers such as interleukin-2, interleukin-1 or leukotrienes in Reye's Syndrome.

20.3.4 Genetic factors

As stated above an increasing range of metabolic/genetic disorders may mimic Reye's Syndrome (Table 20.1). Such metabolic abnormalities may present in one sibling as Reye's Syndrome but in another as sudden infant death syndrome (Roe *et al.*, 1986). Urea cycle defects or organic aciduria defects in fatty acid oxidation may present in an episodic fashion, symptoms often presenting after viral infection and aggravated by fasting (Roe, 1987). In both Reye's Syndrome and these disorders secondary deficiency of carnitine can occur with accumulation of metabolites which form toxic CoA compounds.

There may be an additional load on glycine conjugation, a process which requires ATP and CoA. Aspirin is metabolized by conjugation with glycine. It has a higher affinity for the conjugating enzyme than many of the endogenous products that accumulate in genetic disorders such as valeric acidaemia and can accumulate in Reye's Syndrome particularity if there is relative deficiency of carnitine (Krieger and Tanaka, 1976). Thus it can be speculated that aspirin given to a child with relative carnitine deficiency (carnitine production is increased in Reye's Syndrome) could change what had been a potential Grade 1 Reye's Syndrome into a more severe grade which would be more easily recognizable clinically.

20.3.5 Drugs and Toxins Modifying the Response to Viral Infection

Exogenous chemical factors implicated with varying degrees of frequency include aspirin, aflatoxin, latex paints, pesticides, pesticide emulsifiers, insect repellents, paracetamol (acetaminophen), pteridines, isopropyl alcohol, margosa oil (Azadriachta indica) and products of akee fruits (*Blighia sapida*), including hypoglycin A and 4-pentaenoic acid (Sullivan-Boyla and Corey, 1981; Crocker, 1982; Kilpatrick-Smith *et al.*, 1989). The evidence associating any of these with Reye's Syndrome is at present contentious.

20.4 EVIDENCE LINKING ASPIRIN ADMINISTRATION DURING THE PRODROMAL ILLNESS TO REYE'S SYNDROME

The evidence for this takes four forms.

20.4.1 Epidemiological Evidence

Four case control studies from North America have shown that patients with Reye's Syndrome had taken aspirin significantly more frequently,

Table 20.1 Genetic disorders mimicking Reye's Syndrome

Defects in mitochondrial fatty acid oxidation (Acyl-CoA
  dehydrogenase deficiency) . . . 6 forms
Organic acidurias
Urea cycle defects
Disorders of branch-chain amino acid metabolism
Systemic carnitine deficiency
Fructosaemia
Familial erythrophagocytic reticulosis
Cystic fibrosis

---

prior to, or early in, the illness, than had controls with prodromal illnesses that were similar (Centres for Disease Control, 1980; Starko *et al.*, 1980; Halpin *et al.*, 1982; Waldman *et al.*, 1982). These studies were severely criticized because of bias in case and control selection and in data collection (Brown *et al.*, 1983).

To resolve these difficulties and to determine any implication of medication in Reye's Syndrome, a Task Force was formed by the US Public Health Service with the help of an advisory board from the Institute of Medicine of the National Academy of Sciences. Its remit was to develop and test techniques that would avoid the major methodological defects in these earlier studies. They concluded that a strong statistical association was observed with the ingestion of salicylates, mainly aspirin, in the antecedent illness of Reye's Syndrome. It should be noted, however, that in the pilot study (Hurwitz *et al.*, 1985) there were 30 patients with 145 controls, while in the main study (Hurwitz *et al.*, 1987) there were only 27 patients and 140 controls, although it had been envisaged in the study protocol that 100 or 200 patients would be required. The study was stopped prematurely because of the increasing rarity of Reye's Syndrome in the USA and the consequent expense and difficulty in enrolling additional patients in a reasonable period of time. Even with the skills and resources available to the Task Force, essential biases remain in these studies (Kang *et al.*, 1986). Widespread knowledge of the association may have led to preferential diagnosis and reporting of cases with the diagnostic criteria and a history of aspirin ingestion; parents, guardians, or children themselves may, with litigation in mind, have reported aspirin ingestion once they knew the diagnosis. A further problem is that the diagnostic criteria used in these studies were relatively non-specific and could have led to the inclusion of children with distinct genetic metabolic disorders. This criticism is particularly pertinent since in the two Task Force reports only 15 patients (27%) had histological support for the diagnosis in the form of microvesicular lipid accumulations in the liver, a non-specific finding for which there are many other causes. It is not stated if the specific mitochondrial abnormality was demonstrated on electron microscopy in any of the cases; nor is it clear what steps were taken to exclude genetic disorders.

In a further attempt to confirm the validity of the aspirin/Reye's Syndrome association another even more thorough epidemiological study was undertaken to minimize five potential sources of bias (Forsyth *et al.*, 1989). The investigation showed that case control studies could adhere more closely to the principles of experimental research than had previously been considered possible if given careful planning and much resources. Reporting bias, for example, was assessed by blanket surveillance of 112 non-tertiary hospitals in five New England States over a 10-month period. Clinicians in these hospitals were telephoned every 2 weeks and asked to report any subject under 18 years of age with suspected Reye's Syndrome, profuse vomiting or altered mental status. None of the eight potential cases, when reviewed by experts, met the study's definition of Reye's Syndrome. To minimize diagnostic suspicion bias, 64 distinctive diagnostic codes encompassing all likely clinical presentations of Reye's Syndrome were used in the initial triage of the medical records of subjects 18 years and younger discharged from 27 paediatric units in a 3-month period. In the 282 records retrieved, 150 patients were found to have had vomiting or signs of encephalopathy in the 48 h prior to admission. Three paediatric experts concluded that Reye's Syndrome should have been considered in 13. Eleven of the 13 had ammonia levels or liver transaminases measured. Since only two of 150 had not had appropriate tests for Reye's Syndrome the authors concluded that bias related to differing degrees of diagnostic suspicion was unlikely to be a major source of error in the study. Similarly stringent measures were taken to overcome potential bias due to the severity of the prodromal illness, disease susceptibility, the time of administration of medication and recall of medications used.

Between February 1986 and August 1987, 129 patients meeting the eligibility criteria were reported from 108 paediatric centres with intensive care facilities in North America. Sixty-three of the patients fulfilled the screening criteria. On review of all the clinical data except the drug history, 24 were classified as definite Reye's Syndrome. Only two of the cases were less than 4 years of age. Five had grade 1 disease. Five died. Eight had undergone liver biopsies. Twelve had urine, collected early in the illness, examined by gas chromatography and fast atom bombardment-mass spectrometry. Given the tremendous epidemiological effort of the study it is almost churlish to comment that it is not clear whether these 12 include any of the 8 who had liver biopsies. Nor is it stated how many of the biopsies had the typical electron microscopic or enzymatic studies. Be that as it may, 21 (88%) of the 24 cases had taken aspirin in the prodromal illness as compared with 8 (17%) of the 48 matched controls. Thus an odds ratio (OR) for an association between aspirin use and Reye's Syndrome was calculated as 35. The OR increased to 106 in the 8 who had large doses of aspirin (>70 mg kg^{-1}). In contrast paracetamol (acetaminophen) was used by 38% of cases and 71% of controls (OR 0.16).

In the UK a system of surveillance of Reye's Syndrome was initiated in 1981 with paediatricians notifying cases to the Communicable Disease Surveillance Centre. Active ascertainment was introduced in July 1986. The epidemiology of Reye's Syndrome differs from that in the USA in that the median age of cases was 14 months as opposed to 11 years and there is no clear association with influenza (Hall, 1986). A case-comparison study suggested that an association between Reye's Syndrome and aspirin may exist, 59% of cases having taken aspirin as compared to 26% in the comparison group (Hall et al., 1988). Eighty percent of the cases had taken aspirin in previous febrile illness without ill effect. In contrast, an epidemiological study in Japan failed to confirm the association (Yamashita et al., 1985).

Further data cited as evidence in support of an association between salicylate and Reye's Syndrome include the occurrence of the syndrome amongst children on long-term salicylate therapy for connective tissue disorders (Rennebohm et al., 1985).

In spite of flaws in the epidemiological evidence, government agencies in many developed countries in the mid-1980s took measures to limit the use of aspirin in children aged 12 or less except when specifically indicated for chronic rheumatic disorders. There was little reason to challenge these decisions, since there is equally no evidence that aspirin or any other antipyretic provides anything other than symptomatic relief.

In the USA where surveillance began in 1974 the annual number of reported cases fell from a peak of 550 cases in 1980 to 20 in 1988 (Anon., 1989). In the UK the peak number of 79 cases occurred in 1983/4, falling to 19 in 1988/9 (Porter et al., 1990), during which time the frequency of aspirin use as an antipyretic decreased significantly. In part the fall in the number of cases may be due to improved recognition of metabolic disorders which mimic Reye's. This seems unlikely since the median age of cases reported in 1988/89 is only 8 months. It is more probable that investigations for metabolic disorders are not being performed in these children.

In the USA where the fall in the reported incidence of Reye's

Syndrome was paralleled by a decrease in aspirin use it was suggested that the two observations were directly related. This author suspects that this may be only one factor. It should be noted that a review of autopsy files in major children's hospitals for the years prior to 1960 revealed very few cases (Sullivan-Bolya and Corey, 1981). It is difficult to believe, with the very gross post-mortem findings, that an incidence similar to what it seems to have been in the 1970s and early 1980s when several thousand cases were identified in voluntary notification schemes, could have been completely missed up to then. Did aspirin administration to children increase in the period between 1960 and 1980? There is no evidence that aspirin overdosage became more common then. We should consider the possibility that the degree of exposure to another noxious exogenous agent or agents might better fit the apparent frequency of the disorder.

20.4.2 Histopathological Evidence

The second piece of evidence relating aspirin to Reye's Syndrome was the finding of apparent histopathological similarities between liver changes in Reye's Syndrome and those associated with salicylate poisoning. This was not confirmed in a subsequent study (Partin *et al.*, 1984).

20.4.3 Serum Salicylate Levels

The third piece of evidence, elevated serum salicylate levels in Reye's Syndrome, was based on non-specific techniques and was not confirmed with appropriate methodology (Partin *et al.*, 1982). Cases of fully confirmed Reye's Syndrome do occur in which there is no evidence of aspirin ingestion.

20.4.4 Experimental Studies

The final evidence is derived from experimental studies. An apparent concentration of cases of Reye's Syndrome in an area of Canada that had recently been heavily sprayed with insecticide was followed by an interesting series of experimental studies in young mice (Rozee *et al.*, 1982). An encephalopathy with fatty infiltration of the viscera and similar biochemical changes in the serum to those of Reye's Syndrome was produced in mice to which dicophane (DDT) and fenitrothion (an organophosphate) had been applied topically prior to exposure to sublethal doses of an encephalomyocarditis virus. Subsequent studies showed that pesticide emulsifiers such as polyoxyethylene were the active agent. Neither the agent nor the virus alone caused similar pathological features. Using a similar model, Hug and co-workers (1981) produced a Reye-like lesion with 'Atlox' or with butylated hydroxytoluene, but not with salicylate, fructose or pentachlorophenol.

The pesticide emulsifier Toximul in dilution of 1/10 000 000 increases viral plaque formation in Hela cell culture (Rozee et al., 1979). Using a mouse-adapted human influenza B virus in the presence of surfactant it was possible to produce mitochondrial dysfunction in young mice, but without the fatty liver or the free fatty acidaemia that is characteristic of Reye's Syndrome. If aspirin was added as a co-factor, it caused early death but did not increase the overall mortality (Crocker et al., 1986; Murphy et al., 1986). Studies in mice aged 2 weeks show that pretreatment with either aspirin or paracetamol (acetaminophen) followed by exposure to polyoxyethylene and modified influenza B virus produced a marked increase in mortality compared with those not pretreated. In mice of 5 weeks of age pretreatment did not increase mortality. In a study using one specific genetic strain of mice, pretreatment with paracetamol followed by influenza B infection caused liver cell necrosis, but, when an inducer of mixed function oxidase was given prior to infection, the animals developed fatty livers similar to those of Reye's Syndrome (McDonald et al., 1984). A spontaneous animal model of Reye's Syndrome has been observed in young adult mice with enteritis caused by a coronavirus (hepatitis, minute virus, or rotavirus), but this has not been reproduced experimentally (Brownstein et al., 1984). In 5-week-old chicks a diet high in carbohydrates and low in fats and protein can produce a fatty liver with features similar to Reye's Syndrome (Bannister and Cleland, 1977). In young ferrets with hyperammonaemia due to an arginine-deficient diet, the severity of encephalopathy is increased by both aspirin administration and viral infection (Deshmuk et al., 1983).

Sublethal endotoxin doses given to rats in whom fibronectin has been depleted by fasting or by intravenous gelatin, give rise to the metabolic and histological features of Reye's Syndrome. The addition of aspirin enhances the effect of endotoxin, producing both a fall in ketones and the same pattern of hepatic acyl-CoA esters as seen in Reye's Syndrome. One possible mechanism for this effect of aspirin may be by stimulating the release from macrophages of cytokines, particularly tumour necrosis factor. Both interleukin-1 and tumour necrosis factor inhibit beta-oxidation of fatty acids, causing both an increase in potentially toxic acyl-CoA intermediates and decreased ATP production, particularly in the fasted state (Kilpatrick-Smith et al., 1989). The effect of fasting has also been demonstrated in the response of rats to intraperitoneal injection of pentaenoic acid, an

543

in-vitro inhibitor of mitochondrial fatty acid oxidation (Thayer, 1984). Rats fasted for 48 h develop microvesicular fatty infiltration and *in-vitro* studies on mitochondria are consistent with inhibition of fatty acid beta oxidation at the level of acyl-CoA dehydrogenase. Animals not fasted did not show this response (Deshmuk *et al.*, 1983). In healthy adult volunteers a single dose of aspirin did not decrease blood 3-hydroxybutyrate concentrations either in the fed or fasted state. In contrast a single dose of sodium valproate in healthy fasted subjects caused a 75% decrease in blood 3-hydroxybutyrate concentrations due to an inhibition of beta-oxidation of fatty acids (Williams *et al.*, 1990). In Reye's Syndrome the fatty acid and CoA ester profiles in plasma and liver are compatible with a block in beta-oxidation of fatty acids (Martens and Lee, 1984). Plasma from Reye's Syndrome patients causes inhibition of oxidation of NAD^+-linked substrates by isolated mitochondria. There is a calcium-dependent increase in permeability of mitochondrial membranes with depletion of intramitochondrial NAD^+. Whether these effects are secondary to fasting, vomiting and the marked metabolic derangements of Reye's Syndrome or precede these features, is at present unknown. With intact rat liver mitochondria preparations, allantoin, the oxidation product of uric acid and Ca^{2+}, induced respiratory inhibition with respect to NAD^+-linked substrate. Very low concentrations of salicylate and Ca^{2+} had a similar effect, appearing to induce increased permeability of the inner mitochondrial membrane. Studies using isolated hepatic mitochondria from chinchillas, which lack uricase and thus do not produce allantoin, suggest that the mitochondrial perturbation is caused directly by dicarboxylic acids (Tonsgard and Getz, 1985). Dicarboxylic acids amount to as much as 54% of the total free fatty acids in Reye's Syndrome serum.

Their origin is not clear. They are the products of omega-oxidation in microsomes and appear during starvation and in disorders in which beta-oxidation is impaired. Tonsgard (1985, 1989) hypothesized that dicarboxylic acids, particularly long-chain ones, have a key role in the pathophysiology of Reye's Syndrome by acting as uncouplers of oxidative phosphorylation and thus reducing mitochondrial energy production and those mitochondrial processes depending on it. Both dicarboxylic acids and serum from patients with Reye's Syndrome cause similar enlargement of isolated hepatic mitochondria. Moreover, aspirin is a potent inducer of omega-oxidation (Kundu *et al.*, 1991).

The animal studies referred to above provide examples of the adverse effects of exogenous factors on the response to viral infection in the growing animal, effects that are aggravated by dietary factors and, particularly, by starvation. Just how these chemicals interact with viruses to cause functional or structural changes in mitochondria, either directly or via an effect on the immune system, is at present unclear.

With the above reservations, information from both epidemiological and experimental studies is compatible with the hypothesis that 'cryptogenic' Reye's Syndrome arises from an unusual response to viral infection, possibly determined by host genetic factors but modified by a range of exogenous agents of which aspirin could be one. It must remain an open question whether aspirin acts alone or requires some additional factor such as an emulsifier or insecticide. It is hard to challenge the conclusion of Dr Susan Hall and her co-workers (1988), 'If aspirin has an aetiological role there must be an exceptional unpredictable combination of circumstances that act as trigger'.

ACKNOWLEDGEMENT

The author is grateful to Sue Williams for typing the manuscript.

REFERENCES

Anon. (1982) Reye's syndrome – epidemiological considerations. *Lancet*, **i**, 941–3.

Anon. (1989) Reye's syndrome surveillance – United States, 1987 and 1988. *MMWR*, **18**, 325–7.

Bannister, DW, and Cleland, MA. (1977) The biochemistry of fatty liver and kidney of *Gallus domesticus*, reduced gluconeogenesis from precursors that are independent of pyruvate carboxylase. *Int. J. Biochem*, **8**, 569–75.

Brown, A.K., Fikrig, S. and Findberg, L. (1983) Aspirin and Reye's syndrome. *J. Pediatr.*, **102**, 157–78.

Brownstein, D.G., Johnson, E.A. and Smith, A.L. (1984) Spontaneous Reye's-like syndrome in BALB/cByl mice. *Lab. Invest*, **51**, 386–95.

Centres for Disease Control (1980) Reye's syndrome – Ohio, Michigan. *MMWR*, **29**, 537–9.

Crocker, J.F. (1982) Reye's syndrome. *Sem. Liv. Dis.*, **2**, 240–52.

Crocker, J.F.S., Renton, K.W., Lee, S.H. *et al.* (1986) Biochemical and morphological characteristics of a mouse model of Reye's syndrome induced by the interaction of influenza B virus and a chemical emulsifier. *Lab. Invest.*, **54**, 32–40.

Deshmuk, D.R., Deshmuk, G.D., Shope, T.C. and Radin, N.S. (1983) Free fatty acids in an animal model of Reye's syndrome. *Biochim. Biophys. Acta*, **573**, 153–8.

Ede, R.J. and Williams, R. (1988) Reye's syndrome in adults. *Brit. Med. J.*, **296**, 518–19.

Forsyth, B.W., Horwitz, R.I., Acamora, D. *et al.* (1989) New epidemiologic evidence confirming that bias does not explain the aspirin/Reye's syndrome association. *J. Am. Med. Assoc.*, **261**, 2517–24.

Glasgow, J.F.T. (1984) Clinical features and prognosis of Reye's syndrome. *Arch. Dis. Child.*, **59**, 230–5.

Unwanted effects

Hall, S.M. (1986) Reye's syndrome and aspirin. A review. J.R. *Soc. Med.*, **79**, 596–8.

Hall, S.M., Plaster, P.A., Glasgow, J.F.T. and Hancock, P. (1988) Preadmission antipyretics in Reye's syndrome. *Arch. Dis. Child.*, **63**, 857–66.

Halpin, T.J., Holtzhauer, F.J., Campbell, R.J. *et al.* (1982) Reye's syndrome and medication use. *J. Am. Med. Assoc.*, **248**, 687–91.

Heubi, J.E., Daugherty, C.C., Partin, J.S., *et al.* (1984) Grade 1 Reye's syndrome – outcome and predictors of progression to deeper coma grades. *N. Engl. J. Med.*, **311**, 1539–42.

Hug, G., Bosken, J., Bove, K. *et al.* (1981) Reye's syndrome simulacra in liver of mice after treatment with chemical agents and encephalomyocarditis virus. *Lab. Invest.*, **45**, 89–109.

Hurwitz, E.S., Barrett, M.J., Bergman, D. *et al.* (1985) Public health service study on Reye's syndrome and medications. Report of the pilot phase. *N. Engl. J. Med.*, **313**, 849–57.

Hurwitz, E.S., Barrett, M.J., Bergman, D. *et al.* (1987) Public health service study on Reye's syndrome and medication. *J. Am. Med. Assoc.*, **257**, 1905–11.

Huttenlocher, P.R. and Trauner, D.A. (1978) Reye's syndrome in infancy. *Pediatrics*, **62**, 84–90.

Kang, A.S., Crocker, J.F.S. and Johnson, G.M. (1986) Reye's syndrome and salicylates. *N. Engl. J. Med.*, **314**, 920–1.

Kilpatrick-Smith, L., Hale, D.E. and Douglas, S.D. (1989) Progress in Reye syndrome: epidemiology, biochemical mechanism and animal models. *Dig. Dis.*, **7**, 135–46.

Krieger, I. and Tanaka, K. (1976) Therapeutic effects of glycine in isovalericacidemia. *Pediatr. Res.*, **10**, 25–8.

Kundu, R.K., Tonsgard, J.H. and Getz, G.S. (1991) Induction of omega-oxidation of monocarboxylic acids in rats by acetylsalicylic acid. *J. Clin. Invest.*, **88**, 1865–72.

McDonald, M.G., McGrath, P.P., McMartin, D.N. *et al.* (1984) Potentiation of the toxic effects of acetaminophen in mice by concurrent infection with influenza B virus: a possible mechanism for human Reye's syndrome? *Pediatr. Res.*, **18**, 181–7.

Martens, M.E. and Lee, C.P. (1984) Reyes syndrome. Salicylates and mitochondrial functions. *Biochem. Pharmacol.*, **33**, 2869–76.

Mowat, A.P. (1988) Endogenous factors in Reye' syndrome. In *Reye's Syndrome* – Royal Society of Medicine Round Table Symposium, No. 8 (ed. C. Wood), Royal Society of Medicine, London.

Murphy, M.G., Archambault-Schertzer, L., Ackman, R.G. and Crocker, J.F.S. (1986) Serum lipid abnormalities in a chemical/viral mouse model of Reye's syndrome. *Lipids*, **21**, 37–82.

Partin, J.S. (1988) The ultrastructural changes in the liver, muscle and brain in Reye's syndrome. In *Reye's Syndrome* – Royal Society of Medicine Round Table Symposium, No. 8, (ed. C. Wood), Royal Society of Medicine, London.

Partin, J.S., Partin, J.C., Schubert, W.K. and Hammond, J.G. (1982) Serum salicylate concentrations in Reye's disease. A study of 130 biopsy-proven cases. *Lancet*, **i**, 191–4.

Partin, J.S., Daugherty, C.C., McAdams, A.J. *et al.* (1984) A comparison of liver ultrastructure in salicylate intoxication and Reye's syndrome. *Hepatology,* **4**, 687–90.

Porter, J.D.H., Robinson, P.H., Glasgow, J.F.T. *et al.* (1990) Trends in the incidence of Reye's syndrome and the use of aspirin. *Arch. Dis. Child.,* **65**, 826–9.

Rennebohm, R.M., Heubi, J.E., Daugherty, C.C. and Daniels, S.R. (1985) Reye's syndrome and children receiving salicylate therapy for connective tissue disease. *J. Pediatr.,* **107**, 877–80.

Reye, R.D.K., Morgan, G. and Baral, J. (1963) Encephalopathy and fatty degeneration of the viscera: a disease entity in childhood. *Lancet,* **ii**, 749–52.

Roe, C.R. (1988) Metabolic disorders producing a Reye's like syndrome. In *Reye's Syndrome* – Royal Society of Medicine Round Table Symposium, No. 8, (ed. C. Wood), Royal Society of Medicine, London.

Roe, C.R., Billington, D.S., Maltby, D.A. and Kinnebrew, P. (1986) Recognition of medium chain acyl CoA dehydrogenase deficiency in asymptomatic siblings of children dying of sudden infant death or Reye-like syndromes. *J. Pediatr.,* **108**, 13–18.

Rozee, K.R., Lee, S.H., Crocker, J.F.S. and Safe, SH. (1979) Enhanced virus replication in mammalian cells exposed to commercial emulsifiers. *Appl. Environ. Microbiol.,* **35**, 297–300.

Rozee, K.R., Lee, S.H., Crocker, J.F. *et al.* (1982) Is a compromised interferon response an etiological factor in Reye's syndrome? *Can. Med. Assoc. J.,* **126**, 798–802.

Starko, K.M., Ray, C.G., Dominguez, L.B. *et al.* (1980) Reye's syndrome and salicylate use. *Pediatrics,* **66**, 859–64.

Sullivan-Bolya, J.S. and Corey, L. (1981) Epidemiology of Reye's syndrome. *Epidemiol. Rev.,* **3**, 1–31.

Thayer, W.S. (1984) Inhibition of mitochondrial fatty acid oxidation in pentanoic acid-induced fatty liver. A possible model for Reye's syndrome. *Biochem. Pharmacol.,* **3**, 1187–94.

Tonsgard, J.H. (1985) Urinary dicarboxylic acids in Reye syndrome. *J. Pediatr.,* **107**, 79–84.

Tonsgard, J.H. (1989) Effect of Reye's syndrome serum on the ultrastructure of isolated liver mitochondria. *Lab. Invest.,* **60**, 568–73.

Tonsgard, J.H. and Getz, G.S. (1985) Effect of Reye's syndrome serum on isolated chinchilla liver mitochondria. *J. Clin. Invest.,* **76**, 816–25.

Waldman, R.J., Hall, W.N., McGee, H. and Van Amburg, G. (1982) Aspirin as a risk factor in Reye's syndrome. *J. Am. Med. Assoc.,* **247**, 3089–94.

Williams, F.M., Ferner, R.E., Graham, M. *et al.* (1990) The metabolic effects of aspirin in fasting and fed subjects: relevance to the aetiology of Reye's syndrome. *Eur. J. Clin. Pharmacol.,* **38**, 519–21.

Wood, C. (ed.) (1988) *Reye's syndrome* – Royal Society of Medicine Round Table Symposium, No. 8, Royal Society of Medicine, London.

Yamashita, N.F., Eiichiro, O., Kimura, A. and Yoshida, I. (1985) Reye's syndrome in Asian countries. In *Reye's Syndrome 4* (ed. J.D. Pollack), National Reye's Syndrome Foundation, Ohio, pp. 47–60.

21 *Aspirin-induced asthma*

A. SZCZEKLIK

21.1 DEFINITION AND PREVALENCE

The majority of people tolerate aspirin well. Asthmatics, however, are an exception. Many of them cannot tolerate aspirin or other analgesics. They suffer from a special type of asthma, called aspirin-induced asthma (AIA). Aspirin-induced asthma is a distinct clinical syndrome with a characteristic course and clinical picture. Precipitation of the asthmatic attacks by aspirin and other non-steroidal anti-inflammatory drugs (NSAIDs) is the hallmark of the syndrome.

The reported incidence of AIA in adults varies according to the diagnostic methods used. When oral challenge coupled with spirometry is performed (Fig. 21.1), the frequency among asthmatics is 8% to about 20%. Other surveys relying only on history have found a lower prevalence, for example, 4%. Challenge tests have provided more realistic results than history alone, which is subject to whims of memory. The syndrome is uncommon in children (Stevenson and Simon, 1988). The large majority of patients have a negative family history.

21.2 MAIN CLINICAL FEATURES

The course of the disease and its clinical picture are very characteristic (Samter and Beers, 1968; Virchow, 1976; Settipane, 1983; Szczeklik and Gryglewski, 1983; Stevenson, 1984). In individual cases the onset of symptoms before puberty or after the age of 60 have been well documented. In the majority of patients, however, the first symptoms appear during the third or fourth decade of life. The disease invariably starts suddenly with symptoms of malaise, nasal discharge, nasal obstruction and sneezing. Cough and expectoration without pneumonia are commonly associated with it. All these symptoms resolve within a week or two, except for the rhinitis which is characterized by intermittent,

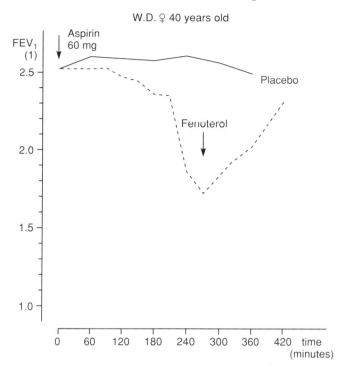

Figure 21.1 Oral aspirin provocation test. Aspirin, contrary to placebo, produced rhinorrhea, shortness of breath accompanied by a fall of FEV_1, which was reversed by fenoterol.

profuse watery rhinorrhea resistant to treatment. The rhinitis persists, nasal polyps often develop, and several months or even years later bronchial asthma and intolerance to aspirin appear. The intolerance presents itself as a unique picture: within an hour following ingestion of aspirin, acute asthmatic attacks develop, often accompanied by rhinorrhea, conjunctival irritation and scarlet flushing of the head and neck. Since many of these patients have taken aspirin in the past with impunity, the initial reaction is usually unexpected and, in fact, quite often not attributed to the drug. These reactions are dangerous; indeed, a single therapeutic dose of aspirin or other anti-cyclo-oxygenase agent can provoke a violent bronchospasm, shock, unconsciousness, and respiratory arrest (Picado *et al.*, 1989). The fully developed clinical syndrome has been termed the aspirin-triad (asthma, aspirin intolerance and nasal polyps). Asthma runs a protracted course despite the avoidance of aspirin and cross-reactive drugs. Opacification of one or more paranasal tissues can be demonstrated with routine roentgenograms. Migraine is a common

549

complaint (Grzelewska-Rzymowska *et al.*, 1985). The eosinophil count is elevated. Skin tests with common aero-allergens are often negative and those with aspirin are always negative.

21.3 INTOLERANCE TO ANALGESICS, OTHER DRUGS AND CHEMICALS

21.3.1 Common Offenders and Safe Alternatives

In patients with aspirin-induced asthma, not only aspirin but several other anti-inflammatory drugs precipitate bronchoconstriction. They are listed in Table 21.1. These drugs are contraindicated in patients with AIA. Not all of them produce adverse symptoms with the same frequency. This depends both on a drug's anti-cyclo-oxygenase potency and dosage, as well as on the individual sensitivity of a patient (Szczeklik *et al.*, 1977a; Stevenson, 1984). Table 21.1 presents also NSAIDs which can be taken safely by patients with AIA. There have been recent developments concerning tolerance to salicylates, paracetamol, pyrazolones and steroids.

21.3.2 Salicylates

In 1968 Samter and Beers in their classical paper concluded that 'intolerance to acetylsalicylic acid is certainly not an intolerance to salicylates'. This notion was subsequently adopted by most clinicians, though a recent report questioned its validity (Stevenson *et al.*, 1988). Differences in tolerance to salicylates by aspirin-sensitive asthmatics might be related to activity of these drugs toward cyclo-oxygenase. None of the salicylates approaches the inhibitory potency of aspirin, but some are weak inhibitors, while others are not. It is, therefore, interesting to note that diflunisal, a moderately active reversible cyclo-oxygenase inhibitor, produced adverse respiratory symptoms in half of 30 aspirin-intolerant patients (Szczeklik and Nizankowska, 1985; Nizankowska, 1988). Salsalate, a somewhat weaker inhibitor, precipitated adverse reactions in two of ten such patients (Stevenson *et al.*, 1988). On the other hand, salicylates deprived of anti-cyclo-oxygenase activity, like sodium salicylate (Rosenkranz *et al.*, 1986; Samter and Beers, 1968), salicylamide (Nizankowska and Szczeklik, 1979) or guaiacolic ester of acetylsalicylic acid (Bianco *et al.*, 1979) were very well tolerated by aspirin-sensitive asthmatics in controlled studies. Choline magnesium trisalicylate can be safely administered to the latter group. This non-acetylated salicylate with strong anti-inflammatory and analgesic activity was shown in a controlled study to be perfectly well tolerated by aspirin-sensitive asthmatics, even on prolonged administration in high therapeutic doses (Szczeklik *et al.*, 1990a).

21.3.3 Pyrazolones

Pyrazolones can precipitate adverse symptoms ranging from urticaria and angioedema to asthma and anaphylactic shock. Patients with these

Table 21.1 Tolerance of anti-inflammatory drugs in aspirin-induced asthma

Precipitate attacks of asthma	Well tolerated (cause no bronchoconstriction)
Salicylates	Sodium salicylate
Aspirin	Choline salicylate
Diflunisal	Choline magnesium trisalicylate
Salsalate (salicylsalicylic acid)	Salicylamide
Polycyclic acids	Dextropropoxyphene
Acetic acids	Azapropazone
Indomethacin	Benzydamine
Sulindac	Chloroquine
Tolmetin	Paracetamol*
Aryl aliphatic acids	
Naproxen	
Diclofenac	
Fenoprofen	
Ibuprofen	
Ketoprofen	
Tiaprofenic acid	
Enolic acids	
Piroxicam	
Fenamates	
Mefenamic acid	
Flufenamic acid	
Cyclofenamic acid	
Pyrazolones	
Aminopyrine	
Noramidopyrine	
Sulfinpyrazone	
Phenylbutazone	
Steroids	
Hydrocortisone hemisuccinate	

* When beginning therapy, give half a tablet of paracetamol and observe patient 2–3 h for symptoms which occur in no more than 5% of patients.

symptoms do not form a homogeneous population, but can be clearly divided into two groups with different pathogenesis.

In the first group, the mechanism responsible for the reactions appears to be allergic. In these patients: (1) noramidopyrine and aminophenazone induce anaphylactic shock and/or urticaria; (2) skin tests with these drugs are highly positive; (3) phenylbutazone, sulfin-pyrazone and several other cyclo-oxygenase inhibitors, including aspi-rin, can be taken with impunity; (4) chronic bronchial asthma is present only in about one fifth of the subjects.

In the second group, the symptoms precipitated do not depend on antigen–antibody reactions, but are due to inhibition of cyclo-oxygenase. Thus, in these patients: (1) noramidopyrine, aminophena-zone, sulfinpyrazone and phenylbutazone, as well as several other inhibitors of cyclo-oxygenase, including aspirin, lead to open asthmatic attacks; (2) skin tests with pyrazolone drugs are negative; (3) all patients have chronic asthma.

The existence of these two groups, first noticed in 1977 (Szczeklik *et al.*, 1977a) and described in detail in later years (Czerniawska-Mysik and Szczeklik, 1981; Szczeklik, 1986) has been confirmed by several authors (Voigtlaender, 1985; Virchow *et al.*, 1986; Fabro *et al.*, 1987). Differential diagnosis of these two groups is presented in Table 21.2.

Azapropazone, a modified benzotriazine, sometimes classified as a pyrazolone drug, can be taken safely by patients with AIA (Szczeklik *et al.*, 1990b).

21.3.4 Paracetamol

Paracetamol can be taken with impunity by a majority of the patients. However, it is safer to give half a tablet first and then observe a patient for 2–3 h for symptoms. We have found only 6% (3/49) of aspirin-sensitive patients with asthma reacting when they were challenged with a provoking dose of paracetamol in the range of 150–600 mg (Szczeklik *et al.*, 1977a). In a recent study, Barles *et al.* (1988) observed mild, though definite, bronchoconstriction in 5 of 32 Spanish patients (15%). Our patients, in whom paracetamol produced obstruction to airflow, experienced the same effect following ingestion of phenacetin which is metabolized to paracetamol.

The dose probably should not surpass 1000 mg. Thus, Delaney (1976) found no cross-reactivity when challenges were performed with 500 mg of paracetamol, but by increasing the provoking dosage to 1000 mg, bronchoconstriction was induced in 12/42 (28%) aspirin-sensitive patients with asthma. Similarly, two patients studied by Settipane and Stevenson (1989), underwent challenges with 500 mg

Table 21.2 Intolerance to pyrazolone drugs (data based on 50 consecutive patients of each group)

	Aspirin-induced asthma %	Pyrazolone allergy %
Adverse symptoms		
Bronchospasm	100	10
Urticaria	2	30
Shock	2	75
Other drugs intolerance		
Aspirin	100	0
Indomethacin	100	0
Positive skin tests		
With noramidopyrine and/or		
aminophenazone	0	75
Clinical history		
Asthma	90	15
Nasal polyps	65	2

dosages without adverse effect, but reacted to 1000 mg provoking dosage. These two subjects tolerated 1000 mg paracetamol well following desensitization with aspirin.

The mechanism of the rare adverse reactions produced by paracetamol in aspirin-sensitive patients is unknown. *In vivo*, paracetamol at a dose <500 mg does not affect cyclo-oxygenase function. *In vitro*, under standard assay conditions with purified enzyme, the drug is deprived of any cyclo-oxygenase activity. However, when the level of lipid peroxides becomes drastically reduced in experiments *in vitro*, paracetamol can become a cyclo-oxygenase inhibitor (Lands, 1981). Whether this unique property of the drug could account for the rare adverse symptoms is unknown. The reactions discussed here should be distinguished from acute hypersensitivity to paracetamol, which is not associated with aspirin intolerance and is presumably mediated immunologically (Stricker *et al.*, 1985; Ellis *et al.*, 1988).

21.3.5 Tartrazine and Other Food Additives

Tartrazine, a yellow azo-dye, is used for colouring foods, drinks, drugs and cosmetics. Unlike aspirin-like drugs, tartrazine does not inhibit

553

cyclo-oxygenase activity (Gerber *et al.*, 1979). In some aspirin-sensitive subjects, bronchoconstriction similar to that caused by aspirin has been observed following tartrazine ingestion. Older reports suggested that such a reaction could be quite common, affecting up to 40% of aspirin-intolerant asthmatics. A critical evaluation of the studies reporting a high incidence of tartrazine intolerance was published by Simon (1984). He pointed out that these studies were either totally non-placebo controlled or the criteria for positive reactions were subjective and vaguely defined. Furthermore, many of the reactions considered positive were merely a product of clinical liability in these patients from whom all symptomatic treatment was usually withheld at the beginning of the test.

In a multicentre, international study we found tartrazine hypersensitivity to be rare. Of 168 Italian, Polish and Swiss patients with well documented AIA, only four had positive reactions when challenged with tartrazine (Virchow *et al.*, 1988). Similarly, Weber *et al.* (1979) were unable to confirm a single case of tartrazine intolerance among 44 patients. Morales *et al.* (1985) observed one questionable case in 47 patients, and Simon (1984) found none among 125 patients.

Occasionally, in a patient with AIA, other food and drug additives, such as benzoates, metabisulphites or monosodium glutamate may produce adverse bronchial effects (Allen *et al.*, 1987; Sabbah *et al.*, 1987). Williams *et al.* (1989) demonstrated that these additives are able to inhibit the cyclo-oxygenase–thromboxane pathway of platelets *in vitro*. They speculated that this weak aspirin-like property may induce intolerance in susceptible patients.

21.3.6 Corticosteroids

Sporadically, hydrocortisone succinate injection might provoke an airflow obstruction and asthmatic attack in a patient with AIA (Partridge and Gibson, 1978; Dajani *et al.*, 1981; Szczeklik *et al.*, 1985). Such patients tolerate injections of sodium phosphate salts of dexamethasone, prednisolone and betamethasone well. The mechanism of these reactions is unknown. Participation of lipocortins seems unlikely, since all the above steroids induce lipocortins. An interesting explanation was recently suggested by Taniguchi and Sato (1988). They confirmed a previous report (Szczeklik *et al.*, 1985) that succinate is well tolerated by patients who respond with bronchoconstriction to hydrocortisone succinate. They went on challenging a group of 20 aspirin-sensitive asthmatics with a variety of glucocorticosteroid esters, and observed cross-sensitivity with succinate esters. Accordingly, bronchoconstriction could be precipitated by succinate salts of both hydrocortisone and methylprednisolone, but not by the phosphate salts.

Irrespectively of its mode of action, hydrocortisone therapy should be used with caution in patients with AIA. In several patients it produced a slight, transient, and clinically irrelevant impairment of airflow, but it can also lead to open bronchoconstriction. It is, therefore, advisable to use other steroids in patients with AIA, preferably non-succinate salts.

21.4 PATHOGENESIS

21.4.1 Genetics

Clustering of aspirin intolerance has been described in a few families (Szczeklik, 1986). However, most patients with aspirin-induced asthma have a negative family history of both asthma and aspirin-intolerance. Out of 600 patients with proven aspirin-induced asthma, treated over the 15-year period 1971–1986 in our Department, there were only two cases of familial intolerance to aspirin. One was a 19-year-old male whose only brother, also asthmatic, died after taking aspirin. The other was a 21-year-old asthmatic woman whose father had never suffered from asthma, but presented a history of angioedema and urticaria without dyspnoea after aspirin ingestion; this was confirmed in a challenge test.

When HLA typing was performed, no difference in class I HLA-A,B and C antigens or in HLA-DR antigens were found (Jones et al., 1984; Mullarkey, et al., 1986). However, there was an increase in HLA-DQw2 in about two-thirds of patients with AIA, as compared to other types of asthma with good tolerance to aspirin (Mullarkey et al., 1986). Whether these genetic findings, observed in a rather small group of patients, are related at all to the pathogenesis of the disease, remains to be established. Theoretically, a genetic repertoire might increase susceptibility to a viral insult that activates rhinitis and asthma.

21.4.2 Allergic Mechanism

Clinical symptoms precipitated by aspirin in sensitive patients with asthma are reminiscent of immediate-type hypersensitivity reactions. Therefore, an underlying antigen–antibody mechanism has been suggested. However, skin tests with aspirin are negative, and numerous attempts to demonstrate specific antibodies against aspirin or its derivatives have been unsuccessful (Schlumberger, 1980). Furthermore, in patients with AIA asthmatic attacks can be precipitated not only by aspirin but by several other analgesics with different chemical structures, which makes immunological cross-reactivity most unlikely.

21.4.3 Complement Activation

Yurchak *et al.* (1970) suggested a direct activation of the complement system by aspirin as the pathogenic mechanism of aspirin intolerance. The adverse reactions could be mediated by complement-derived split products, particularly the anaphylaxins C3a and C5a.

Aspirin, indeed, activates complement both *in vivo* and *in vitro*. Such activation can be demonstrated in healthy subjects and in aspirin-intolerant patients (Schlumberger, 1980). The significance of the above findings is not clear. Voigtlaender *et al.* (1981) did not find any significant complement deficiencies in 40 aspirin intolerant patients with either asthma or urticaria. These authors also noted that *in vitro* sodium salicylate induced about 10-fold higher complement consumption than aspirin. Sodium salicylate is very well tolerated by patients with AIA. The study by Pleskow *et al.* (1983b) who measured both CH50 and C4 activation by rocket immunoeletrophoresis for C4d and C5 in arterial and venous samples of 16 ASA-sensitive patients failed to show any significant changes during and after ASA-provoked bronchospasm.

21.4.4 Discharge of Mast Cell Mediators

It has been proposed (Schlumberger *et al.*, 1974) that non-immunologic triggering of mast cells by aspirin was the initiating event provoking asthmatic reactions in aspirin-sensitive individuals. Blood histamine levels may rise during the attack induced by aspirin (Szmidt *et al.*, 1981; Stevenson and Simon, 1988), but this is not a consistent finding, and occurs in other types of asthma. A multicentre study (Simon *et al.*, 1983) in which histamine, platelet factor 4, and neutrophilic chemotactic factor were measured in plasma and urine, failed to detect significant changes in samples assayed for these mast cell products during and after aspirin-induced reactions. In two other studies an increase in blood neutrophil chemotactic activity roughly paralleled aspirin-induced bronchoconstriction (Hollingsworth *et al.*, 1984; Ortolani *et al.*, 1984). Preincubation with aspirin failed to alter spontaneous or A23187-stimulated histamine release from leukocytes of aspirin-intolerant donors (Bochner *et al.*, 1984).

Thus, there is little evidence to support the hypothesis that release of mast cell mediators plays a leading role in aspirin-precipitated bronchoconstriction. Part of the aspirin reaction, however, is consistent with release of histamine, including flushing or ocular injection. Indeed, pretreatment with an H_1 antihistamine blocks or attenuates these latter symptoms, but not the central event of bronchospasm (Szczeklik and Serwonska, 1979; Phillips *et al.*, 1989).

21.4.5 The Cyclo-oxygenase Theory

Many concepts have been advanced to explain the pathogenesis of AIA. The idea (Szczeklik *et al.*, 1975) that the attacks might result from the specific inhibition of a single enzyme, namely cyclo-oxygenase, in the respiratory tract has been, perhaps, most discussed. It stimulated a number of hypotheses on the mechanism of bronchoconstriction. All these hypotheses operate within the framework of the cyclo-oxygenase theory. Thus, their major assumption, now firmly established, is that inhibition of cyclo-oxygenase triggers specific biochemical reactions which lead to open asthma attacks.

FORMULATION OF THE THEORY

In the early 1970s, allergic mechanisms as an explanation for aspirin intolerance were vigorously pursued. Contrary to these concepts, the cyclo-oxygenase theory proposed that precipitation of asthmatic attacks by aspirin is not based on antigen-antibody reactions, but stems from the pharmacological action of the drug, discovered by John Vane (1971, 1987). The original observations (Szczeklik *et al.*, 1975, 1977a) that the drug intolerance could be predicted on the basis of its *in vitro* inhibition of cyclo-oxygenase, have been consistently reaffirmed during the ensuing years (Stevenson and Lewis, 1987). Evidence in favour of the cyclo-oxygenase theory (Szczeklik, 1990) can be summarized as follows: (1) Analgesics with anti-cyclo-oxygenase activity invariably precipitate bronchoconstriction in aspirin-sensitive patients; (2) analgesics not affecting cyclo-oxygenase are devoid of bronchospastic properties in these patients; (3) there is a positive correlation between the potency of analgesics to inhibit cyclo-oxygenase *in vitro* and their potency to induce asthmatic attacks in sensitive patients; (4) the degree of enzymatic inhibition that is sufficient to precipitate bronchoconstriction is an individual hallmark (thus, if the threshold dose for any anti-cyclo-oxygenase in a particular patient is known, one can predict the threshold doses for other analgesics in that patient); (5) *in vitro* anti-cyclo-oxygenase inhibitors activate platelets to release cytotoxic mediators in aspirin-sensitive asthmatics, but not in atopic asthmatics

Unwanted effects

or healthy subjects (Capron *et al.*, 1985; Ameisen *et al.*, 1986); (6) in patients with AIA inhibition of thromboxane A_2 synthesis, the next step from the cyclo-oxygenase enzyme in the arachidonic acid cascade, neither precipitates asthmatic attacks nor alters pulmonary function (Szczeklik *et al.*, 1987) (Fig. 21.2); (7) after desensitization to aspirin, cross desensitization to other analgesics which inhibit cyclo-oxygenase also occurs (Stevenson and Lewis, 1987). Thus, the inhibition of bronchial cyclo-oxygenase by aspirin-like drugs appears to set off a chain reaction leading to asthmatic attacks in aspirin-intolerant patients. What follows at the biochemical level remains largely unknown.

IMBALANCE IN $PGE_2/PGF_{2\alpha}$ or PGE_2/β-ADRENERGIC SYSTEM

At the time of publication of the cyclo-oxygenase hypothesis (Szczeklik *et al.*, 1975), the only eicosanoids known to be produced by the cells of the respiratory tract were PGE_2 and $PGF_{2\alpha}$. It was presumed (Toogood, 1977) therefore, that although cyclo-oxygenase was inhibited by aspirin, a selective deficiency among the cyclo-oxygenase products must also occur, such that bronchodilator PGE_2 was decreased relative

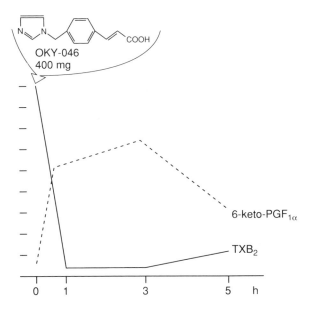

Figure 21.2 In this 38-year-old woman, ingestion of 400 mg OKY 046, the specific thromboxane A_2 synthase inhibitor, produced almost total depression of serum TXB_2, and a distinct rise in serum prostacyclin metabolite, 6-keto-$PGF_{1\alpha}$. However, pulmonary function tests remained unaltered throughout the 5 h observation period (data not shown).

to bronchoconstrictor $PGF_{2\alpha}$. This idea was not universally appealing because, although the efficacy of aspirin and certain other NSAIDs as inhibitors of cyclo-oxygenase was clearly demonstrated, the relative effects on PGH_2-PGE_2 isomerase and PGH_2-$PGF_{2\alpha}$ isomerase were not.

An early explanation (Szczeklik et al., 1975) that aspirin-sensitive asthmatics might rely more on PGE_2 than on the beta-adrenergic system to keep their bronchi unobstructed, seems unlikely today. These patients, indeed, respond better to inhaled PGE_2 than other asthmatics (Szczeklik et al., 1977b) but clinical practice leaves no doubts that their lung function also improves substantially following inhalation of beta-adrenoceptor-mimetics.

PARTICIPATION OF LEUKOTRIENES

The most popular explanation postulates shunting of arachidonic acid from the generation of prostaglandins to the biosynthesis of leukotrienes, with resulting bronchoconstriction, mucosal permeability and secretion, and neutrophil influx into the tissues. Thus, leukotrienes are incriminated as the principal mediators. Their overproduction could be due to: (1) increased bioavailability of arachidonic acid (not being metabolized by cyclo-oxygenase), or (2) enhancement by raised 12-HETE (Maclouf et al., 1982), or (3) removal of the inhibiting control of PGE_2/PGI_2 (Kuehl et al., 1984).

There is some experimental support for the concept of a shift in arachidonic acid metabolism, though clinical evidence is still lacking. In a guinea-pig model of antigen-induced anaphylaxis, pretreatment of animals with indomethacin resulted in an augmentation of the pulmonary mechanical response to intravenous antigen and this was accompanied by an increased generation of LTB_4 (Lee et al., 1986). In the allergic sheep model, cyclo-oxygenase inhibition led to increased production of bronchoconstrictor and lipoxygenase products as detected in broncho-alveolar lavage fluid (Dworski et al., 1989). Pretreatment of passively sensitized human airways with indomethacin resulted in an increased release of leukotrienes from human bronchi in response to both antigen and anti-IgE stimulation (Undem et al., 1987). However, others have found (Vigano et al., 1988) that in normal human lung parenchyma an anti-IgE challenge in the presence of indomethacin does not produce a shift towards leukotriene formation.

In a recent interesting study, Sladek et al., (1989) found that cyclo-oxygenase inhibition, sufficient to suppress systemic formation of TXA_2, was not associated with an alteration of acute allergic bronchoconstriction or abolition of the late response in unselected asthmatic subjects. Urinary levels of the TXB_2 metabolite and of LTE_4 increased

2 h after the challenge, but were not elevated during the late response. Indomethacin significantly reduced urinary 11-dehydro-TB$_2$X levels without affecting the excretion of LTE$_2$ or pulmonary function. Thus, no evidence was obtained for enhanced leukotriene formation during allergic stimulation *in vivo* in the presence of cyclo-oxygenase inhibition. It should be pointed out that in this study the cellular source of LTE$_4$ was unknown, and the asthmatics were not sensitive to aspirin.

Two groups studied the release of leukotrienes into the nasal cavity following aspirin administration to patients with AIA. Ortolani *et al.* (1987) noticed an increase in mean LTC$_4$ concentration in nasal washings of seven aspirin-sensitive asthmatics following nasal spray provocation with aspirin. However, clinical symptoms occurred within a minute or two after the challenge, while LTC$_4$ increase was observed 60 min later. Ferreri *et al.* (1988) used oral aspirin to provoke clinical symptoms in five intolerant patients. During the reactions provoked, LTC$_4$ increased in three patients. In two of five patients a fall in PGE$_2$ preceded the appearance of clinical symptoms. In control subjects, ingestion of higher doses of aspirin (650 mg) resulted in a distinct fall in PGE$_2$ without the release of LTC$_4$ into nasal washings. A recent study by Bisgaard *et al.* (1988) casts serious doubts on the validity of mediator measurement in nasal lavage fluid in relation to symptoms following local nasal challenge.

It is not clear in which cells of the respiratory tract alterations in arachidonic acid metabolism might occur. Leukocytes, especially eosinophils, present in large amounts in nasal and bronchial tissue of aspirin-sensitive asthmatics (Godard *et al.*, 1982; Szczeklik, 1986) could be considered as a source of leukotrienes. Goetzl *et al.*, (1986) suggested a generalized abnormality of the regulation of the arachidonic acid oxidative pathway in peripheral blood leukocytes of patients with AIA. Two recent studies do not support this idea. Nizankowska *et al.* (1988) studied production by polymorphonuclear leukocytes of 5-HETE and LTB$_4$ in 10 aspirin-sensitive asthmatics and 10 matched healthy controls. The blood cells were obtained before administration of the threshold doses of aspirin, and during the aspirin-induced reaction. Initial levels of eicosanoids determined did not differ between the two groups, and remained unchanged following aspirin challenge. Tsuda *et al.* (1988) measured the production of LTB$_4$ and LTC$_4$ in peripheral blood leukocytes stimulated by calcium ionophore A 23187. They compared four groups (controls, AIA, atopic, and intrinsic asthma) before and after indomethacin challenge. All three asthmatic groups produced more LTC$_4$ than the healthy controls, but there was no difference between aspirin-intolerant patients and atopic or intrinsic ones. LTB$_4$ production (as well as PGE$_2$ and TXB$_2$) was similar in all four groups.

Indomethacin did not affect leukotriene generation in any of the groups studied.

The concept of arachidonic acid shunting needs an additional assumption that the airways of aspirin-intolerant patients are more sensitive to leukotrienes than those of other patients with asthma (Szczeklik and Gryglewski, 1983). If not, all asthmatic patients would react with bronchoconstriction in response to aspirin-like drugs.

Three research groups addressed this problem. Vaghi et al. (1985), also Bianco (1986), measured the bronchial response to LTC_4 in 10 aspirin-sensitive asthmatics as compared to 10 controls. They were unable to find any significant difference. Sakakibara et al. (1988a) studied airway responsiveness to methacholine, histamine and LTD_4 in 12 patients with AIA, 13 patients with extrinsic asthma and 12 patients with intrinsic asthma. There were no significant differences in either concentrations of any of the agents producing a 20% fall in FEV_1 or the slope of FEV_1 changes among the groups studied. The only positive finding was a somewhat delayed recovery in FEV_1 following challenge with LTD_4 in the aspirin-intolerant group as compared to the others. These two studies do not support the concept of increased bronchial reactivity to LTC_4 or LTD_4. However, results of Arm et al. (1989) suggest a selective increase in airway responsiveness to LTE_4. They measured a 35% fall in the specific airway conductance (PD35) following histamine and LTE_4 inhalations in five subjects with aspirin-induced asthma and in 15 asthmatics without aspirin sensitivity. The airways of aspirin-intolerant patients had a significant, 13-fold increase in responsiveness to LTE_4 relative to histamine when compared to control asthmatics. Interestingly, this hyper-responsiveness to LTE_4 became abolished after aspirin desensitization.

The concept of the diversion of arachidonic acid metabolism from prostanoids to leukotrienes is hard to accept in view of the likely compartmentalization of arachidonic acid in the lung (Gryglewski et al., 1976). This concept still awaits testing with a powerful, specific leukotriene inhibitor. In a recent trial (Nizankowska et al., 1987), pretreatment of aspirin-intolerant asthmatics with a leukotriene inhibitor failed to prevent aspirin-precipitated bronchospasm. The bioavailability of the inhibitor, administered by inhalation, remained, however, uncertain.

PLATELET INVOLVEMENT

In patients with AIA aspirin challenge may lead to activation of peripheral blood platelets which parallels the time course of bronchospastic reaction. However, the detection of endogenous PAF release has not been a consistent finding leading to the conclusion that aspirin-induced bronchoconstriction is not based on the contracting properties of PAF (Schmitz-Schumann et al., 1987).

Platelets isolated from patients with aspirin-induced asthma were reported (Capron et al., 1985; Ameisen et al., 1986) to react abnormally in vitro to aspirin and other cyclo-oxygenase inhibitors by generating cytocidal molecules that can kill parasitic larvae. No such effect was observed on platelets from normal donors or allergic asthmatics. It was suggested (Joseph et al., 1987) that this abnormality is associated with inhibition of cyclo-oxygenase leading to a defect in binding of prostaglandin endoperoxide PGH_2 to its receptors on the platelet membrane.

Nizankowska et al., (1988) measured 12-HETE production by platelets in 10 aspirin-sensitive asthmatics and 10 matched healthy controls before and after administration of the threshold dose of aspirin. Initial levels of 12-HETE did not differ between the two groups. Following aspirin challenge, 12-HETE rose to similar levels in both groups. These data do not support the concept of a leading role of 12-HETE in AIA (Maclouf et al., 1982) or the concept of a generalized abnormality in arachidonic acid oxidative pathways in platelets of aspirin-sensitive asthmatics. Lack of a protective effect of prostacyclin infusions on aspirin challenge also raises doubts about the participation of platelets in these reactions (Nizankowska et al., 1988).

INCREASE IN TXA_2/PGE_2 RATIO

An interesting hypothesis was recently proposed by Gryglewski (1989). It is based on the idea that arachidonic acid metabolism in the lungs is compartmentalized (Gryglewski et al., 1976). Thus, PGE_2 is generated by smooth muscle of large airways, TXA_2 by contractile elements of lung parenchyma, prostacyclin by vascular endothelium and leukotrienes by leukocytes residing in the lungs and by fibroblasts. In AIA patients cyclo-oxygenase of large airways would be more susceptible to pharmacological inhibition than cyclo-oxygenase of lung parenchyma. In consequence, an ingestion of an anti-cyclo-oxygenase drug would cause an increase in the TXA_2/PGE_2 ratio. The most likely explanation for an augmented selective susceptibility of bronchial cyclo-oxygenase to analgesics is chronic viral infection of the upper airways of patients with AIA (Gryglewski et al., 1977; Szczeklik, 1988). This chronic infection might either change the biochemical characteristics of cyclo-oxygenase in upper airways or make it easily accessible to analgesics. Another possibility is that in AIA we are dealing with a specific retroviral infection which changes genes responsible for the

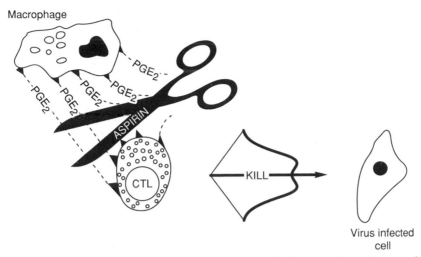

Macrophage

Figure 21.3 The viral hypothesis: aspirin turns off the control mechanism by blocking PGE_2 production. As a consequence, specific cytotoxic T lymphocytes (CTL) attack and kill virus infected cells of the respiratory tract.

assembly of cyclo-oxygenase in bronchial smooth muscle or epithelium. If the hypothesis is right, then simultaneous pretreatment of patients with TXA_2 synthetase inhibitor and TXA_2/PGE_2 receptor antagonist should protect them against the aspirin-induced bronchoconstriction (Fig. 21.2).

VIRAL INFECTION

Viruses have been implicated in the pathogenesis of asthma (Busse, 1989), including aspirin intolerance (Gryglewski *et al.*, 1977; Schlumberger, 1980), though in the latter case no explanation was offered how a virus infection could be linked with cyclo-oxygenase-dependent mechanisms. Such an explanation has been given by a recent hypothesis (Szczeklik, 1988).

The hypothesis postulates that aspirin-induced asthma results from a chronic viral infection. In response to a virus, a long time after the initial exposure, specific cytotoxic lymphocytes are produced. Their activity is suppressed by PGE_2 produced by pulmonary alveolar macrophages. Anti-cyclo-oxygenase analgesics block PGE_2 production, and allow cytotoxic lymphocytes to attack and kill target cells, i.e. virus-infected cells of the respiratory tract. During this reaction, toxic oxygen intermediates, lysosomal enzymes and mediators are released, which precipitate attacks of asthma. These acute attacks can be prevented by

563

avoidance of all drugs with anti-cyclo-oxygenase activity, however, the asthma continues to run a protracted course because of the chronic viral infection (Fig. 21.3).

The hypothesis is based on the following concepts: (1) the clinical course of aspirin-induced asthma is reminiscent of a viral infection (Szczeklik *et al.*, 1990b; Prieto *et al.*, 1988); (2) latency or semi-latency of viruses is being increasingly recognized (Anon., 1989; Routes and Cook, 1989). In man, a notable example is Epstein–Barr virus, causing infection which persists for life, and is subject to reactivations. Interestingly, some of the clinical manifestations of acute Epstein–Barr virus infection, such as Guillain–Barré syndrome, hepatitis or suppression of haematopoiesis may be caused by secondary immune responses to latently infected lymphocytes (Pagano, 1988); (3) cytotoxic T lymphocytes form part of the human immune system in the respiratory tract. Their numbers rise in response to viral infections, and they are highly specific; (4) lung macrophages produce PGE_2 which suppresses immunological responses (Morley, 1974), including cytotoxic activity of lymphocytes (Herberman, 1986; Roitt *et al.*, 1989). This inhibition can be overcome by anti-cyclo-oxygenase analgesics, which deprive macrophages of PGE_2; (5)a virus infection of alveolar macrophages has been associated with an increase in output of some arachidonate metabolites, most notably PGE_2 (Laegreid *et al.*, 1989a). Bacterial killing by virus-infected alveolar macrophages, but not control alveolar macrophages, was significantly enhanced by cyclo-oxygenase inhibitors (Laegreid *et al.*, 1989b).

21.5 DIAGNOSIS BY ASPIRIN-CHALLENGE TESTS

While a patient's clinical history might raise suspicion of aspirin-induced asthma, the diagnosis can be established with certainty only by aspirin challenge. There are no *in vitro* tests suitable for routine clinical diagnosis.

Patients are challenged when their asthma is in remission and their FEV_1 is greater than 1.5/1 or $FEV_1/VC > 65\%$ of predicted values. They continue regular medication, including corticosteroids, but stop sympathomimetics and methylxanthines for 10 h, and antihistamines for 48 h prior to the challenge. Regular intake of sodium cromoglycate and ketotifen should be interrupted 72 h before the challenge. Aspirin reactions can be blocked by ketotifen (Delaney, 1983; Szczeklik *et al.*, 1980; Wuetrich and Fabro, 1981), and modified by H_1-antihistamines (Szczeklik and Serwonska, 1979). Sodium cromoglycate can alleviate aspirin reactions (Basomba *et al.*, 1976) though this has not been a uniform experience (Dahl, 1981; Hollingsworth *et al.*, 1984). Glucocorticosteroids attenuate aspirin-precipitated reactions (Nizankowska and Szczeklik, 1989).

Oral challenge tests are most commonly performed. They consist of administration of increasing doses of aspirin (starting dose is 10–20 mg) and placebo, according to a single-blind procedure and careful monitoring of clinical symptoms, pulmonary function tests and parameters reflecting nasal patency during 6 h following administration of the drug.

The reaction is considered positive if a decrease in $FEV_1 > 15\%$ of baseline occurs, accompanied by symptoms of bronchial obstruction and irritation of nose or eyes. In most patients the threshold dose evoking positive reactions varies between 40 and 100 mg aspirin (Fig. 21.1). Adverse symptoms are relieved by inhalation of a beta$_2$-adrenoceptor agonist; if necessary, aminophylline and steroids can be administered intravenously.

A modification of the challenge tests has been developed in which, instead of giving aspirin by mouth, an aerosol of lysine acetylsalicylate is administered by inhalation (Bianco *et al.*, 1977a; Schmitz-Schumann *et al.*, 1982, 1985; Sakakibara *et al.* 1988b; Phillips *et al.*, 1989). The step-by-step performance of both oral and inhalation challenge tests with aspirin has been recently described (Szczeklik and Nizankowska, 1992; Picado *et al.*, 1992).

In inhalation challenge tests the increase in aspirin dosage is achieved every 30–45 min, and the test is completed in one morning. It is, therefore, faster than oral challenge which often takes 2–3 days. On the other hand, in oral tests there is no need for special equipment and the chances that aspirin will evoke other than bronchial symptoms are higher.

In a few patients only naso-ocular responses are provoked by orally administered aspirin. These patients usually exhibit bronchial asthma at other times. Pleskow *et al.* (1983a) recorded this type of reaction in three of 50 patients with documented aspirin idiosyncrasy and chronic respiratory tract disease.

In the majority of patients, aspirin intolerance once developed, remains for the rest of their lives. Repeated aspirin challenges are, therefore, positive though some variability in intensity and spectrum of symptoms occurs. However, we and others (Simon, 1984) have observed an occasional patient in whom a positive aspirin challenge became negative after a period of a few years.

Provocation tests are the only way of diagnosing aspirin-intolerance and should be performed in any suspected case in order to avoid serious reactions in the future. If performed by an experienced team, they are quite safe. However, since they carry a potential risk, they must not be executed by a general practitioner, and their use, though important, should be limited to specialized centres.

21.6 DIFFERENTIAL DIAGNOSIS

AIA should be clearly differentiated from other forms of aspirin-associated reactions (Szczeklik, 1986). Up to 40% of patients with chronic urticaria develop an obvious increase in weals and swelling after taking aspirin. These reactions occur usually when urticaria is active, and though the reason for them is not known, it appears that different mechanisms may be responsible in different patients. Skin reactions other than exacerbation of chronic urticaria are less common, but may create serious clinical problems.

There is a distinct subgroup of asthmatics who respond favourably to aspirin and other cyclo-oxygenase inhibitors (Szczeklik and Nizankowska, 1983; Nelson et al., 1986; Prieto et al., 1988). It has been suggested that pharmacological removal of a product of arachidonic acid cyclo-oxygenation from the respiratory tract of patients responding favourably to aspirin-like drugs helps them to overcome their airway obstruction (Szczeklik and Nizankowska, 1983). These patients are clinically indistinguishable from those in whom aspirin provokes bronchoconstriction. Although the syndrome is infrequent, and appears to affect less than 1% of adult asthmatics, it is worth bearing in mind by the practising physician since a trial of aspirin can result in improvement.

21.7 TREATMENT

Patients with AIA should avoid aspirin, all products containing it, and other analgesics which inhibit cyclo-oxygenase. They are left with two options. If necessary, they can take safely, even for prolonged periods, certain agents which do not inhibit cyclo-oxygenase, like choline magnesium trisalicylate, dextropropoxyphene, azapropazone or benzydamine. Most patients will also tolerate well paracetamol, at a dose not exceeding 1000 mg daily. Alternatively, they can undergo desensitization.

This can be achieved by giving 4–8 incremental doses of aspirin every 2–3 h under careful observation. The procedure takes 2 days. It starts usually with a dose producing mild adverse symptoms and ends with 600 mg aspirin which is then well tolerated. The state of aspirin tolerance (refractory period) lasts 2–5 days, but in most patients it can be extended over months, if aspirin is administered regularly in a daily dose of 600 mg. At the same time patients can take other anti-cyclo-oxygenase drugs without any adverse effects. Refractoriness to aspirin following indomethacin administration has also been observed (Simon *et al.*, 1983). Desensitization is possible in most (Bianco *et al.*, 1977a, b; Stevenson, 1984), but not all (Baldocchi *et al.*, 1983) aspirin-intolerant patients with asthma.

Some patients noted improvement in their underlying chronic respiratory symptoms after aspirin desensitization and during maintenance of the desensitized state (Chiu, 1983; Lumry *et al.*, 1983). However, Bianco *et al.* (1982) noted no such improvement in their patients. Dor *et al.* (1985), after inducing aspirin tolerance in nine corticosteroid-dependent asthmatics, noted deterioration of lung function in all patients taking aspirin for more than 1 month. According to Stevenson (1984), desensitization, followed by prolonged administration of aspirin, leads to significant improvement in nasal symptoms but not in the clinical manifestations and the course of asthma.

Despite being desensitized to aspirin, all patients remain asthmatic. Methacholine and histamine inhalation challenges before and after aspirin desensitization are unchanged and the patients remain hyperreactive to these agents (Simon, 1984). In addition, patients maintained on aspirin in a desensitized state, still develop asthmatic relapses from all of their prior provoking factors, except for aspirin.

The mechanism of desensitization is unknown. One possible explanation is that during the period necessary for replacement of irreversibly inhibited cyclo-oxygenase the original regulatory mechanisms are removed, and the functional balance in the bronchi is based on a prostanoid-independent regulatory system. Hypersensitivity to aspirin would then re-occur with the return of the tissue capacity to generate prostaglandins after aspirin withdrawal (Kowalski *et al.*, 1984).

There could be another explanation (Szmidt *et al.*, 1987a). Incremental doses of aspirin are quickly biotransformed to salicylate which has been shown to interfere with aspirin inhibitory action on platelet and vascular cyclo-oxygenase (Vargaftig, 1978; Cerletti *et al.*, 1984). Salicylate is believed to bind at a supplementary site, in close proximity to the catalytic centre of cyclo-oxygenase. By anchoring at the cyclo-oxygenase supplementary binding site, salicylic acid could prevent consecutive aspirin molecules from reaching the catalytic site, and thus prevent the sensitivity symptoms (Szmidt *et al.*, 1987b). In nine AIA patients choline magnesium trisalicylate administered at a dose of 3000 mg daily for 3 days, offered a moderate protection against aspirin-induced symptoms; it diminished the severity and/or delayed the appearance of a fall in FEV_1 and attenuated the nasal symptoms (Nizankowska *et al.*, 1990).

Whether desensitized or not, most patients with aspirin-induced asthma need regular therapy to control the symptoms of their disease. The therapy does not differ from that of other types of asthma. Long term treatment with systemic corticosteroids is necessary in at least half of the patients. Dietary fish oil in large quantities should be avoided, because it might worsen the airflow obstruction, possibly through inhibition of the cyclo-oxygenase pathway (Picado *et al.*, 1988).

REFERENCES

Allen, D.H., Delohery, J. and Baker, G. (1987) Monosodium L-glutamate induced asthma. *J. Allergy Clin. Immunol.*, **80**, 530–7.

Ameisen, J.C., Capron, A., Joseph, M. and Tonnel, A.B. (1986) Platelets and aspirin induced asthma. In *Clinical Pharmacology and Therapeutic Progress in Asthma* (ed. A.B. Kay), Blackwell, London, pp. 226–36.

Anon. (1989) Herpes simplex virus latency. *Lancet*, **i**, 194–5.

Arm, J.P., Hickey, S.P., Spur, B.W. and Lee, T.H. (1989) Airways responsiveness to histamine and leukotriene E_4 in subjects with aspirin-induced asthma. *J. Allergy Clin. Immunol.*, **83**, 187 (Abstr.).

Baldocchi, G., Vervloet, G. and Charpin, J. (1983) Acetylsalicylic acid therapy in aspirin-sensitive asthmatics. *J. Allergy Clin. Immunol.*, **71**, 148–53.

Barles, P.G., Duce-Garcia, F., Portillo-Olmo, J.R. *et al.* (1988) Adverse reaction to acetaminophenon as an alternative analgesic in AAS triad. *Allergol. Immunopathol.*, **16**, 321–5.

Basomba, A., Romac, A., Pelaez, A. *et al.* (1976) The effect of sodium cromoglycate in preventing aspirin-induced bronchospasm. *Clin. Allergy*, **6**, 269–75.

Bianco, S. (1986) Asthme et médicaments anti-inflammatoires non-steroïdiens. In *Allergologie* (ed. J. Charpin), Flammarion, Paris, p. 683.

Bianco, S., Robuschi, M. and Petrigni, G. (1977a) Aspirin-induced tolerance in aspirin-induced asthma detected by a new challenge technique. *IRCS J. Med. Sci.*, **5**, 129–30.

Bianco, S., Robuschi, M., Petrigni, G. and Allegra, L. (1977b) Respiratory effects due to aspirin (ASA): ASA-induced tolerance in ASA-asthmatic patients. *Bull. Europ. Physiopath.*, **13**, 123–4.

Bianco, S., Petrigni, G., Felisi, E. and Robuschi, M. (1979) Tolerance of guaiacolic ester of acetylsalicylic acid by patients with aspirin-induced asthma. *Scand. J. Resp. Dis.*, **60**, 350–4.

Bianco, S., Robuschi, M. and Petrigni, G. (1982) Treatment of aspirin idiosyncrasy. *J. Allergy Clin. Immunol.*, **70**, 222.

Bisgaard, H. Robinson, C., Romeling, F. *et al.* (1988) Leukotriene C_4 and histamine in early allergic reaction in the nose. *Allergy*, **43**, 219–27.

Bochner, B.S., Thomas, L.L., Godnik, L. and Samter, M. (1984) Effect of calcium ionophore A23187 and aspirin on histamine release *in vitro* from leukocytes of aspirin-intolerant donors. *Int. Arch. Allergy Appl. Immunol.*, **74**, 104–7.

Busse, W.W. (1989) The relationship between viral infections and onset of allergic diseases and asthma. *Clin. Exp. Allergy*, **19**, 1–9.

Capron, A., Ameisen, J.C., Joseph, M. *et al.* (1985) New function for platelets and their pathological implications. *Int. Arch. Allergy Appl. Immunol.*, **77**, 107–14.

Cerletti, C., Bonati, M., del-Maschio, A. *et al.* (1984) Plasma levels of salicylate and aspirin in healthy volunteers: relevance to drug interaction on platelet function. *J. Lab. Clin. Med.*, **103**, 869–77.

Chiu, J.T. (1983) Improvement in aspirin-sensitive asthmatic subjects after rapid aspirin desensitization and aspirin maintenance (ADAM) treatment. *J. Allergy Clin. Immunol.*, **71**, 560–4.

Czerniawska-Mysik, G. and Szczeklik, A. (1981) Idiosyncrasy to pyrazolone drugs. *Allergy*, **36**, 381–4.

Dahl, R. (1981) Oral and inhaled sodium cromoglycate in challenge test with food allergens or acetylsalicylic acid. *Allergy*, **36**, 161–5.

Dajani, B.M., Sliman, N.A., Shubair, K.S. and Hamzeh, Y.S. (1981) Bronchospasm caused by intravenous hydrocortisone sodium succinate (Solu-Cortef) in aspirin-sensitive asthmatics. *J. Allergy Clin. Immunol.*, **68**, 201–4.

Delaney, J.C. (1976) The diagnosis of aspirin idiosyncrasy by analgesic challenge. *Clin. Allergy*, **6**, 177.

Delaney, J.C. (1983) The effect of ketotifen on aspirin-induced asthmatic reactions. *Clin. Allergy*, **13**, 247–51.

Dor, P.J., Vervloet, D., Baldocchi, G. and Charpin, J. (1985) Aspirin intolerance and asthma induction of a tolerance and long-term monitoring. *Clin. Allergy*, **15**, 37–42.

Dworski, R., Sheller, J.R., Wickersham, N.E. *et al.* (1989) Allergen stimulated release of mediators into sheep bronchoalveolar lavage fluid. Effect of cyclooxygenase inhibition. *Am. Rev. Resp. Dis.*, **139**, 46–51.

Ellis, M., Haydik, I., Gillman, S. *et al.* (1988) Immediate adverse reactions to acetaminophen. *J. Allergy Clin. Immunol.*, **81**, 180 (Abstr. 348).

Fabro, L., Wuetrich, B. and Walti, M. (1987) Acetylsalicylic acid allergy and pyrazole allergy or pseudoallergy? Results of the skin tests and antibody determinations in a multicenter study. *Z. Hautkr.*, **62**, 470–8.

Ferreri, N.R., Howland, W.C., Stevenson, D.D. and Spiegelberg, H.L. (1988) Release of leukotrienes, prostaglandins and histamine into nasal secretions of aspirin-sensitive asthmatics during reaction to aspirin. *Am. Rev. Resp. Dis.*, **137**, 847–54.

Gerber, J.G., Payne, N.A., Oelz, O. *et al.* (1979) Tartrazine and the prostaglandin system. *J. Allergy Clin. Immunol.*, **63**, 289–94.

Godard, P., Chaintreuil, J., Damon, M. *et al.* (1982) Functional assessment of alveolar macrophages: comparison of cells from asthmatic and normal subjects. *J. Allergy Clin. Immunol.*, **70**, 88–93.

Goetzl, E.J., Valacer, D.J., Payan, D.G. and Wong, M.Y. (1986) Abnormal responses to aspirin of leukocyte oxygenation of arachidonic acid in adults with aspirin intolerance. *J. Allergy Clin. Immunol.*, **77**, 693–8.

Gryglewski, R.J. (1989) Eicosanoids in aspirin-induced asthma. *Agents Actions Suppl.*, **28**, 113–21.

Gryglewski, R.J., Dembińska-Kiec, A., Grodzińska, L. and Panczenko, B. (1976) Differential generation of substances with prostaglandin-like and thromboxane-like activities by guinea-pig trachea and lung strips. In *Lung Cells in Disease* (ed. E. Bouhuys), Elsevier, Amsterdam, pp. 289–307.

Unwanted effects

Gryglewski, R.J., Szczeklik, A. and Nizankowska, E. (1977) Aspirin-sensitive asthma: its relationship to inhibition of prostaglandin biosynthesis. In *Prostaglandins and Thromboxanes* (eds F. Berti, B. Samuelson and G.P. Velo), NATO Advanced Study Institute, Series A: Life Science, Plenum Press, New York, pp. 191–203.

Grzelewska-Rzymowska, I., Bogucki, A., Szmidt, M. *et al.* (1985) Migraine in aspirin-sensitive asthmatics. *Allergol Immunopathol. (Madr.)*, **13**, 13–16.

Herberman, R.B. (1986) Natural killer cells in lungs and other tissues and regulation of their activity by suppressor cells. *J. Allergy Clin. Immunol.*, **78**, 566–70.

Hollingsworth, H.M., Downing, E.T., Braman, S.S. *et al.* (1984) Identification and characterization of neutrophil chemotactic activity in aspirin-induced asthma. *Am. Rev. Resp. Dis.*, **130**, 373–9.

Jones, D.H., May, A.G. and Condemi, J.J. (1984) HLA DR typing of aspirin-sensitive asthmatics. *Ann. Allergy*, **52**, 87–9.

Joseph, M., Capron, A., Ameisen, J.C. *et al.* (1987) Plaquettes sanguines et asthme à l'aspirine. *Allergi. Immunol. (Paris)*, **19**, 7–10 (suppl.).

Kowalski, M.L., Grzelewska–Rzymowska, I, Rozniecki, J. and Szmidt, M. (1984) Aspirin tolerance induced in aspirin-sensitive asthmatics. *Allergy*, **39**, 171–8.

Kuehl, F.A., Dougherty, H.W. and Ham, E.A. (1984) Interaction between prostaglandins and leukotrienes. *Biochem. Pharmacol.*, **33**, 1–5.

Laegreid, W.W., Taylor, S.M., Leid, R.W. *et al.* (1989a) Virus-induced enhancement of arachidonate metabolism by bovine alveolar macrophages *in vitro*. *J. Leukocyte Biol.*, **45**, 283–92.

Laegreid, W.W., Liggitt, H.O., Silflow, R.M. *et al.* (1989b) Reversal of virus-induced alveolar macrophage bactericidal dysfunction by cyclooxygenase inhibition *in vitro*. *J. Leukocyte Biol.*, **45**, 293–300.

Lands, W.E.M. (1981) Actions of anti-inflammatory drugs. *Trends Pharmacol. Sci.*, March, 78–80.

Lee, T.H., Israel, E., Drazen, J.M. *et al.* (1986) Enhancement of plasma levels of biologically active leukotriene B compounds during anaphylaxis in guinea-pigs pretreated by indomethacin or by a fish-oil enriched diet. *J. Immunol.*, **136**, 2575–82.

Lumry, W.R., Curd, J.G., Zeiger, R.S. *et al.* (1983) Aspirin-sensitive rhinosinusitis: the clinical syndrome and effects of aspirin administration. *J. Allergy Clin. Immunol.*, **71**, 580–7.

Maclouf, J., Fruteau de Laclos, B. and Borgeat, P. (1982) Stimulation of leukotriene biosynthesis in human blood leukocytes by platelet-derived 12-hydroperoxyeicosatetraenoic acid. *Proc. Natl, Acad. Sci. USA*, **79**, 6042–6.

Morales, M.C., Basomba, A., Pelaez, A. *et al.* (1985) Challenge tests with tartrazine in patients with asthma associated with intolerance to analgesics (ASA-triad). *Clin. Allergy*, **15**, 55–9.

Morley, J. (1974) Prostaglandins and lymphokines in arthritis. *Prostaglandins*, **8**, 315–26.

Mullarkey, M.F., Thomas, P.S., Hansen, J.A. *et al.* (1986) Association of aspirin-sensitive asthma with HLA-DQw2. *Am. Rev. Resp. Dis.*, **133**, 261–3.

Nelson, R.P., Stablein, J.J. and Lockey, R.F. (1986) Asthma-improved by acetylsalicylic acid and other nonsteroidal anti-inflammatory agents. *N. Engl. Region. Allergy Proc.*, **7**, 117–25.

Nizankowska, E. (1988) Aspirin-sensitive asthma and arachidonic acid metabolism. Doctor's thesis, Copernicus Academy of Medicine, Cracow.

Nizankowska, E. and Szczeklik, A. (1979) Keine Bedenken gegen Solosin bei acetylsalicylicsaure-empfindlichen Asthmatikern. *Dtsch. Med. Wschr.*, **104**, 1388–9.

Nizankowska, E. and Szczeklik, A. (1989) Glucocorticosteroids attenuate aspirin-precipitated adverse reactions in aspirin-intolerant patients with asthma. *Ann. Allergy*, **63**, 159–62.

Nizankowska, E., Sheridan, A.Q., Maile, M.H. *et al.* (1987) Pharmacological attempts to modulate leukotriene synthesis in aspirin-induced asthma. *Agents Actions Suppl.*, **21**, 203–13.

Nizankowska, E., Michalska, Z., Wandzilak, M. *et al.* (1988) An abnormality of arachidonic acid metabolism is not a generalized phenomenon in patients with aspirin-induced asthma. *Eicosanoids*, **1**, 45–8.

Nizankowska, E., Dworski, R., Soja, J. and Szczeklik, A. (1990) Salicylate pretreatment attenuates intensity of bronchial and nasal symptoms precipitated by aspirin in aspirin-intolerant patients. *Clin. Expt. Allergy*, **20**, 647–52.

Ortolani, C., Capsoni, F., Restuccia, M. *et al.* (1984) Neutrophil chemotactic factor of anaphylaxis (NCF-A) release in aspirin-induced asthma. *Clin. Allergy*, **14**, 443–52.

Ortolani, C., Mirone, C., Fontana, A. *et al.* (1987) Study of mediators of anaphylaxis in nasal wash fluids after aspirin and sodium metabisulfite nasal provocation in intolerant rhinitic patients. *Ann. Allergy*, **59**, 106–12.

Pagano, J.S. (1988) Epstein–Barr virus. In *Anti-Viral Drug Development. A Multidisciplinary Approach* (eds E. De Clerq and R.T. Walker), NATO Advanced Study Institute, Series A, Life Science, Plenum Press, New York, Vol. 143, pp. 81–90.

Partridge, M.R. and Gibson, G.J. (1978) Adverse bronchial reactions to intravenous hydrocortisone in two aspirin-sensitive asthmatic patients. *Brit. Med. J.*, **1**, 1521.

Phillips, G.D., Foord, R. and Holgate, S. (1989) Inhaled lysine-aspirin as a bronchoprovocation procedure in aspirin-sensitive asthma: Its repeatability absence of a late-phase reaction and the role of histamine. *J. Allergy Clin. Immunol.*, **84**, 232–41.

Picado, C., Castillo, J.A., Shinca, N. *et al.* (1988) Effects of a fish oil enriched diet on aspirin intolerant asthmatic patients: a pilot study. *Thorax*, **43**, 93–7.

Picado, C., Castillo, J.A., Montserrat, J.M. *et al.* (1989) Aspirin-intolerance as a precipitating factor of life-threatening attacks of asthma requiring mechanical ventilation. *Eur. Respir. J.*, **2**, 127–9.

Picado, C., Ramis, I., Rosellò, J. *et al.* (1992) Release of peptide leukotriene into nasal secretions after local instillation of aspirin in aspirin-sensitive asthmatic patients. *Am. Rev. Resp. Dis.*, **145**, 65–9

Pleskow, W.W., Stevenson, D.D., Mathison, D.A. *et al.* (1983a) Aspirin-sensitive rhino-sinusitis/asthma: spectrum of adverse reactions to aspirin. *J. Allergy Clin. Immunol.*, **71**, 574–79.

Pleskow, W.W., Chenoweth, D.E., Simon, R.A. *et al.* (1983b) The absence of detectable complement activation in aspirin-sensitive asthmatic patients during aspirin challenge. *J. Allergy Clin. Immunol.*, **72**, 462–8.

Prieto, L., Palop, J., Castro. J. and Basomba, A. (1988) Aspirin-induced asthma in a patient with asthma previously improved by nonsteroidal antiinflammatory drugs. *Clin. Allergy*, **18**, 629–31.

Roitt, I.M., Brostoff, J. and Male, D. (1989) *Immunology*, Churchill Livingstone, London.

Rosenkranz, B., Fischer, C., Meese, C.O. and Frolich, J.C. (1986) Effects of salicylic and acetylsalicylic acid alone and in combination on platelet aggregation and prostanoid synthesis in man. *Brit. J. Clin. Pharmacol.*, **21**, 309–17.

Routes, J.M. and Cook, J.L. (1989) Adenovirus persistence in man. *J. Immunol.*, **142**, 4022–6.

Sabbah, A., Drouet, M., Bonneau, J.C. and Le Sellin, J. (1987) Adverse reactions to sulfites in aspirin sensitive asthma. *Allerg. Immunol. (Paris)*, **19**, 25–8.

Sakakibara, H., Suetsugu, S., Saga, T. *et al.* (1988a) Bronchial hyperresponsiveness in aspirin-induced asthma. *Jap. J. Thorac. Dis.*, **26**, 612–19.

Sakakibara, H., Tsuda, M., Suzuki, M. *et al.* (1988b) A new method for diagnosis of aspirin-induced asthma by inhalation test with water soluble aspirin (aspirine-D,L,-lysine, Venopirin). *Jap. J. Thorac. Dis.*, **26**, 275–83.

Samter, M. and Beers, R.F. Jr (1968) Intolerance to aspirin. Clinical studies and consideration of its pathogenesis. *Ann. Intern. Med.*, **68**, 975–83.

Schlumberger, H.D. (1980) Drug-induced pseudo-allergic syndrome as exemplified by acetylsalicylic acid intolerance. In *Pseudo-Allergic Reactions. Involvement of Drugs and Chemicals* (eds P. Dukor, P. Kalloś, H.D. Schlumberger and G.B. West), Karger, Basel, pp. 125–203.

Schlumberger, H.D., Lobbecke, E.A. and Kalloś, P. (1974) Acetylsalicylic acid intolerance. *Acta Med. Scand.*, **196**, 451.

Schmitz-Schumann, M., Schaub, E. and Virchow, C. (1982) Inhalative Provokation mit Lysin-Azetylsalicylsaure bei Analgetika-Asthma-Syndrom. *Prax. Klin. Pneumol.*, **36**, 17–21.

Schmitz-Schumann, M., Juhl, E., Costabel, U. *et al.* (1985) Analgetikaprovokationsproben bei Analgetika-Asthma Syndrom. *Atemwegs. Lungenkrankh.*, **11**, 479–86.

Schmitz-Schumann, M., Menz, G., Schaufele, A. *et al.* (1987) Evidence of PAF release and platelet activation in analgesics-asthma-syndrome. *Agents Actions Suppl.*, **21**, 215–23.

Settipane, G.A. (1983) Aspirin and allergic diseases: a review. *Am. J. Med.*, **74**, 102–9.

Settipane, R.A. and Stevenson, D.D. (1989) Cross sensitivity with acetaminophen in aspirin-sensitive subjects with asthma. *J. Allergy Clin. Immunol.*, **84**, 26–33.

Simon, R.A. (1984) Adverse reactions to drug additives. *J. Allergy Clin. Immunol.*, **74**, 623–30.

Simon, R.A. Pleskow, W., Kaliner, M. *et al.* (1983) Plasma mediator studies in aspirin-sensitive asthma: lack of the role for the mast cell. *J. Allergy Clin. Immunol.*, **71**, 146.

Sladek, K., Dworski, R., FitzGerald, G.A. *et al.* (1990) Allergen stimulated release of thromboxane A_2 and leukotriene E_4 in humans: effect of indomethacin. *Am. Rev. Resp. Dis.*, **141**, 1441–5.

Stevenson, D.D. (1984) Diagnosis, prevention and treatment of adverse reactions to aspirin and nonsteroidal anti-inflammatory drugs. *J. Allergy Clin. Immunol.*, **74**, 617–22.

Stevenson, D.D. and Lewis, R.A. (1987) Proposed mechanisms of aspirin sensitivity reactions. *J. Allergy Clin. Immunol.*, **80**, 788–90.

Stevenson, D.D. and Simon, R.A. (1988) Aspirin-sensitivity: Respiratory and cutaneous manifestations. In *Allergy. Principles and Practice*, Vol. II (eds E. Middleton, Jr, C.E. Reed, E.F. Ellis, N.F. Adkinson, Jr and J.W. Yunginger), C.V. Mosby Comp., St Louis, Washington, Toronto, pp. 1537–54.

Stevenson, D.D., Schrank, P.J., Hougham, A.J. *et al.* (1988) Salsalate cross-sensitivity in aspirin-sensitive asthmatics. *J. Allergy Clin. Immunol.*, **81**, 181.

Stricker, B.H., Meyboom, R.H.B. and Lindquist, M. (1985) Acute hypersensitivity reactions to paracetamol. *Brit. Med. J.*, **291**, 938–9.

Szczeklik, A. (1986) Analgesics, allergy and asthma. *Drugs*, **32** (suppl.4), 148–63.

Szczeklik, A. (1988) Aspirin-induced asthma as a viral disease. *Clin. Allergy*, **18**, 15–20.

Szczeklik, A. (1990) The cyclooxygenase theory of aspirin-induced asthma. *Eur. Respir. J.*, **3**, 588–93.

Szczeklik, A. and Serwonska, M. (1979) Inhibition of idiosyncratic reactions to aspirin in asthmatic patients by clemastine. *Thorax*, **34**, 654–7.

Szczeklik, A., and Gryglewski, R.J. (1983) Asthma and antiinflammatory drugs. Mechanisms and clinical patterns. *Drugs*, **25**, 533–43.

Szczeklik, A. and Nizankowska, E. (1983) Asthma improved by aspirin-like drugs. *Brit. J. Dis. Chest*, **77**, 153–8.

Szczeklik, A. and Nizankowska, E. (1985) The effect of diflunisal on pulmonary function in aspirin-sensitive asthma. *J. Allergy Clin. Immunol.*, **75**, 158 (Abstr. 216).

Szczeklik, A. and Nizankowska, E. (1992) Pharmacological agents in bronchial provocation tests. In: *Methods in Asthmology* (eds L. Allegra, P. Braga and R. Dal Negro), Raven Press, New York (in press).

Szczeklik, A., Gryglewski, R.J. and Czerniawska-Mysik, G. (1975) Relationship of inhibition of prostaglandin biosynthesis by analgesics to asthma attacks in aspirin-sensitive patients. *Brit. J. Med.*, **1**, 67–9.

Szczeklik, A., Gryglewski, R.J. and Czerniawska-Mysik, G. (1977a) Clinical patterns of hypersensitivity to nonsteroidal antiinflammatory drugs and their pathogenesis. *J. Allergy Clin. Immunol.*, **60**, 276–84.

Szczeklik, A., Nizankowska, E. and Nizankowski, R. (1977b) Bronchial reactivity to prostaglandins $F_{2\alpha}$, E_2 and histamine in different types of asthma. *Respiration*, **34**, 323–31.

Szczeklik, A. Czerniawska-Mysik, G., Serwonska, M., and Kuklinski, P. (1980) Inhibition by ketotifen of idiosyncratic reactions to aspirin. *Allergy*, **35**, 421–4.

Szczeklik, A., Nizankowska, E., Czerniawska-Mysik, G. and Sek, S. (1985) Hydrocortisone and airflow impairment in aspirin-induced asthma. *J. Allergy Clin. Immunol.*, **76**, 530–6.

Szczeklik, A., Nizankowska, E., Splawinski, J. *et al.* (1987) Effects of inhibition of thromboxane A$_2$ synthesis in aspirin-induced asthma. *J. Allergy Clin. Immunol.*, **80**, 839–43.

Szczeklik, A., Nizankowska, E. and Dworski, R. (1990a) Choline magnesium trisalicylate in patients with aspirin induced asthma. *Eur. Respir. J.*, **3**, 535–9.

Szczeklik, A., Nizankowska, E. and Czerniawska-Mysik, G. (1990b) Tolerance of azapropazone: Allergic and pseudo-allergic reactions and comparison with other nonsteroidal anti-inflammatory drugs. In *Azapropazone* (ed. K.D. Rainsford), Kluwer, Dodrecht, Boston pp. 265–74.

Szmidt, M., Grzelewska-Rzymowska, I., Rozñiecki *et al.* (1981) Histaminemia after aspirin challenge in aspirin-sensitive asthmatics, *Agents Actions* **11**, 105–7.

Szmidt, M. Grzelewska-Rzymowska, J., Kowalski, M.L. and Rozniecki, J. (1987a) Tolerance to acetylsalicylic acid (ASA) induced in ASA-sensitive asthmatics does not depend on initial adverse reaction. *Allergy*, **42**, 182–5.

Szmidt, M., Kowalski, M.L., Grzelewska-Rzymowska, I. and Rozniecki, J. (1987b) Protective effect of sodium salicylate against aspirin (ASA) induced adverse reactions in sensitive asthmatics. *J. Allergy Clin. Immunol.*, **79**, 257.

Taniguchi, M. and Sato, A. (1988) Aspirin-induced asthmatics (AIA) have cross-sensitivity with the steroid succinate esters. *N. Engl. Region. Allergy Proc.*, **9**, 338 (Abstr. 358).

Toogood, J.H. (1977) Aspirin intolerance, asthma, prostaglandins and cromolyn sodium. *Chest*, **72**, 35–7.

Tsuda, M., Sakakibara, H., Kamidaira, T. *et al.* (1988) Arachidonic acid metabolism of peripheral blood leukocytes in aspirin-induced asthma. *N. Engl. Region. Allergy Proc.*, **9** 437 (Abstr. 755).

Undem, B.J. Pickett, W.C. Lichtenstein, L.M. and Adams, G.K. (1987) The effect of indomethacin on immunologic release of histamine and sulfidopeptide leukotrienes from human bronchus and lung parenchyma. *Am. Rev. Resp. Dis.*, **136**, 1183–7.

Vaghi, A., Robuschi, M., Simone, P. and Bianco, S. (1985) Bronchial response to leukotriene C$_4$ (LTC$_4$) in aspirin asthma. Abstracts SEP 4th Congress, Milano, Stresa, p. 171.

Vane, J.R. (1971) Inhibition of prostaglandin synthesis as a mechanism of action for aspirin-like drugs. *Nature*, **231**, 232–4.

Vane, J.R. (1987) The evolution of non-steroidal anti-inflammatory drugs and their mechanism of action. *Drugs*, **33** (Suppl. 1), 18–27.

Vargaftig, B.B. (1978) Salicylic acid fails to inhibit generation of thromboxane A$_2$ activity in platelets after *in vivo* administration to the rat. *J. Pharmacol. Pharm.*, **30**, 101–4.

Vigano, T., Toia, A., Crivellari, M.T. *et al.* (1988) Prostaglandin synthetase inhibition and formation of lipoxygenase products in immunologically challenged normal human lung parenchyma. *Eicosanoids*, **1**, 73–7.

Virchow, C. (1976) Analgetika-Intoleranz bei Asthmatikern (Analgetika-Asthma-Syndrom) vor laufige Mittelung. *Prax. Pneumol.*, **30**, 684–92.

Virchow, C., Schmitz-Schumann, M. and Juhl-Schaub, E. (1986) Pyrazolones and analgesic asthma syndrome. *Agents Actions Suppl.*, **19**, 291–301.

Virchow, C., Szczeklik, A., Bianco, S. *et al.* (1988) Intolerance to tartrazine in aspirin-induced asthma: results of a multicenter study. *Respiration*, **53**, 20–3.

Voigtlaender, V. (1985) Dermatologische Nebenwirkungen von Pyrazolonen. In *100 Jahre Pyrazolone* (eds K. Brune and R. Lanz), Urban Schwarzenberg, München, pp. 261–6.

Voigtlaender, V., Haensch, G. and Rother, U. (1981) Acetylsalicylic acid intolerance: a possible role of complement. *Int. Arch. Allergy Appl. Immunol.*, **66** (Suppl. 1), 154–5.

Weber, R.W., Hoffman, M., Raine, D.A. and Nelson, H.S. (1979) Incidence of bronchoconstriction due to aspirin, azo dyes, non-azo-dyes, and preservatives in a population of perennial asthmatics. *J. Allergy Clin. Immunol.*, **64**, 32–7.

Williams, W.R., Pawlowicz, A. and Davies, B.H. (1989) Aspirin-like effects of selected food additives and industrial sensitizing agents. *Clin. Exptl. Allergy*, **19**, 533–7.

Wuetrich, B. and Fabro, L. (1981) Azetylsalicylsaeure end Lebensmittel additiva-Intoleranz bei Urtikaria, Asthma bronchiale und chronischer Rhinopathie, *Schweiz. Med. Wschr.*, **111**, 1445–9.

Yurchak, A.M., Wicher, K. and Arbesman, C.E. (1970) Immunological studies on aspirin. Clinical studies with aspiryl-protein conjugates. *J. Allergy*, **46**, 245–51.

22 *Other unwanted side effects and drug interactions with aspirin and other salicylates*

M. KUROWSKI and K. BRUNE

22.1 INTRODUCTION

Aspirin (ASS) and the salicylates are generally considered safe drugs, although they can cause a characteristic spectrum of adverse drug reactions (ADR). Since Vane discovered that ASS inhibits prostaglandin synthesis by irreversible acetylation of cyclo-oxygenase, it was assumed that anti-inflammatory effects and unwanted side effects of ASS are based on this mechanism (Vane, 1971). Since then the inhibition of prostanoid production by ASS has been demonstrated in several tissues such as gastric mucosa (Vane, 1971), platelets (Smith and Willis, 1971) and spleen (Ferreira *et al.*, 1971).

In contrast non-acetylated salicylates are believed to cause their effects by reversible cyclo-oxygenase inhibition and should have different inhibitory concentrations and time courses of their pharmacodynamic effects.

In vitro ASS is significantly more active than salicylate in preventing PG synthesis (Vane, 1971). Following oral administration in humans, however, salicylate has a similar anti-inflammatory potency and is almost equipotent in reducing PG concentrations in inflammatory exudates in rats (Higgs *et al.*, 1976). This discrepancy has not yet been satisfactorily explained. Data on the inhibition of PG production by salicylate are scarce (Rosenkranz *et al.*, 1986) and have been put in question by later results (Higgs *et al.*, 1987). If salicylate is not an inhibitor of PG production in other tissues at therapeutic doses this should be reflected in a lower incidence and intensity of unwanted drug effects putatively related to inhibition of cyclo-oxygenase. As far as possible we shall examine this conclusion on the basis of the available epidemiological data. The wide distribution and frequent clinical use of ASS has led to a solid data base on adverse reactions, which allows more exact risk estimations as compared to the non-acetylated salicylates. In the course of its therapeutic use the following adverse

576

drug reactions of different organ systems are of major clinical interest (Cuthbert, 1974).

22.1.1 Gastrointestinal Tract

Upper gastrointestinal tract ulceration with pain, dyspepsia, constipation, diarrhoea, etc.; gastrointestinal haemorrhage; perforation (Chapter 18).

22.1.2 Skin

Hypersensitivity reactions with rashes, angioedema, urticaria and asthma (Chapter 21).

22.1.3 Kidney

Impairment of kidney function with hypertension, electrolyte imbalance, oedema; nephrotoxicity (usually during co-administration with other analgesics/NSAIDs) (Chapter 19).

22.1.4 Liver

Hepatotoxicity, frequently manifested as elevation of certain liver enzymes (predominantly in patients with rheumatic diseases, e.g. SLE or RA) (Prescott, 1986) (section 22.4).

22.1.5 Blood Cells and Cardiovascular System

Blood dyscrasias, e.g. thrombocytopenia, agranulocytosis, aplastic anaemia, pancytopenia; reduction of platelet aggregation (ASS: at low doses) and prolongation of the prothrombin time (ASS doses > 4000 mg) (Miescher and Pola, 1986) (section 22.3.2).

22.1.6 Central Nervous System

'Salicylism': tinnitus, dizziness, confusion, headache, nausea; impairment of vision and hearing (Moll, 1968) (section 22.7)

22.1.7 Other

Among the various rare side effects of ASS, Reye's syndrome has drawn considerable attention because of its severity and high lethality in children (Chapter 20).

Unwanted effects

In addition, the effects of salicylates on pregnancy and teratogenesis as well as acute poisoning with salicylates will be covered in this chapter.

As the number of chemical variations such as different salts and galenic formulations of salicylic acid are substantial, we will concentrate on selected preparations and modifications which are available on the European and North American markets.

As with other drugs the rates of reported ADRs are dependent on various conditions of the drug application and use. In the case of salicylates some of these factors should be analysed with regard to ADR incidences:

(a) Only a small proportion of total salicylate consumption is under the control of practising physicians and clinicians. The majority of salicylate use is subject to self medication. Thus the estimation of the denominator in the calculation of ADR rates is generally imprecise.

(b) In West European countries salicylates are widely available in pharmacies as over-the-counter drugs. In the USA salicylates can be purchased additionally in supermarkets, etc.

(c) Salicylate doses required for anti-phlogistic treatment are markedly higher than analgesic or anti-pyretic doses. The ADR rates observed with anti-inflammatory doses of several grams per day may vary considerably from those obtained during use for other indications. Moreover, the high dosage of salicylates is predominantly utilized in the USA whereas such doses are generally avoided in Europe because of low tolerability. Thus the observed ADR rates have to be considered with respect to the use of these drugs, e.g. analgesic, anti-thrombotic, anti-inflammatory, etc.

Due to the limited quality of the available data, this chapter will concentrate on the following substances:

> salicylic acid and its salts,
> acetylsalicylic acid;
> salicylsalicylic acid (salsalate); and
> diflunisal.

22.2 THE PHARMACOLOGICAL BASIS OF SIDE EFFECTS

Several of the unwanted drug effects of salicylates may be attributable to the inhibition of cyclo-oxygenase, which is almost ubiquitously present in the human body. These side effects are fairly predictable and occur in principle with each NSAID, but with different incidences.

578

Pharmacokinetic properties, namely absorption, distribution and elimination determine onset, intensity and duration of the observed effects (Martin, 1971; Needs and Brooks, 1985). The tissue distribution and selective accumulation in the stomach, kidney and inflamed tissues may be responsible for non-specific therapeutic or toxic effects of acidic NSAIDs (Brune, 1974).

Considerable changes in the actions of ASS occur following the loss of the acetyl moiety, which can be due to hydrolysis or acetylation of the cyclo-oxygenase in some tissues or other proteins (Rainsford et al., 1983), e.g. platelets and gastric mucosa (Trnavska and Zachar, 1975). The cleavage leaves salicylic acid as a weak anti-inflammatory metabolite in concentrations below the in vitro IC_{50} for cyclo-oxygenase inhibition. For a systemic, anti-inflammatory treatment a dose of approximately 8 g of salicylic acid daily is necessary (Stricker, 1876). The analgesic dose appears to be, as with ASS, much lower (Preston et al., 1989).

Many among this type of side effects (e.g. salicylism, impaired kidney function) are related to plasma concentrations and can be observed more frequently at high doses (Moll, 1968). For a number of side effects however the relation of pharmacokinetic and pharmacodynamic properties may not be as simple, e.g. immunological reactions. The most serious side effects are allergic and pseudo-allergic reactions, of which only the latter are dose- or concentration-dependent; both may occur after a single oral dose (Szczeklik, 1987).

In order to avoid side effects by obtaining more tissue specificity the salicylate molecule was modified with subsequent changes in lipophilicity and acidity. However, a tissue specific blockade of cyclo-oxygenase by a particular salicylate has not yet been achieved. The pattern of distribution can be modified by the route of administration, e.g. topical administration may lead to high concentrations in the adjacent soft tissues, rectal administration delivers different pharmacokinetic and pharmacodynamic profiles compared to oral administration due to different absorption of the compounds (Martin, 1971; Connolly et al., 1979; Needs and Brooks, 1985).

The mode of action in the case of acetylsalicylic acid includes acetylation of the cyclo-oxygenase. This irreversible reaction implies a different time course of its pharmacological effects. Some tissues are subjected to high concentrations and rapid de-acetylation, e.g. the stomach wall following oral administration (Brune et al., 1981; Rainsford et al., 1981) In some cell types, e.g. platelets, the effects are reversed solely by physiological formation of new cells.

Other cells can overcome the cyclo-oxygenase blockade by de novo synthesis of the enzyme, e.g. vascular endothelium (Burch et al., 1978). Therefore the different susceptibility and duration of effect in various tissues was attributed either to the distribution of the drug or the ability to overcome the cyclo-oxygenase blockade.

In contrast, at high doses salicylate may inhibit cyclo-oxygenase reversibly (Smith and Willis, 1971). At low oral doses, however, it can be found in higher concentrations in inflammatory exudates than after intake of the same dose (200 mg) of ASS (Higgs *et al.*, 1987). Therefore it was suggested, that salicylate is the active anti-inflammatory species and the authors came to agree with Dreser (1899) in the conclusion that ASS represents a prodrug for salicylate (Dreser, 1899; Higgs *et al.*, 1987; Vane, 1987).

22.3 BLOOD DISTURBANCES

22.3.1 Platelet Aggregation

The aggregability of platelets *in vivo* is regulated, among other factors by the balance between thromboxane A_2 (TXA_2) as a proaggregating and prostacyclin as an anti-aggregating agent (Moncada and Vane, 1978). ASS inhibits the formation of both compounds from arachidonic acid. However, the concentrations required to suppress prostacyclin production are at least 10 times higher than inhibitory concentrations for TXA_2. Thus with single small doses of ASS the TXA_2 can be suppressed effectively without disturbing the subendothelial prostacyclin production in the vessel wall significantly (Wenger and Hull, 1980) (Chapters 5 and 10).

Sodium salicylate, salicylic acid (Ferreira, and Vane, 1974) and salsalate (Estes and Kaplan, 1980) have no measurable effect on platelet aggregation; diflunisal possesses only $1/18$ to $1/35$ of the potency of ASS (Stone *et al.*, 1977). However these compounds have been shown to exhibit anti-inflammatory activity in patients (Aberg and Larrson, 1970; Dieppe and Huskisson, 1978).

In a clinical study, the inhibitory effects of 40 mg and 300 mg of ASS were compared. Both doses inhibited the TXA_2 production for at least 96 h. A dose of 40 mg of ASS had no effect on prostacyclin synthesis, whereas 300 mg reduced the circulating levels for over 48 h (Hanley *et al.*, 1981). In patients with cardiovascular diseases 750 mg of ASS was required in order to reduce completely the generation of thromboxane B_2. The thromboxane synthesis from prostaglandin H_2 was not suppressed in these patients. The significance of these findings is inferred by the assumption that an imbalance between TXA_2 and prostacyclin contributes greatly to conditions such as myocardial infarction and cerebral thrombosis (Matsumoto *et al.*, 1980). The therapeutic use of this pharmacological effect in thrombogenic disorders, however, seems to be successful only in male patients. A protection against deep vein thrombosis (Harris et al., 1977) and a reduction of transient ischaemic attacks, cerebral strokes and mortality (The Canadian Cooperative Study Group, 1978; Fields et al., 1978) could be demonstrated in men only. In 1980 it was concluded from over 10 000 treated patients in six studies, that ASS reduces cardiovascular mortality and myocardial reinfarction (Anon., 1980). For the combination of ASS with other NSAIDs in anti-arthritic doses the establishment of a different equilibrium between TXA_2 and prostacyclin levels can be assumed as compared to ASS alone, which may lead to a different spectrum of cardiovascular effects.

The use of a combination of ASS with dipyridamol has been studied recently in different indications associated with anti-coagulation. In a prospective randomized placebo-controlled trial with 249 patients, who had aortocoronary vein bypass surgery, Pfisterer et al. (1989) compared low-dose ASS plus dipyridamol with conventional anti-coagulant therapy. The desired effect – prevention of early and late graft occlusions – was achieved by both treatments similarly. In the ASS/dipyridamol group adverse reactions such as severe bleeding, myocardial infarction and death occurred significantly less often (Chapter 16). Associated with the beneficial effects of ASS in cardiovascular disorders, the risk of various haemorrhagic events has to be taken into account. In a comparative study with aspirin or aspirin with dipyridamole, Kingham and co-workers found a high incidence of macular haemorrhage in patients over 60 years of age (Kingham et al., 1988). The anti-coagulant therapy with aspirin was assumed to be the cause by exclusion of other factors such as choroidal neovascularization with the use of fluorescein angiography. The administration of aspirin in patients over 60 years of age with ocular macular degeneration should be considered carefully according to the authors.

A single case of a patient with recurrent conjunctival haemorrhage after ocular surgery was reported. This patient had consumed large quantities of aspirin prior to surgery in order to suppress ocular pain (Werblin and Pfeiffer, 1987). Bleeding persisted for over 9 min and was terminated 2 h after transfusion of platelets.

Also ASS contributes to menorrhagia and increased blood loss in childbirth (Dukes, 1988).

22.3.2 Effects on the Haemogram

Among haematological reactions consisting of pathological changes in erythrocyte, leucocyte or platelet counts or disorders, or a combination of these reported to the Committee on Safety of Medicines in Great

Britain (CSM, Great Britain, 1963–76) 15% of the cases, including 22 fatalities, were attributed to the intake of ASS (Vanecek, 1980).

Various forms of anaemia can be observed following ASS ingestion: deficiency of red blood cells is caused predominantly by gastrointestinal blood loss and subsequent decrease in iron. The rate has been estimated to be 1% in analgesic use (Miller and Jick, 1977) and 10–15% in patients on chronic treatment for rheumatoid arthritis (Anon. 1970).

In patients with rheumatoid arthritis and abusers of analgesics, macrocytic anaemia associated with folate deficiency had been described (Williams *et al.*, 1969).

In patients with deficiency of glucose-6-phosphate dehydrogenase or of red-cell glutathione peroxidase, aspirin may cause haemolytic anaemias (Necheles *et al.*, 1970). Furthermore, salicylates are able to reduce red-cell ATP levels and aggravate haemolysis in patients with pyruvate kinase deficiency (Glader, 1976).

During treatment with diflunisal, thrombocytopenia occurred in a patient with rheumatoid arthritis. It was concluded that diflunisal caused peripheral platelet damage by the thrombocyte fluorochromasia cytotoxic assay (Bobrove, 1988). In another study 32 patients with drug-induced thrombocytopenia were studied and an increase in IgG was observed after ingestion of a variety of drugs including ASS. It was suggested that this mechanism may underlie ASS-induced thrombocytopenic purpura (Conti *et al.*, 1984).

The most severe haematological reactions however are pancytopenia and agranulocytosis with a mortality rate of approximately 50%. During the years 1963–76 the British Committee on Safety of Medicines received the following number of ASS-related reports on severe haematological reactions:

> thrombocytopenia: 23 cases
> aplastic anaemia: 20 cases
> agranulocytosis or pancytopenia: 19 cases
>
> (Vanecek, 1980).

Further clarification of the incidence of these severe reactions was obtained from the IAAAS (International Agranulocytosis and Aplastic Anaemia Study). The first report from this population-based case-control study covering 80 million person-years was published in 1986 (IAAAS, 1986). In this trial the use of different peripherally acting analgesics 1 week before the onset of clinical symptoms of agranulocytosis or aplastic anaemia was compared between 221 confirmed cases of agranulocytosis and 1425 hospital controls. The relative risk after salicylate consumption was 1.6 with a borderline statistical significance (lower 95% confidence limit: 1.0).

22.4 LIVER TOXICITY

Many NSAIDs (e.g. benoxaprofen, diclofenac, phenylbutazone, pirprofen, sulindac) have been reported to induce liver toxicity (Prescott, 1986). Although salicylates have been used extensively for decades, their potential to cause liver damage has been recognized only relatively recently. During the period between 1964 and 1974 only 32 cases of hepatoxicity associated with the use of ASS were reported to the CSM (Rainsford, 1984).

The hepatotoxic potential of ASS and the salicylates includes transient, dose-dependent and reversibly elevated serum levels of liver enzymes, namely GOT, GPT, Gamma-GT and alkaline phosphatase. Abnormalities of bilirubin and prothrombin levels may occur, too. Serious hepatic events during correct dosage with NSAIDs are uncommon, a higher risk may be attributable with the use of ASS in children (Bernstein *et al.*, 1977; Prescott, 1981). Secondary CNS effects of ammonia may be observed in patients with severe liver damage (Mäkelä *et al.*, 1980).

Especially in patients treated with aspirin for systemic lupus erythematosus (SLE) (Seaman *et al.*, 1974a), juvenile rheumatoid arthritis (Russell *et al.*, 1971), rheumatoid arthritis (RA) (Chalmers *et al.*, 1969) or rheumatic fever (Manso *et al.*, 1956) case reports and clinical studies revealed higher incidences of liver toxicity. In a retrospective analysis of 80 SLE patients 19 cases of at least transient abnormal liver tests were reported. In two thirds of these patients ASS seemed to be responsible for this condition. In a consecutive clinical trial in 20% (4/20) of RA patients and 44% (7/16) of SLE patients pathological liver conditions were diagnosed (Seaman and Plotz, 1976). The overall rate of mild, dose-dependent liver damage as indicated by clinico-chemical findings among patients taking anti-inflammatory doses of ASS has been estimated to be 50% (Prescott, 1986). Moreover children and younger female patients with connective tissue disorders were identified as a population at risk of these events (Bernstein *et al.*, 1977; Prescott, 1981).

The typical hepatic effects of ASS include intrinsic hepatocellular damage, which is dose dependent and appears after a latent period of approximately 1 week (Zimmerman, 1978, 1981; Lewis, 1984). It was proposed to monitor serum aminotransferase in order to prevent permanent hepatocellular damage.

In a few cases liver biopsies have been obtained. The histological findings were consistent with toxic hepatitis (Seaman *et al.*, 1974b). The generalized hepatocellular damage is characterized by focal vacuolation, degeneration and necrosis of hepatocytes and periportal infiltration of mononuclear cells. Cessation of salicylate therapy resulted in normal liver tests and histology after 1 week (Seaman *et al.*, 1974a, b).

Only a small minority of patients experience severe liver damage including jaundice, prolongation of the prothrombin time and bleeding (Athreya, 1975; Rochanawutanon *et al.*, 1979), intravascular coagulation (Sbarbaro and Bennett, 1977) and CNS symptoms due to elevated blood ammonia levels (e.g. Mäkelä *et al.*, 1980).

The overall incidence of mild and severe liver reactions remains to be investigated more closely in order to quantify the risk. Reye's syndrome, a rare reaction including liver toxicity, is covered in a separate chapter (Chapter 20).

Cholestatic jaundice attributable to administration of diflunisal has been observed by Warren (1978). For salsalate no hepatic adverse reactions have been reported as yet (Singleton, 1980).

22.5 SPECIAL SENSES

22.5.1 Hearing Disorders

In several cases of suicide attempts with doses of 10–50 g of ASS marked ototoxicity has been observed (Oudot, 1979). In this published series of 10 cases, tinnitus, headache, intermittent vertigo and a sensation of pressure occurred. Complete but reversible deafness lasted from 4 to 5 h after ingestion until 48 h after. It was concluded that the observed phenomena were due to depolarization of the cochlear apparatus and because of its reversibility there is no reason to restrict its use in deaf patients. Hearing impairment mainly affects higher frequencies, and occasionally permanent salicylate-induced deafness has been reported (Ballantyne, 1970). In a series of 33 cases of hearing loss a high positive correlation was observed between the risk and the dose of administered ASS (between < 600 and > 1200 mg of ASS) (Porter and Jick, 1977).

In other studies tinnitus, dizziness and impairment of hearing start at plasma concentrations of 25 mg per 100 ml (Moll, 1968).

22.5.2 Visual Disorders

Studies concerning cataract development during treatment with aspirin yielded controversial results. A previous report, that the incidence of the occurrence of cataracts is lower in aspirin users than in non-users could not be verified in a controlled trial (Kewitz *et al.*, 1986). It was demonstrated that aspirin use is no determining or protecting factor for the development of a cataract.

Similar results were obtained by British physicians in a prospective controlled trial. No association between aspirin use and the incidence of cataract development was found. The figures were 77.1 and 86.1 primarily diagnosed cataracts/10 000 man-years in the control and the aspirin group (Antiplatelet Trialists Collaboration, 1988).

With diflunisal, CNS effects such as dizziness and headaches have been observed in approximately 5% of the cases. Tinnitus occurred rarely (Huskisson *et al.*, 1978).

22.6 TERATOGENESIS AND SECOND-GENERATION DISORDERS

Hitherto the question as to the possible teratogenicity of ASS in man has remained unresolved. Because it has been estimated that ASS is taken by approximately 50% of all pregnant women, anecdotal case reports, which attribute congenital malformations to the intake of ASS, do not give a clue. Two studies by Shapiro and Slone did not yield conclusive evidence for an association between malformations, higher perinatal mortality or lower birth weight and the ingestion of ASS (Shapiro *et al.*, 1976; Slone *et al.*, 1976). The intake of 19 g of ASS during the first trimester of pregnancy in a suicide attempt was probably linked to a developmental defect with subsequent failure of both kidneys in the infant. Following kidney transplantation, pathological findings revealed diffuse tubopapillary adenomata, which replaced each kidney (Bove *et al.*, 1979).

Fifty-three cases of intracranial haemorrhage were observed in another study with 108 infants weighing 1.5 kg or less, or born at 34 weeks of gestation or earlier. Among infants with mothers who had taken ASS, the incidence of haemorrhage was significantly higher than in infants with mothers who did not use either ASS or acetaminophen (Rumack *et al.*, 1980).

The risk of congenital cardiac defects due to ASS ingestion during the first trimester of pregnancy has been studied recently (Werler *et al.*, 1989). A group of 1381 cases with any structural cardiac defects was assembled and five groups of selected cardiac malformations were formed: aortic stenosis, coarctation of the aorta, hypoplastic left ventricle, transposition of the great arteries and conotruncal defects (total $n=1265$). The use of ASS during the first trimester was compared to a control group of 6966 infants with different malformations. The authors did not find an increased risk of congenital heart defects as compared to that of other malformations.

In conclusion, an increased risk of teratogenesis as a result of the use of salicylates in man cannot yet be demonstrated. However, due to its pharmacodynamic properties (bleeding, etc.) the use of ASS is highly questionable and probably inappropriate during the whole period of pregnancy.

In previous studies with ASS and salicylate salts the induction of congenital malformations in rodents was reported (Warkany and Takacs, 1959; Larrson *et al.*, 1963, 1964; Larrson and Boström, 1965; Brown and West, 1964; Bertone and Monie, 1965; Takacs and Warkany, 1968). Long term comparative teratogenic studies by Eriksson concluded that foetal damaging effects were not different for salsalate, ASS and sodium salicylate (Eriksson, 1971). The toxicological profiles of ASS and diflunisal in mice and rabbits were similar (Tempero, *et al.*, 1978).

22.7 INTOXICATION AND OVERDOSAGE

Acute intoxication with salicylates can occur as a result of accidental ingestion by young children or due to deliberate self-poisoning by adults. In addition, therapeutic overdosing can lead to chronic salicylate intoxication, when metabolic pathways are saturated and plasma levels of salicylate increase to toxic levels. The problem of overdosage is common because of the frequent use and the believed harmlessness of aspirin. Thus, salicylate poisoning remains a major medical hazard.

Until the early 1970s, salicylates constituted a major cause of death from accidental poisoning in children under 10 years of age. Acute salicylate intoxication and death in children have decreased since the introduction of safety packaging. However, in the 20 years, 1958–77, 23% of all drug-induced deaths in children were caused by salicylates, mostly aspirin (Fraser, 1980).

About 10% of adult hospital admissions in the UK for deliberate self-poisoning involve salicylates (Proudfoot, 1983). This declined from 16% of patients taking salicylates in 1967 to 10% by 1977. During this time the death rate from paracetamol or paracetamol/propoxyphene mixture (distalgesic) overdose has steadily increased and is now more prevalent than that from salicylate poisoning.

Acute toxic manifestations after salicylate poisoning consist of the well-recognized syndrome of 'salicylism' (Smith and Smith, 1966), that is: tinnitus, deafness, nausea, vomiting, abdominal discomfort, hyperventilation, sweating, vasodilatation and tachycardia. These symptoms are associated with plasma salicylate concentrations of 300–500 mg l^{-1}. Severe intoxication, with plasma salicylate concentrations of 800–1000 mg l^{-1}, may also lead to delirium, convulsions, coma, pyrexia, hypertension and cardiac arrest. Other serious toxic effects which have been reported include pulmonary and cerebral oedema, renal failure, metabolic acidosis, tetany, hypoglycaemia and encephalopathy (Prescott, 1984).

The symptoms of salicylate poisoning can be attributed to:

(a) Central nervous system effects beginning with tinnitus, deafness, confusion and vomiting, followed by delirium, convulsions and, ultimately, coma. The respiratory centre is stimulated by salicylates leading to dyspnoea, reduction of partial pressure of CO_2 in the alveolar air and a rise in blood pH. This changes the acid-base balance and causes respiratory alkalosis.

(b) Local gastrointestinal effects including vomiting, haematemesis, and retrosternal and epigastric pain.

(c) Metabolic effects including heat production (hyperpyrexia), increase in oxygen consumption, tachycardia and increased cardiac output. Stimulation of metabolism by salicylates is a consequence of the uncoupling of mitochondrial oxidative phosphorylation. The increased rate of catabolism leads to an increase in CO_2 production. The resultant rise in PCO_2 causes acidosis which is the opposite effect to that produced by stimulation of respiratory centres. The uncoupling of oxidative phosphorylation also leads to an accumulation of metabolic intermediates in the form of organic acids, which contribute further to the metabolic acidosis. In severe poisoning with salicylates, when the respiratory centres are depressed, respiratory alkalosis gives way to metabolic acidosis. Inhibition of glycolysis combined with anoxia finally leads to coma and death. The hyperpyrexia which develops as a result of the uncoupling of oxidative phosphorylation can be a cause of death in young children.

(d) Renal failure may contribute to death from salicylate poisoning, since prolonged inhibition of prostaglandin synthesis can lead to impaired renal function. Thus, salicylate will cause sodium and water retention and some degree of hypokalaemia.

Death occurs with coma, respiratory failure, cardiac and circulatory arrest and kidney failure at plasma salicylate concentrations greater than 900 mg l^{-1} (Moll, 1968).

Treatment of salicylate poisoning is directed towards prevention of further absorption of the drug and increase of the excretion of salicylate from the body. Children are treated with emetics such as ipecacuanha and adults receive gastric lavage to remove unabsorbed drug from the stomach. In addition, children with plasma salicylate concentrations exceeding 350 mg l^{-1} and adults with concentrations greater than 500 mg l^{-1} are subjected to forced alkaline diuresis induced with large volumes of intravenous alkaline fluid. This increases the rate of kidney tubular urine flow and decreases tubular reabsorption of salicylate, since the increase in urinary pH maintains the drug in an ionized state. Haemodialysis and charcoal haemoperfusion are effective methods of removing salicylate from the plasma of severely intoxicated patients or those with cardiac or renal failure (Proudfoot, 1983). A case of pulmonary oedema associated with salicylate poisoning was treated with diuretics and positive end-expiratory pressure (Hrnicek *et al.*, 1974), whereas an infusion of mannitol successfully reversed the encephalopathy and cerebral oedema in two young children overdosed on aspirin (Dove and Jones, 1982).

Poisoning with salicylates other than aspirin is not very common. However, in London during 1980 and 1981, 22 cases of drug intoxication were attributed to the salicylate derivative, diflunisal. The symptoms of overdose were similar to those seen with ASS. Severe symptoms were associated with plasma concentrations of 263 mg l^{-1} and 500 mg l^{-1}, whereas in two fatal cases, plasma diflunisal concentrations of 640 mg l^{-1} and 670 mg l^{-1} were measured (Court and Volans, 1984). A case report of a 38-year-old man, who committed suicide by ingesting 18 diflunisal tablets, was cited by Levine *et al.* (1987).

In spite of the wide prescribing of non-steroidal anti-inflammatory drugs, overdosage with NSAIDs, other than salicylates, is rare. These drugs vary with regard to the severity of their acute toxic effects. Phenylbutazone, oxyphenbutazone and mefenamic acid cause severe toxic symptoms whereas propionic acid derivatives such as ibuprofen have low toxicity in man. However, due to the over-the-counter sales of ibuprofen, most cases of NSAID overdosage are due to this drug (Court and Volans, 1984).

22.8 INTERACTIONS WITH OTHER DRUGS

22.8.1 Pharmacokinetic Interactions

ASS and the salicylates are amongst the most widely used drugs in the world and are administered as co-medication in many disease states. In plasma, ASS and its metabolite salicylic acid are highly protein bound and undergo extensive metabolism, thus a potential for various pharmacokinetic interactions can be expected. In addition pharmacodynamic interactions with some drugs have to be considered.

Salicylates affect mainly the pharmacokinetic properties of drugs, which are extensively bound to plasma proteins themselves. To this class belong not only other non-steroidal anti-inflammatory drugs, but also methotrexate and phenytoin. When co-administered with one of these drugs, displacement from plasma protein binding and subsequent elevation of free plasma concentrations and total plasma

Table 22.1 Pharmacokinetic interactions of salicylates with other drugs

Drug	Mechanism of interaction	Source
NSAID		
Diclofenac	PBD, Cl_{tot} ↑	Muller *et al.*, 1977
Diflunisal	C_{ss} ↓	Schultz *et al.*, 1979
Fenoprofen	Cl_{tot} ↑, $t_{1/2}$ ↓	Rubin *et al.*, 1973
Flurbiprofen	Presumed PBD, Cl_{tot} ↑	Brooks and Khong, 1977
Ibuprofen	Presumed PBD, Cl_{ss} ↓	Grennan *et al.*, 1979
Indomethacin	Absorption, reabsorption ↓	Kwan *et al.*, 1978
	Cl_R ↓, Cl_B ↑, Cl_{tot}	
Isoxicam	PBD, Cl_{tot} ↑	Esquivel *et al.*, 1984
Ketoprofen	PBD, Cl_{tot} ↑	Williams *et al.*, 1981
Naproxen	PBD, Cl_R ↑	Segre *et al.*, 1974
	PBD, Cl_{tot} ↑	Furst *et al.*, 1987
Tolmetin	PBD, Cl_{tot} ↑	Cressman *et al.*, 1976
Zomepirac	PBD, C_u ↑, inhibition of glucuronidation	Desiraju *et al.*, 1984
Other drugs		
Acetazolamide	PBD, C_u ↑, inhibition of renal tubular secretion	Sweeney *et al.*, 1986
Methotrexate	PBD, inhibition of renal tubular secretion	Liegler *et al.*, 1969
Penicillin	PBD	Moskowitz *et al.*, 1973
Phenytoin	PBD	Fraser *et al.*, 1980
		Leonard *et al.*, 1981
		Lunde *et al.*, 1970
Salicylamide	Mutual inhibition of glucuronidation	Levy and Procknal, 1968
Secobarbital	PBD	Moskowitz *et al.*, 1973
Valproic acid	PBD, C_u ↑	Abbott *et al.*, 1986
Warfarin	PBD	Watson and Pierson, 1961

PBD, protein binding displacement; C_{ss}, concentration at steady-state; C_u, concentration of unbound drug; Cl_{tot}, total plasma clearance; Cl_R, renal clearance, Cl_B, biliary clearance; $t_{1/2}$, terminal plasma half-life.

clearance can be seen. A comprehensive survey of pharmacokinetic interactions with ASS and salicylates has been published by Miners (1989). Recently, however, it has been questioned, principally whether displacement from protein binding alone leads to clinically relevant interactions. The author concluded that most interactions attributed to pure displacement occur through the effects of the displacers on the elimination of the displaced drug (MacKichan, 1989). ASS does not

Table 22.2 Drugs affecting the pharmacokinetics of salicylates

Drug	Mechanism of interaction	Source
Caffeine	C_{max} ↑, AUC ↑,	Yoovathaworn *et al.*, 1986
Cimetidine	Inhibition of metabolism?	Trnavska *et al.*, 1985
Contraceptive steroids	Induction of glucuronidation, salicylurate formation	Miners *et al.*, 1986
Corticosteroids	C_{ss} ↓, induction of metabolism?	Baer *et al.*, 1987
Salicylamide	Mutual inhibition of glucuronidation	Levy and Procknal, 1968
Zomepirac	PBD, C_u ↑, inhibition of glucuronidation	Desiraju *et al.*, 1984
Chlorpropamid	Blood levels ↑	Stowers *et al.*, 1959

AUC, area under the plasma concentration versus time curve; PBD, protein binding displacement;
C_{ss}, concentration at steady-state;
C_u, concentration of unbound drug;
C_{max}, maximum plasma concentration.

seem to affect renal lithium elimination significantly (Ragheb, 1987). (For summary of interactions see Tables 22.1–22.3.)

22.8.2 Pharmacodynamic Interactions

ASS should not be co-administered with anti-coagulant drugs because of various interactions. The pharmacodynamic effect of coumarins will be increased by protein binding displacement and the bleeding tendency is potentiated by the drug itself. Gastric haemorrhage will be enhanced and become more severe, when anti-coagulants are given. Ethanol enhances the effect of ASS on the bleeding time until at least 36 h after ASS ingestion (Deykin *et al.*, 1982). The cause is unclear; moreover the use of ethanol alone does not prolong bleeding time.

In a previous study, the use of ASS contributed significantly to the failure of IUD (intrauterine devices) in humans (Poulson *et al.*, 1981). A large case-control study in medical practices recently confirmed this observation. The consumption of ASS was compared between 717 cases of pregnancy during the use of IUD to 717 controls, who did not become pregnant. Women of the case group used NSAIDs, particularly ASS, more frequently than women of the control group ($P<0.001$) (Papiernik *et al.*, 1989).

Table 22.3 Drugs affecting the pharmacokinetics of ASS

Drug	Mechanism of interaction	Source
Activated charcoal	Absorption $\downarrow$ C_{ss} $\downarrow$,	Levy and Tsuchiya, 1972
Antacids	Cl_R $\uparrow$ due to urine pH $\uparrow$	Leonards and Levy, 1969
Cholestyramine	Delayed absorption	Hahn et al., 1972
Dipyridamole	C_{max} + AUC $\uparrow$, inhibition of ASS esterase?	Nitelius et al., 1985
Metoclopramide	Earlier absorption and C_{max} $\uparrow$ in migraine patients	Ross-Lee et al., 1983
Metoprolol	C_{max} $\uparrow$	Spahn et al., 1986

AUC, area under the plasma concentration versus time curve; Cl_R, renal clearance; C_{ss}, concentration at steady-state; C_{max}, maximum plasma concentration.

Interactions of diflunisal with ASS, indomethacin, naproxen, aceno-coumarol, paracetamol, phenprocoumon and thiazide diuretics have been reviewed by Tempero et al. (1979). Data on interactions with salsalate are not available. (For summary of interactions see Table 22.4.)

22.9 CONCLUSIONS

ASS and the non-acetylated salicylates clearly differ from each other concerning their clinical use and their safety profiles. They have to be discussed separately.

Due to its side effect profile ASS has changed its role in present-day medicine during the last decade. Its leading position as an 'every-day analgesic' has been challenged by acetaminophen, the pyrazolones and recently by several NSAIDs, in particular ibuprofen. Low gastric tolerability and the occurrence of rare, but severe side effects (e.g. Reye's syndrome) have contributed to the doubts in the uncritical and unlimited use of ASS.

On the other hand one of the 'side' effects, the inhibition of platelet aggregation, has advanced ASS in another therapeutic area, where it plays an important part in today's medicine. The occurrence of adverse effects depends strongly, as with every medicine, on the dose administered. Although ASS is an old drug, more trials are needed in order to establish efficacious but safe dosages especially for its new therapeutic applications.

In contrast, the non-acetylated salicylates, especially salts of salicylic acid, have been neglected although the few available data and experimental

591

Table 22.4 Phamacodynamic interactions between ASS and other drugs

Drug	Mechanism of interaction	Source
Ascorbic acid	Enhanced drug crystalluria	Sestili, 1983
Cimetidine	Decrease of GI bleeding	Welch et al., 1978
Ethanol	Enhancement of bleeding	Deykin et al., 1982
Food allergens	Potentiation	
Furosemide	Antagonism of the effect	Bartoli et al., 1980
Glucocorticoids	Potentiation of ulcerogenic potential	
NSAIDs	Potentiation of ulcerogenic potential	
Probenecid	Antagonism of the effect	Pascale et al., 1955 Brooks and Ulrich, 1980
Spironolactone	Antagonism of the effect	Labram, 1974
Streptokinase	Potentiation of the effect	Section 22.3
Sulfinpyrazone	Antagonism of the effect	Yu et al., 1963
Sulfonylureas	Potentiation of effect (mechanism unknown)	Limbeck et al., 1965
Warfarin	Potentiation of effect (mechanism unknown)	Watson and Pierson, 1961

NSAIDs: Non-steroidal anti-inflammatory drugs.

results imply superior safety due to a lack of PG-synthesis inhibition at low (analgesic) doses. They deserve a clinical re-evaluation with regard to their risk-benefit ratio.

REFERENCES

Abbott, F.S., Kassam, J., Orr, J.M. and Farrell, K. (1986) The effect of aspirin on valproic acid metabolism. Clin. Pharmacol. Ther., 40, 94–100.

Aberg, G. and Larrson, K.S. (1970) Pharmacological properties of some antirheumatic salicylates. Acta Pharmacol. Toxicol., 28, 249–57.

Anon. (1970) Susceptibility to aspirin bleeding (leading article). Brit. Med. J., 2, 436.

Anon. (1980) Aspirin after myocardial infarction. Lancet, i, 1172.

Antiplatelet Trialists' Collaboration (1988) Secondary prevention of vascular disease by prolonged antiplatelet treatment. Brit. Med. J., 296, 320–31.

Athreya, B.H. (1975) Aspirin-induced hepatotoxicity in juvenile rheumatoid arthritis. Arthritis Rheum., 18, 347–52.

Baer, P.A., Shore, A. and Ikeman, R.L. (1987) Transient fall in serum salicylate levels following intraarticular injection of steroid in patients with rheumatoid arthritis. *Arthritis Rheum.*, **30**, 345–7.

Ballantyne, J. (1970) Iatrogenic deafness. *J. Laryngol. Otol.*, **84**, 967–1000.

Bartoli, E., Arras, S., Faedda, R. *et al.* (1980) Blunting of furosemide diuresis by aspirin in man. *J. Clin. Pharmacol.*, **20**, 452–8.

Bernstein, B.H., Singsen, B.H., King, K.K. and Hanson, V. (1977) Aspirin-induced hepatotoxicity and its effect on juvenile rheumatoid arthritis. *Am. J. Dis. Child.*, **131**, 659–63.

Bertone, L.L. and Monie, I.W. (1965) Teratogenic effect of methyl salicylate and hypoxia in combination. *Anatom. Rec.*, **155**, 143.

Bobrove, A.M. (1988) Diflunisal-associated thrombocytopenia in a patient with rheumatoid arthritis. *Arthritis Rheum.*, **31**, 148–9.

Bove, K.E., Bhathena, D., Wyatt, R.J. *et al.* (1979) Diffuse metanephric adenoma after *in utero* aspirin intoxication. *Arch. Pathol. Lab. Med.*, **103**, 187–90.

Brooks, C.D. and Ulrich, J.E. (1980) Effect of ibuprofen or aspirin on probenecid induced uricosuria. *J. Int. Med. Res.*, **8**, 283–5.

Brooks, P.M. and Khong, T.K. (1977) Flurbiprofen–aspirin interaction: a double blind crossover study. *Curr. Med. Res. Opin.*, **5**, 53–7.

Brown, R. A. and West, G. B. (1964) Effect of acetylsalicylic acid on foetal rats. *J. Pharm. Pharmacol.*, **16**, 563–5.

Brune, K. (1974), How aspirin might work: a pharmacokinetic approach. *Agents Actions*, **4**, 230–2.

Brune, K., Rainsford, K.D., Wagner, K. and Peskar, B.A. (1981) Inhibition by anti-inflammatory drugs of prostaglandin production in cultured macrophages: Factors influencing the apparent drug effects. *Nauny–Schmiedebergs's Arch. Pharmacol.*, **315**, 269–76.

Burch, J.W., Baenziger, N.L., Stanford. N. and Majerus, P.W. (1978), Sensitivity of fatty acid cyclo-oxygenase from human aorta to acetylation by aspirin. *Proc. Natl Acad. Sci. USA*, **75**, 5181–4.

Chalmers, T.M., Kellgren, J.H. and Plat, D.S. (1969) Evaluation in man of fenclozic acid (I.C.I. 54450 Myalex), a new anti-inflammatory agent. II. Clinical trial in patients with rheumatoid arthritis. *Ann. Rheum. Dis.*, **28**, 596–601.

Connolly, K., Lam, L. and Ward, O.C. (1979) Rectal aspirin – absorption and antipyretic effect. *Arch. Dis. Child.*, **54**, 713–15.

Conti, L., Fidani, P., Chistolini, A. *et al.* (1984) Detection of drug-dependent IgG antibodies with antiplatelet activity by the antiglobulin consumption assay. *Haemostasis*, **14**, 480–6.

Court, H. and Volans, G.N. (1984) Poisoning after overdose with non-steroidal anti-inflammatory drugs. *Adv. Drug React. Ac. Pois. Rev.*, **3**, 1–21.

Cressman, W.A., Wortham, G.F. and Plostnieks, J. (1976) Absorption and excretion of tolmetin in man. *Clin. Pharmacol. Ther.*, **19**, 224–33.

Cuthbert, M.F. (1974) Adverse reactions to non-steroidal anti-rheumatic drugs. *Curr. Med. Res. Opin.*, **2**, 600–9.

Desiraju, R.K., Nayak, R K. and Pritchard, J.F. (1984) Zomepirac–aspirin interactions in man. *J. Clin. Pharmacol.*, **24**, 371–80.

Deykin, D., Janson, P. and McMahon, L. (1982) Ethanol potentiation of aspirin-induced prolongation of the bleeding time. *N. Engl. J. Med.*, **306**, 852–4.

Dieppe, P.A. and Huskisson, E.C. (1978) Diflunisal and acetylsalicylic acid: a comparison of efficacy in osteoarthritis; of nephrotoxicity, and of anti-inflammatory activity in the rat. In *Diflunisal in Clinical Practice* (ed. K.Miehlke), Futura Publishing, New York, pp. 57–61.

Dove, D.J. and Jones, T. (1982) Delayed coma associated with salicylate intoxication. *J. Pediatr*, **100**, 493–6.

Dreser, H. (1899) Pharmakologisches über Aspirin (Acetylsalicylsäure). *Pflüegers Arch.*, **76**, 306–18.

Dukes, M.N.G. (1988) Antipyretic analgesics. In *Meyler's Side Effects of Drugs*, 11th edition, (eds. M.N.G. Dukes, J.K. Aronson, B. Blackwell *et al.*), Elsevier Science Publishers B.V., Amsterdam, pp. 156–69.

Eriksson, M. (1971) Salicylate-induced foetal damage during late pregnancy in mice: A comparison between sodium salicylate, acetysalicylic acid and salicylsalicylic acid. *Acta Pharmacol. Toxicol.*, **24**, 250–5.

Esquivel, M., Cussenot, F., Ogilvie, R.I. *et al.* (1984) Interaction of isoxicam with acetylsalicylic acid. *Brit. J. Clin. Pharmacol.*, **18**, 567–71.

Estes, D. and Kaplan, K. (1980) Lack of platelet effect with the aspirin analog, salsalate, *Arthritis Rheum.*, **23**, 1303–7.

Ferreira, S.H. and Vane, J.R. (1974) New aspects of the mode of action of nonsteroid anti-inflammatory drugs. *Ann. Rev. Pharmacol.*, **14**, 57–73.

Ferreira, S.H., Moncada, S. and Vane, J.R. (1971) Indomethacin and aspirin abolish the prostaglandin release from the spleen. *Nature (New Biol.)*, **231**, 237–9.

Fields, W.S., Lemak, N.A., Frankowski, R.F. and Hardy, R.J. (1978) Controlled trial of aspirin in cerebral ischemia. *Stroke*, **8**, 309–18.

Fraser, D.G., Ludden, T.M., Evens, R.P. and Sutherland II, W.E. (1980) Displacement of phenytoin from plasma binding sites by salicylate. *Clin. Pharm. Ther.*, **27**, 165–9.

Fraser, N.C. (1980) Accidental poisoning deaths in British children 1958–1977. *Brit. Med. J.*, **280**, 1595–8.

Furst, D.E., Sarkissian, E., Blocka, K. *et al.* (1987) Serum concentrations of salicylate and naproxen during concurrent therapy in patients with rheumatoid arthritis. *Arthritis Rheum.*, **30**, 1157–61.

Glader, B.E. (1976) Salicylate-induced injury of pyruvate-kinase deficient erythrocytes. *N. Engl. J. Med.*, **294**, 916–18.

Grennan, D.M., Ferry, D.G., Ashworth, M.E. *et al.* (1979) The aspirin–ibuprofen interaction in rheumatoid arthritis. *Brit. J. Clin. Pharmacol.*, **8**, 497–503.

Hahn, K.-J., Eiden, W., Schettle, M. *et al.* (1972) Effect of cholestyramine on the gastrointestinal absorption of phenprocoumon and acetylsalicylic acid in man. *Eur. J. Clin. Pharmacol.*, **4**, 142–5.

Hanley, S.P., Bevan, J., Cockbill, S.R. and Heptinstall, S. (1981) Differential inhibition by low dose aspirin of human venous prostacyclin synthesis and platelet thromboxane synthesis. *Lancet*, **i**, 969–71.

Harris, W.H., Salzman, E.W., Athanasoulis, C.A. *et al.* (1977) Aspirin prophylaxis of venous thromboembolism after total hip replacement. *N. Engl. J. Med.*, **297**, 1246–9.

Higgs, G.A., Harvey, E.A., Ferreira, S.H. and Vane, J.R. (1976) The effects of antiinflammatory drugs on the production of prostaglandins *in vivo*. *Adv. Prostaglandin Thromboxane Res.*, **1**, 105–10.

Higgs, G.A., Salmon, J.A., Henderson, B. and Vane, J.R. (1987) Pharmacokinetics of aspirin and salicylate in relation to inhibition of arachidonate, cyclo-oxygenase, and anti-inflammatory activity. *Proc. Natl Acad. Sci.*, **84**, 1417–20.

Hrnicek, G., Shelton, J. and Miller, W.C. (1974) Pulmonary edema and salicylate intoxication. *J. Am. Med. Assoc.*, **230**, 866–7.

Huskisson, E.C., Williams, T.N., Shaw, L.D. and Kerry, J. (1978) Diflunisal in general practice. *Curr. Med. Res. Opin.*, **5**, 589–92.

IAAAS (International Agranulocytosis and Aplastic Anemia Study) (1986) Risks of agranulocytosis and aplastic anemia. A first report of their relation to drug use with special reference to analgesics. *J. Am. Med. Assoc.*, **256**, 1749–57.

Kewitz, H., Nitz, M. and Gaus, V. (1986) Aspirin and cataract. *Lancet*, **ii**, 689.

Kingham, J.D., Chen, M.C. and Levy, M.H. (1988) Macular hemorrhage in the aging eye: The effects of anticoagulants. *N. Engl. J. Med.*, **318**, 1126–7.

Kwan, K.C., Breault, G.O. and David, R.L. (1978) Effects of concomitant aspirin administration on the pharmacokinetics of indomethacin in man. *J. Pharmacokinet. Biopharm.*, **6**, 451–76.

Labram, C. (1974) Spironolactone et aspirin. *Concours Med.*, **96**, 211.

Larrson, K.S., Boström, H. and Ericson, B. (1963) Salicylate-induced malformations in mouse embryos. *Acta Pediatr.*, **52**, 36–40.

Larrson, K.S., Ericson, B. and Boström, H. (1964) Salicylate-induced skeletal and vessel malformations in mouse embryos. *Acta Morphol. Neerl. Scand.*, **6**, 35–44.

Larrson, K.S. and Boström, H. (1965) Teratogenic action of salicylates related to the inhibition of mucopolysaccharide synthesis. *Acta Pediatr. Scand.*, **54**, 43–8.

Leonard, F.G., Knott, P.J., Rankin, G.O. *et al.* (1981) Phenytoin–salicylate interaction. *Clin. Pharmacol. Ther.*, **29**, 57–60.

Leonards J.R. and Levy, G. (1969) Reduction or prevention of aspirin-induced occult gastrointestinal blood loss in man. *Clin. Pharmacol. Ther.*, **10**, 571–6.

Levine, B., Smyth, D.F. and Caplan, Y.H. (1987) A diflunisal related fatality: A case report. *Forens. Sci. Int.*, **35**, 45–50.

Levy, G. and Procknal, J.A. (1968) Drug biotransformation interactions in man. 1. Mutual inhibition in glucuronide formation of salicylic acid and salicylamide in man. *J. Pharm. Sci.*, **57**, 1330–5.

Levy, G. and Tsuchiya, T. (1972) Effect of activated charcoal absorption in man. Part 1. *Clin. Pharmacol. Ther.*, **13**, 317–22.

Lewis, J.H. (1984) Hepatic toxicity of nonsteroidal antiinflammatory drugs. *Clin. Pharm.*, **3**, 128–38.

Liegler, D.G., Henderson, E.S., Hahn, M.A. and Oliverio, V.T. (1969) The effect of organic acids on renal clearance of methotrexate in man. *Clin. Pharmacol. Ther.*, **10**, 849–57.

Limbeck, G.A., Ruvalcaba, R.H.A., Samols, E. and Kelly, V.C. (1965) Salicylates and hypoglycemia. *Am. J. Dis. Child.*, **109**, 165–7.

Lunde, P.K.M., Rane, A., Yaffe, S.J. *et al.* (1970) Plasma protein binding of diphenylhydantoin in man. *Clin. Pharmacol. Ther.*, **11**, 846–55.

MacKichan, J.J. (1989) Protein binding drug displacement interactions – fact or fiction? *Clin. Pharmacokin.*, **16**, 65–73.

Mäkelä, A.-L., Lang, H. and Korpela, P. (1980) Toxic encephalopathy with hyperammonaemia during high-dose salicylate therapy. *Acta Neurol. Scand.*, **61**, 156–66.

Manso, C., Taranta, A. and Nydick, I. (1956) Effect of aspirin administration on serum glutamic oxaloacetic and glutamic pyruvic transaminases in children. *Proc. Soc. Exp. Biol. Med.*, **93**, 84–8.

Martin, B.K. (1971) The formulation of aspirin. *Adv. Pharm. Sci.*, **3**, 107–71.

Matsumoto, M., Nukada, T., Uyama, O. *et al.* (1980) Thromboxane generation in patients with essential hypertension or cerebrovascular disease and effect of oral aspirin. *Thromb. Haemostasis*, **44**, 16–22.

Miescher, P.A. and Pola, W. (1986) Haematological effects of non-narcotic analgesics. *Drugs*, **32** (Suppl. 4), 90–108.

Miller, R.R. and Jick, H. (1977) Acute toxicity of aspirin in hospitalized medical patients. *Am. J. Med. Sci.*, **274**, 271–9.

Miners, J.O. (1989) Drug interactions involving aspirin (acetylsalicylic acid) and salicylic acid. *Clin. Pharmacokin.*, **17** (5), 327–44.

Miners, J.O., Grgurinovich, N., Whitehead, A.G. *et al.* (1986) Influence of gender and oral contraceptive steroids on the metabolism of salicylic acid and acetylsalicylic acid. *Brit. J. Clin. Pharmacol.*, **22**, 135–42.

Moll, J. (1968) Synopsis der Rheumatherapie. In *Progress in Drug Research, Vol. 12*, (ed. E. Jucker)., Birkhäuser, Basel, pp. 165–291.

Moncada, S. and Vane, J.R. (1978) Unstable metabolites of arachidonic acid and their role in haemostasis and thrombosis. *Brit. Med. Bull.*, **34**, 129–35.

Moskowitz, B., Somani, S.M. and McDonald, R.H.Jr (1973) Salicylate interaction with penicillin and secobarbital binding sites on human serum albumin. *Clin. Toxicol.*, **6**, 247–56.

Muller, F.O., Hundt, H.K. and Muller, D.G. (1977) Pharmacokinetic and pharmacodynamic implications of long-term administration of non-steroidal anti-inflammatory agents. *Int. J. Clin. Pharmacol. Biopharm.*, **15**, 397–402.

Necheles, T.F., Steinberg, M.H. and Cameron, D. (1970) Erythrocyte glutathione-peroxide deficiency. *Brit. J. Haematol.*, **19**, 605–12.

Needs, C.J. and Brooks, P.M. (1985) Clinical pharmacokinetics of the salicylates. *Clin. Pharmacokin.*, **10**, 164–77.

Nitelius, E., Melander, A. and Wahlin-Boll, E. (1985) Pharmacokinetic interaction of acetylsalicylic acid and dipyridamole. *Brit. J. Clin. Pharmacol.*, **19**, 379–83.

Oudot, J. (1979) Intoxication aigue a l'aspirine et surdite: a propos de 10 cas. *J. Fr. Oto-Rhino-Laryngol.*, **28**, 687–93.

Papiernik, E., Rozenbaum, H., Amblard, P. *et al.* (1989) Intra-uterine device failure: relation with drug use. *Eur. J. Obstet. Gynecol. Reprod. Biol.*, **32**, 205–12.

Pascale, L.R., Dubin, A., Bronsky, D. and Hoffman, W.S. (1955) Inhibition of the uricosuric action of benemid by salicylate. *J. Lab. Clin. Med.*, **45**, 771–7.

Pfisterer, M., Burkart, F., Jockers, G. *et al.* (1989) Trial of low-dose aspirin plus dipyridamole versus anticoagulants for prevention of aortocoronary vein graft occlusion. *Lancet*, **ii**, 1–7.

Porter, J. and Jick, H. (1977) Drug-induced anaphylaxis, convulsions, deafness, and extrapyramidal symptoms. *Lancet*, **i**, 587–8.

Poulson, A.M., Naisbett, J.P. and Chamberlain, P.D. (1981) Aspirin use in women who become pregnant with an intra-uterine device. *Fertil. Steril.*, **36**, 421.

596

Prescott, L.F. (1981) Salicylate hepatitis. In *Drug reactions and the liver* (eds M. Davis, J.M. Tredger and R. Williams), Pitman Medical, London, pp. 267–83.

Prescott, L.F. (1984) Clinical features and management of analgesic poisoning. *Human Toxicol.*, **3**, 75S–84S.

Prescott, L.F. (1986) Effects of non-narcotic analgesics on the liver. *Drugs*, **32** (Suppl. 4), 129–47.

Preston, S.J., Arnold, M.H., Beller, E.M. *et al.* (1989) Comparative analgesic and anti-inflammatory properties of sodium salicylate and acetylsalicylic acid (aspirin) in rheumatoid arthritis. *Brit. J. Clin. Pharmacol.*, **27**, 607–11.

Proudfoot, A.T. (1983) Toxicity of salicylates. *Am. J. Med.*, **75** (suppl. 5A), 99–103.

Ragheb, M.A. (1987) Aspirin does not significantly affect patients' serum lithium level. *J. Clin. Psychiatry*, **48**, 425.

Rainsford, K.D. (1984) Side effects and toxicology of the salicylates. In *Aspirin and the Salicylates* (ed. K.D. Rainsford), Butterworth and Co. Ltd., London, pp. 148–271.

Rainsford, K.D., Schweitzer, A. and Brune, K. (1981) Autoradiographic and biochemical observations on the distribution of non-steroid anti-inflammatory drugs. *Arch. Int. Pharmacodyn. Ther.*, **250**, 180–94.

Rainsford, K.D., Schweitzer, A. and Brune, K. (1983) Distribution of the acetyl – compared with the salicyl – moiety of acetylsalicylic acid. *Biochem. Pharmacol.*, **32**, 1301–8.

Rochanawutanon, M., Bunyaratvej, S. and Israngkura, P. (1979) Salicylate-induced hepatotoxicity in juvenile rheumatoid arthritis – a case report. *J. Med. Ass. Thail.*, **62**, 646–51.

Rosenkranz, B., Fischer, C., Meese, C.O. and Frolich, J.C. (1986) Effects of salicylic and acetylsalicylic acid alone and in combination on platelet aggregation and prostanoid synthesis in man. *Brit. J. Clin. Pharmacol.*, **21**, 309–17.

Ross-Lee, L.M., Ecdie, M.J., Heazlewood, V. *et al.* (1983) Aspirin pharmacokinetics in migraine. The effect of metoclopramide. *Eur. J. Clin. Pharmacol.*, **24**, 777–85.

Rowland, M., Riegelman, S., Harris, P.A. and Sholkoff, S.D. (1972) Absorption kinetics of aspirin in man following oral administration of an aqueous solution. *J. Pharm. Sci.*, **61**, 379–85.

Rubin, A., Rodda, F., Warrick, P. *et al.* (1973) Interactions of aspirin with non-steroidal anti inflammatory drugs in man. *Arthritis Rheum.*, **16**, 635–45.

Rumack, C.M., Guggenheim, M.A., Rumack, B.H. *et al.* (1980) Neonatal intracranial hemorrhage and maternal use of aspirin. *Obstet. Gynecol.*, **58**, 52S–65S.

Russell, A.S., Sturge, R.A. and Smith, M.A. (1971), Serum transaminases during salicylate therapy. *Brit. Med. J.*, **2**, 428–9.

Sbarboro, J.A. and Bennett, R.M. (1977) Aspirin hepatotoxicity and disseminated intravascular coagulation. *Ann. Intern. Med.*, **86**, 183–5.

Schultz, P., Perrier, C.V., Ferber-Pcrret, F. *et al.* (1979) Diflunisal, a new-acting analgesic and prostaglandin inhibitor: effect of concomitant acetylsalicylic acid therapy on ototoxicity and on disposition of both drugs. *J. Int. Med. Res.*, **7**, 61–8.

Seaman, W.E. and Plotz, P.H. (1976) Effect of aspirin on liver tests in patients with RA or SLE and in normal volunteers. *Arthritis Rheum.*, **19**, 155–60.

Seaman, W.E., Ishak, K.G. and Plotz, P.H. (1974a). Aspirin-induced hepatotoxicity in patients with systemic lupus erythematosus. *Ann. Intern. Med.*, **80**, 1–8.

Seaman, W.E., Ishak, K.G. and Plotz, P. H. (1974b) Aspirin and hepatotoxicity: addendum. *Ann. Intern. Med.*, **80**, 279.

Segre, E.J., Chaplain, M., Forchielli, E. *et al.* (1974) Naproxen–aspirin interactions in man. *Clin. Pharmacol. Ther.*, **15**, 374–9.

Sestili, M.A. (1983) Possible adverse effects of vitamin C and ascorbic acid. *Sem. Oncol.*, **10**, 299–304.

Shapiro, S., Siskind, V. and Monso, R.R. (1976) Perinatal mortality and birth-weight in relation to aspirin taken during pregnancy. *Lancet*, **i**, 1375–6.

Singleton, P.T. (1980) Salsalate: Its role in the management of rheumatic disease. *Clin. Ther.*, **3**, 80–102.

Slone, D., Siskind, V. and Heinonen, O.P. (1976) Aspirin and congenital malformations. *Lancet*, **i**, 1373–5.

Smith, M.J.H. and Smith, P.K. (1966) *The Salicylates. A Critical Bibliographic Review*, Interscience Publishers, John Wiley and Sons, London.

Smith, J.B. and Willis, A.L. (1971) Aspirin selectively inhibits prostaglandin production in human platelets. *Nature (New Biol.)*, **231**, 235–7.

Spahn, H., Langguth, P., Kirch, W. *et al.* (1986) Pharmacokinetics of salicylates administered with metoprolol. *Arzneim.-Forsch.*, **36**, 1697–99.

Stone, C.A., Van Arman, C.G., Lotti, V.J. *et al.* (1977) Pharmacology and toxicology of diflunisal. *Brit. J. Clin. Pharmacol.*, **4** (Suppl. 1), 19S–29S.

Stowers, J.M., Constable, L.W. and Hunter, R.B. (1959) Clinical and pharmacological comparison of chlorpropamide and other sulfonylureas. *Ann. NY Acad. Sci.*, **74**, 689–95.

Stricker, S. (1876) II. Aus der Traube'schen Klinik. Ueber die Resultate der Behandlung der Polyarthritis rheumatica mit Salicylsäure. *Ber. Klin. Wochenschr.*, **13**, 1–2, 15–16.

Sweeney, K.R., Chapron, D.J., Brandt, J.L. *et al.* (1986) Toxic interaction between acetazolamide and salicylate: case reports and a pharmacokinetic explanation. *Clin. Pharmacol. Ther.*, **40**, 518–24.

Szczeklik, A. (1987) Adverse reactions to aspirin and nonsteroidal antiinflammatory drugs. *Ann. Allergy*, **59**, 113–8.

Takacs, E. and Warkany, J. (1968) Experimental production of congenital cardiovascular malformations in rats by salicylate poisoning. *Teratology*, **1**, 109–18.

Tempero, K.F., Cirillo, V.J. and Steelman, S.L. (1979) Diflunisal: chemistry, toxicology, experimental and human pharmacology. In *Diflunisal: New Perspectives in Analgesia* (eds. E.C. Huskisson and A.D.S. Caldwell), Royal Society of Medicine, International Congress and Symposium Series, No. 6, pp. 1–20.

The Canadian Cooperative Study Group (1978) A randomized trial of aspirin and sulfinpyrazone in threatened stroke. *N. Engl. J. Med.*, **299**, 53–9.

Trnavska, Z., Trnavsky, K. and Smondrk, J. (1985) The effect of cimetidine on the pharmacokinetics of salicylic acid. *Drugs Exp. Clin. Res.*, **11**, 703–7.

Trnavsky, K. and Zachar, M. (1975) Correlation of serum aspirin esterase and activity and half-life of salicylic acid. *Agents Actions*, **5**, 549–52.

Vane, J.R. (1971) Inhibition of prostaglandin synthesis as a mechanism of action for aspirin-like drugs. *Nature (New Biol.)*, **231**, 235–7.

Vane, J.R. (1987) The evolution of non-steroidal anti-inflammatory drugs and their mechanism of action. *Drugs* (Suppl. 1), 18–27.

Vanecek, J. (1980) Antipyretic analgesics. In *Meyler's Side Effects of Drugs*, 9th ed. (ed. M.N.G. Dukes), Excerpta Medica, Amsterdam, pp. 123–40.

Warkany, J. and Takacs, E. (1959), Experimental production of congenital malformations in rats by salicylate poisoning. *Am. J. Pathol.*, **35**, 315–31.

Warren, J.S. (1978) Diflunisal-induced cholestatic jaundice. *Brit. Med. J.*, **2**, 736–8.

Watson, R.M. and Pierson, R.N. (1961) Effect of anticoagulant therapy upon aspirin induced bleeding. *Circulation*, **24**, 613–16.

Welch, R.W., Bentch, H.L. and Harris, S.C. (1978) Reduction of aspirin-induced gastrointestinal bleeding with cimetidine. *Gastroenterology*, **74**, 459–63.

Wenger, T.L. and Hull, J.H. (1980) Aspirin dosage for cardiovascular effects. *N. Engl. J. Med.*, **303**, 1121.

Werblin, T.P. and Pfeiffer, R.L. (1987) Persistant hemorrhage after extracapsular surgery associated with excessive aspirin ingestion. *Am. J. Ophthalmol.*, **104**, 426.

Werler, M.M, Mitchell, A.A. and Shapiro, S. (1989) The relation of aspirin use during the first trimester of pregnancy to congenital cardiac defects. *N. Engl. J. Med.*, **321**, 1639–42.

Williams, J.O., Mengel, C.E., Sullivan, L.W. *et al.* (1969) Megaloblastic anaemia associated with chronic ingestion of an analgesic. *N. Engl. J. Med.*, **280**, 312–3.

Williams, R.L., Upton, R.A., Buskin, J.N. and Jones, R.M. (1981) Ketoprofen--aspirin interactions. *Clin. Pharmacol. Ther.*, **30**, 226–31.

Yoovathaworn, K.C., Sriwatanakul, K. and Thithapandha, A. (1986) Influence of caffeine on aspirin pharmacokinetics. *Eur. J. Drug Metab. Pharmacokinet.*, **11**, 71–6.

Yu, R.F., Dayton, P.G. and Gutman, A.B. (1963) Mutual suppression of the uricosuric effects of sulfinpyrazone and salicylate: a study in interactions between drugs. *J. Clin. Invest.*, **42**, 1330–9.

Zimmerman, H.J. (1978) Anti-inflammatory and other effects of drugs employed in the treatment of rheumatic and musculoskeletal diseases. In *Hepato toxicity: the Adverse Effects of Drugs and other Chemicals on the Liver.*, Appleton-Century-Crofts, New York, pp. 418–35.

Zimmerman, H.J. (1981) Effects of aspirin and acetaminophen on the liver. *Arch. Intern. Med.*, **141**, 333–42.

Index

Index

Index

Red blood cell aspirin esterase, 79
Red blood cell glutathione peroxidase
    deficiency, 582
Refractory angina, 406–7
Renal effects of aspirin, 510–24
    chronic aspirin therapy, 521–2
    electrolytes, 520–21
    glomerular filtration rate, 518–19
    prostaglandin synthesis, 510–13
        animal studies, 514–17
        cortical, 511
        medullary, 511–12
        production *in vivo* assessment,
            512–13
    renal blood flow, 518–19
    renal/cardiovascular subjects,
        519–20
    tubular damage, 517–18
    water excretion, 520–21
Renal failure, chronic, 265
Renal ischaemia, 49
Renal papillary necrosis, 49
Renin, 513
Reye's Syndrome, 458–9, 531–45
    aetiology, 538–9
    animal model, 543
    aspirin association, 538–45
        epidemiology, 538–42
        experimental studies, 542–4
        histopathology, 542
        serum salicylate levels, 542
    biochemistry/metabolism, 536–7
    cerebral lesions, 533–4
    clinical features, 353–4
    dicarboxylic acids in, 545
    epidemiology, 535–7
    hepatic pathology, 533
    skeletal muscle, 534
Rheumatic fever, 305
Rheumatoid arthritis, 50, 186, 298
    aspirin treatment, 295–303
        assessment measurement,
            301–302
        chronic, 521–2
    disease activity measurement, 300
    inflammation measurement,
        298
    juvenile, 304, 583
    macrocytic anaemia/folate
        deficiency, 582
    pain threshold, 296

liver toxicity, aspirin associated,
    583
Ribonucleic acid, viral, 238
Roll-over test, 453

Salacetamide, 108, 110 (table), 123
    (fig), 125
Salicin, 4
Salicyl acyl glucuronide, 80
Salicylamide, 109 (table), 122–3,
    125 (fig)
    interactions, 589 (table), 590 (table)
    prodrugs, 123 (fig)
    tolerance by aspirin-sensitive
        asthmatics, 550
Salicylates, 108–9
    absorption, 75–7
    adverse effects in pregnancy, 455–7
        blood clotting, 456
        foetal circulation, 456–7
        foetal lung, 456
        inhibition of labour, 456
        teratogenesis, 455
    disposition, 77–9
    enzyme inhibition, 154
    esters, *vs* acidic NSAI drugs,
        312–14
    free carboxyl substituents
        modifications, 473
    intolerance, 550–51, 551 (table)
    intoxication, 586–8
    mechanism of action, 154–5
    models tested, 145–8 (table)
        adjuvant, 148 (table)
        cell migration, 147 (table)
        paw oedema, 146–7 (table)
        pleural inflammation, 146 (table)
        sponge, 148, (table)
        thermal injury, 146 (table)
    non-acetylated, 313, 522–4
    overdosage, 586–8
    pharmacodynamic interactions,
        590–91, 592 (table)
    pharmacokinetic interactions,
        588–90
    protein binding, 77–8
    theories, 152–7
        pre-prostaglandin era, 152–4
        prostaglandin era, 155–7
    unwanted effects *see* Unwanted
        effects

610